TEXTBOOK OF ORTHOPAEDIC MEDICINE
1. Diagnosis of Soft Tissue Lesions

This book is due for return on or before the last date shown below.

TEXTBOOK OF
Orthopaedic
Medicine

VOLUME ONE

Diagnosis of
Soft Tissue Lesions

JAMES CYRIAX

M.D. (Cantab.), M.R.C.P. (Lond.)
Orthopaedic Physician
St. Thomas's Hospital, London

Fifth Edition

LONDON
Baillière Tindall & Cassell

BAILLIÈRE TINDALL & CASSELL LIMITED
7 & 8 Henrietta Street, London WC2

First published as *Rheumatism and Soft Tissue Injuries* 1947
Second edition   1954
Third edition   1957
Fourth edition   1962
Fifth edition   1969

SBN 7020 0286 0

Published in the United States of America by
the Williams & Wilkins Company, Baltimore

Made and printed in Great Britain
by Cox & Wyman Ltd.
London, Fakenham and Reading

Contents

List of Plates

Preface

One of the commonest symptoms, ranking second only to neuroses and respiratory infections as a major cause of industrial disablement, is pain felt at a moving part of the body. Not all such symptoms stem from a local disorder, but a great many do, and everybody suffers from this kind of trouble at intervals throughout life. Thus, joints are sprained or become arthritic; muscles, tendons and ligaments are strained; bursae become inflamed. Nerve-trunks, nerve-roots and the dura mater are liable to compression. Joints, especially spinal joints, are prone to internal derangement. These disorders of the moving parts of the body, so long neglected, deserve exact diagnosis. Many require treatment by non-surgical orthopaedic measures, e.g. induction of local anaesthesia (which is also important diagnostically), infiltration with hydrocortisone, manipulation, traction or massage.

Who is to cater for this huge mass of patients? They wander from doctor to doctor, from one hospital department to another—finally visiting all sorts of lay healers—in the vain hope of finding the right man. Most of their disorders are not 'rheumatic' (although often misnamed so by the patient), since they are seldom connected with rheumatic fever or rheumatoid arthritis, and they do not often call for surgery. Hence, they are not the primary concern of the rheumatologist or the orthopaedic surgeon.

Orthopaedic medical disorders are the only major cause of human suffering and industrial sickness for which the Health Service makes scarcely any provision. In consequence, many patients linger on in pain and off work (and, if they are athletes or sportsmen, off games) for indefinite periods, not for lack of the relevant medical knowledge, but for lack of doctors trained in the relevant discipline. This neglect has led to the irruption of numerous laymen into the void we have left gaping. Their number and success, together with the esteem which the public accords them, serve to indicate the large numbers of people who have been compelled finally to look outside the ranks of the medical profession for relief . . . and have found it at lay hands.

But the picture has another side; for treatment without prior diagnosis entails great waste of time and money. Recourse to laymen, though it has its successes, involves many patients in repeated visits for futile treatment. Disorders easy to put right by the alternative measures of orthopaedic medicine, are given routine manipulation in vain by enthusiastic laymen who, for lack of proper medical training, cannot know when or when not to apply their ministrations. This indefensible situation is common knowledge; doctors and patients alike are aware that they must take their chance with unqualified people on their own initiative and at their own expense—all this at a time when the State has assumed responsibility for every type of medical care.

The hiatus must be closed on financial no less than on humanitarian grounds. If the Health Service can save itself money *and* help patients at the same time, there seems little reason for delay. Yet a hundred years ago Sir James Paget gave a lecture entitled 'Cases that Bonesetters Cure', and the state of affairs he deplored then remains little altered today. During this century the deficiency has become increasingly obvious, and for the last thirty years has been taken seriously at St. Thomas's Hospital. The fruits of the work done there have been set out in successive editions of this book.

The present vacuum has led to so much avoidable sickness and frustration that mounting pressure is calling the requisite speciality into being—Orthopaedic Medicine. An orthopaedic team comprising surgeon and physician covers the whole field within one department, and ensures that each patient comes under the care of the appropriate expert. Sixty years ago, orthopaedic surgery was branching off from general surgery to the accompaniment of some scoffing, Robert Jones being appointed to the first lectureship in orthopaedic surgery in 1909. Just as it seemed redundant to a past generation to make a separate speciality of bone and joint surgery, so will the suggestion of a medical colleague to deal with the non-surgical aspect of the locomotor disorders meet with some resistance. Yet this division already exists in several other sections of medicine, e.g. neurologist and neurosurgeon; gastroenterologist and abdominal surgeon. The birth of this separate province will not be without pangs, though in fact it relieves surgeons of non-surgical work for which most have little liking. Resistance to new ideas is to be expected; it delays but does not affect the eventual outcome since the needs of the sick have always proved paramount in the end.

It has been my life's work to devise, and as far as possible to perfect, a method of clinical examination that leads to accurate diagnosis in locomotor disorders, enabling the physician to ignore the ubiquitous, misleading phenomena of referred pain and referred tenderness. It consists of assessing in turn the function of each moving tissue, the positive and negative responses to examination by selective tension forming a pattern. This pattern is then interpreted on a basis of applied anatomy. Logical conclusions of incontestable validity are drawn (but have aroused much controversy). Since doctors receive little or no undergraduate tuition in how to examine the moving soft parts, they have been apt to look askance at such simple deductions, regarding them as more clear-cut than such obscure clinical material warrants. However, now that the basic research has been carried out the stage is set for immediate impact on contemporary medical thought, diagnosis (since it is purely clinical and requires none of the apparatus that only hospitals possess) coming within the scope of every interested medical practitioner. At present, the number of doctors and physiotherapists trained in this discipline remains so small that the methods of orthopaedic medicine are available to only a tiny fraction of all patients who need them. Moreover, so long as St Thomas's unwillingly retains its present monopoly, the size of this fraction perforce remains stationary.

Since displacements within the spinal joints are so common, and one aspect of orthopaedic medicine involves their reduction, I have become known as that odd and scarcely respectable phenomenon: a doctor who manipulates and, worse still, teaches these techniques (together with the indications and contra-indications) to physiotherapists. Nothing annoys me more; for, though true up to a point, it is a gross error in emphasis. I am a medical man who has spent his graduate days in elaborating clinical methods of examining the non-osseous moving parts (radiography takes care of the bones themselves). Based on these new concepts, I have gone on to as exact an assessment as possible of the position, nature, size and stage of each soft-tissue lesion. This has led to the discovery of scores of hitherto undescribed conditions within the sphere of orthopaedic medicine and of some outside it, e.g. irritation of the median nerve at the wrist (1942), and intermittent claudication in the buttock (1954). It has also led to a good deal of iconoclasm, 'sacro-iliac strain' being debunked in 1941 and 'fibrositis' in 1948. The discal pathology of lumbago, regarded as a muscular affliction since 1904, was set out in 1945, together with the concept of pain arising from the dura mater. All these theories have been confirmed since by workers all over the world.

Logical extension of these clinical findings has led me to adapt, and where feasible improve upon, methods of treatment already in existence, but previously based either on empiricism or on false hypotheses. When no treatment existed, or the disorder had never been recognised, mere palliation was abandoned and methods of treatment were investigated in the light of our new-found diagnostic precision until, as far as possible, an effective measure was discovered. All successful manoeuvres were taught to our physiotherapists; for they were there to treat the patients, especially by the use of their hands. This delegation proved very satisfactory, since it enabled me to get on with my diagnostic work and carried the further advantage of affording physiotherapists a rewarding series of dramatic successes. On the one hand they were sent patients who had been found suitable for such procedures by a medical man; on the other patients were no longer asked to attend for the ephemeral palliation that even today goes by the name of 'orthodox treatment'. (How could it ever be orthodox to treat a displacement by heat and exercises?) Neither was the patient left to the vagaries of fortune, nor to the hits and misses of lay-manipulators. Naturally, this policy enhanced students' interest in this part of their work. The good repute that manipulation by laymen enjoys from some people now began to be transferred to manual methods obtainable within the Health Service, with a corresponding increase in the esteem in which physiotherapists were held. Nevertheless manipulation, emotionally charged treatment though it is, has always provided only a minor part of the work, constituting merely one remedy called for by the major compulsion—an accurate diagnosis. Manipulation is easily learnt; diagnosis is a lifetime's study.

I did not invent massage, which has existed since time immemorial as an extension of the urge to rub a sore spot. Indeed, the first mention of a professor of physiotherapy dates from 585 A.D. when one was appointed under the Sui dynasty in China. I merely devised the method of giving deep massage penetrating to the lesion. I insisted that the structure at fault should alone be treated, avoiding areas of normal tissue in the neighbourhood that happened to be the site of referred pain and tenderness. This turned out very fortunately; for, when the Medical Research Council allowed me hydrocortisone in 1952, the way to identify each lesion and the posture that made it easiest to palpate had already been established. It was thus merely a question of substituting the needle for the physiotherapist's finger. I did not invent manipulation or traction, both of which were practised by Hippocrates; a *scamnum* (bench for traction and reduction) made to his design and four hundred years old stands today in the Wellcome Historical Museum in London. My endeavour has been to codify the application of these measures, placing equal emphasis on 'when not' as on 'when', in an attempt to fit each into its due place in therapeutics. In particular, I have tried to steer manipulation away from the lay notion of a panacea—the chief factor delaying its acceptance today.

My only important discovery, on which the whole of this work rests, is the method of systematic examination of the moving parts by selective tension. By this means, precise diagnoses can be achieved in disorders of the radio-translucent moving tissues. If in years to come I am to be remembered as an original worker at all, it is with this fundamental study that I should like posterity to link my name.

JAMES CYRIAX

I

General Concepts

The disorders with which this book deals are universal. It is a rare individual indeed who does not suffer one or more lesions of his moving parts in the course of his life. Although diagnosis is considered difficult or impossible, it is in fact the reverse; it is merely a matter of applied anatomy. The function of every moving part has been established for years and clinical testing is no more than an informed, anatomical exercise. Function is assessed indirectly, like a series of simultaneous equations, and the pattern of movements—painful, painless; full range, limited range— elicited and interpreted in the light of the known behaviour of these tissues. Care is taken to avoid prejudice towards any particular hypothesis on the disorder likely to be present or on the causation of disease. The physical signs are paramount throughout. I have spent my life working out how best to ascertain the physical signs in soft-tissue lesions, and how to interpret the pattern thus brought to light. This devotion to physical signs is essential to the orthopaedic physician, for none of his patients dies in hospital and he is therefore denied the salutary discipline of the post-mortem room. Nor are X-rays of appreciable value when the radio-translucent tissues are at fault, and in general other objective tests, e.g. on the blood, are of little assistance. Hence, he must take great trouble to be right; for contrary evidence is not often available to bring an error to his notice. Constant self-criticism is thus the hall-mark of the orthopaedic physician, who has, with due humility, to approach the truth contained— better, perhaps, to say concealed—within each patient.

All pains have a source; the diagnosis names it. In visceral disease, abnormality is often difficult and sometimes impossible to demonstrate. With the moving parts the situation is reversed; function is obvious and easy to test clinically. A joint moves within certain known limits; a voluntary muscle contracts and relaxes to known effect. The examination of these structures thus presents little difficulty and interpretation of the findings is based on uncontroversial anatomical facts. The basis of this book is therefore a painstaking search for physical signs, positive and negative, and their interpretation on agreed grounds, unarguably valid. This extreme simplicity is apparently controversial and hard to accept.

'RHEUMATISM'

Nomenclature in medicine is important, for it is by words that we convey our meaning to others. 'Rheumatism' is a word often used by patients and doctors, but with many different meanings. To the layman it implies pain that he associates with the moving parts of the body, appearing for no clear reason. To some medical men it includes every disorder of the moving parts, whatever the cause—arthritis, tendinitis, teno-synovitis, ligamentous and muscle strain, post-traumatic adhesions and internal derangement, especially at the spinal joints. Others confine the term to the collagen diseases; yet others to chorea and rheumatic fever and its cardiac sequels.

The only useful way to employ 'rheumatism' is for the chorea-rheumatic-fever group of diseases. Then it refers to well-defined clinical entities and has a clear aetiological significance. But when a variety of other disorders of diverse aetiologies is grouped together under this name the result is a logical morass. By common consent, arthritis is rheumatic; osteoarthritis with a loose body, impaction of which is causing the symptoms, and neuropathic and pulmonary arthropathy are probably not; tuberculous and gouty arthritis are certainly not. Monarticular rheumatoid arthritis is rheumatic; the locally identical condition occurring in serum sickness is not, because its allergic origin is obvious. Gonococcal and Reiter's arthritis are rheumatic only so long as their urethral origin remains undetected. Tabes, localized neuritis, or displaced fragments of intervertebral disc cause pain felt in muscles and joints; these conditions are regarded as rheumatic only when the true nature of the condition is overlooked. A familiar example is lumbago; until recently it was regarded to be the result of fibrositis caused by rheumatic toxins settling in the lumbar muscles; now that it is known to be caused by internal derangement of a lumbar joint it has ceased to be rheumatic. Tennis-elbow and supraspinatus tendinitis were thought of as rheumatism of the elbow and shoulder only so long as the traumatic cause of these two types of tendinitis was not realized. When the aetiology of rheumatoid and spondylitic arthritis is ultimately discovered, these disorders also will cease to be caused by 'rheumatism'. The medical use of the word can then cease (apart from rheumatic fever). Thereafter 'rheumatic' would remain a useful evasion, but it would no longer carry any medical significance.

The word 'rheumatism' has another disadvantage. Since it is applied to all sorts of painful conditions, it means quite different things to different patients. Thus one patient may be deeply relieved to know that his pain is 'only rheumatism'; another is appalled, because a relation of his is crippled by 'rheumatism' in every joint.

Primary Fibrositis

In this condition, pain and tenderness are experienced in the trunk. Since the trunk is covered by muscles, the patient complains of pain felt in the tissue he knows to lie there, i.e. the muscle. This provides no evidence that the pain arises from the muscle, and when resisted movement of the muscle alleged to be at fault proves strong and painless, the non-muscular origin of the pain becomes evident. In fact, primary fibrositis (the disorder, not the symptom) is an imaginary disease. This has been amply borne out by post-mortem experience, for many pathologists have sought for evidence of 'fibrositis', and though almost every patient in the country has had this label applied to one or other of his symptoms, no evidence pointing to the real existence of primary fibrositis has ever come to light. Indeed, the conditions once ascribed to such inflammation in the soft structures of the body, e.g. acute torticollis, pleurodynia, lumbago, can be shown by proper interpretation of the physical signs to result from internal derangement of a spinal joint. 'Rheumatic' inflammation of the soft tissues was postulated as a pathological entity and the cause of lumbago by Sir William Gowers in 1904. He offered no evidence, but his bare statement was accepted for forty years until it was challenged for the first time in *The Lancet* (Cyriax, 1945).

'Primary' fibrositis is in fact a secondary phenomenon. When the dura mater is compressed, usually *via* the posterior ligament by a protruding disc, pain is felt in the neighbourhood, but not necessarily at the site of pressure. Within this painful area there is always a tender spot at a point where no lesion exists at all. It is a remarkable finding, but it does not mislead those who test the function of the tissue containing the tender spot. When such a spot is found in a structure, the function of which can be shown to be normal, its referred nature becomes evident. The irony of the situation lies in the fact that disc lesions, which do not result in inflammation of muscle but merely referred tenderness, are often called 'fibrositis', whereas when traumatic inflammation of fibrous tissue *is* present, e.g. in supraspinatus tendinitis, tennis-elbow, a sprained ligament, this word is seldom used.

Various efforts have been made to relate referred tenderness to metabolites formed locally as the result of nervous impulses. That no such reaction occurs is clearly demonstrated by watching the changes in an area of referred tenderness during manipulative reduction of a displaced portion of cervical disc. At first, the patient has an area of tenderness which he

B

fingers himself and regards as the source of his symptoms. As reduction of the displacement proceeds, this area moves abruptly from place to place; as a rule, the pain and tenderness in the lower scapular area shift closer towards the midline and move upwards from the mid-thorax towards the lower neck. The tenderness follows the pain, and a tender spot, a minute later, entirely ceases to be painful on pressure; but another tender spot appears in a new position. Clearly, metabolites produced locally could not move from one muscle to another in a few seconds merely because the neck was manipulated. When a full and painless range of movement has been restored to the cervical joints the final tender point disappears.

Electromyography has shown that lower motor neurone lesions lead to fasciculation in the relevant muscles. It was once thought that this might explain the referred tenderness so frequently present in spinal nerve-root compression. In sciatica the facts fit quite well, for the tenderness is usually found in the gluteal muscles (which are derived from the correct roots). But at the neck, in seventh cervical root-compression, the tenderness lies in the trapezius, levator scapulae or spinatus muscles, none of which is supplied by this root. Electromyography reveals, as would be expected, that the scapular and vertebro-scapular muscles are free from fasciculation in a disorder at this level; hence referred tenderness cannot be correlated with the muscular fasciculation due to partial denervation.

Secondary Fibrositis

There is no important controversy about the existence of five categories of this disorder: traumatic, rheumatoid, infectious, parasitic and myositic.

1. Traumatic Fibrositis

This may show itself as a painful scar. The cause may be overuse or a single strain. Perhaps the best example is a tennis-elbow. A minor rupture occurs at the origin of the common extensor tendon from the lateral humeral epicondyle. Very little aching occurs at first, but, as the torn edges begin to unite and are pulled apart again each time the muscle is used, excess scar tissue is laid down in the healing breach. Within one to three weeks the elbow becomes quite painful from the development of chronic traumatic fibrositis at the site of the tear.

Scarring in an intercostal or in the gastrocnemius muscle, golfer's elbow, tendinitis at the shoulder, adherence of a ligament after a sprain, periarticular adhesions after an injury, capsular contracture after immobilization, crepitating teno-synovitis caused by overuse, olecranon bursitis after a blow, ischaemic contracture—all these and a number of similar conditions could be regarded as caused by post-traumatic fibrositis. But they are better described under their proper names.

2. Rheumatoid Fibrositis

Rheumatic inflammation occurs, of course, in rheumatic fever and chorea. A similar type of inflammation has been found in rheumatoid arthritis. In the U.S.A., Curtis and Pollard (1940) carried out biopsies on skin and muscle from patients with this disease and demonstrated small foci of round cells of the chronic inflammatory type. In 1942 Freund *et al.* demonstrated similar nodules on the nerve-sheaths. In England, Gibson, Kersley & Desmarais (1946 and 1948) confirmed these findings, and further proved that they were absent in patients suffering from ankylosing spondylitis. They showed that local degenerative changes affected the axons and medullary sheaths of the nerves close to these lesions, and they also demonstrated an increase in the interstitial connective tissue accompanied by extreme thinning of the muscle fibres. These findings were again confirmed by Morrison *et al.* at Harvard in 1947. Electromyographic studies (Steinberg & Parry, 1961) on patients with rheumatoid arthritis showed evidence of polymyositis in 85 per cent of such cases. These changes bore no direct relation to the degree of muscular weakness or of wasting, or to the use of steroid therapy.

Lately rheumatoid neuropathy has attracted increasing attention. This begins, most often in both lower limbs, with paraesthesia; later, motor weakness often supervenes. Patients with gross articular disease are liable to neuropathy; one-fifth of all such patients die within a year (Hart, 1960; Steinberg, 1960). There is thus no doubt that rheumatoid inflammation can affect a number of the fibrous tissues of the body. This fully accords with the clinical findings, which show that, in addition to the joint lesions, the tendon-sheaths thicken, the tendons become rough and nodular (particularly in the palm), and the bursae swell and fill with fluid. 'The inference may be drawn that rheumatoid arthritis is a generalized affection of the fibrous tissues of the body in which the chief and most obvious incidence is on the capsule of the joints.' (Cyriax, 1947.)

Polymyalgia rheumatica, a disorder of elderly people, was considered an entity allied to fibrositis until Coomes and Sharp (1961) pointed out that, although it is characterized by pain felt in the muscles, the muscular, symptoms are in fact referred from the joints. Arteritis, especially of the temporal vessels, is a common accompaniment and the sedimentation rate is raised, usually over 60 mm. in the first hour. Hamkin *et al.* (1964) prefer the term 'polymyalgia arterica'.

3. Infectious Fibrositis

Epidemic myalgia (Bornholm disease) is an infectious disease due to a virus which has been identified. It is characterized by fever, severe pain in the abdominal and thoracic muscles, and speedy recovery.

4. Parasitic Fibrositis

Infestation with *Trichina spiralis* causes fever and painful swelling of the affected muscles, and the overlying skin may become red; the tendons may also be invaded. The disease occurs about ten days after eating infected pork. Active contraction of the affected muscle increases the pain. The symptoms and signs subside in some weeks, and the patient becomes completely unaware of the foreign bodies in his muscles.

5. Myositis

This is a diffuse inflammatory disease of muscle. There is no pain; the muscle wastes progressively and marked weakness develops, which can be halted only by steroid therapy. The affection is often bilateral and symmetrical and is seldom distinguishable from myopathy except by biopsy.

Generalized Fibrositis

Rheumatoid arthritis is the only condition to which the term 'generalized fibrositis' properly applies. By contrast, the disorder to which this name is often given is disc lesions at several spinal levels. This may lead to considerable aching over part or the whole of the trunk—areas, where muscular crepitus and fatty nodules are commonly detectable. Unrecognized osteitis deformans or ankylosing spondylitis is repeatedly called fibrositis.

Another disorder often called 'generalized fibrositis' is psychoneurotic pain. The idea of generalized fibrositis has led to such concepts as 'the psychological basis of rheumatism'—a notion in which the cart is put before the horse. Clearly, psychogenic pain is not rheumatism, and the discovery of the real cause should lead to revision of that ascription, not to an attempt to fuse two incompatible diagnoses.

MUSCLE TONE

Postural Tone

Feldberg (1951) points out that acetylcholine is released not only as a result of a nerve-impulse, but also at a very low level when the muscle is at rest. So long as the mechanism for the destruction of acetylcholine is intact, the amount liberated is too small to cause muscular contraction and the electromyograph cannot therefore detect its presence. It is probable that this phenomenon is more marked in trained than untrained muscles; tone may well be affected by variation in the subliminal level of acetylcholine production. In mammals it appears that tone is served by what is now known as the small motor-nerve-fibre system. The anterior roots have long been known to contain a distinct group of small diameter fibres (Eccles and Sherrington 1930), as well as the large fibres. The function of these fibrils remained unknown until it was recently shown to serve the maintenance of sustained muscular contraction.

Kremer (1958, *Brit. med. J.* ii, 123) has summarized the results of Merton and his colleagues' work on the maintenance of postural bone, thus:

'A muscle is brought into action by motor impulses, but the degree of that contraction is estimated by sensory receptors in the muscle, and in the light of this information, called the "feedback", it modifies the rate of motor discharge. It is true that visual information may modify the motor discharge, as may cutaneous impulses, but it is the muscle sense organs which play the major part in assessing or monitoring the performance of the muscles themselves.

'The muscle spindles are the sensory organs of muscles. They lie among the main muscle fibres, having the same attachments and therefore altering in size with contraction or relaxation of the muscle itself. It must be remembered that the poles of these muscle spindles are contractile and receive very fine-fibred efferent supply, the γ fibres, whereas the main muscles receive large or α fibres. The reflex connections of the muscles are such that impulses set up by stretching the spindles excite the muscles' own motor neurones. Thus extension of the muscle results in an augmented contraction which tends to resist the extension. This is the stretch reflex of Liddell and Sherrington (1924). This has the properties of a closed loop self-regulating mechanism using information from the spindles to maintain a constant muscle length. It is clear that this has enormous advantages over a straight-through system in which posture is maintained by a steady stream of motor impulses without sensory modification or feedback, in that it automatically compensates for changes in load or for fatigue.

'This type of stretch reflex would maintain a fixed posture well, but it is clearly inflexible and needs modification for ease of changing muscle-lengths while maintaining postural tone. This modification is carried out by means of the contractile poles of the muscle spindles. The sensory portion of the spindle lies between these poles, hence shortening the poles by impulses along the efferents will stretch the sensory spindle so that the stretch reflex will be activated just as if the muscle itself had been stretched. The muscle will then shorten reflexly until the increased rate of spindle discharge has been offset, and that will be when the muscle has shortened to the same extent as the contractile poles of the spindle.

'Merton and his associates have named the loop mechanism of the simple stretch reflex the "length-servo" mechanism and the modification next mentioned the "follow-up servo".'

Joseph (1964) has shown that the maintenance of the upright position needs very little energy. The only muscles in constant action are the calf muscles and those over the maximum convexity of the trunk—i.e. mid-thorax; only slight activity can be detected in the lumbar and cervical regions. The knees are kept straight by the tautening of their posterior ligaments, not by quadriceps action. Provided the vertical dropped from the centre of gravity falls through the ankles, there is little difference between the energy consumption of a person erect or lying down, irrespective of different degrees of curvature of the spine.

Athletic Tone

Electromyography has demonstrated that the concept of muscle tone as a state of slight neurogenic sustained muscular contraction is false. This is not surprising, for training increases what used to be called tone. Obviously, if use of a muscle caused it to relax less readily than before, training would defeat its own object and a highly trained runner would have to walk on tiptoe. Training clearly enhances the function of muscle, i.e. it contracts *and* relaxes more efficiently. Joseph (1964) states that it is difficult to eradicate the idea that a relaxed muscle still possesses tone. This idea was first put forward by Müller in 1838 and has proved most tenacious, in spite of clear demonstration by even the most delicate electromyography that no contracting motor units exist in relaxed muscle. Joseph suggests that the term 'muscle tone' should be abandoned and 'response to stretch' substituted. Hypertonic and hypotonic states would then refer to excessive or reduced stretch response respectively. Muscles, he states, which cannot be completely relaxed are contracting, and should not be regarded as hypertonic. A spastic muscle is not just hypertonic; it is a muscle undergoing a continuous contraction easily demonstrated electromyographically.

This fact has an important practical bearing. For example, if a patient suffering from the thoracic outlet syndrome is given exercises to the elevator muscles of the scapulae, no advantage accrues; for however strengthened these muscles become, they relax perfectly as soon as voluntary movement ceases, and the scapulae then occupy the same position as before.

Neurogenic Hypertonus

Muscular spasm secondary to painful lesions is unconnected with the hypertonus that accompanies neurological disease. In the former, when movement is limited at an arthritic joint a certain amount of mobility is painless, but at a constant point muscular spasm brings it to an abrupt stop and no forcing without anaesthesia can take it beyond this point. By contrast, neurogenic hypertonus results in an early resistance to passive movements until, suddenly, the resistance to stretch of the muscles is overcome and a full range of painless movement is revealed. Initial resistance, later giving way, also occurs in hysteria.

Cramp

This may result from hyperventilation, hypocalcaemia, tetanus, strychnine poisoning, salt deprivation or pyramidal lesions, and can be very painful. It is also common in healthy people, usually occurring only at night. The pain is in the calf, possibly in the foot also, the foot and toes becoming fixed in full flexion or full extension. The disorder is un-connected with tetany, but it is apt to affect the calf muscles on the same side as a past attack of sciatica and is a common sequel to a posterior radicotomy at the fifth lumbar or first sacral level. The fact that several muscles of one limb are affected in a co-ordinate way suggests a nervous aetiology; it may be due to a discharge of impulses from the spinal cord, analogous to the mechanism of epilepsy—a concept supported by the electromyographic studies of Norris, Gasteiger & Chatfield (1957) who regard the cramp as being initiated in the central nervous system. Cer-tainly, in cramp, it is the muscles that hurt. Cramp does not spontaneously affect a muscle; it is brought on by a voluntary contraction. Hence patients soon discover that it is most quickly abolished by passively stretching the affected muscle.

Muscle Spasm

The notion of 'fibrositis', with its emphasis on alleged primary disease of muscle, has led to further misconceptions. One is painful muscle spasm fixing a joint. The spasm is thought to be primary, but it is merely called into being by a protective reflex originating elsewhere. Capener (1961) has lent his authority to the idea of painful muscle spasm in 'acute derangements of the lower spine'. In his view, the muscle spasm over-shadows everything else and as soon as it is controlled the trouble begins to subside. The converse is the case, as can be proved by epidural local anaesthesia which cannot reach the lumbar muscles. When the disc-displacement recedes, the pain, felt in the muscles but not originating from them, abates.

In orthopaedic disorders, the muscle spasm is secondary and is the result of, not the cause of, pain; of itself it causes no symptoms. It is only cramp and neurogenic spasms that hurt muscles. Muscle spasm is thought to require treatment, as evidenced by the many muscle relaxants that are advertised for the cure of, e.g. lumbago, osteo-arthritis of the hip. The treatment of muscle spasm is of the lesion to which it is secondary; it never of itself requires treatment in lesions of the moving parts.

The main function of muscle is to contract. This function is evoked by any important lesion in the vicinity of the muscle, whether it involves a moving tissue or not. For example, appendicitis or a perforated ulcer leads to spasm of the abdominal muscles, although this has no effect on the mobility of the viscus at fault. It is true that muscles spring readily into spasm to protect a moving part, but they also contract about lesions whose behaviour they cannot influence. Spasm is thus the reaction, indeed the only reaction of which a contractile structure is capable, to any lesion of sufficient severity in its neighbourhood. Although spasm (neurogenic apart) originally evolved as a protective mechanism, it is not always beneficial. It is clearly useful in acute arthritis, preventing movement at the joint; it is equally obviously harmful after the disorder has become chronic. If manipulation under anaesthesia does good, the spasm was clearly militating against recovery.

Spasm in Arthritis

The muscles are not in constant spasm about an arthritic joint. When the joint is at rest in a neutral position, spasm is absent. It springs into being to prevent movement beyond a certain point, and even then only one group of muscles contracts. When the capsule of the joint is stretched to a certain limit, involuntary spasm of the muscles that oppose that movement is elicited; the movement stops instantly. However often this movement is repeated, it always ceases at exactly the same point. If movement in a different direction is attempted, that too is restricted by spasm of another group of muscles. Such contraction of muscle is no more painful nor greater than if the patient had voluntarily used his muscles to arrest movement at that same point. For example, the muscle spasm that limits movement at the wrist in carpal fracture is no more intense than if the movement were stopped voluntarily. Moreover, at the extreme of the possible range, the pain is felt at the wrist, not in the upper forearm where the contracting bellies lie. It would have been reasonable to suppose that this muscle guarding would give them more to do; yet muscles waste about a damaged joint.

Though muscle spasm in arthritis is protective, and in bacterial arthritis most beneficial, it is excessive in less grave articular disorders. For example, the marked traumatic arthritis in the knee after sprain of a ligament causes far more limitation of joint movement than is required merely to prevent further overstretching of the ligament. Indeed, there is no muscle at the knee which can limit the valgus mobility that would result in further stretching in medial ligament strain. The prompt abatement of the arthritis by hydrocortisone applied at the point where the ligament is torn greatly hastens recovery. It is clear, therefore, that the arthritic reaction to the injury, and the consequent restriction of movement by muscle spasm, serve no useful purpose. The same may or may not apply to a chronic articular lesion. An adhesion may have formed, and may prove incapable of rupture because of muscle spasm limiting the therapeutic movement. After rupture under anaesthesia, the joint remains mobile and painless. In this instance, the spasm is harmful. Yet in rheumatoid arthritis the same joint with the same degree of limitation of movement would flare up severely if anaesthesia were employed to abolish spasm and to permit manipulation. In this case the spasm is beneficial. When an abcess forms in the bone near a joint, arthritis with limited movement maintained by muscle spasm results. Such sympathetic arthritis serves no purpose, for no lesion of the joint exists at all. Immobility of, say, the temporo-mandibular joint does not hasten the healing of a septic tooth socket. A similar situation exists in the lung, where commencing erosion of the ribs by a neoplasm may set up spasm of the pectoralis major muscle, such that the arm cannot be raised above the horizontal.

It is clear that the defences of the body cannot distinguish between lesions in which spasm is beneficial (e.g. bacterial and rheumatoid), in which it is useless (e.g. visceral), and in which it is harmful (e.g. post-traumatic adhesions). The lesion, whatever type it is, merely engenders spasm in neighbouring muscles, as a uniform reaction to various stimuli.

Spasm in Bursitis

In bursitis, although limitation of movement occurs, involuntary muscle spasm is absent. For example, when the subdeltoid bursa is acutely inflamed, movement of the arm is so painful that the patient brings it to a halt by voluntarily contracting the relevant group of muscles. If he is asked to allow a little more movement disregarding pain, he can do so. This is a situation quite different from arthritis where the patient cannot be cajoled into permitting greater range, since this is limited by involuntary muscle spasm.

Spasm in Internal Derangement

Internal derangement blocks a joint, partly mechanically, partly as a result of protective muscle spasm. This is beneficial when it prevents the ligamentous overstretching which would result if the blocked movement were forced, but a disadvantage when it impedes reduction of the displacement. When the meniscus is displaced at the knee, both mechanisms arise. The hamstrings go into beneficial spasm to prevent the ligamentous overstretching that full extension of the joint would produce; but this militates against manipulative reduction, which therefore has often to be carried out after the spasm has been abolished by general anaesthesia. The same applies in lumbago with considerable lateral deviation at the deranged spinal joint; side-flexion towards the convex side is prevented by muscle-guarding. The spasm is often on the painless side, thus proving that it is not the muscle that hurts. Lying down diminishes the compression strain on the lumbar joint and consequently the degree of protrusion. The list to one side visible on standing may therefore disappear so long as the patient remains recumbent. Manipulative reduction abolishes the pain and the deviation *pari passu*. This is quite a different situation from arthritis where, for example, the amount of limitation of movement at the knee or a tarsal joint is the same whether the patient bears weight on the joint or not. The patient whose lumbar spine tilts sideways may be told of his awkward posture and see it in a mirror, but he does not feel asymmetrical. The position which his lumbar spine adopts because of muscle spasm is involuntary and painless.

Spasm in Nerve-root Compression

Muscle spasm comes into play to protect the nerve-roots from the third lumbar to the third sacral from painful stretching. This occurs only when the mobility of the dural sleeve of these six nerve-roots is impaired. When the third lumbar nerve-root loses its mobility, prone-lying knee-flexion may be limited. When the other nerve-roots are compressed, straight-leg raising is nearly always restricted. Spasm of the quadriceps or hamstring muscles is responsible; it is involuntary and painless. The pain on stretching originates from the nerve-root, not the muscle. This can be shown by lifting the straight leg as far as it will go; in sciatica, this hurts. The patient is then asked to bend his head forwards, and the sciatic pain is often sharply increased. Whereas the nerve-root can be stretched *via* the dura mater by neck flexion, the hamstring muscles cannot.

Though straight-leg raising may have remained limited for many years, no contracture of the hamstring muscles results. Even in chronic cases, epidural local anaesthesia often restores a full range of straight-leg raising within a few minutes, by abolishing the sensitivity of the nerve-root whence the stimulus to the hamstrings to contract originates.

Spasm in Fracture and Dislocation

Spasm is constant about a recent fracture, immobilizing the broken ends, not necessarily in a good position. Reduction may prove impossible until the spasm is abolished. This can be accomplished by general anaesthesia, which inhibits the cerebral maintenance of muscle contraction, or by stopping the afferent impulses to which it is due, i.e. by local anaesthesia induced at the broken surfaces. Immobilization in a special position is often required, so that after reduction the broken piece is not pulled out of place again when muscle spasm returns after anaesthesia ceases.

Dislocation makes the muscles go into spasm and often prevents reduction, which has therefore to be carried out under general anaesthesia.

Spasm in Partial Rupture of Muscle Belly

Partial rupture of a muscle belly causes localized spasm, protecting the breach from tension. This spasm is localized; for example, when some fibres of the gastrocnemius muscle are torn, the muscle shortens centrally only. In consequence, the foot can be moved down and up by contraction and relaxation of the unaffected upper and lower parts of the muscle, but full dorsiflexion is limited by the contracture and the patient has to walk on tiptoe for the first few days. In partial rupture of the quadriceps and hamstring muscles, prone-lying knee-flexion or straight-leg raising is often limited by the muscle shortening owing to localized muscle spasm about the breach. This spasm does not hurt, but tension on the ruptured fibres, when exerted by passive stretching or resisted contraction of the damaged muscle, is painful.

When a tendon ruptures, the muscle belly does not go into spasm but, in due course, develops a contracture. No limitation of passive movement at the joint can result, although active movement may no longer be possible. Even if the belly shortens, since it is no longer attached to bone, the passive range at the joint remains unaltered.

Muscle Spasm protecting the Dura Mater

The dura mater is stretched in flexion of the neck and is at its shortest in full extension. An early sign in meningism is limitation of neck-flexion, and in severe meningitis intense muscle spasm fixes the neck in full extension, thereby relaxing the dura mater to the maximum. This, of course, does not help therapeutically. A minor manifestation of this phenomenon is theracic or lumbar pain on flexion of the neck when the mobility of the dura mater is impaired by a postero-central disc-protrusion. Occasionally, the movement is limited by slight muscle guarding.

In lumbago, muscle spasm also comes into play to protect the lower extent of the dura mater from being stretched. In a postero-central disc-protrusion of any size, straight-leg raising is bilaterally limited by spasm of the hamstring muscles. This restriction protects the theca from the pull of the sciatic nerve-roots, when its mobility is impaired at a low lumbar level.

Spasm in Sepsis

Sepsis in the region of a joint (e.g. staphylococcal olecranon bursitis) causes swelling and limited movement, the result of muscle spasm. Any inflammatory focus within the abdomen causes maintained spasm of all the anterior muscles. The board-like abdominal wall in peritonitis is the extreme example. Even a mere inflamed gland in the neck lying in contact with the scalene muscles may set up enough spasm to fix the neck in side-flexion towards the painful side for a week or two. Such spasm has no virtue; the gland recovers at its own speed.

Spasm of unstriated muscle within the abdomen is of itself painful as sufferers from biliary, renal or intestinal colic know well. Such inter-mittent contraction of the circular fibres provokes no secondary contrac-tion of the abdominal muscles.

Arterial Spasm

Damage to an artery leads to spasm of the circular coat but, as in spasm of the bronchioles, no pain is caused; it is a beneficial phenomenon which arrests the bleeding when the artery is cut or torn. However, it is dan-gerous when the artery is badly enough bruised to go into spasm while it is still intact. At the elbow, ischaemic contracture in the flexor muscles of the forearm results when the brachial artery is affected, usually after a supracondylar fracture of the humerus.

Should Muscle Spasm be Treated?

Except in cramp, no. In the lesions with which this book deals, muscle spasm is a secondary phenomenon and its treatment is that of the primary disorder. No one treats by relaxants the muscle spasm due to appendicitis. Similarly, if an arthritis or a degree of internal derangement can be abated, the protection given to the joint by the muscles becomes unnecessary. Muscle spasm takes care of itself; all that is necessary is to treat the lesion. This is important, since the wide vogue for relaxant drugs for 'rheumatism', 'fibrositis', lumbago, etc., is based on the fallacy of painful muscle spasm.

Muscle Wasting

The bulk and strength of a muscle depends on three factors: use, nerve supply and the integrity of the joint it spans. The more the patient uses his muscles, the stronger they become. Disuse, especially immobilization in plaster, prevents a muscle working and quickly leads to wasting. If nerve conduction is impaired, a number of muscle-fibres no longer contract since they receive no impulse; they waste. Use and a normal nerve supply do not suffice. For example, the gluteal and quadriceps muscles are given plenty of work by a man with a normal knee and osteoarthritis of the hip, who walks about with a fairly good range of movement. Yet these muscles will have lost much of their bulk. The fact that the muscles waste unduly in rheumatoid arthritis has been noted for many years, and this wasting is much greater than the joint involvement warrants. Steinberg and Parry's (1961) electromyographic findings have demonstrated polymyositis in 85 per cent of cases of established rheumatoid arthritis.

The integrity of the joint, even if the patient is unaware of any disease, is an important factor governing the state of the muscles. This is well illustrated by the following case:

A man of 66 had spent six months in bed at the age of 40 with gonorrhoeal arthritis of the hip joint. The W.R. was negative. After apparent recovery he used the leg normally, and stated that for 25 years he had walked as far as he liked without discomfort, apart from some feeling of tiredness in the thigh. He complained of some weeks' aching in the left thigh. Examination revealed gross wasting in quadriceps, gluteal and hamstring muscles, but, surprisingly, a full range of movement at the hip joint. However, his discomfort was reduced by forcing rotation at the hip joint. X-ray examination revealed complete destruction of articular cartilage and large osteophytes (Plate 1). A week later the pain ceased spontaneously.

This extreme instance of symptomless arthritis, accompanied by many years' full use of the muscles about the joint, shows how dependent muscle bulk is on the integrity of the joint as such. The wasting is not the result merely of disuse, because years of full function through the full range does not restore the muscle atrophy.

No structure of the body is so quickly altered by influences outside itself as muscle. Once a muscle has wasted considerably, even though no disease of the muscle itself has ever occurred, it may never regain full bulk. It is not uncommon, for example, to see, in a patient who had the meniscus removed, a full range of movement at the knee, which has given no trouble for years; yet the quadriceps muscle is noticeably and permanently wasted.

Exercise and Exertion

When a patient is asked to 'take exercise', he thinks in terms of exertion. When he is asked to 'do exercises', he is more likely to think in terms of movement. 'Exercise' is an ambiguous term, which should not be used without further explanation when speaking to patients; otherwise, they are apt to follow instructions incorrectly. From the therapeutic point of view, exercise and exertion are quite distinct, and often have contrary results. Consider a patient who has recently undergone meniscectomy. He now needs to restore the range of movement at his knee by *exercises*, i.e. gentle, voluntary increase in range each day. He also needs to strengthen his quadriceps muscles by *exercises*, i.e. exertion without weight-bearing at first, so as not to overstrain the joint. Were he to exert his knee joint and gently move his muscles, the result would be disastrous.

It is also an exercise to keep a joint still against a force tending to move it, but the layman does not appreciate this. When a patient with a lumbar disc lesion without displacement is shown how to avoid recurrence by maintaining his lordosis by muscular effort, he is using his muscles to keep the joints motionless in a good position. In this way, the muscles are exercised and the joints are not. None of these differences is clear to patients, on account of the many interpretations of the word 'exercise'. Hence, many people with a stiff shoulder decide to dig, thus subjecting a painful joint to overuse and consequent increase in pain. By contrast, benefit may well follow gentle active movements of increasing amplitude without load. A footballer's knee muscles need exertion for final re-habilitation after injury, but no one (I hope) would make a patient bend to lift heavy weights in order to keep him free from lumbago. The lesion present and the aims of rehabilitation determine the type of exercises that are required.

Limited Movement in Arthritus

It is frequently taught and believed that in arthritis movement is necessarily limited in every direction. This is not so. For example, in early arthritis at the shoulder, lateral rotation may at first be the only movement to be limited, and even some time later medial rotation may be of full range, though painful. At the knee and elbow, in even moderately advanced arthritis, both rotations remain of full range and painless; even gross arthritis often leaves the hip with a full range of lateral rotation; an arthritic talocalcanean joint fixes in full valgus. The idea that movement is necessarily limited in every direction in arthritis deserves revision, for it leads to long delay in reaching a correct diagnosis at those joints where the capsular pattern happens to be selective. It also prevents correct ascription in joints that are supported purely by ligaments and possess no muscles about them to control movement, e.g. the acromio-clavicular or sacro-iliac joints. Here, no limitation of movement can result however severe the arthritis, for muscle spasm limiting movement at a certain point cannot occur, since no such muscles exist.

It is also taught and believed that arthritis is visible radiographically. Advanced degeneration of a joint involving the bones does show, but in many instances this never happens. Even long-standing arthritis at the shoulder, for example, may produce no radiographic change at all. I have waited five years for an arthritic sacro-iliac joint to show sclerosis, and in early gout, rhematoid or Reiter's arthritis, the X-ray appearances are of no help. Complete fixation of the lumbo-thoracic joints in spondylitis precedes visible ossification by many years, and spondylitic hips, even though movement is grossly limited during a flare-up, do not at first show any radiographic change. Traumatic arthritis at finger, elbow or knee, and even the meniscus displaced within the knee, are invisible on the X-ray photograph.

Arthritis is present when the capsular pattern (see Chapter 6) is found on clinical examination, whatever the X-ray and other ancillary examinations may or may not show.

Menopausal Arthritis

I regard this term as a misnomer. Women develop a number of painful disorders at one joint or another, amongst other times, between the ages of forty and sixty. These disorders do not differ from the same conditions occurring at other ages, or in men. In fact, the commonest condition to which the label menopausal arthritis is erroneously applied, is an impacted loose body in the knee joint.

In my view it is not reasonable to label a condition menopausal unless it occurs only in female patients at the climacteric, and I have been unable to identify any joint disease peculiar to this sex and this epoch.

Panniculitis

In middle-aged women, symmetrical fatty deposits develop, especially at the buttocks and thighs. They lie just under the skin, superficial to the muscles. If pain in the buttocks or thigh arises in such a patient, the association of pain with the presence of sensitive deposits in the same area can be deceptive, but only if the examiner relies on palpation alone. If he finds, as might be expected, that some movement of the trunk or limb affects the pain, he knows that the pain arises from a moving part. Fat lying between skin and muscle cannot interfere with movement, as examination of the other limb—equally tender but painless—will show. Nor can it give rise to referred pain, for it lies too superficially.

Relapsing non-suppurative nodular panniculitis (Weber-Christian disease) is of course a real entity. It is characterized by the periodic appearance of crops of tender subcutaneous fatty nodules with fever. This was regarded as an incurable disorder until Benson and Fowler (1964) found that Tanderil (oxyphenbutazone) was effective in a dose of 200 mg. three times a day for three days followed by 100 mg. three times a day for a month.

ECONOMIC CONSIDERATIONS

The economic effect of different ways of treating disease is a subject to which little attention has so far been paid. When it is a matter of life and death, money does not matter, for the relief of lethal disease and the prevention of crippledom carry benefits beyond price. However, progress in medicine and surgery has been so great that many common and potentially serious disorders have ceased to be much of a financial burden. As a drain on the nation's purse, their place has been taken by conditions medically unimportant but industrially disabling, e.g. lumbago. For example, thanks to penicillin, large numbers of patients no longer spend six months off work with pneumonia followed by empyema. But large numbers are still off work today for a similar period with sciatica due to a disc lesion, just as they were in previous decades. As a result of the recently acquired control of dangerous illness, the less serious causes of disablement

Millions of days per year

52·27 Neurosis, psychosis	15·39 Tuberculosis
40·18 Arthritis, rheumatism	12·13 Stomach trouble
35·42 Influenza	4·21 Allergy
29·53 Bronchitis	2·58 Hernia
16·51 Accidents	2·21 Pneumonia
16·28 Heart and blood- vessel disease	0·55 Cancer

Days lost to industry through illness 1956–7. Note that disorders of the moving parts (rheumatism) are outnumbered only by neurosis.

have reached a new prominence. Lesions of the soft moving parts now constitute a major cause of inability to work, taking second place only to psychoneurosis. Since so much of this invalidism is avoidable, attention should be concentrated on these lesions, not only on humanitarian grounds but also to save the National Health Service and employers from paying out large sums unnecessarily.

Let us take a simple example. A man spends a fortnight in bed with lumbago. Our figures show that 50 per cent of such cases can be relieved in one treatment. Were each such patient treated, and every other one successfully, a saving of five-sevenths of his weekly salary would be made in money paid out for work not done. This figure is reached by assuming that the patient is off work for two days instead of two weeks. If 20,000 such sufferers exist each week and receive a salary of £1,000 a year, this implies a weekly loss of £300,000 to industry. Two hundred doctors could see these patients at the rate of twenty a day, and their cost to the country (at £3,000 a year each) would be a mere £11,540 a week in salary and perhaps a similar sum for accommodation in hospital. Hence, from lumbago alone a profit to the nation of thirteen times the outlay would accrue.

This figure takes no account of the many other lesions of the moving parts which keep a patient off heavy work for months instead of days or weeks, nor of the cases of neglected lumbago that become sciatica and lead to months of bed rest. One American firm (quoted anonymously in the *Sunday Citizen* for 20th June, 1965) for fifteen months compared the effect of the manual treatment of backache with the figures for the previous fifteen months, when traditional treatment only was given. They found that the total of days lost from work dropped from 1,203 to 119, and that compensation payments fell from $20,000 to $2,500. This fits in very well with the thirteenfold saving arrived at in the above calculation. The President of the British Rheumatism and Arthritis Association stated (1965) that 10 per cent of working time lost through illness was due to locomotor disorders, with an estimated loss to the nation of £100 million a year. It may well be argued that this figure includes rheumatoid arthritis, osteoarthritis and even mitral stenosis, and the significance of these figures would be clearer if it could be ascertained what proportion of these patients had each type of illness. Help is given by an investigation carried out in Sweden (Edstrom, 1945), in which every doctor in the country was asked to report on the incidence of rheumatic disorders. Sixty-two thousand statements were collated, with the following results:

Sciatica, backache, myalgia and similar disorders	42·2 per cent
Chronic arthritis	26·8 per cent
Osteoarthritis	17·9 per cent
Rheumatic fever and acute polyarthritis	13·3 per cent

Since so much cervical and lumbar disc-trouble is attributed to 'osteo-arthritis' if the patient is no longer young, it is reasonable, from the figure quoted above, to add to the number of cases of sciatica etc. half the number of cases of osteoarthritis. This implies that half of all these patients suffered from disc trouble. Hence, the annual loss from this cause of disablement may well run into 13 million days a year. Since most people in this country earn at least £3 a working day, the minimum figure for money paid for work not done is nearly £40 million a year. As skilled treatment of disc lesions reduces the period off work by about nine-tenths, the saving on this score alone would amount to £36 million. Confirmatory statistics were published by H.M.S.O. in 1965. During that year there were 21 million people in Britain covered by National Insurance. They made 9 million claims in a year and 300 million working days were lost. Of this number, 20 million days were lost because of arthritis and rheumatism, of which Edstrom's reckoning suggests half are disc lesions. Ten million days a year are thus lost on this account: a thirtieth of the total. During that year benefit was paid to the tune of £220 million, and a thirtieth of that is £7·3 millions. Nine-tenths of that is £6·6 millions and represents the saving that orthopaedic medicine offers to the Sickness Funds, in this part of its scope alone.

Further data were put forward at a symposium held at Glasgow in 1966, derived from a study of 6·5 million periods of absence from work. The analysis showed that 5·1 per cent of absence in men was due to back troubles, and 2·4 per cent in women, the total number of back lesions causing absence from work amounting to 500,000. In men drawing injury benefit, the proportion rose to 11·4 per cent, in women to 6·2 per cent. Nearly 8 per cent of all injuries involving time off work were due to the back. Extraordinary figures emerged for the average length of time off work with back troubles. Although only 45,720 out of 342,720 cases were labelled sciatica (which after all can last some time), the remaining 87 per cent complained of backache only. Yet the average periods of 'incapacity' reported in this survey were: 13 weeks in men and 17 weeks in women under twenty-five years of age. After the age of 45, these periods rose to 22 and 24 weeks respectively. Moreover, the figures ignored 'short' cases lasting only three or four weeks, so that the actual figures are much larger. At St. Thomas's Hospital, backache causing absence from work for as long as four weeks would be regarded as most unusual. If these long periods of idleness are countenanced over large parts of the country, and are at all representative of the general situation, the benefit accruing from the provision of an orthopaedic medical service throughout the country far surpasses anything previously envisaged.

This sum, however, represents only a fraction of the potential saving. For example, the prevention of months off work with brachial neuritis by manipulative reduction of the cervical disc lesion responsible, at the time when it presents no difficulty—namely, during the stage of only scapular pain—would produce another large saving. Then there are the painful shoulders, tennis-elbows, sprained wrists and knees, which may keep men off heavy work for months and yet are often quickly relievable by orthopaedic medical means. Moreover, the system of diagnosis outlined in this book singles out cases of psychogenic pain and of malingering —the former a common, undetected cause of prolonged absence from work.

The treatment offered by orthopaedic medicine has nothing in common with the contemporary attitude in which radiography, reassurance that the bones are intact and no important disease is present, followed by routine physiotherapy, are considered adequate treatment for arthritis, a displacement, a damaged ligament or a strained tendon. It is in vain that doctors assure patients that nothing serious is amiss medically, when the patient finds he cannot work; for that to him *is* serious. The trouble is that lasting harm does not accrue to a patient's health if he is unable to go to work as the result of, say, backache; he suffers economic disability rather than any damage to his bodily health. The disadvantage to the patient of withholding effective treatment is social and financial; again, these are matters regarded as not strictly medical. The doctor may say to himself that the patient receives the same salary whether on the job or not; he returns, at the end of however many weeks it may be, to work neither better nor worse for having recovered slowly with the passage of time rather than quickly as the result of adequate treatment. If he is self-employed, he has suffered economic loss, pain and anxiety beyond the minimum, and if he has a tendency to neurosis, this has been encouraged. If he is a salaried worker, the loss is to the nation. Since so much of the damage is economic, it is the Insurance Companies, the Federation of employers and the National Health Service that would benefit from the practice of orthopaedic medicine as much as would the patients themselves. Educated patients know this; hence, informed people often themselves patronize, and insist on valued employees visiting, osteopaths for conditions suitable and unsuitable alike. They prefer to pay private fees in the hope of getting well quickly, even though the State has assumed the entire responsibility for the medical care of the nation. The existence of some 3,000 lay manipulators in this country—one to each eight family doctors—affords some measure of the degree to which one aspect only of orthopaedic medicine is lacking from the medical facilities offered to the nation.

This is a unique hiatus. No matter what disease a patient may develop, under the National Health Service he will be competently treated on lines basically similar at all hospitals throughout the country. For this reason there are no penicillinopaths or insulinopaths, and no one with heart disease would dream of consulting a cardiopath, for the simple reason that from the first his illness will be properly treated within the medical aegis, and he knows this to be so. The only exceptions are the disorders that come within the scope of orthopaedic medicine, for which few facilities exist and the patient often feels—unfortunately with justification—that nothing, or nothing constructive, is being done.

2

Trauma to Soft Tissues

REST AND PAIN

An important landmark in medical history was the appearance, in 1863, of Hilton's book on the value of rest in the treatment of pain. This book has held sway over medical thought until recently, although perusal shows that nearly all the cases on which Hilton based his recommendations would now be recognized as tuberculous. When pain is due to bacterial inflammation, Hilton's advocacy of rest remains unchallenged and is today one of the main principles of medical treatment. When, however, somatic pain is caused by inflammation due to trauma, his ideas have required modification. When non-bacterial inflammation attacks the soft tissues that move, treatment by rest has been found to result in chronic disability later, although the symptoms may temporarily diminish. Hence, during the present century, treatment by rest has given way to therapeutic movement in many soft tissue lesions. Movement may be applied in various ways: the three main categories are (1) active and resisted exercises; (2) passive, especially forced, movement; (3) deep massage.

Hilton spoke of pain generically; whereas inflammation causing pain is nowadays divided, from the point of view of treatment, into that which *is* caused and that which *is not* caused by bacteria. In either case it is pain and loss of function that the patient experiences; for the symptoms of, say, a bacterial or rheumatoid or a traumatic arthritis may be identical. Hence the patient cannot decide for himself whether his pain is due to a lesion requiring rest or movement for its alleviation. How can he understand that a sprained shoulder or ankle should be moved, but a sprained elbow or back rested? Indeed, a patient normally takes the view that pain is Nature's danger signal, and regards any activity that causes pain as harmful. This theorizing is perfectly logical, and sometimes correct; but sometimes it is not, even when it at first appears confirmed when avoidance of activity is found initially to ease the pain. Once more the false conclusion is reached that rest is the treatment of all pain. Only the medical man can decide whether the patient's symptoms arise from a lesion requiring treatment by rest or by movement. It depends on the diagnosis, and is different for different joints and different tissues.

It is becoming increasingly clear that the reaction of the body to noxious stimuli, whatever their nature, is the same. Physical and chemical agents set up the same stereotyped inflammation as do bacteria. Menkin's series of experiments has left no doubt on this point.

The excessive reaction of tissues to an injury is conditioned by the over-riding needs of a process designed to limit bacterial invasion. If there is to be only one pattern of response, it must be that suited to the graver of the two possible traumata. However, elaborate preparation for preventing the spread of bacteria is not only pointless after an aseptic injury, but is so excessive as to prove harmful in itself. The principle on which the treat-ment of recent post-traumatic inflammation is based is that the reaction of the body to an injury unaccompanied by infection is always too great. The most recent view of inflammation, now generally accepted, is that the noxious agent plays a smaller part in maintaining the defensive reaction than do the products elaborated by the injured tissues. These increase capillary permeability and encourage diapedesis of leucocytes: reactions of no advantage in an aseptic injury.

'Endothelial cells are much involved in the development of the phenomena of inflammation and it seems established that the great leakage of plasma during acute inflammation is due to the substantial separation of one endothelial cell from another at the interendothelial junctions and not to increased activity of the caveolae'. (Florey, 1966)

This is a far cry from previous ideas on the endothelial lining of the vascular system, which he likens to a sheet of nucleated cellophane. Obviously, local or distant oedema possesses no virtue in hastening the healing of a tear; on the contrary, since the tension it exerts causes pain and impedes movement, its effect must be damaging. Fluid in the joint ob-viously does no good either. The hindrance to movement set up by muscular spasm to the degree that often occurs is pointless. If the spasm were confined to protecting the torn structure from further overstretching it would be useful, but in fact it is great enough to cause more limitation of movement at the joint than is needed to fulfil this requirement. Apart from the synthesis of collagen, fibroblasts, new blood-vessels, nerves and lymph channels grow in from adjacent intact structures. Union is accompanied by contracture. Tension within the granulation tissue lines the cells up along the direction of stress. Hence, during the healing of mobile tissues, excessive immobilization is harmful. It prevents the formation of a scar strong in the important directions by avoiding the strains leading to due orientation of fibrous tissue, and also allows the scar to become unduly adherent, e.g. to bone. However, Rundles *et al.* made the surprising discovery that 2 mg. of zinc sulphate taken three times a day led to marked acceleration of the union of wounds, especially in the speed of consolidation. This opens a way of so treating athletic injuries that sound union is obtainable in a shorter time and it is now under investigation at St. Thomas's Hospital.

The rational basis for the use of movement in the treatment of recent injury still rests on the original work of Stearns (1940). Using a special technique, she watched the development of fibrous tissues under the microscope. Her main conclusion on the mechanics of the formation of scar tissue was that external mechanical factors, *not* a previous organization of the intercellular medium, were responsible for the development of the fibrillary network into orderly layers. Within four hours of applying a stimulus, an extensive network of fibrils was already visible round the fibroblasts; during the course of forty-eight hours this became dense enough to hide the cells almost completely; and in twelve days a heavy layer of fibrils had appeared. At first the fibrils developed at random, but later they acquired a definite arrangement apparently as a direct result of the mechanical factors mentioned above. Of these factors, movement is obviously the most important; and equally obvious it is most effective and least likely to cause pain before the fibrils have developed an abnormal firm attachment to neighbouring structures. *Gentle passive movements do not detach fibrils from their proper formation at the healing breach but prevent their continued adherence at abnormal sites.* The fact that the fibrils rapidly spread in all directions provides a sufficient reason for beginning movements at the earliest possible moment; otherwise they develop into the strong fibrous scars (adhesions) that so often cause prolonged disability after a sprain.

Since the intensity of the inflammatory response to trauma leads to secondary effects that impair mobility, the immediate endeavour is to inhibit inflammation to the greatest degree possible, so as to facilitate early movement. A localized lesion is therefore infiltrated with hydrocortisone as soon as the patient is seen. In diffuse lesions this approach is impractical, and deep massage and passive movement have to be substituted, whereby the tissue is moved manually in imitation of its normal behaviour. Suffusion of tissues with blood and unwillingness of muscles to move is overcome passively. A haematoma or haemarthrosis calls for aspiration. Some ligaments, e.g. the coronary ligaments at the knee, can be kept adequately moving only by the physiotherapist's finger. The fact that bone and ligament move in relation to each other provides the way in which mobility is maintained; the agency is immaterial. It is the muscles about a joint, not the joint itself, that are differently affected by different types of movement; the ligament moves over the bone during a passive movement exactly as much as it does during an active movement of equal range, and it is no good giving exercises, i.e. treating the *muscle*, for an *articular* lesion. If the joint can be quickly put right, the muscles do not have time to waste appreciably.

SELF-PERPETUATING INFLAMMATION

Fibrous tissue appears capable of maintaining an inflammation, originally traumatic, as the result of a habit continuing long after the cause has ceased to operate. This is particularly apt to happen after minor injury to a tendon, the scar that forms remaining painful whenever tension is put upon it, perhaps for decades. Occasionally a ligament at the knee or ankle is affected in the same way. Tendinitis at the shoulder has no time limit and cases of twenty and more years' standing are not rare. It seems that the inflammatory reaction at the injured fibres continues, not merely during the period of healing, but for an indefinite period afterwards, maintained by the normal stresses to which such tissues are subject. If this habit of chronic inflammation is broken for only a fortnight by inhibition at its exact site with local infiltration of hydrocortisone, the scar becomes painless and usually remains so. Obviously there has been no change in structure, only in habit.

The same applies in rheumatoid arthritis. Patients are encountered who have had one or two joints chronically inflamed for years. A few injections into the joint serve to inhibit the rheumatoid inflammation. This may not return and the joint remains sign and symptom free for years. Again, nothing has been done to alter the bodily state that causes the inflammation in the joint capsule; the only result is the temporary cessation of a habit, which remains reversed.

Many lesions with which orthopaedic medicine deals are due to scarring that remains unwarrantedly painful, alternatively to rheumatoid inflammation. If, as seems evident, many such lesions are the result of a habit, an attempt to discover the mechanism of such self-perpetuation would form an interesting piece of research.

TREATMENT OF TRAUMATIC INFLAMMATION

The aim of treatment in non-specific inflammation of moving parts is the formation of a strong and *mobile* scar; of static parts, the attainment of strong *immobile* union. Thus, in the former case, healing must take place in the presence of movement: in the latter case, in the absence of movement. For a joint or a muscle, therefore, treatment is designed to reduce the normal reaction in the injured part to as small proportions as possible, the patient being encouraged to ignore whatever discomfort remains. In bone, on the contrary, firm union is encouraged by immobilization of the fracture, taking care that movement elsewhere is interfered with as little as possible.

Minor Muscular Tears

The chief function of muscle is to contract; as it does so it broadens. The other function of muscle is to elongate; from the therapeutic point of view this movement appears less vital. Intramuscular scarring is apt to limit full broadening of a muscle. Treatment must therefore be directed chiefly to the maintenance of such mobility as allows full painless contraction of a muscle. Whereas active exercises cannot fail to secure the fullest possible stretching of any muscle—for this is a purely passive movement so far as the injured muscle is concerned—they may not be able to restore the full capacity to broaden, especially when a muscle spans a rigid part or is affected close to its bony attachment.

Recent Injury

Normal movement of the uninjured part of a damaged muscle can usually be obtained by the immediate induction of local anaesthesia at the site of the lesion, since the cessation of impulses arising from the damaged area allows muscle spasm at each side of it to abate for the time being. The sooner this is done after a minor rupture the better; the injection is given when the diagnosis is made, followed by off-weight exercises.

Deep massage given transversely imitates its normal behaviour and restores the mobility of muscle towards broadening; it is therefore indicated in all recent muscular injuries and is begun the day after the infiltration. After-treatment follows; the limb is put into the position that best fully relaxes the muscle and voluntary or faradic contractions are carried out. This ensures movement of the muscle without tension on the healing breach such as might re-rupture the uniting fibres, and so ensures healing with full mobility.

Established Scarring

Interference with mobility of moving tissues may arise from macroscopic or microscopic adhesions. It seems that the traumatic adhesions which form about a partial tear in a ligament are macroscopic; they bind the ligament down and part audibly when manipulatively ruptured. By contrast, the adhesions that diminish muscular mobility appear to be microscopic and to mat the fibres together. These cause pain when the muscle is called upon to contract, i.e. to broaden. Such adhesions also require manipulative rupture, not by stretching, which merely approximates the muscle-fibres, but by teasing them apart with deep transverse massage; for it is not possible to broaden out muscles artificially in any other way. Active exercises or faradism with the muscle in the fully relaxed position broadens the muscle and serves to maintain the passive effect of the localized transverse friction.

The efficacy of treatment depends on the site of the lesion in the muscle belly (Fig. 1). If the minor rupture occurs in the centre of the belly, active exercises without resistance can restore the range of broadening, although they have this effect slowly. When the tear lies fairly close to the insertion of the muscle into tendon or bone, the local mobility towards broadening is diminished and active exercises become powerless, whereas transverse massage and local anaesthesia remain effective. When a muscle is affected very close to its insertion, the adjacent rigid structure markedly limits the increase in width possible and only massage can restore the range of broadening.

Gross scarring of a muscle is often unaccompanied by pain, for example in ischaemic or post-septic contracture, or when the belly adheres to the site of a fracture, or after division and suture during operation. In muscles, therefore, it is not so much diffuse fibrosis or one thick scar with normal tissues on either side of it that appears to cause symptoms, as localized areas of microscopic adhesion. The explanation is that small scars within the elastic tissue result in local variations in tension when the muscle contracts, with pain resulting from overstretching at the junction between normal muscle and scar-tissue. Such local variations in tension do not arise if the scar reaches right across the muscle belly or if the whole muscle is diffusely affected, e.g. in ischaemic contracture. The pull on the muscle is then evenly distributed.

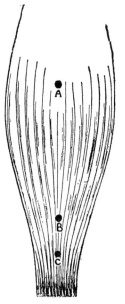

FIG. 1. Different sites of lesion in a muscle

At point A, treatment by active exercises, local anaesthesia and deep massage are all effective. At point B, treatment by local anaesthesia and deep massage are effective. At point C, only treatment by deep massage is effective.

Myosynovitis

This appears to be the best name for pain arising from a muscle as the result of overuse, with crepitus on movement. In severe cases, crepitus may be felt over a large extent of muscle belly (Cyriax, 1941). It occurs in the upper limb in the extensor muscles of the forearm. In the lower limb it is found in the tibialis anterior muscle only. Massage is quickly curative.

Tendinous Lesions

Tendinous lesions have six sites: roughening of the gliding surfaces of a tendon in its sheath (teno-synovitis); painful scarring in the body of a tendon (tendinitis); painful scarring at a teno-periosteal junction; painful scarring at the musculo-tendinous junction; primary thickening of a tendon-sheath (teno-vaginitis); a spindle-shaped enlargement of the tendon that jams in the sheath (the trigger phenomenon).

Teno-synovitis

This is a primary lesion of the gliding surfaces of the external aspect of a tendon and the internal aspect of a tendon-sheath. Pain is set up as the roughened surfaces move against each other; if the disorder is at all severe crepitus is clearly palpable. Fine crepitus results from teno-synovitis caused by overuse; coarse crepitus is due to rheumatoid disease or tuberculosis (not dealt with below).

The principle of treatment is to restore painless movement of the tendon within its sheath. This can be attained in three ways: (1) by injection of hydrocortisone, (2) by slitting open the tendon-sheath, and (3) by deep massage. Immobilization is the traditional treatment, but is slow to take effect, and splintage is so cumbersome and uncertain in its results that it should be forgotten. During friction, the inner aspect of the sheath is moved repeatedly to and fro across the external aspect of the tendon and the surfaces are smoothed off. The second method enlarges the sheath, so that it no longer fits the tendon, thus bringing about immediate cure. Since the gliding surfaces are no longer in contact, the roughening ceases to matter.

However, hydrocortisone introduced into the plane between the tendon and its sheath is so quickly and uniformly effective that neither massage nor operation have much application today. Until well the patient must, so far as possible, avoid all activities that cause pain. Exercises are contra-indicated, since the disorder is the result of exertion.

Tendinitis

The function of tendons that do not possess a sheath is merely to transmit power from muscle belly to bone. For this purpose they must bear stress equally throughout their substance.

Strain occurs both at a teno-periosteal junction and in the substance of a tendon. Minor rupture occurs at either site, leading to a small scar which often remains lastingly painful, as the result of voluntary movement imposing a series of pulls on the early fibroblasts. Each muscle contraction is apt to renew the rupture in the healing breach; later on, it further irritates the painful scar. Treatment consists of: (1) disinflaming the painful scar by local infiltration of hydrocortisone; or (2) getting rid of the scar-tissue by deep massage to the exact spot. The former is quicker, less painful and preferable, but reduction of inflammation is less radical than wearing down the scar by deep friction; hence the incidence of recurrence is higher.

Teno-vaginitis

This is a primary lesion of the tendon-sheath, usually with considerable thickening. It may follow repeated strains but is often apparently causeless. In rare instances, rheumatoid disease, gout, gonorrhoea or xanthomatosis is responsible. Crepitus never occurs in this condition.

In non-specific teno-vaginitis, hydrocortisone, deep massage or incision of the tendon-sheath are curative, but again hydrocortisone is preferable for its simplicity and speed. One or two infiltrations suffice. Till well, the patient should avoid exerting the affected tendon.

Localized Tendinous Swelling

Any of the digital flexor tendons may develop a rounded swelling on its course in the palm or within the carpal tunnel. It may engage and become fixed within a constricted part of its sheath—the trigger phenomenon—or press on an adjacent nerve.

Sprains at a Joint

The function of a joint capsule is to hold the bone ends together while allowing free movement at the joint. Ligaments reinforce the capsule at points of special stress; they have a large range of movement over bone, which has to be maintained after a sprain. Ligaments are not appreciably elastic; hence overstretching leads to permanent laxity, which in due course becomes painless. Those ligaments, the tension on which is not controlled by muscles, are particularly liable to such lengthening with consequent instability of the joint.

Recent Articular Sprain

The principles of treatment depend on whether movement at a joint is, or is not controlled by muscle.

(1) *Joints at which Movement is under Voluntary Control*

As soon as the patient is seen hydrocortisone should be injected at the site of the ligamentous or capsular lesion. Traumatic inflammation is thus reduced, and so far as possible structural and reflex changes are prevented. There is considerable after-pain for twelve to twenty-four hours requiring analgesics. Next day, if there is oedema, effleurage diminishes swelling and pain, thereby lessening both local and voluntary obstruction to movement. If the sprained point lies within reach of the physiotherapist's finger, a short period of friction then moves the damaged structure to and fro over subjacent bone. Since there is no question of breaking down strong scars but merely of preventing young fibroblasts from forming unwanted points of adherence, the deep massage need last only a minute or two and should be as gentle as is compatible with securing adequate movement of the damaged tissue. The physiotherapist then puts the injured joint or joints through the greatest possible range of movement without causing appreciable pain.

Before hydrocortisone existed, the best immediate treatment was to induce local anaesthesia at the lesion. It did not affect the local response to trauma, but enabled the patient to move the part better for two hours and temporarily abolished the afferent impulses that set up reflex oedema, fluid in the joint, muscle spasm, etc. Physiotherapy to the lesion followed the next day (as above).

(2) *Joints at which Movement is not under Voluntary Control*

The important joints are the acromio-clavicular, sterno-clavicular, sacro-iliac, sacro-coccygeal, symphysis pubis, cruciate ligaments at the knee, and the inferior tibio-fibular ligament. Since no muscles span the joint effectively, healing in the absence of enough movement need not be feared. Adhesions limiting movement cannot form since the patient cannot use his muscles to keep the joint too still. On the contrary, such capsular and ligamentous overstretching as may have taken place is permanent, although it does not necessarily cause symptoms. The principle of treatment is thus to avoid movement, as far as possible, by protection of the joint and hydrocortisone infiltration of the area of traumatic inflammation. If this is thus abated and the joint kept as immobile as possible, recovery takes only a few days. Painful chronic laxity can be converted to painless chronic laxity by local infiltration with hydrocortisone. Painless laxity is compatible with excellent function. If it causes sufficient symptoms, at some sites it can be corrected by operation.

Chronic Ligamentous Sprain

In such cases, adhesions have been allowed to form because of inadequate treatment in the acute stage; they now limit the play of the ligament over bone, and each time the patient uses his joint vigorously, he resprains the adherent ligament. The object of treatment is restoration of full, painless mobility. Forced movement ruptures adhesions about a joint and is curative; carried out gently it stretches the adhesion to no purpose. However, there are three sites where manipulative rupture of adhesions is impossible and the attempt harmful: at the coronary ligaments, at the ligaments of the wrist and at the deltoid ligament of the ankle. In the first two, deep massage is quickly curative, but the deltoid ligament requires relief from tension and infiltration with hydrocortisone.

Internal Derangement of Joints

This is far commoner than was formerly supposed. At the knee-joint, apart from the well-known subluxation of a torn meniscus, another type of internal derangement caused by an impacted loose body, has lately been recognized as of frequent occurrence (Cyriax, 1954; Helfet, 1963). At the elbow and wrist joints internal derangement is not uncommon. Moreover, a large number of obscure pains in the trunk and limbs are now known to result from displacements within the intervertebral joints, quite apart from fully developed briachial root-pain and sciatica.

Treatment varies from joint to joint, but in essence is:

(1) Inducing the displaced intra-articular structure to return to its bed. For this purpose manipulation, usually during traction, is often required and may yield an immediate happy result. At the spinal joints reduction by sustained traction provides an alternative.

(2) Once obtained, the maintenance of reduction is equally important; for in all disorders caused by loose-body formation within a joint liability to recurrence is pronounced. The avoidance of certain activities, postural training or retentive apparatus may be required.

(3) Removal of the loose fragment. This is the normal procedure at the

knee, and less often at other peripheral joints, especially in young people in whom the loose body has an osseous nucleus and its position can be ascertained radiologically. At the spinal joints, if reduction proves impracticable and the symptoms warrant, removal is indicated.

Manipulation — Set and Not Set

Set

In a 'set' manipulation, the physician knows what he intends to do. For example, reduction of a fracture or a displaced meniscus at the knee continues until the fragment is felt to click back. No cooperation from the patient is required; indeed, it is best if he is unconscious.

Not Set

By contrast, manœuvres exist based on quite a different principle. The manipulator does not know what he will have to do and is guided by the result of each measure as he proceeds. General anaesthesia is contraindicated since it destroys the necessary cooperation. These manœuvres are not 'set'.

When, say, reduction is attempted for disc lesions, one technique may do good, another harm. Only by examining the patient between each manœuvre does the manipulator know what to do, what to avoid, when to stop and when to go on.

DIMETHYL SULPHOXIDE

Great hopes were raised in 1965 by the discovery that a well-known industrial solvent, dimethyl sulphoxide, when placed on a patient's skin, penetrated, carrying drugs dissolved in it. This raised visions of introducing procaine or hydrocortisone into the area of, say, a strained ligament at the knee or ankle by merely applying the appropriate solution at the site. It was quickly discovered that the solvent was toxic to eyes in experimental animals and the death of one patient was reported after using dimethyl sulphoxide. The Food and Drugs Committee in the U.S.A. forbad its use on human beings, but the restrictions were relaxed in September 1968, short-term topical use being regarded as 'reasonably safe'.

3

Referred Pain

It is important that referred pains should be designated as such; for the phrase invites the question—referred from where? When a referred pain has by common consent been given a name, e.g. sciatica, it is easy to suppose that a diagnosis has been reached. In consequence, the search for the origin of the pain ceases. Realization that 'sciatica' describes a symptom, common to many lesions placed at the upper part of the fourth lumbar to second sacral segments, avoids this error. Recognition that a pain, even if it has been given a name, is referred is essential to any organized search for its origin.

The chief obstacle to correct diagnosis in painful conditions is the fact that the symptom is often felt at a distance from its source. Diffusion of pain is a phenomenon common to all aspects of medicine, but in the strictly medical and surgical fields the pain is usually accompanied by constitutional signs that help to identify the lesion, or at least give rise to unequivocal signs of disease. In the disorders of soft tissues and joints with which the orthopaedic physician deals the complaint is often merely of pain, local and general signs being conspicuously absent. The diagnosis in such cases turns on the assessment of the site and nature of the pain and the manner in which it is projected and elicited—in other words, on a clear understanding of 'referred pain' and of the conditions favouring its reference. Moreover, this knowledge enables an otherwise misleading phenomenon to be turned to diagnostic advantage. In deep-seated soft tissue lesions the symptoms are often very deceptive and, taken at their face value, lead to incorrect diagnosis and treatment applied in the wrong place. Such symptoms are particularly common among patients sent to the orthopaedic physician.

Pain felt elsewhere than at its true site is termed 'referred'. Familiar examples are pain in the shoulder accompanying diaphragmatic disorders, pain in the knee in arthritis of the hip, the sacral pains of childbirth, and pain in one or both arms in angina pectoris.

Referred pain is an error in perception. This was well known to John Hunter who explained it as a disorder occurring in the mind (1835 edition, vol. 1, p. 363). But this was forgotten and referred pain became known as 'neuritis' or 'fibrositis' until the fact that it was an error in perception was pointed out again (Cyriax, 1941; Lewis, 1942). On all previous occasions in the patient's lifetime, a stimulus reaching certain cells in the sensory cortex has meant to him that damage was being inflicted on a certain area of skin. When the same cells receive a painful stimulus arising from a deep-seated structure, naturally the sensorium interprets this message on a basis of past experience, i.e. refers the pain to the area of skin connected with those particular cortical cells, but with the important difference that the pain is felt deeply, not in the skin itself. Hitherto, all painful stimuli reaching the cortex have arisen by an external agency affecting primarily the skin—the tissue of which an individual is most aware. When, for the first time pain arises from a structure within the body, the cortical cells 'feel' the pain at the area whence it has always arisen before, i.e. in the relevant dermatome: the dermatome corresponding to the segment that contains the lesion. The distance the pain can travel from its source is dependent upon the size of the dermatome. The curious situation thus arises that the shape of the dermatome determines the extent of the distal radiation of pain; yet, the sensory cortex perceives a deep-seated pain, felt not in the skin itself. The dermatome limits the distal extent of a pain, not its depth.

The crucial experiment in this sphere was made by Sir Thomas Lewis in the autumn of 1936. Wishing to investigate muscular pain, he injected an irritant deeply into the lower lumbar region. He found that a diffuse pain running down the lower limb resulted and that the subject experienced little or no discomfort at the site of the injection. In 1938, Kellgren published the results of a systematic examination of the phenomena of referred pain, showing them to radiate segmentally and not to cross the mid-line.

Until this time, wide radiation of pain had been regarded as evidence of involvement of nerves, whereas this research showed that many soft tissues could be the source of diffuse symptoms. Thus, to approach the problem of referred pain with an open mind, the reader must consciously divest himself of the idea that projection of pain necessarily follows a nerve. This idea has proved most tenacious, in spite of experimental proof that the pain is merely interpreted by the cerebrum as occupying part or the whole of an embryological segment. It has presented the chief obstacle to a logical approach to the problems arising when the origin of a diffuse pain is sought. The source of this confusion may be that the nerve-supply to all structures is distributed on a segmental basis. This arrangement by no means warrants the notion that pains are projected down nerves.

c

There are many relevant clinical phenomena which any doctor can investigate for himself. One of the most common and obvious is tennis-elbow. When pain from this lesion diffuses so far as the hand, it is nearly always felt in the long and ring fingers. No single nerve runs from the elbow with such a distribution, whereas this area represents the distal part of the seventh cervical segment. Rarely the pain is referred to the ring and little fingers; yet it is inconceivable that a lesion at the *lateral* humeral epicondyle could affect the ulnar nerve. Again, down what nerve can pain diffuse from the subdeltoid bursa or the supraspinatus tendon to the arm and forearm? How can a posterior cervical pain radiate to the area supplied by the trigeminal nerve in the forehead? What nerve stretches from the heart or diaphragm to the arm, from the appendix to the umbilical area, from the shoulder-joint to the wrist, from the sacro-iliac ligaments to the heel?

It might be argued that an axon reflex is involved and that sensory fibres carry the impulses to the cord, whence they are projected down the limb. Proof that this is not so is the fact that section of the supposed efferent trunk to this reflex does not affect reference of pain. Even amputation distal to the focus from which the pain starts is without effect, pains being felt to run along an absent limb, because *the cells corresponding to it in the sensory cortex remain,* and it is here that the stimulus spreads. Destruction of the ganglion of the trigeminal nerve, for example, does not affect the patient's capacity to perceive pain the forehead referred from the cervical joints. Myocardial and diaphragmatic pains are projected down an absent upper limb and referred pain may occur in an area rendered anaesthetic from a peripheral nerve palsy. This finding was confirmed by Harman (1951) who found anginal pain in the arm to be unaltered by a brachial plexus block. Sciatica occurs in an absent limb, because the source of the pain lies at a low lumbar joint and the pathway from there to the cerebrum is in no way altered by amputation of the lower limb.

It has been suggested that root-pain and referred pain are in some way different. This is not so; for pressure exerted on a nerve-root leads to pain extending along the relevant dermatome and pain arising in any other tissue deeply placed at the proximal end of a segment also sets up pain felt in any part of the relevant dermatome. There is thus no difference in the nature or the extent of the pain, merely in which movements evoke it. Of course, paraesthesia does not appear unless a nerve-root is affected and severe pain of recent onset is more characteristic of root-pain. However, the fact remains that the extent of the pain is no different when it is referred from a nerve-root than when it arises in some other tissue derived from the same segment.

THE SEGMENTS

Plates 2 and 3 give a general impression of the embryological origin of the skin (dermatomes) but do not allow for the overlap. This is so considerable that division of one posterior spinal root causes little interference with cutaneous sensibility, and the changes after the division of two adjacent roots are sometimes barely perceptible. These figures do no more than represent the central parts of each segment and indicate the type of arrangement. Much more accurate knowledge of the shape of each dermatome is required of the practitioner of orthopaedic medicine if he is to derive assistance in diagnosis therefrom.

When the foetus is a month old, division into about forty segments starts. The final ten are coccygeal and by a fortnight later all but two of these have disappeared. In due course each segment becomes differentiated into dermatome (skin), myotome (muscles and other soft tissues) and sclerotome (bone and fibrous septa). The extent of the relevant dermatome governs the distance that pain arising from any point in the myotome may travel distally. Since the dermatome often projects further distally than the myotome, pain may be felt to occupy an area more extensive than the myotome in which it arises. For example, the pain of supraspinatus tendinitis may reach the radial border of the hand, whereas the fifth cervical myotome does not extend below the elbow. By contrast, in some places the myotome extends further proximally than the dermatome. For example, the fifth cervical dermatome ends at the shoulder; but the scapula and its muscles, and the pectoral muscles at the trunk, form part of the fifth cervical myotome.

Dermatomes

These vary somewhat in shape from person to person. Judging by the distribution of paraesthesia in known root-lesions in the neck, there are marked individual discrepancies. If, for example, patients with a cervical disc lesion leading to a seventh-root paresis (as judged by the pattern of muscular weakness) are questioned about the site of the pins and needles that they experience in their fingers, a few state that all five digits are affected; some all the four fingers but not the thumb; most the index, long and ring fingers; some the index and long finger; some the long and ring fingers, and some only the index or only the long finger. Yet in each case the pattern of muscle weakness shows that the seventh cervical root is compressed. Hence, it is deduced that the distal cutaneous area supplied by one nerve-root is very variable. One reason for this variability was

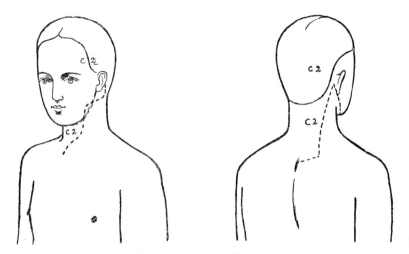

FIG. 2. Second cervical dermatome

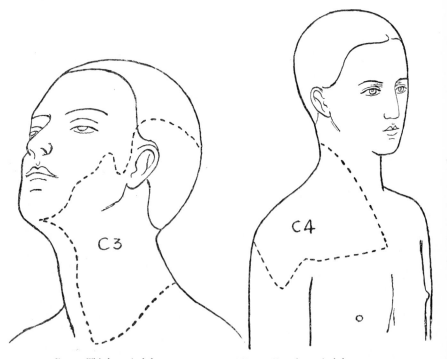

FIG. 3. Third cervical dermatome   FIG. 4. Fourth cervical dermatome

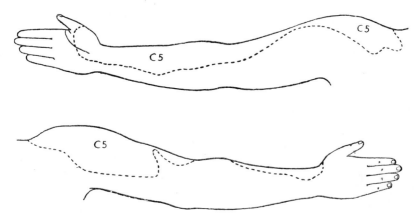

FIG. 5. Fifth cervical dermatome

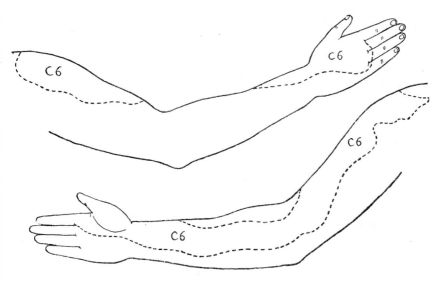

FIG. 6. Sixth cervical dermatome

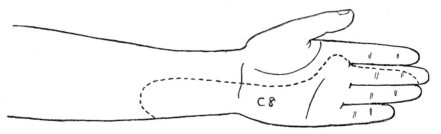

FIG. 7. Eigth cervical dermatome

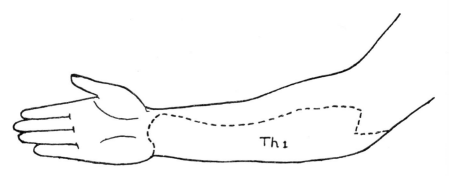

FIG. 8. First thoracic dermatome

put forward by Schwartz (1956). At cervical laminectomy he noticed rootlets running to join the posterior root of the adjacent segment. He therefore dissected thirteen normal necks and found such anastomotic rootlets in each. The sixth and seventh roots were those most often connected.

Foerster's (1933) painstaking work accords very well with clinical findings and is, therefore, set out below in detail.

Cervical 1. Uncertain. (Probably the vertical area of the skull.)

Cervical 2. The whole occiput, the chin and the medial parts of the front and back of the neck (Fig. 2).

Cervical 3. The entire neck, the posterior half of the mandible and the ear (Fig. 3).

Cervical 4. The shoulder area, the front of the upper chest, the lower half of the neck (Fig. 4).

Cervical 5. The shoulder, the front of the arm the forearm as far as the base of the thumb (Fig. 5).

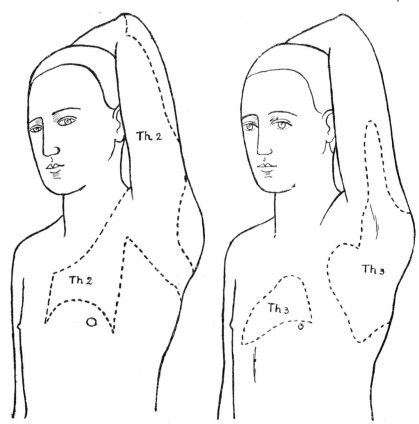

FIG. 9. Second thoracic dermatome   FIG. 10. Third thoracic dermatome.

Cervical 6. The outer aspect of the arm and forearm, the thenar eminence, thumb and index finger (Fig. 6).

Cervical 7. Uncertain. (Probably the back of the arm, the outer side of the forearm and the index, long and ring fingers.)

Cervical 8. The inner aspect of the forearm, the inner half of the hand, third, fourth and fifth digits (Fig. 7).

Thoracic 1. The inner side of the forearm as far as the wrist. The upper margin of the dermatome is uncertain (Fig. 8).

Thoracic 2. A Y-shaped area stretching from the inner condyle of the humerus up the arm and then dividing into two areas reaching to the sternum anteriorly and the vertebral border of the scapula behind (Fig. 9).

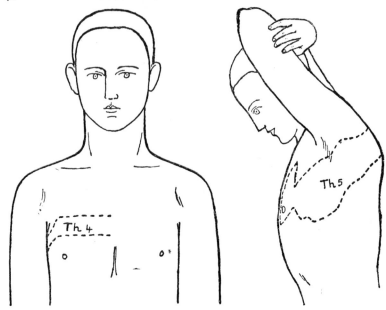

FIG. 11. Fourth thoracic dermatome FIG. 12. Fifth thoracic
dermatome

Thoracic 3. An area on the front of the chest, and a triangular patch in the
axilla (Fig. 10).

Thoracic 4, 5 and 6. These encircle the trunk reaching the level of the
nipple (Figs. 11 and 12).

Thoracic 7 and 8. These encircle the trunk reaching to the lower costal
margin.

Thoracic 9, 10 and 11. These encircle the trunk reaching the level of the
umbilicus (Fig. 13).

Thoracic 12. Uncertain. (Probably reaches to the groin.)

Lumbar 1. The lower abdomen and groin; the lumbar region from the
second to fourth vertebrae; the upper and outer aspect of the buttock
(Fig. 14).

Lumbar 2. Two discontinuous areas. The lower lumbar region and upper
buttock (Fig. 16). The whole of the front of the thigh (Fig. 17).

Lumbar 3. Two discontinuous areas. The mid-buttock (Fig. 16). The
inner aspect (sometimes the front) of the leg as far as the medial
malleolus (Fig. 18).

Lumbar 4. The anterior and medial aspects of the leg according to Foerster;

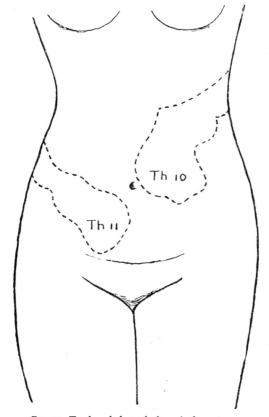

FIG. 13. Tenth and eleventh thoracic dermatomes

the postero-medial part of the upper calf; the medial side of the dorsum of the foot; the whole hallux (Fig. 19). *N.B.* Experience of the distribution of pain in fourth lumbar root-pressure suggests that the dermatome occupies the outer rather than the inner aspect of the thigh and leg, crossing to the inner border of the foot at the tarsus.

Lumbar 5. The outer aspect of the leg; the dorsum of the whole foot and the first, second and third toes (Fig. 20). The inner half of the sole (Fig. 20). *N.B.* the fourth and fifth lumbar dermatomes are all but identical.

Sacral 1. The sole of the foot, the two, three or four outer toes and the lower half of the posterior aspect of the leg (Fig. 21). *N.B.* During the treatment of chronic sciatica Sicard and Leca (1954) divided the sensory part of the fifth lumbar nerve-root in 49 patients and the first sacral root in 83 patients. They found a narrow band of cutaneous analgesia along the posterior aspect of the thigh in each case, and that the first and second toes became numb after section of the fifth lumbar posterior root, and the outer two toes after section at the first sacral level. This

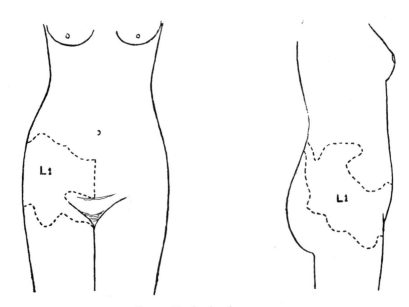

FIG. 14. First lumbar dermatome

fits in extremely accurately with the usual distribution of pain in sciatica and affords the first experimental evidence of a posterior crural extension of these two dermatomes.

Sacral 2. The back of the whole thigh, leg, sole and the plantar aspect of the toes (Fig. 22).

Sacral 3. Uncertain. Certainly a circular area around the anus. Probably a narrow strip following the inguinal ligament and running down the inner side of the thigh to the knee. If this is correct, the analogy with the second thoracic dermatome is close. Bohn, Franksson and Petersen (1956) state that stimulation of the second and third sacral roots sets up pain in the groin; and of the fourth sacral root, pain in the coccyx and rectum.

Sacral 4. Saddle-area, anus, perineum, scrotum and penis, labium and vagina, inner uppermost thigh.

EMBRYOLOGICAL DERIVATION

The dermatomes do no more than represent the original relationship to the trunk of the limb-buds at the earliest stage of development of the embryo. At the end of a month's development the limb-buds appear as raised papules at each side of the neck and caudal region. During growth, these projections draw out into themselves the segments from which they start, thereby deforming at these areas the original circular shape of each

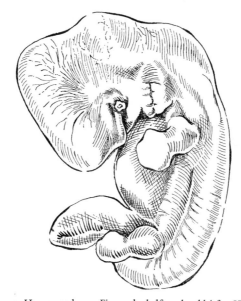

FIG. 15. Human embryo. Five and a half weeks old (after Hill).

segment.

Thus, some segments are largely missing from the trunk in the lower-cervical-upper-thoracic and in the lower-lumbar-upper-sacral regions; they have gone to form the limbs. If the upper limb is held out horizontally, thumb upwards, the original position of the bud is recreated. Thus, the base of the thumb represents the end of the elongated fifth cervical dermatome, the thumb and index the sixth, the long and ring fingers the seventh, the ring and little fingers the eighth cervical, and the ulnar border of the wrist and forearm the first thoracic dermatome. The third to twelfth thoracic segments suffer no comparable deformation; the lower merely come to slope obliquely downwards anteriorly to form the abdominal wall.

The original position of the bud for the lower limb is recreated by abduction of the thigh to 90 degrees and lateral rotation until the big toe points vertically. The second and third lumbar segments now lie uppermost, i.e. the adductor and quadriceps muscles covered by the second and third dermatomes, the former extending from groin to patella, the latter covering the same crural area but extending down the front of the leg to just above the ankle. The lower part of the quadriceps muscle and the

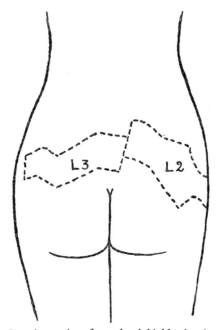

FIG. 16. Posterior portion of second and third lumbar dermatomes

front of the leg form the fourth lumbar myotome, which is also represented in the buttock by the gluteus medius and minimus muscles. The dermatome occupies the outer leg, the dorsum and inner border of the foot as far as the big toe. Of course, each segment also takes part in the sacrospinalis muscle at the appropriate level. The fifth lumbar segment reaches to the hallux, forming, together with the first sacral segment, the foot and calf. The dermatome ends at the three inner toes. These two myotomes are also represented in the gluteus maximus and take a small share in the other two gluteal muscles. The hamstring and upper calf muscles are formed from the upper two sacral myotomes except for the biceps femoris muscle which is chiefly derived from the third sacral segment. The fourth sacral segment forms the perineum and anus; where the myotome and dermatome once more correspond exactly.

Visceral Embryology

For the convenience of those faced with thoracic or abdominal pain, a list of the approximate segmental derivations of the viscera is appended.

Heart	C8–T4
Lungs	T2–5
Oesophagus	T4–5
Stomach and duodenum	T6–8
Liver and gall-bladder	T7–8 right
Pancreas	T8 left
Small intestine	T9–10
Appendix and ascending colon	T10–L1
Epididymis	T10
Ovary, testis, and suprarenal	T11–12, L1
Bladder fundus ⎫ Kidney ⎬ Uterine fundus ⎭	T11–L1
Colonic flexure	L2–3
Sigmois and rectum ⎫ Cervix* ⎬ Neck of bladder, prostate, and urethra ⎭	S2–5

Discrepancies between Dermatomes and Myotomes

There are eight areas where the skin and the structure it covers have different embryological derivations. They are the head, the scapular, pectoral, and intrathoracic regions, and the hand, buttock, thigh and scrotum. Discrepancies also occur within the abdomen but do not appreciably concern the practitioner of orthopaedic medicine.

1. The Head

When the embryo is about four weeks old, the projection that will form the head turns twice in the course of growth until it is folded forward on itself like an inverted J. Meanwhile the future mandibular region has appeared as an anterior fold. These two protuberances then fuse about the gap that forms the buccal cavity. In other words, the whole of the head and face as far as the mouth is developed from the back of the neck, and

* Theobald (1966) does not agree that the cervix uteri refers pain to the lower sacral dermatomes. He has provoked pain from the cervix by electric stimulation and finds that it is felt at first 4 cm. above the symphysis pubis. It spreads to the whole hypogastrium, occupying the triangle formed by a horizontal line joining the anterior superior iliac spines and the inguinal ligaments. This corresponds to a reference within the tenth thoracic to first lumbar dermatomes.

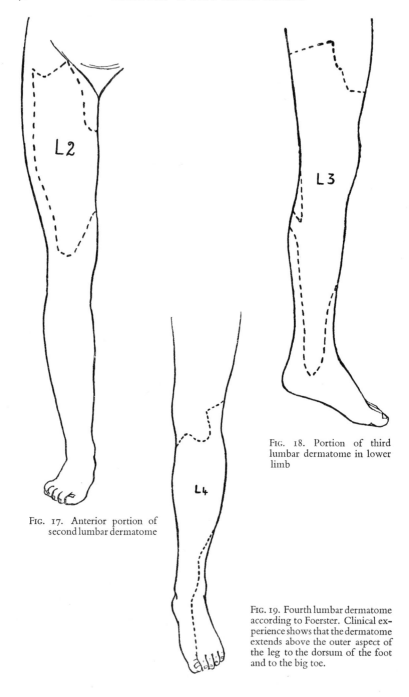

Fig. 17. Anterior portion of
second lumbar dermatome

Fig. 18. Portion of third
lumbar dermatome in lower
limb

Fig. 19. Fourth lumbar dermatome
according to Foerster. Clinical experience shows that the dermatome
extends above the outer aspect of
the leg to the dorsum of the foot
and to the big toe.

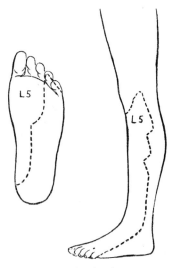

FIG. 20. Fifth lumbar dermatome

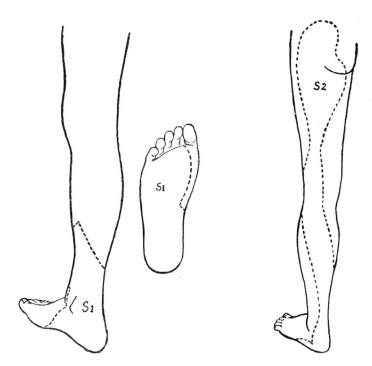

FIG. 21. First sacral dermatome   FIG. 22. Second sacral dermatome

only the lower jaw region develops from the front of the neck. The head and face are formed from the upper two cervical segments.

The nerve that conducts sensory impulses from the skin of the face and scalp as far back as the vertex is the fifth cranial. There is, then, no nerve along which a pain could run from the back of the neck to the forehead. Since such reference of pain is common, it illustrates that a referred pain does not run down a somatic nerve but represents an error in perception. The patient feels a pain somewhere within, or, when the strength of the stimulus is great enough, diffused all over the segment in which it arises.

2. The Scapular Region

The growth of the bud that is to become the upper limb draws the lower cervical and uppermost thoracic segments out into itself. The scapula and its muscles (including the latissimus dorsi) are derived from the middle and lower cervical segments, yet the skin overlying, and the ribs beneath them are formed from thoracic segments. Hence, pain in the upper posterior part of the thorax has a cervical or scapular origin if it radiates to the shoulder and upper limb, and an upper thoracic origin if it radiates to the front of the chest.

3. The Pectoral Region

The interposition is the same as at the scapula. The intercostal muscles, the ribs and the overlying skin form part of the thoracic segments, whereas the pectoral muscles are developed from the lower part of the neck.

4. The Intrathoracic Region

The diaphragm is developed largely from the third and fourth cervical segments. The heart forms part of the upper three thoracic segments. Pain from either structure may, therefore, radiate to the shoulder. From the myocardium it may also spread to the arm as far as the ulnar border of the hand, i.e. to the end of the first thoracic dermatome. Hence, pain referred from the diaphragm, heart or the pectoral muscles may have the same quality and may all cause pain at the shoulder; from the heart or the pectoral muscle the pain may spread along the upper limb. Since all three are thoracic structures, the local pains to which they may give rise are indistinguishable to the patient.

5. The Hand

The skin of the radial side of the hand is developed from the fifth and sixth cervical segments, whereas the thenar and interosseous muscles form part of the eighth cervical and first thoracic myotomes.

6. *The Buttock*

The skin of the outer buttock is derived from the first lumbar dermatome, overlapping the second and third segments at a small area at the upper inner quadrant (see Fig. 16). The gluteal muscles, however, are formed within the fourth lumbar to first sacral segments. Hence, at the upper buttock, these muscles extend further proximally than their relevant dermatomes and come to lie beneath skin of first lumbar provenance.

7. *The Thigh*

Patients suffering from fourth and fifth lumbar nerve-root pressure repeatedly describe their pain as spreading to the buttock, then to the thigh. Seldom does the patient say that the pain jumps from buttock to calf omitting the thigh. Yet the fourth and fifth dermatomes begin at, or just above, the knee. It is thus theoretically impossible for pain to be felt in the thigh in sciatica; yet that is, in fact, the common site for severe pain. This phenomenon remained unexplained until Sicard and Leca's findings (1954) after posterior radicotomy at the fifth lumbar and first sacral levels. They were able to demonstrate a narrow band of cutaneous analgesia running along the back of the thigh when either posterior root was divided. Hence, a hitherto unsuspected part of the dermatome has been charted, and accounts for the well-known crural radiation of the pain in sciatica.

8. *The Scrotum*

The scrotum is derived from the fourth sacral dermatome, yet it encloses the testicles, which are derived from the two lowest thoracic and first lumbar segments. Hence pain felt within the scrotum may have two sources. On the one hand, lesions at the eleventh or twelfth thoracic levels, or at the first lumbar, by pressing on the origin of the genito-femoral nerve, may give rise to pain felt in one or both testicles. On the other hand, when pressure is exerted at a low lumbar level on the intraspinal course of the fourth sacral nerve root, pain or paraesthesia felt in one or both testicles also results. Oddly enough, the patient never mentions the scrotum. There are thus two levels from which testicular pain may be referred, since skin of fourth sacral provenance covers structures of lowest thoracic and first lumbar origin.

Exception to Segmental Reference

For reasons that remain obscure, the dura mater does not obey the rules of segmental reference at all. For example, patients with cervical root pressure are frequently encountered, the level of whose lesion is clearly indicated by, say, a seventh root-palsy. Yet they often complain of pain running up the neck and through to the forehead (C2, 3) and down towards the lower scapular area (T3, 4, 5, 6). The latter is often the first symptom, interscapular pain transferring itself to the whole of one scapular area before the radiation to the upper limb begins. Thus, in the stage first of central, then of lateral dural pressure, the pain is usually felt in areas derived from a segment quite other than that in due course found to contain the lesion. Once the protrusion has reached the nerve-root, the pain radiates in the expected way; hence it is irritation of the dura only, not its investment of the nerve-root, that sets up pain felt at the wrong level. The reverse phenomenon may be experienced during gradual manipulative reduction at the neck; pain and referred tenderness at the lower scapular area can be made gradually to move upwards and proximally as the displaced fragment is shifted bit by bit towards its bed.

Extrasegmental reference is also common in the lumbar region. Backache caused by pressure on the dura mater at a low lumbar level often radiates to the abdomen or up to the back of the chest. Patients may even state that their lumbago is accompanied by a headache that comes and goes with the lumbar symptoms. In acute lumbago due to a lower lumbar protrusion the pain often radiates to one or both groins, or one or both iliac fossae, thus encroaching on lower thoracic segments. Since the possibility of such segmental transgression has never been described and results in pain whose pathway is anatomically inexplicable, suspicion of renal calculus or appendicitis or neurosis may easily arise, and the removal of the appendix for discogenic pain referred extrasegmentally from the dura mater is by no means uncommon.

Other structures in the neighbourhood of the dura mater do not share its independence from segmental reference of pain; hence the mere fact that the patient describes a reference of pain that is theoretically impossible should at once focus attention on the dura mater. Thus the site of pain, taken alone, cannot necessarily differentiate between a cervical or an upper thoracic disc lesion, or a lower thoracic and a lumbar disc lesion.

Extrasegmental reference is also met with in disorders outside the sphere of orthopaedic medicine. For example, in angina the pain is often referred from the myocardium (T1, 2, 3) to the neck and jaw (C3) as well as to the upper limb.

Referred Tenderness ('Fibrositis')

The fact that a painful area, though it contains no lesion, is often *diffusely* tender was noted by Lewis in 1942. However, a different type of referred tenderness also exists (Cyriax, 1948). When pressure is exerted on the dura mater, usually by a small displaced fragment of disc bulging out of the posterior longitudinal ligament, a *localized* tender spot forms within the painful region, and when pressed is instantly identified by the patient as the source of his symptoms. It is a genuine, unilateral, deep tenderness, and not associated with cutaneous hyperalgesia. It is the result of pressure on the dura mater, i.e. a secondary phenomenon, but has been, and still sometimes is, regarded as the primary lesion, the more so since the patient insists that it is the origin of his symptoms. Formerly, 'fibrositis of the trapezius' when it got worse was regarded as leading to 'brachial neuritis', despite the fact that no lesion of this muscle (C2, 3, 4) can refer pain down the upper limb. Today, this localized tender spot in a neck or scapular muscle still leads to concepts such as 'trigger points' and 'myalgic spots'. These are thought of as primary lesions rather than as a secondary effect of pressure on the dura mater, leading to pain and tenderness felt at a level inconsistent with the segmentation of the body. The formation of metabolites at the muscle has been brought in to explain the tenderness (Weddell *et al.*, 1948) and fatty lobules had a vogue for a time. The simple experiment, whereby the tender spot can be made to shift from place to place in a few seconds, can be confirmed by any physician who manipulates the neck of a sufferer from alleged 'scapular fibrositis'. Moreover, he will find that, when a full and painless range of movement has been restored to the cervical joint, the pain and tenderness in the muscle cease together. Nevertheless, 'fibrositis' has proved a most enduring idea. It was coined by Gower in 1904 to explain the pathology of lumbago and even now the word remains semi-respectable. The amount of misdirected massage and injections that this secondary tender spot has attracted beggars calculation, and the resulting advantage to lay-manipulators has been equally large.

Referred Pain as a Clue to Segmental Origin

The knowledge that pain is referred segmentally, apart from being employed clinically to estimate the limits within which the source of pain must lie, may also be used experimentally to demonstrate the embryological origin of the tissue concerned.

The capsule of the hip-joint provides a good example. Pain originating in this structure may be felt as a local pain in the groin and buttock referred to the front of the thigh and the knee, and often to the anterior aspect of the leg almost to the ankle. It follows that the capsule of the hip joint is developed from the third lumbar segment. Again the sacro-iliac ligaments were regarded by me as developed within the first and second sacral segments. This was confirmed when pain from these ligaments was found to radiate to the posterior thigh and calf.

CONDITIONS FAVOURING REFERENCE OF PAIN

The erroneous perception of the site of a pain depends on four factors: (1) the strength of the stimulus, (2) the position of the painful structure, (3) the depth from the surface, and (4) the nature of the structure.

1. The Strength of the Stimulus

The stronger the stimulus, the less can the patient tell where it originates. For example, arthritis at the shoulder starts as a pain at the shoulder. If it becomes more severe, the pain spreads to the arm and forearm, possibly leaving the shoulder area altogether. When the arthritis regresses the reverse phenomenon takes place. In other words the position of slight pain is often correctly appreciated by the patient; intense pain radiates widely.

The mechanism of this phenomenon remained obscure until 1941. On general grounds it could be assumed that the error lay centrally rather than peripherally; for a larger number of sensory nerve fibres would clearly not be stimulated by an increase in the severity of a lesion unaccompanied by an increase in its extent. The mechanism by which pain is referred was revealed by the experiments of Woolsey, Marshall and Bard on monkeys. Electro-encephalography showed that stimulation of a given area of skin gave rise to an electrical reaction in a fixed and minute area of cortex. Increase in the intensity of the stimulus led to a corresponding increase in the number of cortical cells affected. Such spread to adjacent cells would obviously be interpreted by the patient as an enlargement of the painful area.

The mosaic forming the sensory cortex is arranged dermatome by dermatome, and the extensive reaction resulting from a strong stimulus is confined within the limits of the piece of cortex corresponding to that dermatome. The absence of spread beyond the limit of each piece of cortex is demonstrated most clearly at the two points in the sensory cortex where the arrangement departs from the normal sequence. The region of sensorium corresponding to the fifth cranial nerve adjoins that corresponding to the eighth cervical segment, and the second cervical and first thoracic areas also lie next to each other. Cerebral spread beyond a dermatome would, in these two situations, give rise to bizarre distributions.

Clinical experience shows that this type of reference to symptoms (e.g. from the face to the ulnar side of the hand) does not in fact take place. The fact that the diffusion occurs at the cells of the sensory cortex also explains why amputation distal to the lesion does not prevent the radiation of pain to the absent part; for this is still represented—just as before the amputation—in the sensory cortex. The phenomenon that electroencephalography fails to explain is the replacement of an original pain by referred pain, symptoms being no longer experienced at the site of the lesion but distally only.

2. The Position of the Painful Structure

Pain will be referred a long way only where elongated segments exist, i.e. in the limbs. The longest segments are the first and second sacral which stretch from mid-buttock to foot.

As a rule, pain is referred only distally, and it is therefore from the proximal ends of the longer segments that diffuse pains usually arise. The structures about the knee and elbow stand almost alone in setting up pain felt to radiate equally in both directions, but the patient seldom fails to realize where his symptoms arise. Pain originating about the wrist or tarsus may also set up an ache in the forearm or leg, but never enough to deceive the patient as to its source. Thus, a diffuse pain may be expected to spring from a structure placed towards the upper end of the painful segment, but by no means necessarily within the area outlined by the patient.

Conversely, the further the lesion lies from the trunk, the more accurate are the patient's sensations. Thus, although there is no theoretical reason why a pain in the foot should not be felt to travel to the buttock, just as a pain arising in the buttock is felt to reach the foot, in fact this does not occur.

3. The Depth from the Surface

The more superficially a soft structure lies, the more precise is its localizing ability (Kellgren, 1938). One of the most important protective functions of the skin is accurately to localize tactile stimuli. Pains are therefore not referred from its surface; even so, the fingers can localize to within a millimetre, whereas the skin of the back can only do so to within two centimetres. It is no part of the ordinary function of deep structures like muscle to localize stimuli accurately. Up to a point, the more deeply a soft structue lies, the greater is its capacity for giving rise to diffuse pains. Lewis (1942) says: 'We assume that a unit area of skin must transmit, by its special path, sensory impulses to the sensorium which is able to recognize this unit as the source of the message . . . Tissues supplied by deep pain nerves may be regarded as endowed with a similar but simpler form of mechanism, the tissues being represented more in bulk and collectively. The coarsest form of such representation would be that in which tissues in a given segment were represented in such a way that no fine distinctions would be possible in localization.'

While the concept of referred pain as no more than an error in perception on the part of the cerebrum is clear enough, the fact that pain arising from the proximal part of a segment is usually felt diffusely over a much larger area than when its source lies distally gives rise to difficulty. For example, the pain of sacro-iliac arthritis may radiate to the calf, but calf pains are very seldom projected as far as the buttock. Further research is required to elucidate the paradox formed by these two conflicting observations—namely, that the buttock and calf possess both common and separate representation in the sensory cortex.

4. The Nature of the Structure

When different parts of the nervous system are subjected to pressure no symptoms whatever need be felt at the point of impact.

Pressure on the spinal cord results in extrasegmental distribution of pins and needles, just as pressure on the dura mater leads to extrasegmental reference of pain. They may be felt in the trunk, all four limbs, the lower limbs or only the feet. Not an uncommon symptom in pressure on the spinal cord in the neck is paraesthesia felt bilaterally from the front of the knee to all the toes, i.e. all the dermatomes from L2 to S1.

Pressure on the dural investment of a nerve-root leads to pain, often severe, felt throughout, or in any part of the relevant dermatome. Pain from neck to hand or from lumbar region to foot is commonplace, but it is equally possible for pain of spinal origin to be felt in, say, the arm or thigh only, or the forearm or leg only. Pins and needles are often, but not invariably, felt distally and occupy the digits appropriate to the dermatome, not to the territory of a nerve-trunk.

Pressure on a nerve-trunk, by contrast, causes no pain, only distal paraesthesia in an area corresponding to the known cutaneous distribution of that nerve. The symptoms are therefore much the same at whatever point along the main nerve the pressure is exerted. The reason is that a stimulus applied direct to the sensory fibres of a nerve-trunk sets up an impulse travelling proximally—an impulse which the sensory cortex interprets as originating from the area of skin supplied by these fibres. Hence no pain is felt at the point of impact. Thus, the spinal cord and nerve-trunks refer pain more deceptively than any other structure and much more misleadingly than pressure on a nerve-root. This is curious; for the perineurium is not concerned with conduction, and it might have been supposed that pain arising from pressure on a nerve-trunk would be felt no more diffusely than those from other fibrous structures in the same neighbourhood.

Pain is apt to be referred from joint-capsule, ligament, muscle and bursa in an indistinguishable manner. Bone and periosteum, although the deepest structures of a limb, set up pain that hardly radiates at all. Thus fractures and uncomplicated bony abnormalities due to infection or new growth give rise to pain felt close to their site. There is no obvious reason for this discrepancy between hard and soft structures.

DIAGNOSIS OF REFERRED PAIN

Referred pain should always be suspected when a patient complains of a deep burning or ache along a limb, from the back of the trunk to its anterior aspect, of 'neuritis', or indeed of any deep pain of large extent and indefinite boundaries. Furthermore, if the painful area presents no physical signs of disorder and there is no disturbance of function of the painful part, the probability is very high that the pain is referred.

Of the structures from which pain is referred, the following concern the orthopaedic physician; joint-capsule, tendon, muscle, ligament and bursa, in order of descending importance. To these must be added dura mater and nerve-sheath; for it is the orthopaedic physician who is commonly called upon to deal with pressure on dura mater, nerve-root or nerve-trunk.

There is a great diversity of lesions that can give rise to referred pain, and it is essential to consider each case as an isolated problem on the lines described in Chapter 6. Although these pains are often called 'neuritis' by the patient, they are not due to pain arising in, travelling along, or even dependent on the integrity of the nerve-paths distal to the site of the lesion. They pass upwards from the site of the stimulus by the ordinary sensory paths, but they do not run *down* any structure; their site is merely erroneously localized by the patient's brain, and can be felt in an absent limb, or one deprived of its nerve supply.

Practical Considerations

Referred pain can be relieved only by treatment to its source. Patients often unwittingly draw attention away from the right spot by insisting that they know from their feelings exactly where the lesion lies, and by rubbing what they maintain is the tender place. Palpation of a tender spot discovered and regarded as relevant by the patient provides a very poor substitute for diagnosis by selective tension. Palpation for tenderness of the structure found to be at fault follows only if the tissue lies within fingers' reach.

It is in difficult cases with referred pain only, without any discomfort felt near the lesion itself, that diagnosis by selective tension is particularly important. Local anaesthesia is then most useful to confirm or disprove the suspected site of the lesion.

Treatment is exactly the same whether a lesion gives rise to referred pain or to local pain only. The diagnostic difficulties are sometimes increased in the former case; but once the right structure has been singled out, it is treated on standard lines. Moreover, since referred pain does not arise from superficial structures, superficial treatment cannot affect its source. Whatever therapeutic measure is employed, it must have a penetrating effect.

4

Neuritis and Pressure on Nerves

The layman often uses the word 'neuritis' to designate pain running along a limb. The same pain, when felt at the back of the trunk, is often called 'fibrositis'. The medical profession is apt to use the word 'neuritis' when pain is accompanied by pins and needles. However, paraesthesia, though indicating that some part of the nervous system is at fault, are common to extrinsic and intrinsic disease. External pressure on a normal nerve sets up pins and needles no less than does parenchymatous degeneration. These two disorders require radically different treatment and must be distinguished.

Pressure on a nerve from without occupies the territory where the neurologist and the practitioner of orthopaedic medicine meet. The nerves may conduct normally; hence no involvement of the nervous system appears to be present. Examination of the somatic structures may exclude any lesion affecting a moving part of the body. The patient may, therefore, fall between two stools, neither type of examination revealing the existence of a lesion. In fact, the pain results from pressure on a nerve-root or nerve-trunk insufficient to impair conduction. This possibility has thrown doubt on the view that, for the examination of the peripheral nervous system, estimation of conduction along it suffices (Cyriax, 1942).

PINS AND NEEDLES DUE TO COMPRESSION

This feeling is a most interesting phenomenon; for it appears to provide the only example of a pathognomonic sensation. Lesions of visceral, skeletal or muscular provenance all give rise to identical pains, indistinguishable by the patient. The pains may behave differently (e.g. in colic) but they are identical in quality. Pins and needles, by contrast, arise only from lesions of the nervous, especially the peripheral nervous, system. The different origins of this sensation are set out below.

1. Small Nerve

When pressure is applied to a nerve close to its distal extremity, some pins and needles are felt, but the main symptom is numbness. This occupies the cutaneous area supplied by that nerve; the edge is well defined and towards the centre of the area full anaesthesia is often demonstrable. The analgesic area occupies one aspect of the part. Meralgia paraesthetica is a well-known example of this type of paraesthesia; the numb area lies at the antero-lateral aspect of the thigh, the edge is clear, the centre of the region is often anaesthetic, and the numbness more evident to the patient than pins and needles.

2. Nerve-trunk—the Release Phenomenon

Minor pressure on the trunk of a nerve sets up pins and needles rather than numbness. They occur as a *release* phenomenon. Faint tingling and numbness appear momentarily when a nerve-trunk is first compressed; then nothing is noted until the pressure on the nerve has been released. Painful paraesthesia then comes on some time after the pressure on the nerve-trunk ceases. The interval bears a close relationship to the duration of the original pressure. Thus, after five minutes' pressure, the paraesthesia will appear after perhaps thirty seconds; after release from twelve hours' compression, they may not be felt for two to three hours. It is common knowledge that pressure on the sciatic nerve while sitting causes no symptoms; the pins and needles come on when the subject relieves the pressure by standing up. Active movement of the affected digits or stroking the analgesic area of skin usually brings on a shower of pins and needles. This is so wherever along the nerve the point of pressure lies, and has no localizing significance. Thus, if moving the fingers provokes pins and needles, it must not be thought that the lesion lies in the forearm or hand. By contrast, if they are elicited by a distant movement, this constitutes the important diagnostic finding. For example, if keeping the shoulders shrugged makes the fingers tingle, it becomes clear that raising the lower trunk of the brachial plexus off the first rib has evoked the release phenomenon.

When a nerve-trunk is compressed at the distal part of the upper limb, the release-phenomenon ceases to operate. For example, pressure on the ulnar nerve at the elbow causes paraesthesia in the two fingers, which stops a few moments after the pressure is released. Again, when the median nerve is irritated in the carpal tunnel, work involving repeated hand movements is apt to bring on the pins and needles. Curiously enough, this distal change does not occur in the lower limb. If different parts of the sciatic nerve are compressed by, say, sitting on the lower buttock, crossing the knees or applying the outer side of one ankle to the lower thigh, the paraesthesia is felt after the posture has been changed.

In any event the pins and needles are felt only in the distal part of the cutaneous area supplied by that peripheral nerve, no matter at what point in its course the impact occurs; hence *clinical examination must include the full length of the nerve.*

Constant pressure on a nerve-trunk causes a painless lower motor neurone lesion; there is no paraesthesia.

3. Nerve-root—the Compression Phenomenon

The pins and needles are a *pressure* phenomenon, continuing more or less so long as the pressure is sustained. They are abolished instantly by relief from the pressure. Pins and needles in the hand, of however long standing, that result from a cervical disc protrusion often cease as soon as traction is applied to the neck, and return when the traction is released. It is very odd that pins and needles should come on with *pressure* on a nerve-root and with *release of pressure* on a nerve-*trunk*. In root-pressure, they are felt in the distal extremity of the dermatome, often conspicuously occupying an area not supplied by any one nerve-trunk. For example, when a cervical disc protrusion compresses the seventh nerve-root, the paraesthesia occupies the index, long and ring fingers—fingers supplied by no one nerve-trunk. The paraesthesia has neither edge nor aspect, being felt within the fingers. Stroking the skin may, as in nerve-trunk pressure, provoke the pins and needles. However, moving the digits is no longer effective, and this finding may prove helpful when, in a difficult case, distinction must be drawn between pressure on a nerve-trunk and a nerve-root.

In pressure on a nerve-root the pins and needles tend to disappear when the numbness comes on; especially in the lower limb they tend to follow each other rather than coincide—major pressure on the root causing analgesia; minor, pins and needles.

Another major difference exists between pressure on a nerve-trunk and on a nerve-root. Pressure on a nerve-trunk, though it may cause paraesthesia distally, causes no local pain at all. When the pressure is applied to the dural sleeve investing a nerve-root, severe pain occupying all or any part of the dermatome results. A nerve is insensitive to pressure along its entire length except at the dural investment of the nerve-root (Cyriax, 1957). Hence, disc protrusion, since it impinges against the dural sleeve, usually causes severe pain, whereas the same degree of pressure applied another inch distally along the nerve would have produced no local pain at all. Pain felt in the relevant dermatome has, therefore, a clear significance in distinguishing where along a nerve the impact falls.

At cervical laminectomy, Frykholm (1951) showed that stimulation of the anterior division of the nerve-root gave rise to deep pain associated with muscle tenderness, thus confirming the views (Cyriax, 1948) on the phenomena that had given rise to the idea of 'fibrositis'. He also found that stimulation of the posterior division brought on a more peripheral pain associated with paraesthesia. Since disc-protrusions may impinge against one aspect only of a nerve-root, they may compress the inferior aspect only and thus affect the motor fibres alone. Or the pressure may come from above, and affect the sensory fibres alone. In consequence, a protruded disc may cause a partial root-lesion, sensory or motor, depending on which aspect of the root receives the main impact. Only in the former event are pins and needles brought on.

4. Spinal Cord

When the cord is compressed the pins and needles are apt to be bilateral and to ignore the segmentation of the body, occupying areas beyond the cutaneous supply of any one trunk- or nerve-root. There is no pain and neither moving the digits nor striking the skin evokes pins and needles. For example, the patient may complain of pins and needles from both patellae to all the toes in each foot, thus spanning five dermatomes. Another interesting complaint is pins and needles in both big toes on neck-flexion which ceases after manipulative reduction at the neck.

One cause of pins and needles felt in all four limbs or in the upper or the lower limbs only, is a minor degree of pressure on the spinal cord in the neck. When the cord is compressed at its thoracic extent, the paraesthesiae are felt solely in the lower limbs, often only in the feet. Neck-flexion is usually the only way to bring the pins and needles on. In central cervical and thoracic disc-lesions pins and needles may be felt in the lower limbs, their extrasegmental distribution often providing the diagnostic clue.

STRETCHING THE NERVE-ROOT

Stretching a nerve-root whose mobility is impaired may be painful and is sometimes limited in range. The common cause is a disc-protrusion and limitation of range occurs only at the lower lumbar levels.

The different ways of stretching the root are:

1. Straight-leg Raising

When there is impaired mobility of any root between the fourth lumbar and the second sacral, the movement stretching the nerve-root is usually painful and restricted in range; moreover, at its extreme, paraesthesia may be evoked at the distal end of the dermatome. Not only is straight-leg raising painful and limited, but neck-flexion after the leg has been raised as far as it will go may increase the pain and elicit a shower of pins and needles in the appropriate part of the foot.

2. Prone-lying Knee-flexion

This movement stretches the third lumbar nerve-root. If a disc-protrusion encroaches on the intervertebral foramen, the mobility of this root becomes impaired. In consequence, the movement may be restricted or unilaterally painful at the extreme. Rarely, in addition to the pain, pins and needles are provoked in the anterior tibial area.

3. Neck-flexion and Scapular Approximation

When the neck is flexed it is 3 cm. longer than in full extension. Hence, when the mobility of the dura mater is impaired at a thoracic or lumbar level, neck-flexion often brings on or increases the pain in the lower back or the posterior (seldom the anterior) aspect of the thorax.

Scapular approximation pulls on the eighth cervical and first thoracic nerve-roots, thus drawing the dura mater upwards in the same way as does neck-flexion. Hence, in thoracic intraspinal lesions the pain at the back or the front of the chest is brought on not only by neck-flexion, but also by scapular approximation (Cyriax, 1950). (In lumbar disc lesions, scapular approximation does not alter the pain.) The fact that movement of the scapula has induced posterior thoracic symptoms is apt to be mis-interpreted, and is thought to incriminate muscles such as the rhomboid and lower trapezius. In fact, the resisted scapular movements do not hurt and, when the active movement already found painful is repeated passively by the examiner, this does hurt. In this way it can be shown that the muscles moving the scapula are not themselves involved.

4. Neck Movements

When a cervical nerve-root is compressed, one or other of the neck movements may increase the root pain in the upper limb and also provoke pins and needles in the fingers of the appropriate dermatome. In osteo-phytic root-palsy this movement is likely to be side-flexion towards the painful side. Sometimes a neck movement evokes pain and paraesthesia only if the upper limb is placed in a special position first, most often held out forwards.

Since neck-flexion stretches the dura mater down the whole length of the vertebral column, the fact that this hurts must not be regarded as showing the lesion to lie in the neck.

NOMENCLATURE

Neuritis

Conduction along a nerve can suffer in two ways: from primary degeneration of the parenchyma or from pressure exerted on the nerve from without. The term 'neuritis' should be reserved for cases in which neurological examination discloses signs of diminished conduction along a peripheral nerve as the result of lesions confined to the parenchyma. In neuritis the lesion does not affect the mobility of the nerve; hence stretching it causes no pain and the movement is not limited.

Peripheral Neuritis

This disease is characterized by both sensory and motor paresis; hence pins and needles, numbness, loss of reflexes and muscular weakness all ensue.

The causes are:

1. Drugs: e.g. isoniazid, thalidomide.
2. Toxins: e.g. diphtheria.
3. Metals: e.g. lead.
4. Vitamin B deficiency: secondary to alcoholism or pernicious anaemia, beri-beri, pellagra.
5. Carcinoma: without invasion of the nerve itself. The tumour secretes an antigen provoking an autoimmune reaction.
6. Myopathy: e.g. peroneal atrophy (motor only).

Ascending polyneuritis is a serious disease, coming on after influenza, or with serum sickness, or as a virus disease. The disorder begins in the lower limbs, which soon show flaccid paralysis. Within a few days the trunk and arms may also suffer. The myocardium often becomes affected. The patient may at any moment need a respirator urgently, hence he must be nursed in hospital until the extent to which the paralysis will progress becomes clear, and so long as the heart is severely affected. The paralysis remains static for some weeks and recovery may take one, even two years.

Mono-neuritis

One part of a nerve, then another part of another nerve may become affected in an erratic way. The common causes are primary arterial inflammation, rheumatoid arthritis and diabetes. Miller (1966) states that polyartheritis nodosa leads to multiple areas of infarction, causing ischaemic spots along the nerve trunk. In diabetes the legs are the main site; the feet burn and shoots of pain in the calves are experienced, both chiefly at night. A painful partial lesion of one ulnar or one lateral popliteal nerve is apt to complicate diabetes.

Infectious Neuritis

Isolated painful neuritis also affects two other nerves; the long thoracic and suprascapular. It is a puzzling disease, lying half-way between herpes zoster and anterior poliomyelitis, presumably caused by a virus. It is distinguishable from the former by the absence of vesicles and from the latter by (1) the absence of fever or any constitutional symptoms, (2) the absence of extension of the paralysis to muscles outside the thoraco-brachial area, and (3) the presence, as a rule, of pain. So far as my experience goes, infectious neuritis attacks only the scapular muscles.

The first symptom is unprovoked, unilateral, continuous pain in the upper thorax day and night, unaffected by rest, exertion or movement of the neck, scapula or upper limb. At the end of three weeks, the pain ceases. At no time are pins and needles felt. After the first few days, the patient notices a vague weakness of the arm. If the suprascapular nerve is affected, the two spinatus muscles become weak, as shown by testing abduction and lateral rotation at the shoulder against resistance. If the serratus anterior muscle becomes weak, the patient cannot perform the final 45 degrees of elevation of the arm. Rarely a long thoracic neuritis may develop painlessly. Paralysis of the trapezius following a spinal accessory neuritis has been described; it is stated to come on painlessly. The prognosis is good and in cases occurring in England spontaneous recovery of the affected muscles in three to six months is the rule, but when contracted in the Middle East eventual spontaneous recovery of muscle power is much less certain. No treatment is effective or required, except for analgesics during the first three weeks.

Infectious neuritis involving the muscles of the lower limb, analogy suggesting the buttock, appears not to occur.

Neuralgic Amyotrophy

The nerve itself becomes acutely inflamed. The lesion must be peripheral, since one muscle may be paralysed; others supplied by the same nerve or nerve-root remain unaffected. Several unconnected muscles in one limb may be affected in this random way.

The disease nearly always affects the arms only. It begins with sudden pain in the neck, spreading within hours to both arms. In most cases, it leaves one upper limb but the other remains painful for three or four months. In minor cases random paralysis of several muscles is found, in severe cases, nearly all the muscles of both upper limbs may be very weak. The paralysis is maximal from the outset; the pain is severe, gradually diminishing after the first two months. In minor cases, the muscles may recover in six months; in severe cases up to two years are required. Numbness and pins and needles are seldom experienced except in severe paralysis, and then only at the cutaneous area of the nerve most affected.

Neuralgia

This term is used for pains arising, apparently spontaneously, within the cutaneous area supplied by a sensory nerve. Paroxysms of superficial pain occur at intervals with periods of complete freedom. The short sharp repeated stabs of facial neuralgia elicited by touching a trigger spot or by movement, e.g. eating, are quite different from the continuous ache, for example, of temporal arteritis or of pressure on a nerve-root, and should not be confused with the sharp twinge on movement characterizing subluxation of a loose body within a joint. When, as is usual, the fifth cranial nerve is affected, conduction along the nerve never becomes impaired, no matter how long the neuralgia lasts. Patients with multiple sclerosis are prone to this disease. The lightning pains of tabes dorsalis also represent a type of neuralgia; here the neurological deficit is obvious.

Post-herpetic neuralgia may arise after infection of a posterior spinal ganglion with herpes zoster virus. This is a continuous ache, punctuated by stabbing pains, felt in the area where the vesicles appeared. Occasionally conduction along the relevant part of the nervous system is temporarily or permanently impaired. When segmental muscular palsy complicates post-herpetic neuralgia, it is clear that the inflammatory process, instead of remaining confined to the posterior root ganglion, has spread to some of the anterior horn cells of the same segment.

In *migrainous neuralgia*, the pain is severe and continuous; it lasts for hours and several attacks come on within some days; then there are long pain-free periods.

For trigeminal neuralgia, the best treatment appears to be Tegretol (carbamazepine) 100 mg. twice a day, increasing up to 500 mg. until relief

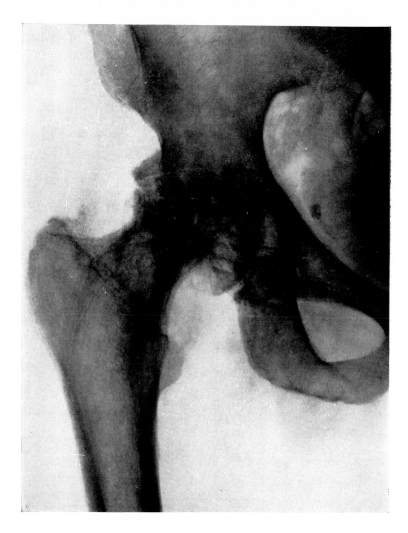

PLATE I

Gonococcal arthritis of the hip. Twenty years previously this patient, now aged 66, had spent six months in bed with gonococcal arthritis at his hip. The contrast is striking between the X-ray appearances and the fact that a full and painless range of movement at the joint was present. The muscles were considerably wasted.

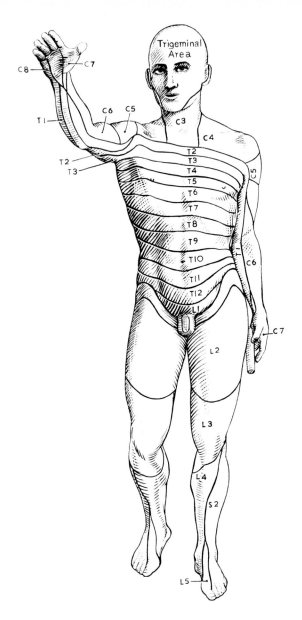

Plate 2

The dermatomes. Anterior view of the embryological segmentation of the skin (after Déjerine). Note how the circular arrangement at the trunk has suffered deformation at the lower cervical and lower lumbar regions where the dermatomes have been drawn out into the limbs.

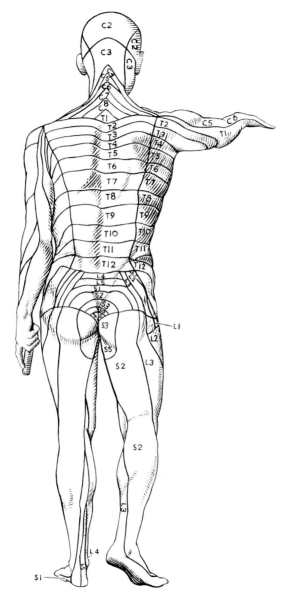

PLATE 3

The dermatomes. Posterior view of the embryological segmentation of the skin (after Déjerine). These two diagrams give an adequate impression of the general arrangement, but do not allow for the considerable overlap. Only the central portion of each dematome is outlined.

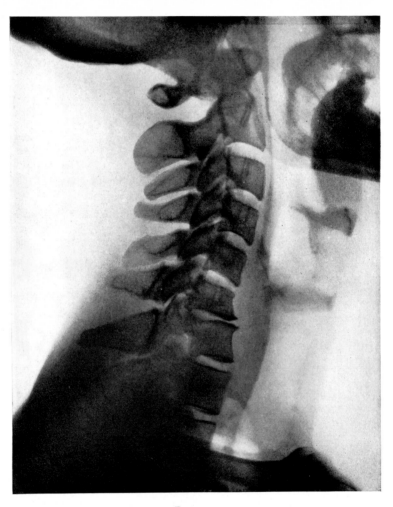

PLATE 4

Sixth cervical disc lesion. Lateral view of cervical spine showing marked narrowing and tilt at the sixth cervical joint. This contrasts with the normal spaces above and below. The patient had a seventh-root palsy.

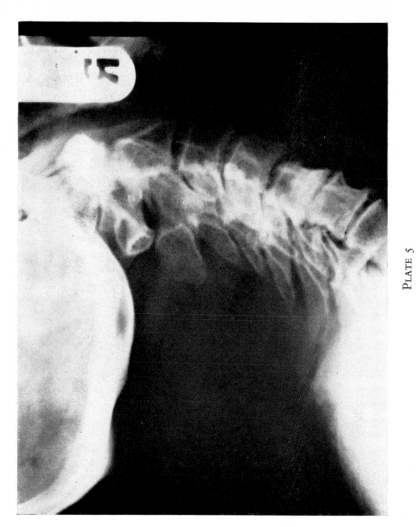

PLATE 5

Osteophytic compression. A man of 68 had had three years' tingling at the right thumb due to compression of the sixth cervical root. No root paresis was detectable.

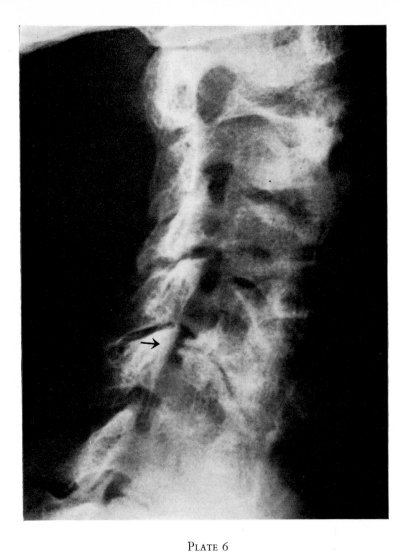

PLATE 6

Osteophytes encroaching on the fifth cervical foramenn. The patient, aged 68, had a sixth cervical root palsy.

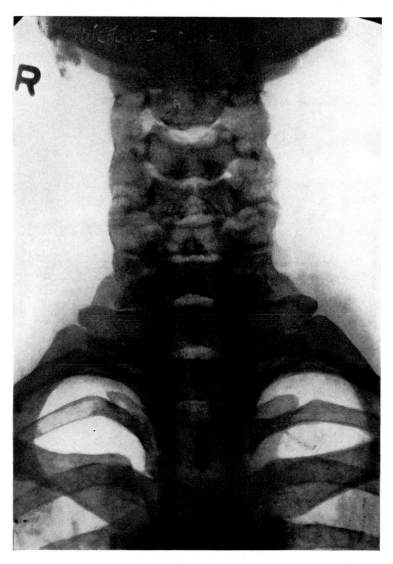

PLATE 7

Cervical spine. Radiograph taken before traction. Compare with Plate 8.

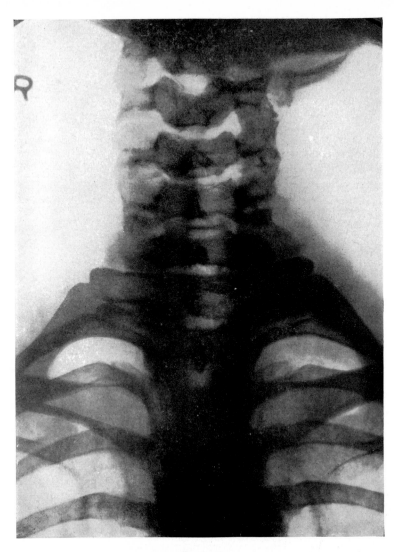

PLATE 8

Cervical spine. Radiograph of the same subject (see Plate 7) taken after several seconds' manual traction. The distance between the upper border of the first thoracic vertebra and the lower border of the fourth cervical has increased by 1 cm, i.e. by 2·5 mm per joint.

results. The patient still feels minor twinges in the face; when these cease he knows he is in remission and can stop treatment for the time being. Half to two-thirds of patients do well; in the others, or if toxic reactions ensue, Gasserian section should not be delayed.

Tegretol has been reported as unsuccessful in post-herpetic neuralgia and migrainous neuralgia (Henderson, 1967). Tabes calls for phenytoin.

Causalgia

The use of this term should be confined to cases in which the following criteria are satisfied: (a) a history of injury involving a nerve; (b) long-standing constant burning pain involving the distal part of a limb, aggravated by changes in temperature or attempted movement; (c) trophic change distally, coming on some time after the injury.

Lewis regards the pain as arising from the peripheral release of a chemical substance that excites the sensory nerve endings. More recently, vasomotor studies have revealed a persistent increase in blood-flow in the whole limb; a condition best described as capillary hypertension. Indeed the capillaries can be seen on microscopy to be dilated and pulsating. In 1944 Granit et al. showed that nerve impulses set up in a motor-root are transmitted to the sensory fibres at the point where a nerve has been severed, tied or crushed. Causalgia has been attributed to such trans-axonal excitation.

The pain is severe, even agonizing, and, although often requested by the patient, amputation brings no relief. Neither dividing the spinal cord vertically into two halves, thereby severing the pain-carrying fibres of the spino-thalmic tract, nor any other operation on the somatic nervous system appears to have any effect. However, cure often follows removal of the appropriate autonomic ganglion. If the pain disappears for the duration of anaesthesia after a stellate ganglion block or after an injection of tetraethylammonium bromide, removal of this ganglion is indicated. Slessor (1947) in a review of twenty-two cases confirms the benefit of ganglionectomy and states that relief had lasted for over three years. As in other forms of intractable pain, leucotomy offers a final resort.

Pain in a Phantom Limb

M. A. Falconer (1953) put forward an interesting theory to explain pain in a phantom limb. He adduced evidence that in some cases the cells of the secondary neurones in the spinal cord are themselves responsible for the pain. He has found the symptoms relievable by antero-lateral chordotomy, without impairing awareness of the phantom itself. In his

D

view, the cells, deprived of the continuous stimuli that normally reach them, discharge either spontaneously or as a reaction to aberrant impulses, causaglia resulting. This theory serves to explain how percussion of neuromata affords relief. The hammering restores the lacking afferent stimuli to an intensity high enough to abolish the pain of excessive quiescence.

Radium Neuritis

This is usually the result of excessive radiation reaching the brachial plexus during treatment of carcinoma of the breast and causes severe pain starting about six months later and lasting many months, even years. Sometimes a considerable and permanent palsy of the whole upper limb results.

Traumatic Palsy

If a nerve is severely overstretched, conduction may cease for some months. Familiar examples are obstetrical traction-palsies of the brachial plexus, and paralysis of the deltoid muscle as the result of tension on the axillary nerve when the shoulder dislocates. The continuity of the nerve is maintained and spontaneous recovery is invariable.

PRESSURE ON A NERVE

Pressure on a nerve-root causes pain felt in the whole, or any part of the relevant dermatome. Pressure on a nerve-trunk is painless; only distal paraesthesia results. Neuritis and neuralgic amyotrophy hurt, although they too affect peripheral nerves. The situation is very confusing, and a most difficult task is to distinguish between painful and painless nerve-lesions and their differentiation from the similar pains that arise from disorders of the moving parts.

When the external aspect of a nerve or a nerve-root is compressed, none of the classical signs of neurological disease is necessarily detectable. The first paper on affections confined to the external aspect of nerves appeared twenty-five years ago (Cyriax, 1942). A book describing the same entities more fully under the name of 'Peripheral Entrapment Neuropathy' appeared in 1963 (Kopell and Thompson).

Pain may originate from pressure on a nerve-root, but conduction along it may remain normal. No pins and needles or numbness need be experienced. Stretching the nerve-root may leave the pain unaltered and its range full. Nothing in such cases suggests pain arising from any part of the nervous system. However, the possibility arises when the joints, muscles, etc., comprising the same segment as the painful area are entirely normal. This finding draws attention to pressure on a nerve-root insufficient in degree to impair either conduction or mobility. Obviously, interference with the external aspect of the root need not be great enough to be transmitted to the conducting element. Secondary parenchymatous change may, of course, develop in due course, if the pressure increases. When these neurological signs appear the label 'neuritis' might seem warranted, but leads in fact to an error in emphasis, focusing attention on the secondary, rather than the primary organic process.

Rheumatoid Perineuritis

The careful pathological studies of Freund, Steiner, Leichentritt and Price (1942) have shown that long-standing rheumatoid arthritis is often complicated by sharply-defined inflammatory nodules in the perineurium. These authors suggest that the paraesthesiae and trophic cutaneous changes occurring in chronic cases are due to irritation of the conducting fibres of the nerve by such nodules, since microscopy revealed no abnormality of the nerve parenchyma. Gibson, Kersley and Desmarais (1946) showed that nodular polymyositis also occurs in advanced rheumatoid arthritis. The nodules in muscle and nerve-sheath are absent in ankylosing spondylitis. Arteritis of the vasa nervorum may lead to peripheral nerve palsies, chiefly in patients with severe generalized rheumatoid disease. The event carries a bad prognosis, a quarter of such patients dying within twelve months.

SIGNS OF PRESSURE ON A NERVE

The signs fall into seven groups, but are seldom all present in one case. Occasionally, no physical signs can be detected, the diagnosis being established on the history, the patient's sincerity, the manner of onset and subsequent migration of the symptoms, the quality of the pain and the absence of signs of any other disorder or of psychogenic pain.

It is noticeable that in almost every case nerve-sheaths are affected where they lie in close contact with bone or cartilage or traverse a foramen.

1. Pain on Stretching the Nerve

This is the outstanding sign only when the dural sheath of the lower two lumbar and upper two sacral nerve-roots is affected; the movement that stretches the nerve, i.e. straight-leg raising, is often limited. The hamstrings go into spasm when traction is exerted via the sciatic nerve-trunk on the compressed and therefore immobile root. In third-root compression full straight-leg raising is painful only at its extreme, and pronelying knee-flexion may be limited and is nearly always painful at full range. Full extension of the wrist occasionally hurts when the elbow is extended but not when this is kept fixed in cases of compression of the median nerve in the carpal tunnel. Movement of the scapula may painfully stretch the first and second thoracic nerve-roots in disc lesions at these two levels, and the trapezius may contract to keep the scapula involuntarily elevated to prevent further traction on a recently overstretched axillary nerve.

2. The Provocation of Pins and Needles

Unless pressure is applied on a nerve from without, no movement provokes the paraesthesia. All movements, except those of the digits in which the pins and needles are felt, have diagnostic value. For example, when elevation of the scapulae brings on a patient's nocturnal pins and needles in the hands, the lower trunk of the brachial plexus has clearly been lifted off the first rib. If neck-flexion evokes pins and needles in the lower limbs, pressure is being exerted on the cervical extent of the spinal cord. If straight-leg raising causes a shower of pins and needles in the foot, a low lumbar nerve-root is compressed at the intervertebral foramen.

3. Tenderness and Swelling of the Nerve-sheath

Both are presumably present in every case and, where practicable, the point should be sought where pressure on the nerve reproduces the distant pain. Swelling occurs at the ulnar nerve in the groove at the elbow and the median nerve in the carpal tunnel. A neuroma, discoverable only at operation, is always found in the late stage of Morton's metatarsalgia.

4. Postural Deformity

In severe sciatic and cervical disc lesions, lateral deviation of the spine develops from adopting the posture best calculated to relieve pressure on the nerve-root. Cubitus valgus, whether developmental or the result of mal-union of a fracture near the elbow, often results in pressure on the ulnar nerve.

5. Evidence of Secondary Parenchymatous Change

Interference with conduction occurs if pressure on the nerve-sheath is sufficient also to interfere with the parenchyma of the nerve. At the facial nerve only when palsy supervenes does the condition become apparent at all. If conduction becomes impaired later, a diagnosis of pressure on the external surface of a nerve is clearly correct.

6. Cessation of Symptoms for the Duration of Local Anaesthesia

This is the best method of confirming a tentative diagnosis. If this is correct, and the anaesthetic solution reaches the nerve-sheath, relief is achieved within a minute or two, and lasts for about an hour and a half. In many cases, a lasting therapeutic effect is also achieved; hence local anaesthesia should always be employed in a doubtful case.

7. Relief Following Topical Hydrocortisone

An injection of hydrocortisone into the carpal tunnel is almost always followed by weeks or months of, or even permanent, relief. Hence it provides a good diagnostic test in uncertain cases.

Individual Lesions

These are merely listed, since they are dealt with in the appropriate chapters of this book. They also appear in Kopell and Thompson's book, where my original descriptions have been considerably expanded.

1. Facial nerve-palsy (not dealt with)
2. Cervical disc-lesion
3. Thoracic outlet syndrome
4. Axillary nerve palsy
5. Ulnar nerve palsy at the elbow
6. Carpal tunnel syndromes
7. Ulnar nerve palsy at the pisiform
8. Contusion of the radial nerve at the wrist
9. Pressure on the digital nerve in the palm
10. Thoracic disc lesion
11. Meralgia paraesthetica
12. Compression of the anterior cutaneous nerve of the thigh
13. Compression of the obturator nerve
14. Lumbar disc lesion
15. Pressure on the tibial nerve at the knee
16. Pressure on the long saphenous nerve at the knee
17. Pressure on the common peroneal nerve at the fibula
18. Pressure on the superficial peroneal nerve at mid-leg
19. Tarsal tunnel syndromes
20. Bruising of the first plantar digital nerve
21. Morton's metatarsalgia

Treatment

In slight cases, prevention of the causative strain may suffice. Thus, avoidance of prolonged flexion of, or pressure on, the elbow allows irritation of the ulnar nerve at the medial condyle to subside. If mild symptoms of pressure on the lower trunk of the brachial plexus from the first rib appear late in life, prohibition against carrying weights and keeping the scapulae elevated often secure relief.

If simple measures fail, and the symptoms are severe, operation is indicated, thus:

1. Removal of the cause of pressure. When a cervical rib, an osteoma, or a protruded intervertebral disc causes pressure on nervous tissue, it may be excised. Intra-articular displacements are often amenable to manipulative reduction. Ganglia can often be aspirated or digitally burst.

2. Elongation of the structure maintaining the position of the skeletal projection. This applies to division of the scalenus anterior muscle in cases of cervical rib. The rib can then sink away from the nerve-trunks.

3. Alteration of the course of the nerve. If neuritis is developing, anterior transposition of the ulnar nerve at the elbow is indicated.

4. Enlargement of the foramen by which a nerve pierces a ligament or fascia. This applies especially to meralgia paraesthetica where incision of the foramen of exit of the lateral cutaneous nerve of the thigh may afford relief.

5. Division of the ligament confining the nerve. This applies particularly to division of the transverse carpal ligament in median nerve pressure.

6. Removal of the nerve. This may be required at the sole of the foot and in meralgia paraesthetica.

5

Rheumatological Aspects of Soft Tissue Lesions

by D. A. H. Yates, M.D., M.R.C.P., D.Phys.Med.

Physician, Department of Physical Medicine, St. Thomas's Hospital

A large variety of diseases can present with musculo-skeletal pain and in this chapter it will not be feasible to provide a detailed description of the numerous rheumatic syndromes. Emphasis will be placed on the modes in which the common chronic rheumatic diseases can present as relatively isolated soft tissue lesions, or mimic them.

The painful conditions affecting joints and connective tissues fall into two main categories, inflammatory and degenerative.

INFLAMMATORY ARTHRITIS

An inflammatory response may be evoked in a joint by a specific infecting organism as in septicaemia or tuberculosis, by uric acid crystals as in gout, by trauma, or by a loose body in the joint. In many of the common rheumatic conditions, including rheumatoid arthritis, psoriatic arthritis, ankylosing spondylitis and Reiter's disease, the exact cause of the inflammatory response is unknown. Evidence is accumulating that some form of auto-immune reaction is responsible for the inflammation as well as for the generalized systemic disturbance which is indicated by a rise in erythrocyte sedimentation rate (ESR) and often by a mild pyrexia.

The first pathological change within affected joints is a thickening and proliferation of the synovial membrane, which is infiltrated by chronic inflammatory cells. If this process continues, the hypertrophied synovium forms a pannus which proliferates over the articular cartilage. The superficial layers of articular cartilage rely for their maintenance on the diffusion of synovial fluid into the interstices, so that the interposition of this pannus interferes with nutrition, producing thinning and in due course complete destruction of the cartilage. The juxta-articular bone has already become hyperaemic as a result of the inflammation, and porotic as a result of disuse. Once it has been exposed, pockets of pannus invade the bone, impelled by the pressures developed within the joint on movement. This produces the characteristic radiological changes of inflammatory arthritis, namely, joint erosions and juxta-articular osteoporosis.

Infiltration with chronic inflammatory cells also occurs in other tissues, particularly those with a high collagen content such as fascial septa, ligaments, tendon-sheaths and muscle insertions. Localized granulomata may cause attrition of the affected structures, sometimes causing elongation with laxity of ligaments and rupture of tendons.

The common chronic rheumatic disorders will be briefly described, with an outline of their differential diagnoses and management, and following this the commonly associated soft-tissue lesions will be considered on a regional basis.

Rheumatoid Arthritis

Rheumatoid arthritis is characterized by a symmetrical arthritis mainly involving the peripheral joints, the formation of nodules and the development of abnormal serum proteins. Females are affected more frequently than males, predominantly in middle age, but the disease can present at any time from infancy to old age. The onset is usually insidious in the hands and feet, characteristically sparing the terminal interphalangeal joints. Occasionally the disease is heralded for several years by so-called 'palindromic arthritis', i.e. recurrent short episodes of acute arthritis in single joints which settle spontaneously in a few days leaving no residua. In juveniles (Still's disease) the onset is often mono-arthritic and more florid, with fever, splenomegaly and a mascular rash, while later the sacro-iliac joints are sometimes involved. As the disease progresses the shoulders, elbows, knees, and sometimes the hips, are symmetrically involved and nodules develop, particularly over the elbows. The cervical joints are frequently affected, but characteristically there is little evidence of involvement of the rest of the spine. Non-articular lesions are common, particularly affecting bursae, tendon sheaths and ligamentous insertions. Pathologically, rheumatoid arthritis can be distinguished from other forms of inflammatory arthritis by biopsy of the nodules and by serological tests. The nodules consist of a central necrotic area surrounded by a layer of chronic inflammatory cells which have a typical radial arrangement giving the appearance of a palisade, and this zone is surrounded by granulation tissue.

During the course of the disease most cases develop an abnormal macroglobulin, rheumatoid factor, which is capable of combining with denatured gamma-globulin. In the sheep cell agglutination test (SCAT) rheumatoid factor is demonstrated by agglutination of sheep erythrocytes coated with rabbit globulin. In the latex fixation test (LFT) latex particles, on to which heated human gamma-globulin has been adsorbed, are clumped in the presence of rheumatoid factor. The SCAT is slightly more specific, but less sensitive, than the LFT. Methods of performing the tests differ slightly between laboratories but a positive titre (usually more than 1:16) is found in more than 80 per cent of cases with erosion and nodules. In juveniles and in early disease in adults the tests are often negative.

The natural history of the disease varies considerably between individuals. Up to 80 per cent of juveniles experience spontaneous arrest of the disease with only moderate residual joint damage. In adults the process is more insidious, but only approximately one-third of patients become severely disabled.

Treatment

During severe phases of the disease bed-rest is helpful, providing that the joints are kept supple by passive movements; gentle static exercises, particularly to the quadriceps, serve to prevent wasting of muscle. Various antirheumatic agents are available, but the patient should be warned at the outset that only partial suppression of symptoms is likely to be achieved. Calcium or enteric-coated aspirin up to 4 g., indomethacin up to 150 mg. or phenylbutazone up to 300 mg. daily often provide satisfactory suppression of the disease. Gold administered weekly as intramuscular injections of 50 mg. gold aurothiomalate (Myocrisin) to a total dose of 0·5 g. may induce a worthwhile remission. If these methods used in sequence do not enable the patient to return to modified employment or domestic independence, systemic corticosteroid therapy may be justified if there are no complicating factors, such as peptic ulceration, hypertension, cardiac failure, tuberculosis or diabetes. Prednisone is the most suitable preparation but the risk of exceeding a total daily dose of more than 10 mg. is rarely justified. The use of intra-articular therapy is discussed later. Antimalarial compounds, such as chloroquine, are better avoided because of the risk of inducing a degenerative retinopathy if dosage continues for some years. Detailed attention to each individual's needs as regards physiotherapy and appliances, as well as help in domestic and industrial resettlement, are essential parts of management.

Psoriatic Arthritis

Some patients with chronic psoriasis develop an arthropathy distinct from rheumatoid arthritis. Characteristically there is asymmetrical involvement of proximal joints, such as the hips and knees, while the feet and hands may show symmetrical involvement, particularly of the terminal interphalangeal joints. The cervical spine is frequently affected, sometimes producing ankylosis, and the sacro-iliac joints may be involved. The SCAT remains negative but the ESR is often elevated. Non-articular lesions are sometimes encountered, particularly affecting bursae, tendon-sheaths and ligamentous insertions but nodules do not occur.

Treatment

The joint symptoms tend to fluctuate with the degree of skin involvement, and during a relapse bed-rest may be beneficial. Salicylates, phenyl-butazone or indomethacin are helpful, but systemic steroid therapy is rarely justified. Although qnite severe destructive changes may occur in individual joints, the disability is seldom severe. Therapy with chloro-quine or gold is contra-indicated as these agents may induce severe exacerbation of the skin condition.

Ankylosing Spondylitis

This condition usually presents in early adult life as an intermittent sacro-iliitis (see Chapter 22) affecting males approximately three times more often than females. If the disease progresses, the lumbar, thoracic and cervical spinal joints become involved by a progressive arthritis with increasing stiffness leading to complete ankylosis. The costovertebral joints also stiffen, limiting chest expansion, and occasionally the hips and knees may be involved, but the peripheral joints are usually spared. Recurrent iridocyclitis is an occasional complication. Apart from the ligamentous lesions related to the spine, non-articular lesions are not a frequent feature. The SCAT remains negative but the ESR is often raised. The earliest radiological changes are sclerosis and irregularity of the sacro-iliac joint margins although these may not be detectable for at least a year from the onset of symptoms. Later progressive ossification of the para-vertebral ligaments produces the typical 'bamboo-spine' appearance.

Treatment

Although no specific cure is available, early recognition of the disease is important, firstly to obviate fruitless attempts to relieve the spinal pain and stiffness by physical treatment and osteopathy, which may exacerbate the symptoms, and secondly to ensure that the patient is trained to adopt an upright posture before ankylosis occurs. Activities that involve recurrent jarring of the spine such as rugby and horse-riding should be avoided. Either phenylbutazone 300 mg. or indomethacin 150 mg. daily usually produce dramatic relief of pain and should be administered intermittently during exacerbations. Oral therapy is precluded by peptic ulceration or severe indigestion, but these drugs can then be given as suppositories. Radiotherapy to the spine, which contains bone marrow, carries a risk of inducing leukaemia and is only justified if incapacitating pain is not relieved by drugs.

Reiter's Disease

Reiter's disease is characterized by the triad of polyarthritis, genital discharge and conjunctivitis; it occurs predominantly in males. Sometimes a pustular rash, keratodermia blennorrhagica is seen mainly on the hands and feet. The precipitating factor of the initial attack, and sometimes of recurrences, appears to be a non-gonococcal urethritis, which is not necessarily venereally acquired. Sometimes inflammation of the bowel such as dysentery, ulcerative colitis or Crohn's disease may precipitate a similar form of arthritis. The arthritis affects predominantly the sacro-iliac, the cervical and lumbar spinal joints. There can be asymmetrical involvement of the limb joints, particularly the knees and the distal interphalangeal joints in the hands and feet. The commonest non-articular lesion is plantar fasciitis manifested by heel pain, which used to be called 'gonococcal heel'. Lesions of tendons and bursae also occur. The SCAT remains negative but the ESR is usually elevated. Radiographs may show, in addition to erosive changes, a characteristic periostitis affecting particularly the phalanges, calcaneus and pelvic bones.

Treatment

No specific treatment is available, but a gonococcal element in the infection must be excluded by the study of urethral smears. A broad-spectrum antibiotic such as tetracycline and prostatic massage may reduce the symptoms arising from the urethritis. Often the systemic illness and the arthritis respond to phenylbutazone or indomethacin in standard dosage, but sometimes the disease runs a protracted course with intermittent exacerbations particularly when irregular sexual habits give rise to recurrent urethral infections.

Gout

Prolonged elevation of the serum uric acid leads in some individuals to the deposition of uric acid crystals in connective tissue and joints. This hyperuricaemia may result from over-production of uric acid due to an inherited metabolic abnormality, to chronic alcoholism or to increased bone marrow activity as in leukaemia. Retention of uric acid may also result from impaired renal excretion in chronic kidney disease, or from the side-effects of drugs such as the thiazide diuretics and salicylates in small doses.

Acute gout most commonly affects the first metatarsophalangeal joint, but any large joint may be affected. Microscopy of synovial fluid aspirated from an acutely inflamed joint shows it to contain numerous microcrystals of monosodium urate, some of which have been phagocytosed by leucocytes.

Treatment

The affected joint should be rested and vigorous therapy with an anti-inflammatory agent begun at once. Colchicine tablets 1 mg. at hourly intervals for up to eight hours are usually effective, but in some subjects vomiting and diarrhoea are induced before relief begins. Phenylbutazone has less unpleasant acute side-effects and can be given either in tablet form 200 mg. six-hourly or, for rapid relief, by deep intramuscular injection of 600 mg. with procaine added to the solution to diminish the local irritant effect. Indomethacin 50 mg. six-hourly is also very effective. Whichever drug is used, these high dosage schedules should not be maintained for more than two days because of the risk of toxic effects, administration at half-dosage being continued for several days afterwards to prevent a relapse.

Chronic gout produces a chronic polyarthritis with acute exacerbations; eventually destructive changes take place in affected joints. Tophaceous deposits also occur in the non-articular soft-tissues, i.e. bursae, tendon-sheaths and muscle insertions. These lesions may prove particularly resistant to local treatment. If chronic gout is producing either frequent disabling acute attacks, or tophaceous deposits with destructive joint changes, or if there is evidence of renal disease, the hyperuricaemia must be corrected. This can be achieved either by promoting increased renal excretion of uric acid with a uricosuric agent, such as probenecid 1–2 g. daily, or by inhibiting the formation of uric acid by allopurinol 200–400 mg. daily. Both drugs are initially likely to precipitate acute gout; hence it is advisable to increment the dosage slowly and to give small suppressive doses of phenylbutazone or colchicine during the first month.

Analgesics containing salicylate antagonize the uricosuric effect of probenecid; hence paracetamol is a suitable alternative. Allopurinol acts by inhibiting the action of xanthine-oxidase which promotes the metabolism of purines to uric acid. Allopurinol is indicated if uricosuric therapy has failed, or if gout is complicated by the formation of uric acid calculi, or if there is severe renal failure. Since the underlying biochemical defect in gout is usually permanent, once therapy with either drug is begun it should be continued indefinitely.

Polymyalgia Rheumatica

This rather vague term has been coined to describe a syndrome occuring in elderly patients who complain of pain and stiffness affecting the neck and the limb-girdle joints and musculature. In addition there is malaise and sometimes fever with night sweats. Clinically there is an arthritis of central distribution with moderate restriction of movement of the cervical spine, shoulders, hips and sometimes the knees, but often these signs are not commensurate with the degree of stiffness of which the patient complains. It will be noted that this distribution of joint involvement is quite distinct from the peripheral distribution described for rheumatoid arthritis. A variety of unrelated diseases can present in this way, including polyarteritis nodosa, temporal arteritis, myeloma, the reticuloses and secondary carcinomatosis. However, in a large proportion of patients, after painstaking investigation, a specific cause cannot be found for the marked elevation of the erythrocyte sedimentation rate, often up to 80 mm. per hour (Westergren). Usually the illness runs a self-limiting course with intermittent exacerbations over several years. Phenylbutazone in small doses may give adequate symptomatic relief. If not, therapy with prednisone is justified at the lowest dosage that will suppress the symptoms and the elevated ESR. The cause remains obscure, but there is some evidence for believing that it may be due to a form of arteritis affecting the larger arteries, which are not readily available for biopsy. All cases need thorough investigation and a close follow-up until the disease becomes inactive.

DIFFERENTIAL DIAGNOSIS

In everyday practice two decisions must be made in treating soft tissue lesions: firstly, the exact anatomical site of the lesion, and secondly whether the lesion is isolated and primary or a local manifestation of an underlying disease process. A complete medical history and careful physical examination will go a long way towards elucidating these two points.

When soft-tissue lesions are detected in a patient who already has arthritis in one or more joints, it is obvious that diagnosis and treatment of the underlying disease process is necessary in addition to the purely local treatment of the presenting lesion. Suspicion of an underlying inflammatory process should be aroused if multiple non-articular lesions are detected or if individual lesions remain resistant to local treatment or recur frequently.

The ESR provides a very useful, simple and cheap screening test for underlying systemic disease. It is usually moderately raised early in the course of the inflammatory polyarthritides and also in skeletal pain caused by sepsis or malignant infiltration. Some patients with early rheumatoid arthritis show an abnormal SCAT test, which is not usually detectable in other forms of inflammatory arthritis. Radiographs may be of some help in reaching an early diagnosis by showing the distribution of articular erosions, but more often their real value is to exclude bone disease. If recurrent non-articular soft-tissue lesions occur, particularly in the male, it is advisable to exclude gout by estimating the serum uric acid level. Analgesics containing salicylate must have been avoided for twenty-four hours before the blood is taken, since these can artificially elevate the serum level.

REGIONAL INCIDENCE OF SOFT TISSUE LESIONS

Having outlined the general principles of differential diagnosis the more common diagnostic problems can be reviewed on a regional basis.

Spine

Although acute pain arising from the spine is most frequently due to intervertebral disc disease other conditions can simulate this. At any level of the spine carious vertebral disease can present acutely and, although typically all spinal movements are grossly restricted by muscle spasm, sometimes some movements are found more restricted than others suggesting a mechanical block to movements, i.e. a disc protrusion. Moreover, diagnosis is complicated by the fact that often in sepsis or malignant disease standard radiographs may show no abnormality for several months. Although the ESR is not invariably raised in these cases, it is most exceptional to find both the ESR and the X-rays normal at the onset of symptoms.

If radiographs reveal diffuse loss of bone density, this should be regarded as a contra-indication to treatment by manipulation or traction. Osteoporosis, defined as the loss of the protein matrix of bone, is common in post-neopausal women but can also be caused by prolonged corticosteroid therapy. In these conditions the serum calcium and alkaline phosphatase levels are normal. Less often, similar radiological changes are produced by osteomalacia due to defective calcium absorption, characterized by a low serum calcium and a raised alkaline phosphatase level. Currently the commonest cause of osteomalacia is steatorrhoea following partial gastrectomy.

Cervical Region

Rheumatoid disease, psoriatic arthritis and Reiter's disease can occasionally present as an acute cervical spondylitis before the disease is manifest elsewhere. Although the more severe forms of acute cervical disc lesion may, at the onset, give rise to gross limitation of spinal movement in all directions, this subsides after a day or so leaving the typical signs of a mechanical block to movement. If pain and severe stiffness last longer, the cause is likely to be either an acute inflammatory spondylitis or carious vertebral disease and in both instances the ESR will probably be elevated. Occasionally patients with long-standing cervical spondylitis, due to rheumatoid arthritis or ankylosing spondylitis, develop severe neck pain radiating to the occiput. This is sometimes the result of subluxation of the odontoid peg of the axis backwards from the anterior arch of the atlas, demonstrated by lateral radiographs in flexion. Since the cervical portion of the spinal cord is in jeopardy in these cases, both traction and manipulation are strongly contra-indicated. Indeed, if symptoms are severe, the upper spinal joints should be stabilized either by a plastic cervical brace or by spinal fusion.

In elderly patients degenerative changes in the apophyseal joints give rise to osteophytic proliferation, which may encroach on the vertebral foramina within which the vertebral artery runs upwards to supply the spinal cord and hind brain. If the lumen of these arteries is already partially obstructed by arteriosclerotic changes, sudden changes of posture may cause transient ischaemia of the brain stem leading to drop attacks or postural vertigo. A history of such episodes is another contra-indication to manipulation or traction. Testing the plantar reflexes for an extensor response which indicates a lesion of the pyramidal tracts should be part of the routine examination of all patients with cervical pain.

Manipulation of the neck is best avoided in juveniles: not only do they find the procedure distressing, but it seems more likely that torticollis in this age group is due to a traumatic arthritis of an intervertebral joint rather than a disc lesion. In children, and also occasionally in adults, acute torticollis can also arise from inflamed deep cervical glands and apical pneumonia.

In the elderly, cranial arteritis can present with painful and limited neck movements caused by inflammation of the occipital arteries. In addition, there is evidence of systemic illness with fever and malaise; the ESR is markedly elevated and the temporal arteries are usually thickened and tender.

Thoracic Region

Ankylosing spondylitis involving the costovertebral joints can give rise to acute episodes of unilateral spinal pain exacerbated by rotation in one direction more than the other, thus simulating a disc protrusion. However, the lumbar region has nearly always been affected already by the disease, so that the patient complains of preceding intermittent low back pain and restriction of movement is noted. The X-ray photographs of the sacro-iliac joints may show sclerosis and the ESR may be elevated.

Lumbo-sacral Region

Here involvement of the sacro-iliac joint, which is a common presenting feature of ankylosing spondylitis and sometimes of Reiter's disease, psoriatic arthritis and Still's disease must be distinguished from a lumbar disc protrusion. The clinical features of sacro-iliitis, described in Chapter 22 are evident at the onset, whereas radiological changes may take some time to develop.

Shoulder

Although an accurate anatomical diagnosis can usually be made (see Chapter 12) the lesion may be the first sign of rheumatic disease. Rheumatoid and psoriatic arthritis can give rise to sub-deltoid bursitis, supraspinatus or infraspinatus tendinitis or an inflammatory capsulitis, simulating a frozen shoulder. Typically a frozen shoulder shows little response to intra-articular hydrocortisone, whereas early mono-articular rheumatoid disease is greatly improved. A frozen shoulder may be associated with disturbance of the neuro-circulatory reflexes in the arm causing osteoporosis and painful swelling of the wrist and hand, termed the shoulder-hand syndrome. Although superficially this condition simulates rheumatoid arthritis, clinical examination reveals trophic changes in the skin of the hands and radiography shows a diffuse osteoporosis without joint erosions. If the hand is allowed to remain inactive, disabling contracture of the joints and flexor tendons may occur during the year or so before spontaneous resolution begins.

Elbow

Resistant or relapsing tennis-elbow may be an early manifestation of gout, and will respond to reduction of the hyperuricaemia by uricosuric drugs.

Wrist and Hand

Extensive proliferation of the synovial membrane at the wrist, carpus and interphalangeal joints, together with granulomatous infiltration of the tendon-sheaths is characteristic of rheumatoid arthritis. The extensor, long abductor and long flexor tendons of the thumb, and occasionally the finger flexors, can develop a simple tenosynovitis due to overuse (p. 331). Lesions affecting other tendons in the region, such as flexor carpi ulnaris, are sometimes early manifestations of rheumatoid disease, and rupture, particularly of the extensor tendons, may result. Compression of the median nerve in the carpal tunnel (p. 333) by rheumatoid granulation tissue is common. The distal interphalangeal joints of digits other than the first are characteristically spared in rheumatoid arthritis, but are frequently affected by osteo-arthritis, psoriatic arthritis and Reiter's disease.

Manubrio-sternal Joint

Inflammation of this joint, which can occur in both ankylosing spondylitis and rheumatoid arthritis, gives rise to a burning deep sternal pain, mimicking pain from the intrathoracic viscera. The joint shows marked local tenderness and the symptoms are relieved by an intra-articular steroid injection.

Hip

Juvenile rheumatoid arthritis often presents as an isolated arthritis of the hip joint. In adults, although involvement of the hip may occur in all the chronic rheumatological disorders, it is rarely the presenting disorder.

Ankle and Foot

No satisfactory explanation has yet been advanced to explain why the ankle joint is so frequently spared while the talo-calcaneal and mid-tarsal joints are so often affected in all forms of chronic inflammatory arthritis. Pain at the back of the heel arising from involvement of the Achilles bursa or erosion of the calcaneum at the insertion of the Achilles tendon can be the first manifestation of rheumatoid arthritis or of Reiter's disease. Plantar fasciitis may result from purely mechanical foot strain, but is also a common presenting symptom in Reiter's disease.

Metatarsalgia can arise from chronic foot deformities, but is also a common early manifestation of rheumatoid arthritis. Episodic arthritis of the first metatarsophalangeal joint, particularly in men, should raise the suspicion of gout. As in the hands, involvement of the terminal interphalangeal joints is suggestive of psoriasis or Reiter's disease.

Local Treatment

The importance of recognizing an underlying disease process and the methods for suppressing this have been outlined. If the local lesion is causing significant symptoms, then local treatment is justified. Non-articular soft tissue lesions will usually respond to accurate infiltration with hydrocortisone. Although the crystalline suspension of hydrocortisone acetate produces more discomfort than the soluble hydrocortisone preparations, the results are more predictable, presumably as the result of slower clearance from the injection site.

In the local treatment of inflamed joints, several principles must be observed. In the acute phase rest is necessary: in the upper limb this can be achieved by a sling or splinting. The weight-bearing joints of the lower limbs can be rested adequately only in bed, but since contractures can develop rapidly during immobilization, these must be prevented by gentle passive movements of the joints by a physiotherapist or a relative who has been suitably instructed. Contractures that have already developed may respond to the application of serial plasters. Muscle wasting can occur rapidly, particularly in the quadriceps, and the patient should be instructed to perform static contractions at regular intervals. Once the acute phase has subsided, reactivation of the patient should begin gradually, but must be modified if a joint flares. If laxity of ligaments or loss of articular cartilage causes instability of a joint, particularly at the knee, permanent splintage may be desirable.

Intra-articular injection of hydrocortisone acetate, in conjunction with the measures outlined, can help to suppress the synovial inflammation.

Massive doses and frequent repetition should be avoided, particularly into unstable joints, since further joint destruction may be caused thus. The injection of smaller volumes of a more concentrated preparation, such as methyl prednisolone acetate, is preferable when small joints are affected. Diseased joints are prone to sepsis; hence it is essential to observe a rigorous aseptic technique. The use of disposable needles and syringes enables injections to be performed safely in domiciliary practice.

DEGENERATIVE JOINT DISEASE

Degenerative changes occur in articular cartilage, joint capsules and ligaments with advancing age or as a result of previous damage by trauma or inflammation. No systemic effect results and the joints do not show any sustained inflammation, although minor trauma may evoke a transitory synovial reaction.

The mechanism of ageing in articular cartilage is not clearly understood. At first localized areas of softening occur and small fissures develop. Gradual erosion of the degenerate cartilage occurs with progressive denundation of the underlying bone and increased friction on movement. The affected joints become stiff, particularly after rest, and secondary capsular contracture occurs, further restricting the range of movement. The juxta-articular bone thickens and may proliferate to form osteophytes. Once the articular cartilage has worn through in some areas, friction at the moving surfaces increases further and is felt as bone-to-bone crepitus. The characteristic radiographic appearances consist of loss of joint space, sclerosis of juxta-articular bone and osteophytic outcrops from the joint margins. Some joints at this stage are the site of continuous discomfort at rest, probably due to increased vascularity of the bone ends or from a secondary low-grade traumatic synovitis.

The nomenclature of degenerative joint disease is still confused, but many authors prefer the use of the term osteoarthrosis to signify that the condition in the joint is not predominantly due to an inflammatory response. Two main patterns of joint involvement are encountered which can be termed primary generalized osteoarthrosis and secondary osteoarthrosis.

Primary Generalized Osteoarthrosis

This syndrome occurs most frequently in women between the fourth and sixth decades. In many subjects, but not all, painful osteophytic nodes appear at the terminal interphalangeal joints (Heberden's nodes) and occasionally at the proximal interphalangeal joints (Bouchard's nodes). A familial tendency to the formation of these nodes is often noted. The hands feel stiff and painful, particularly in the mornings, and this is later followed by aching in other joints particularly the first carpo-metacarpal joints, the shoulders, cervical spine, hips and knees. The patient, who is frequently also undergoing the stresses of the menopause, becomes depressed and fearful that she is developing a crippling disorder. No evidence of a systemic disturbance can be found, the ESR is normal and the SCAT test is negative. Radiographs show only minor degenerative changes, nodes on the fingers and no erosions. Usually the disorder runs a self-limiting course over several years leaving behind only minor restriction of movement, particularly in proximal joints, and nodal proliferation on the fingers. After complete examination the patient can be reassured as to the outcome. For symptomatic treatment mild analgesics suffice, and steroid therapy is never necessary. Elaborate physiotherapy is not justified, indeed local heat may increase the joint discomfort. The patient should modify daily activities to reduce unnecessary strain on affected joints, but gentle use will help to preserve mobility. Dietary restriction may be necessary to avoid a gain in weight.

Secondary Osteoarthrosis

In this condition the degenerative changes occur in a joint which is the site of some previous defect. Taking the hip joint as an example, this defect may be the result of a congenital dysplasia, incongruence of the joint surface as in Perthes' disease, trauma or a previous inflammatory arthritis in the joint. The methods of treatment are described in the chapters devoted to individual joints but the principles will be briefly summarized. In the early stages, joint function can often be improved and pain diminished by stretching out contractures in the joint capsule and redeveloping wasted muscles about the joint by resisted exercises. The patient's daily activities should be modified to diminish unnecessary strain on the affected joints and, when weight-bearing joints are involved, the body-weight should be reduced as much as possible.

If pain at rest is a predominant feature, this may be due to a low-grade traumatic synovitis; if so intra-articular steroid injections may be helpful. These should be used sparingly since too many injections may cause further joint damage. Local steroid injections are contra-indicated in unstable weight-bearing joints.

6

The Diagnosis of Soft Tissue Lesions

The clinical work of the orthopaedic physician consists largely in the diagnosis and treatment of soft tissue lesions. Lesions in the moving parts occur frequently, throughout the body, and at all ages, and the symptoms may mimic a number of visceral or neurological diseases. In purely orthopaedic and neurological cases diagnosis is exact: there is no doubt about the site of a fracture, or the nature of operative intervention, or of the type of a nerve-lesion. It is therefore mainly in the non-surgical conditions affecting the soft tissues, i.e. the fibrosis in moving parts that follows overuse or injury, the various disorders affecting joints, and pressure on the sheath of nerves, nerve-roots and dura mater, that the orthopaedic physician exercises his diagnostic capacity.

One of the two main characteristics of deeply-seated lesions is the discrepancy between the site of the pain and the site of the lesion. Hence the physician must define the source of the identical diffuse pains that may arise from muscle, tendon, joint-capsule, ligament, bursa, dura mater or nerve-root. The other outstanding feature of such pains is the paucity of objective physical signs to which they may give rise; hence diagnosis may rest largely on the correlation of a series of subjective data. This elicitation and interpretation of physical signs requires practice. No effort must be spared to localize exactly the source of each pain, before treatment can usefully begin. For example massage, unless applied to the exact site of a lesion, can do no good. No less accuracy is essential when local injections are employed, since the solution must be introduced at some definite spot. Likewise, when manipulative measures are contemplated, the site and type of the lesion determine whether they are indicated and what form they shall take. If pain arises in a moving part, some movement or some posture must bring it on. This complex is explored and interpreted in the same way as a simultaneous equation.

This chapter describes the principles of a system of diagnosis that reveals the origin of a pain in a high proportion of cases no matter where the symptoms happen to be perceived. Since pain in lesions of the moving parts is brought on largely by tension, diagnosis depends on applying tension in different ways to different tissues and asking the patient to report the result. (Anoxia and local pressure are the other ways of eliciting or aggravating these pains.) The approach is purely mechanical and leads to full anatomical—though not always pathological—definition of the site of a painful lesion. A complex of painful movements is logically resolved into a number of simple components, each of which is then tested separately. Importance is laid equally on what movements prove painful and/or limited and what movements are of full range and/or painless. This is an approach almost mathematical in its precision and is suited to the mechanical function of the structures under examination.

The patient's co-operation is essential. He is asked to state which activities hurt and which do not, disregarding where the pain is felt and what sort of pain it is. This makes diagnosis more difficult when there is pain in the absence of movement; it is hard for a patient to tell what movement hurts him when he is already in constant pain. In such cases he is apt, unless the nature of the question is explained carefully, to state that all movements hurt when he merely means that the constant pain continues unabated; he must realize that the examiner is looking for movements that *alter* the symptoms. To get a patient to perform a series of movements at several joints, to say which bring on or increase the pain and which do not, and to let the responses build up a pattern; to perform special tests for certain structures; to search for tenderness of the structure identified; if it is accessible, to induce local anaesthesia at the chosen spot and to await the patient's verdict—all this takes time and patience.

Positive signs must always be balanced by corroborative negative signs. If a lesion appears to lie at, or near one joint, this region must be examined for signs identifying its site. It is equally essential for the adjacent joints and the structures about them to be examined so that, by contrast, their normality can be established. These negative findings then reinforce the positive findings emanating elsewhere; then only can the diagnosis be regarded as established.

At any examination of which the patient's co-operation forms part, the opportunities for deception are many. Since in many cases the only final criterion of a correct diagnosis is the induction of local anaesthesia—the response to which is often also a subjective phenomenon—the physician should be on his guard against feigned illness; for patients have learned that the symptoms least capable of objective evaluation are those with which the orthopaedic physician most often deals. Thus, while it is no substitute for a diagnosis to regard all patients with obscure pains as having a minor or neurotic disability, a balance must be maintained between credulity and excessive scepticism.

The *Correct* Pain

It is often not enough to discover that a certain movement evokes pain; care must be taken to make sure that it reproduces the very pain of which the patient complains. For example, a patient with slight backache and a pain in his thigh, or some scapular discomfort and pain in his upper limb, may well have a minor spinal disc lesion responsible for the ache in his trunk but severe arthritis in the hip or shoulder joint causing his important symptoms. In this type of case, the spinal movements do cause some local discomfort, i.e. they set up *a* pain, but inquiry will reveal that it is not the patient's pain. When the hip or shoulder is examined, the movements elicit the symptoms that the patient recognizes, i.e. *the* pain.

When pain in separate areas is evoked in this way, the situation must be clarified by giving greater weight to the movement provoking the recognized symptom. This must appear obvious, but the point is made since lay-manipulators take the opposite view. Osteopaths, ever anxious to inculpate the spine as the source of any symptom, regard discomfort on a spinal movement, or even painless limitation of movement at an intervertebral joint, as a good reason for insisting that the distant pain originates from the spine which, by corollary, requires manipulation. Consequently many patients, especially those with arthritis at shoulder or hip, receive endless osteopathy to the unaffected spinal joints, without avail.

OBJECTS OF DIAGNOSTIC MOVEMENTS

Diagnosis in soft tissue lesions must be approached indirectly. No physician would regard palpation of the chest as the chief method of diagnosis in heart disease; even less would he regard an area of intercostal tenderness as indicating which viscus was affected. Palpation of the spine plays little part in assessing the integrity of the spinal cord. Function is tested by remote signs: e.g. feeling the pulse, ascertaining the blood pressure, noting the plantar response, testing urine and so on. For the same reason, immediate palpation of a painful area must be avoided in locomotor disorders. The state of a joint, muscle or nerve is assessed by discovering how well it functions; palpation may or may not follow, and is confined to the tissue identified as at fault, and then only if it lies within reach of the finger.

The object of the diagnostic movements described here is to discover where, i.e. about or at which joint, the symptoms arise. This is not as easy as might be expected; indeed, to tell whether a pain in the buttock has a lumbar, a sacro-iliac or a gluteal origin can prove extremely difficult.

This object is best achieved by carrying out a swift review from end to end of the tissues forming the relevant segment. For example, a patient with obscure pain in the arm should receive a preliminary gross examination from neck to fingers in an endeavour to ascertain roughly the relevant area. This part is then examined in detail, in the sure knowledge that the lesion lies within known limits.

Contractile and Inert

This is a vital distinction. When a voluntary movement is performed, the joint moves and the muscles move it; both are involved. Hence, if an active movement hurts, either tissue may be involved. Lesions, therefore, in these two types of tissue must be separated on the lines of a simultaneous equation in mathematics.

Contractile

By 'contractile' is meant those structures that form part of a muscle— namely the belly itself, the tendon, and their bony insertions. From such structures pain may be elicited both by active contraction and by passive stretching in the opposite direction. But neither of these tests applies much tension to a muscle and both may prove misleadingly negative. The real test for a muscle is contraction against resistance, whereby strong tension is applied to the lesion.

It can be argued academically that neither a tendon nor the bone adjacent to a muscular insertion is a contractile structure; this is true. But in so far as they are attached to the belly of a muscle, they remain contractile clinically, in the sense that contraction of the muscle belly applies tension to them, thus evoking pain. Pain on resisted contraction is caused also when (1) a fracture lies close enough to a muscular insertion for the strain to move the broken ends on each other; (2) when an inflamed lymphatic gland, bursa or abscess lies directly under a muscle.

If the movements show the lesion to lie in a contractile structure, auxiliary tests exist that disclose which one of several possible muscles or tendons is involved, sometimes even which part of it.

Inert or Non-contractile

This term describes those tissues that possess no inherent capacity to contract or relax. The agency for movement lies outside themselves. Joint capsule and ligaments allow movement to reach a certain point and then stop it. Many bursae supply synovial surfaces facilitating movement of one tissue on another. The dura mater and nerve-roots scarcely move at all. From inert tissues pain can be provoked only by stretching. Confusion arises from the fact that a patient can use his own muscles to stretch an inert tissue painfully, e.g. in arthritis at the shoulder active elevation of the arm hurts when the extreme of the possible range is reached, not because of any fault in the elevator muscles, but because the joint capsule is stretched. Hence pain produced at the extreme of an active movement must not be thought to arise from a contractile tissue. It is only when the stretching is carried out for the patient, i.e. passively, that it has diagnostic significance, since the response to active movement is ambiguous. For this reason active movements are best used in the rough preliminary examination that outlines the region at fault and best avoided in the subsequent detailed examination. For the orthopaedic physician the inert tissues are: joint capsule, ligament, bursa, fascia, dura mater and nerve-root.

If the movements show the lesion to lie in an inert structure, it must be decided whether all the structures limiting movement at a joint are involved (i.e. a diffuse capsular lesion), or only a small part of them (e.g. a ligament), or whether an intra-articular block exists (e.g. a displaced part of the meniscus at the knee). If a single inert structure is at fault, its position, whether articular or extra-articular, requires definition.

Finally, correlation of the symptoms and signs determines the stage that the lesion has reached. In some conditions, e.g. internal derangement of a joint or a minor muscular rupture, treatment is the same whether the condition is acute, subacute, or chronic, whereas at other sites treatment on very different lines is required (e.g. arthritis or ligamentous strain).

HISTORY

Since the orthopaedic physician deals with largely subjective disorders, the patient's account of his symptoms is of great importance. So is his manner of recounting his story. In general, straightforward patients, asked to give a chronological report on their symptoms, do so, and are visibly pleased to talk to an interested physician. They do not digress much and can easily be brought back to the point. Patients with unfounded pains are not sure how their symptoms should have behaved and resent being asked for their exact site, manner of reference and of aggravation. They offer a garbled story with internal contradictions and become restive during questions about the symptom responsible for the disablement described.

Objects of Listening

Every patient contains a truth. He will proffer the data on which diagnosis rests. The doctor must adopt a conscious humility, not towards the patient, but towards the truth concealed within the patient, if his interpretations are regularly to prove correct.

1. To find out what the symptoms are, in what chronological order they appeared and how long they have continued, and to compare the patient's account with the examiner's mental map of the dermatomes and his knowledge of the likelihoods. It is well to realize that many patients have given no thought to what their symptoms are before they are actually seated in front of the doctor. Leading questions must be avoided, and all questions must be neutral; e.g. 'What happened after that?' 'Does anything bring the pain on?' Time for reflection and recollection must be given and allowance made for those who do not possess a vocabulary which includes descriptive terms for various sensations or even accurate names for different parts of the body.

2. To discard the irrelevant, and to pursue in detail the pertinent parts of the patient's story, in particular relating to such activity, posture or function as evokes or increases pain. What eases the pain is seldom helpful diagnostically.

3. To piece the symptoms together (some sequences are quite characteristic) and roughly localize the lesion. Such a tentative diagnosis enables relevant questions to be asked in as neutral a way as possible on points that the patient has omitted. Some questions have diagnostic importance; others help to determine treatment or management.

4. To discover the past behaviour of a lesion. For example, whether a fragment of disc is stable or unstable, whether an arthritic shoulder is getting better or worse can be discovered only by listening to the history. Prognosis and treatment may depend almost entirely on the assessment afforded by the progress of symptoms. Is the disorder recurrent; if so, what provokes an attack?

5. To find out what sort of patient sits before the examiner, what is his reaction to pain and how his disorder affects his life and work. Do disablement and symptoms tally? His account of his symptoms suggests the diagnosis, but the patient's digressions and reactions often indicate what sort of person he is.

6. To find out what treatment he has already had, and its results.

7. To decide what sort of examination to conduct and to note pointers suggesting that considerable care or reserve should be exercised.

The history is at its most informative in disorders of the knee and spinal joints, which can be examined only with a clear idea of how the symptoms arose. With the shoulder, by contrast, the history matters little; it is the examination that counts. *The best approach is chronological*, the patient being asked about the events leading up to the onset of the symptoms, what they were then, and then to recount week by week, or year by year, what has happened since.

Findings Based on History

The patient's age is important, for many diseases affect only certain age groups. Consider hip-trouble in childhood, adolescence, early adult life or old age—entirely different diagnoses suggest themselves. Sex is not very relevant in locomotor disorders since both sexes have much the same moving parts; but it may make considerable difference to treatment and management. Occupation has considerable bearing on diagnosis and prevention in industrial hazards, but in orthopaedic medicine it governs chiefly management.

In cases of trauma, the patient should be asked for a description detailed enough to enable the examiner to picture his posture at the moment of the accident and thus to deduce the direction of the strains operating on the injured parts. The events immediately following the accident must be ascertained, especially in patients claiming compensation. The presence of swelling and bruising is considered; blood fills a joint in a few minutes, clear fluid takes hours. The events of that and the succeeding days help to afford ground for giving or withholding credence to the story. Tendinous disorders often follow overuse; hence the activities of the previous few days, or the duration and nature of the work done become relevant.

Recurrence is to be expected in internal derangement, whether caused by a torn meniscus, a damaged disc or a loose body. Since cartilage is avascular, a crack in it cannot unite, and, if it has shifted once, the fragment can shift again. Recurrence is characteristic also of rheumatoid arthritis, gout and ankylosing spondylitis. If internal derangement is suspected, the question of locking, unlocking, twinges and giving-way arises. In what position the joint locks is material, and whether or not it unlocks suddenly. In dislocation of part of the meniscus at the knee, and in lumbago, the joint is locked in flexion. Sudden twinges, often associated with giving way of the lower limb, occur when a loose body subluxates momentarily—i.e. out-in. Painful twinges occur in three disorders:

1. A loose body in a joint. There are then articular signs on examination.

2. A tendinous lesion. The patient describes attacks of painful momentary loss of power in the part, so that he drops what he is holding or lifting.

This is quite common in tennis-elbow, less so in tendinitis at the shoulder. In either case the appropriate resisted movement hurts.

3. Neurological twinges. The lightning pains of tabes, the stabbing pains of post-herpetic neuralgia or trigeminal tic provide familiar examples.

A history of trouble arising for no apparent reason is just as important, since it suggests lesions such as gout or rheumatoid arthritis in which trauma plays no part. It is well to realize that many, if not most, disc lesions come on without an obvious causative strain preceding the moment that the symptom appeared.

The length of time that a symptom has been present has diagnostic significance. A constant pain of some years' standing cannot be caused by cancer or tuberculosis, which must in the end make its presence clear. Where the pain is first felt is often close to the lesion; but there are marked exceptions, such as pins and needles (which are felt distally wherever the nerve is compressed) and in disc lesions with primary postero-lateral evolution (the pain starting distally in a limb and possibly never reaching the trunk).

There are important differences in significance between (a) reference of pain; (b) shifting pain; (c) expanding pain. (a) Reference of pain increases in extent as the lesion, though static in position, becomes more severe, and recedes as the trouble abates. Such reference (except in pressure on the dura mater) outlines the dermatome affected and shows in which segment the symptom originates. Hence an important question is always 'Where was the pain originally and where has it spread since?' For example, in minor arthritis at the shoulder or hip, the pain is felt chiefly at upper arm or groin. Should the arthritis become severe, spread to the wrist or ankle is to be expected. (b) Shifting pain results from a shifting lesion. For example, a renal calculus passing down the ureter gives rise to pain felt first in the loin, then in the iliac fossa, finally in the genitals; as the lesion moves, the pain moves. If a patient states that when his sciatica came on, his central backache went away, he describes a lesion projecting centrally that has now moved to one side. Being of constant size, it had to stop pressing centrally when it moved laterally, and the pain followed suit. This account is typical of a disc-protrusion altering its position within a central cavity, i.e. the intervertebral joint. (c) If, on the other hand, he states that, as his backache got worse, it spread down one and later both lower limbs, he is describing the result of an expanding lesion, e.g. neoplasm.

The relation to rest, posture, activity and exertion provides much information. In difficult cases, especially suspected thoracic disc lesions of primary postero-lateral development (when the pain may remain strictly confined to the anterior trunk for years), it is best also to approach the problem from the other side and inquire into the effect of visceral function on the pain. The rhythmic increase and subsidence of colic, unrelated to any bodily movement, or even making the patient writhe, is characteristic, for trunk pain of spinal origin makes the patient lie still. The effect of eating, hunger and defaecation (which may hurt also in a lumbar disc lesion or in coccygodynia) should be noted, together with any symptoms suggesting a disorder of the urinary tract, or, in women, of the pelvic organs. The fact that a patient declares her backache to be more severe at the time of menstruation does not prove that her pain springs from the uterus, since, uterine referred pain may merely superimpose itself indistinguishably on a backache arising from the back. Backache at period times *only* is a different matter. Pain in the trunk on coughing suggests an intraspinal lesion but occurs also in pleurisy. If pain in a limb is induced by breathing or coughing, the lesion almost certainly lies in contact with the dura mater, but a momentary rise in intra-abdominal pressure also distracts the sacro-iliac joints. Alleviation of pain during rest is not often significant, but if a certain posture or activity brings it on or increases it, it is highly probable that a lesion of the moving parts is present. (The main exceptions are angina and intermittent claudication.) The nature of the aggravating activity may indicate where to look for the source. Pain at rest may contra-indicate active treatment when a joint is at fault.

Whether the symptoms are unilateral or bilateral is sometimes significant. Patients may of course develop osteoarthritis in both hips and the thoracic outlet syndrome is usually bilateral; however, bilateral symptoms point to central origin. Central symptoms do not arise from a unilateral structure—an axiom that is often disregarded. The pain in patients with central backache is so often ascribed to a torn lumbar muscle, sacro-iliac strain or lateral facet syndrome that clearly this discrepancy is ignored by those who wish to make a favourite diagnosis.

There is also the question of pins and needles (dealt with in Chapter 4). The most important points are: what brings them on and which part of the skin they occupy—(1) the known cutaneous area of a small nerve; (2) the skin supplied by a nerve-trunk; (3) the distal part of a dermatome; (4) extra-segmental distribution. In this way the distinction between a peripheral lesion, affection of a nerve-trunk, pressure on a nerve-root or on the spinal cord can be made. Vague tingling is also caused by circulatory disturbance, but if this is so the distal part of the limb changes colour.

In joint lesions, inquiry should always be made for involvement, past or present, of other joints. This may bring to light information helpful in arriving at a diagnosis of rheumatoid, spondylitic, gouty or Reiter's arthritis. In gout, the family history may be suggestive.

In spinal nerve-root pressure the pain may be constant day and night and is sometimes unrelated to exertion; such movements of the limb as do not stretch the affected root are apt if anything to relieve the symptoms for a short time. Heat diminishes most pains but often aggravates that caused by root-pressure or intermittent claudication.

Another virtue of a full history is the warning that it gives to the examiner about when to be careful. Patients with common disorders give an account of their vicissitudes with little variation. The physician recognizes the familiar story, and confirms the diagnosis by examination; but he cannot, especially in an out-patient clinic, always investigate every system in the body. A history noted to differ markedly from the typical arrests the listener's attention and puts him on his guard—partly against psychoneurosis or feigned illness, partly against disorders with which orthopaedic medicine does not deal, and partly against a condition, properly sent to his department, with which the physician is so far unfamiliar.

INSPECTION

This reveals the attitude in which the part is held; some positions are in themselves characteristic, e.g. the hand supporting the other elbow in fracture of the clavicle. Bony deformity, e.g. genu varum and abnormal postures such as torticollis or scoliosis or a short leg, become evident. The presence of general or local swelling, of muscular wasting and of changes in colour of the skin are noted. Colour changes can be induced by dependence or elevation in claudication and post-traumatic osteoporosis.

Inspection also discloses the type of gait, at times a most important finding especially in internal derangement at the knee, arthritis at the hip, spastic diseases and hysteria.

Inspection of the patient's facies may help to decide how severe his pain has been; severe pain leading to sleepless nights shows on the patient's face. The well-covered individual who, with a bland countenance, describes months of intolerable symptoms is quickly identified.

PALPATION

The Joint is Stationary

The dorsum of the examiner's hand detects variations in temperature better than the palm. Localized warmth should be sought, and care taken that the recent removal of a bandage or the application of a rubefacient ointment does not deceive. The detection of heat means that, whatever the lesion, it is in the active stage. Heat is present, therefore, after an operation on a joint, during the stage of active healing of the divided tissues. Heat unaffected by rest is present after a ligamentous sprain, or over a broken bone, if it lies superficially, so long as active healing continues. If adhesions exist, or an impacted loose body lies displaced in a joint subjected to weight-bearing, heat ensues which is quickly abolished by rest. Haemarthrosis is always accompanied by heat, and, if the joint is tense with blood, gross limitation of movement. In all these conditions, there is no synovial thickening. In active Reiter's, gouty, rheumatoid, septic or spondylitic arthritis, heat is present in conjunction with synovial thickening. A superficial malignant deposit eroding bone (e.g. a rib) may feel warm. Sympathectomy produces a warm foot and arterial thrombosis a cold one.

Palpation reveals the size, behaviour and consistency of any swelling and whether there is fluctuation. Bony enlargement results from callus, osteitis deformans or neoplasm. Oedema may pit. Loose bodies may be made to move about inside a joint cavity or a tendon-sheath. Localized swelling of a tendon, osteophytes, a thickened bursa, a cyst, a haematoma or a ganglion are all readily felt. A gap at the point of rupture in a muscle or tendon may be palpable, as is the hard swelling of a muscle belly suffused with blood. Palpation discloses the presence or absence of pulsation in an artery; the extremity of the limb may feel cold to the touch. Any lesion of the lower limb causing muscle weakness in the leg (e.g. sciatica with a root palsy) may make the foot cold. In iliac thrombosis the foot becomes colder than its fellow after exertion only; hence there is often no difference if the patient is examined in bed.

The Joint is Moved

Crepitus indicates the state of the gliding surfaces. Fine crepitus at a joint indicates minor roughening of the joint surfaces; coarse crepitus indicates considerable superficial fragmentation of cartilage; the intermittent creaking of bone against bone shows articular cartilage to have been wholly eroded. Teno-synovitis due to overuse may give rise to fine crepitus as the inflamed tendon moves within its close-fitting sheath. In rheumatoid or tuberculous teno-synovitis the crepitus is much coarser. A fracture may crepitate.

A click may be felt as one bone moves suddenly against another. A partly-detached intra-articular body may also click to and fro on movement.

Palpation of Joint Mobility

At the spinal joints, each may be moved in turn passively, in order to discover at what level the symptoms are best reproduced. A series of extension pressures may demonstrate, for example, that greater discomfort is evoked at the fourth than at the third and fifth lumbar levels. Another approach is to ascertain lack of mobility at a spinal joint. This is difficult to be sure of, and in any case there is no certainty that a joint found hypermobile is not the source of symptoms rather than the joint found too stiff. At the spine feeling for muscle guarding is not very satisfactory either, since this always extends over several joints. For example, in tuberculosis or neoplasm in one lumbar vertebra, gross limitation of movement is visible and palpable at every lumbar joint. Again, in the radiograph of a fourth lumbar disc lesion causing marked lateral deviation (Plate 4), the reader can see that the correcting deviation in the opposite direction starts only at thoracic levels.

Finally, there is the osteopathic and chiropractic claim that palpation can detect one vertebra to be tilted or rotated on its fellow or on the sacrum. This contention I do not regard as valid; and the experiments of Schiotz (personal communication, 1967) showed that when this was carried out by two separate individuals on the same series of cases, their alleged deviations did not tally at all.

DIAGNOSIS BY SELECTIVE TENSION

Five different aspects of this examination have to be considered, though not all are necessarily relevant to any one case.

1. The Active Range of Movement

Active movements indicate a combination of three things—namely, the patient's ability and willingness to perform the movements requested, the range of movement possible and muscular power. Their chief value is to indicate quickly the region whence symptoms originate, and which set of tissues to test in detail. They must be carried out first and then compared with the findings on passive and resisted movements. Since passive range and muscle-power are assessed separately later, a strong contrast between what the affected part can in fact perform and what the patient is prepared to do shows will-power to be defective, involuntarily (neurosis) or voluntarily (malingering). The way a patient moves informs the examiner how gently to conduct his subsequent examination.

The active range may be normal, limited or excessive. If limited, it may be limited in every direction, in some directions but not in others, or in one direction only. If in only one direction, the limitation may be of the proportionate or disproportionate type (see below).

2. The Passive Range of Movement

The passive range of movement indicates the state of the inert tissues. The patient relaxes his muscles while the range of movement in each direction is ascertained; thus the effect of conscious control and muscular effort are eliminated. The patient states whether or not pain is provoked. In cases of doubt the examiner may have to push fairly hard to arrive at a true assessment. Five degrees of limitation of movement carries a quite different significance from full-range with pain and the exact situation *must* be ascertained. Moreover, it may take some persuasion to get beyond a painful arc and to find out that at full range the pain has ceased. Again, the beginning of pain may not correspond with the extreme of range; for example, straight leg-raising may start to hurt at 45 degrees but continue to 90 degrees without increased discomfort. The examiner must note what the resistance is like at the extreme of range—i.e. the end-feel—and if the appearance of pain and the extreme of range are reached together or separately.

Each primary movement of the joint must be tested passively, so as to allow emergence of a pattern, i.e. the relation between the degree of movement obtainable in one and in the other directions. This distinguishes capsular from non-capsular limitation of movement. Any discrepancy between the range of movement obtained actively and passively should be noted. Often accessory movements exist that test single inert structures one at a time.

3. Resisted Movements

These provide clear information on the state of each muscle group about a joint. The patient contracts his muscles forcibly against resistance strong enough to prevent all articular movement while the joint is held somewhere near mid-range, so that all the inert structures are equally relaxed. No movement takes place at the joint; the only tension that alters is within the muscle. A resisted movement may provoke pain, or demonstrate weakness, occasionally both.

The examiner should pay considerable attention to where he stands and how to apply his hands. When strong muscles are tested, minor weakness cannot be detected unless his hands are well placed for resistance and counter-pressure, and his body is properly poised.

E

4. A Painful Arc

This means pain felt at the central part of a range of movement, disappearing as this point is passed in either direction. It may or may not reappear at the extreme of range; so long as pain ceases on each side of the arc, it is significant. A painful arc implies that a tender structure is pinched between two bony surfaces.

5. Abnormal Sensations

These should be studied both when the joint is stationary and when it is moved (see above).

Commentary

The information gained by studying the nature, degree and direction of the movements which cause pain or are weak is the basis of diagnosis in soft tissue lesions. The further discovery that many other movements are painless and strong provides the negative half that emphasises the positive findings. Usually this information is obtainable in no other way; for it may relate to structures inaccessible to the finger and translucent to X-rays, or to places where every structure is sensitive to deep pressure in the normal individual, or to areas too small for differential palpation. *Omission of part of this examination, because the diagnosis seems obvious or to save time, is the common source of error.*

Experience in performing diagnostic movements is required so that the examiner may adopt a routine for each joint. He must be careful to use pure movements that test only one tissue at a time, and pay attention to where he places his hand on the patient's limb, to ensure that he is testing only that particular muscle. For example, if lateral rotation at the shoulder is tested by resistance applied at the dorsum of the patient's hand, instead of at the lowest forearm, resisted extension at the wrist is unwittingly included in the diagnostic movement. Hence, the infraspinatus muscle may receive treatment in a case of tennis-elbow. The physician must therefore consider the purity of each diagnostic movement that he uses. Even so, there exist common, but avoidable, misinterpretations, to be mentioned later. Unless all the relevant movements are tried, and the responses noted and correlated, an uncommon condition that happens to give rise to common symptoms may be overlooked. Unless a great number of movements is tested, there is not enough data to enable him to assess the patient's sincerity, since the examiner is largely dependent on the discovery of an incongruous pattern and on inconsistencies in the patient's replies to recognize gross exaggeration or pain devoid of organic basis.

Errors in localization are easy enough to make in soft tissue lesions examined under the best conditions; in hospital practice, where patients may be slow to grasp what is wanted of them or inexplicit in their answers, the temptation to shirk some part of the examination may be great and must be resisted. The patient must not be flustered; for time is lost, not gained, by hurry and an unsympathetic manner. In this field diagnosis depends largely on correlating the history (a subjective statement) with the responses to a series of movements (again subjective). Unless the patient realizes what is required of him, there is little hope of reaching a correct diagnosis in other than simple cases.

The least reliable way to diagnose in soft tissue lesions is to palpate immediately for tenderness in the area outlined by the patient. Though this may give occasional success, it is most unsatisfactory, partly on account of misleading referred tenderness, partly because the region outlined by the patient does not necessarily contain the lesion, partly because many spots are normally tender, partly because many lesions lie beyond fingers' reach and therefore no relevant tenderness can exist, and partly because successful deception by allegations of feigned symptoms then becomes inevitable. Hence, it must again be emphasized that indirect examination by assessing function is the most important element in localizing a soft tissue lesion.

The orthopaedic physician must be ready to examine patients repeatedly. If diagnosis is uncertain he can seldom hope for appreciable assistance from a colleague or from ancillary methods such as radiography, blood tests, etc. If an apprently relievable lesion fails to improve, either the diagnosis is wrong or treatment has been imperfectly given. If this is given by the physiotherapist, it is my practice to ask her if she has any reason to offer for the lack of progress and whether she agrees with the diagnosis. If this remains in doubt, local anaesthesia is induced in her presence to settle the matter, and we await the result together. If I have ordered manipulation and, though it has failed so far, it still looks as if it ought to succeed, I carry out the manipulation myself. If I succeed, it provides the physiotherapist with a spur to do better; if I fail, it shows that was my judgement that was at fault, not her technique.

SIGNIFICANCE OF DIAGNOSTIC MOVEMENTS

1. *Active and Passive Movements are each Painful in the same direction, and the Pain appears as the limit of Pain is approached. The Resisted Movements do not hurt. An Inert Structure is at fault.*

Diffuse Capsular Lesion

If all the passive movements are painful at their extremes—even more, if the range of movement is limited—the whole inert cuff about the joint is shown to be involved. The clinical picture is arthritis, and the cause of the signs is diffuse capsular irritation in the early stage and actual contracture later on. Arthritis, capsulitis and synovitis all possess identical meanings: that the entire joint is affected. Periarthritis is a misnomer; for it can logically be used only when a tissue (unnamed) in the vicinity of, but not forming part of, the joint is involved. Since all the periarticular structures have names, the word is meaningless and a label stating which periarticular structure is at fault should be substituted. In fact, periarthritis is usually used when arthritis is present, but the radiograph reveals no bony abnormality, because it is wrongly supposed that such evidence of normality precludes arthritis. Periarthritis, synovitis and capsulitis are all terms best abandoned and arthritis maintained alone. The meaning of 'arthritis' is clear; an affection of the whole joint. In early arthritis the whole synovial membrane and capsule of the joint at first resents stretching; later on the capsule shortens. Hence nearly every movement, since it stretches some part of the capsule, hurts towards its extreme and, in all but the slightest cases, is limited in range. In recent arthritis, muscle spasm protects the irritated synovial membrane; in subacute arthritis the limitation results from muscular spasm coming into play to protect the capsule from being stretched; in osteoarthritis it is the capsular contracture itself, hardly guarded by muscular spasm, that restricts range; in advanced disorganization of the joint, the bony outcrops engage. Clearly, the day after an injury leading to gross limitation of joint movement, no capsular contracture exists as yet; the limitation of movement is wholly due to muscle spasm, protecting the synovial membrane; it can be felt to spring into action on gentle forcing. Capsular contracture has a different end-feel. Purists may argue that all limitation of movement at a joint results from muscular spasm. This is not so clinically; indeed the difference is not only clear but carries diagnostic and therapeutic significance. When abrupt muscle spasm limits movement, stretching is contra-indicated, whereas capsular contracture, with its softer stop resembling leather being stretched, invites forced movement in treatment. Whatever the cause of the arthritis, and whether it is acute or chronic makes no difference to the capsular pattern, only to the end-feel. That limitation of movement at the cervical joints is not caused by muscle spasm was proved by Lewit (1967), who examined ten patients' necks before an operation at which complete muscle relaxion was induced by one of the curare group of drugs. During full muscle-relaxation, he re-examined their necks and detected no change in the range of movement. There is thus a series of disorders in which articular contracture is the limiting factor, muscle spasm playing no part; and another in which muscle spasm is the active agent. This fits in very well with the different end-feels that are clinically detectable.

Arthritis, i.e. capsular irritation or contracture, is often spoken of as always causing 'limitation of movement in every direction'. Indeed, this remains the universal belief today, and is standard teaching; but this orthodoxy is not always justified (see Chapter 1).

Arthritis is present when limitation of movement in the capsular pattern (see below) for that joint is revealed by clinical examination, and can perfectly well co-exist with a full range of movement in one direction. For example, severe arthritis at the hip is compatible with a full lateral rotation. At the talo-calcanean joint, only the varus range is restricted, the joint eventually fixing in full valgus. Not very severe arthritis at the elbow and knee is accompanied by a full and painless range of rotation. Whether the examiner stretches the patient's capsule or the patient repeats this movement by using his own muscles, the degree of stretching, and therefore the amount of pain produced, are the same.

End-feel

When the examiner tests passive movement at a joint, different sensations are imparted to his hand at the extreme of the possible range. They possess great diagnostic importance.

Bone-to-bone

This is the abrupt halt to the movement when two hard surfaces meet, e.g. at the extreme of passive extension of the normal elbow. Bone felt to engage against bone in this way is not only diagnostic but affords an important pointer in manipulation; for, once this sensation has emerged, further forcing in that direction is clearly vain.

Spasm

Muscle spasm coming actively into play with a vibrant twang indicates acute or subacute arthritis. It can be felt particularly clearly when movement at the wrist is tested in recent carpal fracture or when secondary deposits have invaded a cervical vertebra. Spasm of this order leads to the 'hard' end-feel that accompanies a severe and active lesion and is a strong contra-indication to manipulation.

Capsular Feel

This consists of a hardish arrest of movement, with some give in it, as if two pieces of tough rubber were being squeezed together or a piece of thick leather were being stretched. It is the way the normal shoulder or hip stops at the extreme of each rotation. This feeling, appearing before normal full range is reached, suggests non-acute (not necessarily minor) arthritis. The arthritis may have been 'chronic' from the onset (if the reader will forgive the word being used in this way), or have become so after a more severe stage.

Springy Block

When an intra-articular displacement exists, a rebound is seen and felt at the extreme of the possible range. This is most obvious at the knee when the torn part of the meniscus engages between the bone ends, blocking extension. A springy block indicates internal derangement.

Tissue Approximation

This is the normal sensation imparted at full passive flexion of a normal elbow or knee. The joint cannot be pushed farther because of engagement against another part of the body, but would clearly move farther as far as the joint itself is concerned. The range of movement is full and no pain is provoked at the extreme.

Empty Feel

If movement causes considerable pain before the extreme of range is reached, and yet the sensation imparted to the examiner's hand is 'empty', i.e. lacking in organic resistance with the patient nevertheless begging the examiner to desist even though he can feel that further movement is in fact possible, important disease is present. Acute bursitis, extra-articular abscess, or neoplasm should be strongly suspected.

This sensation is also imparted to the examiner's hand when the restriction of range is caused by hysteria or neurogenic hypertonus. In such cases there is initial strong resistance to movement, which yields to sustained pressure, disclosing a full range of movement at the joint. In organic disease of a joint the farther the movement is pushed, the greater the resistance, and, of course, full range is unobtainable.

Sequence of Pain and Limitation

Another important point emerges when a passive movement approaches the extreme of the possible range—whether the pain and the resistance to movement come on together or not. The experienced physiotherapist faced with stretching a painful tissue is guided—often unconsciously—by what she feels the joint will accept.

Pain before Resistance

The pain comes on well before the extreme of possible range has been reached. This suggests an active lesion or extra-articular limitation of movement, each unsuitable for stretching.

Pain Synchronous with Resistance

Capsular feel: gentle stretching can be cautiously attempted. Hard feel: postpone stretching a little longer.

Resistance before Pain

The resistance that signals the approach of the extreme of range is felt, but little pain is elicited at this point. Greater pressure moves the joint a little farther, and discomfort begins. This sequence suggests that quite strong stretching will be well tolerated and is particularly noticeable at those lesions of the shoulder and hip joints that benefit from stretching out.

The Capsular Pattern

The capsule of a joint is lined by synovial membrane. In a lesion of either of these structures, limitation of movement of characteristic proportions results. It does not matter if the irritation in synovial only, as in a recent sprain or haemarthrosis, capsular only as in osteoarthritis, or both, as in rheumatoid arthritis; the same pattern results. This varies from joint to joint, but scarcely at all in different patients; in other words, all shoulders, say, are alike, but the pattern of restriction at the shoulder is not the same as that at the hip. At every joint, the proportion that the limitation of movement in one direction bears to that in other directions conforms to a standard which indicates whether arthritis is present or not. To arrive at a diagnosis of arthritis it is not essential—it is merely usual—for movement to be limited in every direction. For example, at the shoulder lateral rotation is the movement most restricted, and in early arthritis it may prove the only movement to be limited. Again, in advanced arthritis, the hip joint may fix in full lateral rotation. Should movement prove limited in quite other than the capsular proportions, one of the disorders other than arthritis capable of causing limited movement has to be considered. *For the concept of arthritis as characterized by limitation of movement in every direction must be substituted the concept of limitation conforming with the capsular pattern for that particular joint.* The presence of the capsular pattern does not indicate what type of arthritis is present; for the pattern is the same whatever the cause of the arthritis. Troisier's (1957) accurate goniometric measurements have shown that the capsular proportions of limitation of movement are precisely the same whether arthritis at the shoulder is post-traumatic, freezing or rheumatoid. This further differentiation rests on extraneous factors: e.g. a history of trauma, the discovery of a raised uric acid level, or of arthritis elsewhere. The reason for the capsular pattern appears merely to be that separate aspects of synovial membrane and joint capsule, when in an irritated state, resent stretching in different degree.

Limited movement in arthritis is maintained in three ways:

(1) *In the early case,* synovial irritation exists without capsular contracture and it is then muscle spasm, springing into play to prevent synovial stretching beyond a certain point, that protects the joint. This is an involuntary reaction, and it always appears at exactly the same degree of stretching. It is destroyed by local anaesthesia applied to the lesion, or general anaesthesia, or by the curare group of drugs. It is a purely secondary phenomenon, and contrary to general belief the muscle spasm that protects a joint is entirely painless. (We all know the widespread belief that muscle spasm causes the pain in lumbago, and the huge sale of drugs alleged to relieve muscle spasm that results from this misconception.) In fact, the muscle involuntarily contracting at a certain point in the range of the attempted movement causes no more pain than if a patient with a normal joint chose to prevent that movement by voluntary muscle action. It is not the protective spasm that hurts in arthritis, but the synoviocapsular stretch. No one supposes that in appendicitis the symptoms are due to the resultant spasm of the abdominal muscles; this is recognized as merely a secondary phenomenon—of diagnostic value but causing no pain. The same applies to arthritis. Judging by the fact that hydrocortisone, introduced into the joint cavity where it lies in contact with synovial membrane rather than capsule, has a marked effect on early arthritis, it would seem that at first synovial irritation is the main factor in evoking the muscle spasm that mediates the limitation of movement.

The bearing of this concept of muscle spasm on treatment is considerable. Since muscle spasm in arthritis is secondary to the synovio-capsular lesion, the treatment of muscle spasm is not to the spastic muscle, but to the lesion causing it. To physiotherapists accustomed to stretching out muscles in the site of neurogenic hypertonus, and to doctors who think in terms of painful muscle spasm in e.g. frozen shoulder or lumbago, treatment by passive movement administered to the joint appears misplaced. It is therefore important to discard the notion of muscle spasm as either the primary lesion or the cause of pain; for treatment must be applied to the cause not the effect. This is universally accepted in e.g. appendicitis; no one treats the muscles in that disorder. But the same does not apply in lumbago, where heat or massage to the muscles, exercises to the muscles, or prescribing muscle-relaxant drugs is as widespread as it is illogical.

(2) *In the later case*, capsular contracture takes over and muscle spasm becomes much less evident. At some joints during mobilization under anaesthesia, the contracture can be felt and heard to rupture; this finding precludes a purely synovial lesion.

(3) *Finally*, osteophyte formation and gross capsulo-ligamentous contracture supervene and prevent movement, even under anaesthesia. Throughout this progression the capsular proportions of limitation of movement are retained.

Arthritis and Radiography

Since evidence of arthritis is often sought by X-rays, it is easy to think of arthritis as an affection of cartilage and bone, and to adopt the view that, if the radiograph reveals no abnormality, arthritis must be absent. This attitude leads to grievous error. Erosion of cartilage, osteophyte formation and changes in the density of the bones characterize advanced arthritis, but are not of themselves painful. Cartilage is devoid of nerve supply and no lesion in cartilage can of itself give rise to pain. Equally, muscle spasm about a joint, osteophyte formation and rarefaction of bone are not of themselves painful. These are secondary phenomena, and are not vital to the clinical concept of arthritis, which displays itself primarily as a capsular contracture, which can continue for many months or years without giving rise to any radiological evidence of disease.

The Capsular Pattern Listed

The capsular pattern exists at only those joints that are controlled by muscles. These spring into action to prevent further movement when the tension on the capsule of the joint and on its synovial lining is about to cause pain. There is no capsular pattern, therefore, at joints that rely for their stability purely on their ligaments, e.g. the acromio-clavicular or the sacro-iliac. Here the degree of arthritis is shown by the severity of the pain brought on when the joint is strained, but no mechanism for involuntary prevention of mobility exists.

Neck

Side-flexion and rotation are equally limited; flexion is usually of full range and painful, extension limited. The common cause of a non-capsular pattern is internal derangement, i.e. subluxation of a fragment of disc.

Sterno-clavicular and Acromio-clavicular Joint

Pain at the extremes of range.

Shoulder

So much limitation of abduction, more limitation of lateral rotation, less limitation of medial rotation. The common cause of a non-capsular pattern is acute subdeltoid bursitis.

Elbow

Rather more limitation of flexion than of extension. In the early stage of arthritis, rotation remains full and painless. The common cause of a non-capsular pattern is internal derangement, i.e. a loose body.

Lower Radio-ulnar Joint

A full range of movement with pain at both extremes of rotation. The common cause of limitation of only pronation is malunion of a Colles's fracture.

Trapezio-first-Metacarpal Joint

Limitation of abduction and of extension; full flexion.

Thumb and Finger Joints

Rather more limitation of flexion than of extension.

Thoracic and Lumbar Joints

The difficulty is to determine, except in gross arthritis, whether the range is limited or not, taking into account the patient's age and habitus. Comparison between the amounts by which extension and side-flexion are limited is scarcely possible. By contrast, the non-capsular pattern is very easy to detect, e.g. gross limitation of side-flexion one way, full range the other way; or full extension accompanied by markedly limited flexion. Again, at the thorax, a full range of rotation in one direction may be matched by 45 degrees limitation in the other. The cause of this type of non-capsular pattern is internal derangement, i.e. displacement of a fragment of disc.

Sacro-iliac, Symphysis Pubis and Sacro-coccygeal Joints

Pain when stress falls on the joint.

Hip Joint

Gross limitation of flexion, abduction and medial rotation. Slight limitation of extension. Little or no limitation of lateral rotation. The common causes of a non-capsular pattern are bursitis or a loose body in the hip joint.

Knee Joint

Gross limitation of flexion (e.g. 90 degrees), slight limitation of extension (e.g. 5 degrees or 10 degrees). In the early stages of arthritis rotation remains full and painless. The common cause of a non-capsular pattern is internal derangement (displaced loose body or meniscus).

Tibio-fibular Joints

Pain when contraction of the biceps muscle stretches the upper tibio-fibular ligaments; pain when the mortice is sprung at the ankle. Normally there is no appreciable movement possible at either joint.

Ankle Joint

If the calf-muscles are of adequate length, rather more limitation of plantiflexion than of dorsiflexion is present. If these muscles are short, they limit dorsiflexion (soft end-feel) before the arthritic limitation (hard end-feel) can be reached. If so, clinically, limitation of plantiflexion is present alone.

Talo-calcanean Joint

Limitation of varus range increasing until, in gross arthritis, the joint fixes in full valgus. In early cases, the extreme of such varus movement as is possible is painful.

Mid-tarsal Joint

Limitation of dorsiflexion, plantiflexion, adduction and medial rotation. Abduction and lateral rotation of full range.

First Metatarso-phalangeal Joint

Marked limitation of extension (e.g. 60 degrees to 80 degrees); slight limitation of flexion (10 degrees to 20 degrees).

Other Four Metatarso-phalangeal Joints

Variable. They tend finally to fix in extension with the interphalangeal joints flexed.

The Non-capsular Pattern

When limitation of movement is discovered in proportions not corresponding to the capsular pattern, arthritis is absent and lesions capable of causing restriction of range, but not involving the whole joint, have to be considered. They fall into three categories: ligamentous adhesions, internal derangement and extra-articular lesions.

Ligamentous Adhesions

Ligaments reinforce the capsule of a joint. When adhesions form about a ligament after an injury, those movements that require a fully mobile ligament for their painless performance resprain the ligament whose mobility is impaired. Hence pain, usually localized, is brought on only by those movements that stretch the adherent structure. Thus some movements are painful, perhaps one movement is slightly limited, and some movements are pain-free in a manner characteristic of the affected ligament, not of the whole capsule of the joint. In ligamentous adhesions movement is restricted in the *proportionate* way, i.e. slight limitation exists in one direction but a full, painless range is present in the other directions.

Internal Derangement

This need be considered only in joints apt to develop intra-articular loose fragments of cartilage or bone. These are the knee, jaw and spinal joints commonly; the elbow, hip and tarsal joints occasionally.

When a loose fragment becomes displaced within a joint, the onset is sudden. A localized block is formed which occupies only one part of the joint. Hence the pain is localized, often at one aspect only of the joint, and those movements that engage against the block are limited, while those that do not are of full range. Examination thus discloses the partial articular—i.e. non-capsular—pattern characteristic of internal derangement.

In minor cases the restriction of movement is often proportionate, but the sudden onset with the limitation coming on immediately shows that ligamentous adhesions cannot be present, for they have not yet had time to form. A major block produces gross *disproportion*; for example, in torticollis or lumbago the spinal joint may possess a full range of side-flexion in one direction and no range at all in the other, deformity and pain appearing simultaneously. A large displacement causes the disproportionate type of non-capsular pattern, a small displacement the proportionate type. It is merely a question of the size of the loose body and the degree and site of the displacement. By contrast, in spinal arthritis the degree of limitation of side-flexion is equal in the two directions. The disproportion is very obvious at the knee when the torn part of a meniscus shifts, blocking extension but not flexion.

Extra-articular Lesions

These can limit movement in two ways:

Disproportionate Limitation

When, for example, the quadriceps muscle is adherent to the shaft of the mid-femur, 90 degrees of limitation of flexion at the knee joint is associated with a full and painless range of extension. Such gross limitation of movement in one direction only, combined with full painless range in all other directions indicates that the joint itself is normal, and that an extra-articular contracture will not permit that one movement. For example the muscle spasm about the breach in a partly torn gastrocnemius muscle grossly limits dorsiflexion at the ankle joint, whereas passive plantiflexion remains of full range and painless.

The same effect can be produced by a large haematoma or cyst in the popliteal space; again the knee will not bend far though it will extend fully, this time because of a swelling that will not allow itself to be compressed beyond a certain point.

In acute subdeltoid bursitis, limitation of movement at the shoulder joint is obvious, but it is gross towards abduction, slight towards the rotations. This disproportion between the range of abduction and lateral rotation, reversing the capsular pattern at the shoulder joint, shifts attention from the joint to the extra-articular structures.

The Constant-length Phenomenon

If the amount of limitation of movement at one joint depends on the position in which another joint is held, the restricting tissue must lie outside any joint. This relationship indicates that the lesion lies in a structure that spans at least two joints, thus clearly excluding any articular tissue. A good example is straight-leg raising. Limitation of hip-flexion (when compared with the other side) when the knee is held straight, but not when the knee is allowed to bend, indicates that the structure which will not stretch runs from below the back of the knee to above the posterior aspect of the hip joint. Now, if neck-flexion during straight-leg raising further increases the pain in the back or lower limb, it becomes clear that the tissue whose mobility is impaired runs from the neck to the calf; and there is only one such tissue—the dura mater and its continuation as the sciatic nerve.

Volkmann's ischaemic contracture provides another example of the constant-length phenomenon. In this condition, the fingers cannot be extended unless the wrist is flexed first. In other words, the amount of movement of which his fingers are capable depends on the position of the wrist—again, a possibility only if the lesion is extra-articular.

★   ★   ★

2. *Passive Movement is Painful in one direction and Active Movement is Painful in the opposite direction*

This indicates a contractile structure to be at fault, i.e. a muscle belly, a tendon, or the attachment of either to periosteum. Since tension is the cause of pain, passively stretching the muscle hurts; active contraction in the opposite direction also hurts. This finding leads to immediate trial of the resisted movements (see below).

The direction of the painful movement indicates which group of muscles is involved. Accessory movements, picking out the various members of the group individually, define the affected muscle, and may even show which part of it is affected. When a muscle spans two joints, e.g. the muscles of the arm or thigh, special tests can be devised.

Exception

In acute teno-synovitis at the wrist, pain is set up when movement occurs between the roughened tendon and its sheath. Hence not only such movements as stretch the tendon, but also those that relax it, set up a painful friction; in the latter case by pushing the tendon down the sheath. The occurrence of pain on those two passive movements might suggest a lesion of an inert structure at the wrist joint. The diagnosis becomes clear only when the resisted movements are tried; these cannot set up pain in an articular lesion.

★   ★   ★

3. *Resisted Movement Reveals Pain or Weakness*

Resisted movement discloses the state of the muscles that perform that movement. Strictly speaking, a resisted movement is not a movement at all, and is a contradiction in terms. It is really a forcible frustrated attempt at movement. Some would prefer to say 'static contraction'. However, this term is not without ambiguity, since static contraction is often used voluntarily to fix a joint and then involves all the muscles controlling the part. 'Resisted movement' is merely short for 'attempted movement against resistance'.

Precautions must be observed to obtain a correct response to this type of testing.

(1) The joint must be held near mid-range. In this position all the ligaments and the capsule itself are equally relaxed, no tension falling on them when the muscle contracts.

(2) The resistance must be so strong that the joint is prevented from moving. Hence, the tension on one muscle group alters as the patient pushes, but the tension on the articular structures does not alter.

(3) The examiner must apply resistance at a point that ensures that only one group of muscles is being tested. For example, testing resisted lateral rotation of the shoulder by pressing against the dorsum of the patient's hand would elicit pain also if the patient had a tennis-elbow, whereas resistance applied to the dorsum of the lower forearm unambiguously singles out the infraspinatus muscle.

(4) The main muscle groups should be tested one by one and the patient asked each time if his discomfort is evoked or increased. If one resisted movement hurts and the others do not, and a full range of passive movement is present at the relevant joint, it is a virtual certainty that a muscle lesion is present. If the resisted movement found painful involves more than one muscle, accessory movements can usually be devised that identify which one within that set of muscles is at fault. For example, if resisted medial rotation of the shoulder hurts, the trouble might lie in the pectoralis major, latissimus dorsi, teres major or subscapularis muscles. The first three are also strong adductors of the arm; hence, if this resisted movement proves painless (as is to be expected), the subscapularis muscle is singled out.

If two congruous movements hurt (e.g. resisted flexion and supination at the elbow in a bicipital lesion), a muscle lesion is present in the muscle that combines these two actions—i.e. not the brachialis.

If several resisted movements, or two incompatible movements, hurt, a muscle lesion is improbable.

If *all* the resisted movements hurt, the last thing to suspect is a muscle lesion. This finding suggests either the exaggeration that denotes psychogenesis or a severe lesion lying close by proximally, to which any movement transmits stress. For example, every resisted movement of the arm often hurts in acute torticollis and of the thigh in acute lumbago, since the patient has to brace his spinal muscles before attempting to move the limb.

In tendinous lesions a full passive range of movement always exists at the relevant joint, and even a lesion in a muscle belly can limit only that passive movement which stretches the healing breach. Many muscles span more than one joint and tests based on the constant-length phenomenon can then be employed to confirm the presence of such a lesion.

There exist two conditions not directly connected with muscle that nevertheless give rise to pain when muscle is tested against resistance. The first is fracture of bone close to the attachment of belly or tendon. Naturally muscle-pull tends to move the fractured ends on each other painfully. For example, anterior fracture of a rib may give rise to pain when the pectoralis major muscle is tested, or fracture of one pubis may hurt on testing resisted adduction of that thigh. The second is compression by the muscle belly of a tender structure. As the muscle hardens and broadens, any adjacent tender structure is squeezed and pain may then be evoked. This phenomenon is met with chiefly in the buttock, where for example a tender gluteal bursa can be compressed by contraction of the gluteus medius muscle.

Interpretation

When the resisted contraction of muscle groups is tested, the possibilities are:

(a) Strong and Painful

This designates a minor lesion of some part of a muscle or tendon. The damage is not gross enough to cause weakness, but a strong contraction hurts, thus indicating that the structural integrity of the muscle-tendon complex is impaired.

Tennis-elbow provides a good illustration of a diagnosis that can be made adequately only by examination of resisted movements. In this condition, the passive movements of the elbow or wrist, and the resisted movements at the elbow, cause no pain. However, when the movements at the wrist are tested against resistance, extension causes pain at the elbow. The diagnosis can be further refined by resisting this movement while the patient keeps his fingers flexed. This also hurts, although the extensor digitorum muscle is now out of action. Hence, one of the extensor muscles of the carpus is involved. When ulnar and radial deviation movements of the hand are resisted, only the latter hurts. By this means the lesion at the elbow can be shown to lie at the upper extent of the radial extensor muscles of the carpus. Mere palpation of so small an area could not have demonstrated whether the fault lay in the ulnar, the digital or the radial extensor muscles.

(b) Weak and Painless

There is often constant pain, but making the weak muscle contract against resistance does not alter the symptoms. This finding may indicate a complete rupture of the relevant muscle or tendon, but much more often a disorder of the nervous system. Impaired conduction along a nerve leads to muscle weakness, but, since the structural integrity of the muscle is maintained, no pain arises when as strong a contraction as possible takes place. It is important to ensure that a patient in constant pain does not merely allude to this fact, but is clear that what the examiner is asking about is an *increase* in his symptoms during the resisted movement.

(c) *Weak and Painful*

This indicates a gross lesion, i.e. the resisted movement proves weak and the attempt increases pain. In, say, fracture of the patella or olecranon resisted extension at knee or elbow is naturally weak and painful. Second ary deposits at the head of the humerus set up pain and weakness when the resisted movements are tested, together with marked restriction of passive joint range.

This finding always suggests serious trouble, even if the first X-ray photograph reveals no abnormality.

(d) *All Painful*

The resisted movements have another quite different virtue. They provide a rough measure of individual variation in sensitiveness to pain. When resisted movements are performed at a joint, the muscles about which are normal, all persons perceive the altered tension on the muscle, but find it in no sense disagreeable. There are patients whose degree of perception is so heightened, usually by fatigue or emotional stress, that they interpret changes in muscular tension as painful. For example, when a patient with backache elicited by lumbar movements also experiences an equal amount of pain at the shoulder—or even in the back!—on resisted arm movements, it is highly probable that he is describing as painful those feelings that do not hurt ordinary individuals. Trial of resisted movements at joints remote from the seat of the patient's pain, helps enormously to indicate whether the symptoms arise from emotional hypersensitivity or pain generated organically.

(e) *All Painless*

If all the resisted movements prove strong and painless, there is nothing the matter with the muscles.

Were this simple and logical concept accepted, the idea of fibrositis would never have arisen. For example, if patients with 'fibrositis of the trapezius' are examined, elevation of the scapula even against the strongest resistance is painless. This shows the muscle to be normal; hence nothing is to be gained by looking for a tender spot within it. Even if one is found, it cannot be relevant to the patient's referred trapezial symptoms.

(f) *Painful on Repetition*

The resisted movements can also be used to provide a measure of arterial patency. If the movement is strong and painless but is found to hurt after a number of repetitions, intermittent claudication is present.

*   *   *

4. *The Elicitation of Pain by Internal Squeezing*

Internal squeezing elicits pain in two ways, one very helpful (a painful arc) and the other misleading (at the extreme of range).

Painful Arc

By this is meant pain appearing near the mid-range of a movement, ceasing as this point is passed. The pain may reappear at the extreme of range, *but it must cease on each side of the arc*. If elevation of the arm begins to hurt when the horizontal is reached, and then continues until full elevation is complete, no painful arc is present. If the pain comes on at the horizontal, ceases above it and then returns (or not) at full elevation, a painful arc has been elicited. This phenomenon is best evoked by active movement, and may appear only on the upward movement of the arm, or only on the downward, or both. In any case, the significance is the same; the lesion lies in a pinchable position. If a tender structure is painfully squeezed when a moving part passes a certain point, anatomical considerations can be used to deduce where the lesion must lie. A painful arc at the shoulder is common and indicates that the tender tissue can be pinched between the acromion and one or other of the humeral tuberosities. This finding therefore incriminates the supraspinatus, infraspinatus or subscapular tendon, or the subdeltoid bursa. Accessory tests then define which is at fault. Once the structure has been singled out, the fact that a painful arc exists indicates which part of it is affected. A painful arc on a spinal movement indicates that the lesion moves suddenly when the tilt on the joint alters from lordosis to kyphosis, i.e. it lies squeezed between the vertebral bodies. A painful arc on straight-leg raising indicates that a small protrusion exists over which the nerve-root slides. At the knee, a painful arc suggests a loose body or a transverse crack in the meniscus; at the hip, bursitis.

Pain at One Extreme of Range

This may prove puzzling; for if pain appears at the extreme of range the examiner is apt to think in terms of stretching and to forget the occasional occurrence of pinching. If he is fortunate, other movements also hurt that identify the structure at fault. For example, when the arm is fully elevated, the greater tuberosity of the humerus engages against the glenoid rim and squeezes the supraspinatus tendon. Hence full passive elevation of the arm may elicit tenderness in supraspinatus tendinitis. This is not the same thing as finding that full *active* elevation of the arm hurts. During the active movement, the supraspinatus muscle is contracting, and pain is therefore to be expected wherever in the tendon the lesion lies. Full passive elevation relaxes the muscle and, in supraspinatus tendinitis, pain can thus result only from squeezing; hence it is a useful localizing sign. Similarly, full passive medial rotation of the arm presses the subscapular tendon against the glenoid rim and full adduction presses the subscapular tendon against the coracoid process. When a lesion lies at the teno-periosteal junction of the biceps tendon at the radial tuberosity, this point is pressed against the shaft of the ulna at the extreme of full passive pronation of the forearm. Both the psoas bursa and rectus femoris tendon can be squeezed by full flexion with adduction of the hip. The bursa lying in front of the tendo Achillis is squeezed between the tibia and the calcaneus on full passive plantiflexion at the ankle joint.

Great diagnostic difficulties arise when only one movement hurts; for example, if, in a painful shoulder only full passive elevation proves painful, is this a pinch or a stretch? The differentiation between early osteoarthritis and psoas bursitis or a loose body in the hip joint is obscured by the same phenomenon.

★   ★   ★

5. *The Passive Range of Movement is Full but there is Inability to Perform One or More Movements Actively*

This shows one or more muscles to be out of action, either from intrinsic defect such as a cut tendon or myopathy, or from interference with nervous paths, e.g. peripheral neuritis, anterior poliomyelitis, cerebral vascular accident or psychogenic disorder. In partial palsies or when only one of several muscles that can perform a movement is affected, trial of the resisted movements is needed to disclose the weakness. In both neurogenic hypertonus and hysteria, inability to perform a voluntary movement is associated with considerable resistance when the movement is attempted passively, greatest at the first moment of forcing.

★   ★   ★

6. *An Excessive Range of Movement Exists*

This results from capsulo-ligamentous laxity at joints whose stability is not under full muscular control. The structures most often concerned are the acromio-clavicular, sterno-clavicular, sacro-iliac and sacro-coccygeal joints, the symphysis pubis, the collateral and cruciate ligaments at the knee joint, the inferior tibio-fibular and the calcaneo-fibular ligaments. The liability to subluxation is noted when too much movement is found, sometimes on active movement but always on passive testing. Permanent laxity of any of these ligaments may follow a severe sprain.

★   ★   ★

7. *A Bony Block Limits Movement*

When a joint is felt to come to a dead stop at a point short of its full range of normal movement, a bony block is present. If no pain is elicited on forcing a neuropathic arthropathy is almost certain; if forcing is uncomfortable the cause is probably large osteophytic outcrops of bone, myositis ossificans or a mal-united fracture close to the joint.

8. *No Movement is Possible*

This may result from the intense muscular spasm set up by bacterial arthritis, or fibrous or bony ankylosis. Absence of movement at the shoulder and hip joints is somewhat masked by scapular and pelvic mobility.

★   ★   ★

9. *A Snap Occurs*

This results when a tendon catches against a bony prominence and then slips over it. Such a sequence of events occurs at the shoulder (long head of biceps) and ankle (peroneal tendons); but if a joint is painful and also snaps, it does not necessarily follow that the pain is the result of a frictional tendinitis. At the hip, the greater trochanter may catch against the edge of the gluteus maximus muscle. An osteoma may first declare itself by catching against a tendon. A small semi-membranous bursa may snap as it jumps from one to the other side of the tendon as the knee is flexed. In trigger-finger, a swelling of the digital flexor tendon jams inside the tendon-sheath and holds the finger fixed in flexion until the engagement is passively released with a snap.

★   ★   ★

10. *A Crack is Heard*

This is a normal phenomenon, occurring when traction is applied to a joint, especially of the fingers. Roston and Haines (1947) showed that traction up to 6 kg. resulted merely in slight separation of the bony surfaces at a man's metacarpo-phalangeal joint. When the traction reached 7 or 8 kg. the bones sprang apart with a loud crack, the distance between them suddenly becoming doubled. Radiography demonstrated that, at that same moment, a bubble of air appeared in the joint. This was doubtless derived from gas dissolved in the intra-articular synovial fluid evaporating as the result of the subatmospheric pressure created by the traction. It was absorbed again in twenty minutes; before this had happened no amount of tension would make the joint crack again.

★   ★   .★

11. *A Click is Palpable*

When a loose body lies inside a joint, it may be felt to move from one position to another by both examiner and patient. This is a commonplace at the knee, and often occurs also at the jaw, spinal and elbow joints. Sometimes it may prove possible digitally to manœuvre a loose body about inside the knee joint. If the knee joint contains fluid, the patella may be clicked down on to the femur.

Laxity of the ligaments may enable a bone to click as it moves in relation to its fellow. This is common at joints unsupported by muscles, e.g. the acromio-clavicular, and after capsular overstretching at the shoulder. Painless clicking of a costal cartilage occurs. The patella often clicks on active extension of a perfectly normal knee.

★   ★   ★

12. Crepitus is Felt

The state of the gliding surfaces of a joint is best assessed by palpation of the moving joint. Fine crepitus means slight roughening of the cartilaginous surfaces; coarse crepitus, considerable surface fragmentation. The intermittent creaking of bone against bone clearly indicates that the articular cartilage has wholly worn through.

In the same way, palpation reveals the state of gliding surfaces in those tendons that possess a close-fitting sheath. Fine crepitus characterizes acute traumatic roughening of the surfaces; coarse crepitus, chronic rheumatoid or tuberculous teno-synovitis.

There are two situations where muscular crepitus occurs. When the extensor and abductor pollicis tendons are affected in the lower forearm, crepitus is expected locally. However, it is sometimes felt throughout the muscle bellies, almost as far up as the elbow (Cyriax, 1941: Thompson, Plewes and Shawn, 1951). Again, when the musculo-tendinous junction of the tibialis anterior suffers strain just above the point where the muscle crosses the tibia, a small area of crepitus is usually palpable.

★   ★   ★

13. No Movement Hurts

When there is full and painless passive movement at a joint and no resisted movement hurts either, the pain felt in that region is clearly referred. If this finding is repeated on examination of all the joints and muscles whence pain might spring, the inference is that a tissue outside the sphere of orthopaedic medicine is at fault, most often part of the nervous system but sometimes a viscus. In this connection it should be remembered that in nerve-sheath lesions ordinary neurological examination may disclose no fault, since it estimates only conduction along the nerve. The external surface of nerve-trunks and nerve-roots suffer painful interference, often insufficient in degree to affect the parenchyma.

Normal function of a tissue precludes its containing a painful lesion. Hence the discovery of tenderness at part of a structure, whose function is normal, is devoid of pathological significance.

OTHER DIAGNOSTIC PROCEDURES

Four other diagnostic procedures may prove useful, but they do not involve testing movement at a joint.

Localization of Lesion in Two Overlapping Tissues

When a muscle overlies another muscle or some other structure, it may be important to decide which of the two is at fault. Tenderness is estimated by applying equal degrees of pressure when the superficial muscle is first relaxed, then taut. If the pain is greater in the latter event, the more superficial of the two tissues is affected. This method can be used to demonstrate whether the fault lies, for example, in the pectoralis major, an intercostal muscle or rib. Again, visceral tenderness may be distinguished in this way from tenderness of the actual abdominal wall.

Test for Distant Pain

When a lesion lies in a long bone, pressure applied distantly may cause pain at the site of the trauma. Thus, pressure on the sternum may set up pain at the site of injury if a rib is broken, or an intercostal muscle torn, or a costo-vertebral joint arthritic.

Diagnostic Traction

If a structure is painfully squeezed, it may prove possible to abolish the symptoms for the time being by traction. This is a very valuable sign, especially in difficult cases of suspected cervical or thoracic articular derangements. For example, pain and/or paraesthesia due to root-pressure caused by a cervical disc lesion may disappear for as long as head suspension or manual traction is maintained. Conversely, compression of a joint may increase symptoms, but is a most unreliable sign.

Aspiration

It is often important to ascertain whether the fluid in a joint is clear liquid or blood. Aspiration provides an immediate answer and is a safe diagnostic method suitable for out-patient use. Radiography after air has been injected into a joint occasionally reveals a loose body otherwise invisible.

Misleading Phenomena

1. *Referred Tenderness*

The phenomenon of localized 'referred tenderness' can be extremely deceptive, and has been considered in Chapter 3.

2. *Associated Tenderness*

This phenomenon is even more misleading; for the tender area is sharply localized and very close to the site of the lesion. The tenderness is undoubtedly connected with the lesion, for both disappear together.

Associated tenderness appears to occur at only two sites; the radial styloid process as the result of tenovaginitis of the abductor longus and extensor brevis muscles at the carpus; and the posterior aspect of the lateral humeral epicondyle just above the radio-humeral joint-line in the teno-periosteal variety of tennis-elbow. No explanation can be offered for this curious phenomenon.

3. Joint Signs in Root Lesions

In cervical and lumbar disc-protrusion leading to root-pressure, a highly misleading phenomenon may be found on examination. In the case of a cervical root, each extreme of movement at the shoulder joint may hurt when tested passively; at times one or more of the resisted movements also prove painful. This distracts attention from the neck, focusing it on the shoulder. As the pain in disc-protrusion may be entirely brachial, real confusion easily arises. Limitation of passive movement is not of course possible in the absence of a local lesion, but patients with acute torticollis often genuinely cannot actively raise the arm on the painful side. When pressure is exerted on a lower lumbar nerve-root, testing the hip joint on the same side may reveal that the extremes of movement are of full range but cause unilateral pain. It might well be supposed that the mechanism is the unavoidable transmission of movement to the lumbar joints when the pelvis moves with the hip joint. This is not so; for movement of the other hip tilts the lumbar spine just as much, and does not hurt. I regard the hip movements as capable at their extreme of altering the tension on the sciatic nerve-roots in a minor way, analogous to straight-leg raising.

This phenomenon adds considerably to the diagnostic difficulties in spinal nerve-root pressure. It also serves to explain how patients mistakenly thought to be suffering from lesions in the shoulder, hip or sacro-iliac joint have been cured by manipulation of the spine.

THE RADIOGRAPH

In soft-tissue lesions the radiograph is uninformative except negatively. It shows fractures, and sooner or later must also show lesions involving bone such as abscess formation, tuberculosis or neoplasm. In fracture work, or in the investigation of pulmonary or abdominal visceral disturbances, it provides the greatest assistance. Contrast media can be introduced into any cavity, a blood vessel, the theca, etc., and produce diagnostic appearances. By contrast, only a few simple lesions within the orthopaedic medical orbit, such as osteoarthritis of the hip joint, show up regularly on the radiograph. Apart from small areas of calcification, not always relevant, the X-ray picture is uniformly negative. For example, whatever is the matter with the shoulder joint, the radiograph shows no abnormality except in cancer, tuberculosis and such rarities as synovial chrondomatosis; diseases which provide between them not more than 1 per cent of all non-traumatic painful shoulders. By contrast, a minor radiographic deviation from the normal is often given diagnostic import-ance when it bears no relation to the patient's trouble. On the strength of visible osteophytes, osteoarthritis of the spinal or sacro-iliac joints is often mistakenly thought to be the cause of symptoms. Osteoarthritis of the knee—an uncommon disorder—is frequently diagnosed through mis-interpretation of radiographic appearances, and any middle-aged 'patient suffering from monarticular rheumatoid arthritis or persistent subluxation of a cartilaginous loose body at the knee is apt to be given this label merely on the strength of changes, present indeed bilaterally, to be expected at that age.

Attempted diagnosis by radiography is proceeding apace nowadays. An elderly patient with say tendinitis, bursitis or arthritis at the shoulder (none of which shows on the X-ray photograph), or even with a tennis-elbow, is very apt to have radiography at the site of pain and at the neck. Since the lesion lies in the soft tissues the local photographs reveal no abnormality, but at that age marked trouble is seen at the neck—osteo-phytosis, one or more diminished joint-spaces, etc. If patients old enough to have angina had their necks X-rayed, it could equally unreasonably be alleged that cervical spondylosis caused coronary disease. No doctor would fall for such a facile lack of logic; yet, it is very common to find that patients with disease in an upper limb have received months of treatment to the neck, because the radiographs were inspected without previous clinical examination.

The locomotor disorders that do show up radiologically are usually gross and therefore easy to detect clinically. Surprises are a rarity. But osteitis deformans with involvement of one shoulder or hip might well be mistaken for ordinary osteoarthritis without X-ray help; and when, say, neoplasm of the ilium, sacro-iliac arthritis or secondary deposit at a vertebral body is suspected, radiography, if necessary repeated, is essential. Nevertheless, the radiograph need not reveal early disease and must not be taken as excluding such diseases, if the symptoms are of recent date. Five years have elapsed for sclerosis to show at an arthritic sacro-iliac joint and eighteen months for both spinal tuberculosis and myeloma to become radiologically apparent.

On the whole, in orthopaedic medical disorders, irrelevant radiographic appearances must be resolutely ignored. I regard it (but am probably alone in doing so) as far more dangerous to the patient—not to the physician—to omit a proper clinical examination and to rely on radio-graphy, than to do the reverse. Negligence in clinical examination is scarcely capable of proof, whereas failure to X-ray is a simple fact; hence, undue prominence has been given by the Courts to this omission. Hindsight makes it clear that in this particular case an X-ray photograph would have helped, but the Courts ought to take into account the thousand other useless radiographs that would have had to be ordered to prevent the one error. In consequence, doctors nowadays fear not to have a patient X-rayed, since large sums are awarded in damages. But many mistakes, some quite ludicrous and just as culpable medico-legally, were proof to hand, result from attempts at diagnosis in soft tissue lesions mainly by radiography. Moreover, the lulling effect of a normal X-ray picture in early serious disease may prove disastrous. The strength to ignore both a positively and a negatively misleading radiograph comes only from proper clinical examination.

Welcome support for revolt against excessive routine radiography has lately stemmed from the National Hospital, Queen Square. There Bull and Zilkha (1968) carried out a retrospective survey of 410 patients and a prospective study of 200 more. Their conclusion was that radio-graphy in 'migraine or headache, pain in the neck, vertigo or Ménière's disease, and epilepsy, in the absence of physical signs, does not contribute materially to the diagnosis.'

EXAMINATION OF THE NERVOUS AND ARTERIAL SYSTEM

This should never be neglected in cases of obscure pain. The search is not for the gross signs that characterize advanced neurological disease, but for minor deviations from the normal. In nerve-sheath lesions the patient may complain of pins and needles and numbness; yet examination reveals that cutaneous sensibility at the area felt to be numb is either normal or so little impaired as to leave the issue in doubt. Alternatively, a small degree of muscular weakness or an area of analgesia rather than of anaesthesia are the most that can be expected in the lesions primarily affecting a nerve-sheath that so often find their way to the orthopaedic physician.

When a neurological symptom identifies one cutaneous area, *the whole length of the corresponding nerve must be examined*; for the symptoms are felt distally no matter where the nerve-trunk suffers compression. For example, ulnar paraesthesia may result from pressure on the eighth cervical root, on the lower trunk of the brachial plexus where it crosses the rib, on the ulnar nerve at the back of the elbow, or at the wrist. Signs of a relevant somatic disorder must be sought at each of these four levels, and the whole attainable stretch of nerve should be palpated as well. Again, paraesthesia of median distribution can arise from fifth cervical disc lesions, the thoracic outlet syndrome, and compression in the carpal tunnel; search from neck to wrist is required. When the paraesthesia occupies, say, every digit of the hand, it is clear that the lesion lies above the differentiation of the brachial plexus, and a much shorter stretch of nerve need be examined, i.e. from the spinal cord to the axilla.

Pins and needles felt in the feet are often an early symptom of pressure on the spinal cord, and may be experienced many years before the plantar response becomes extensor.

PALPATION

Interpretation of the pattern that emerges when the patient is examined in the manner set out in this chapter nearly always enables the tissue at fault to be singled out. Accessory signs may then disclose at what point in its extent it is affected; if so, palpation is unnecessary. Alternatively, if the structure containing the lesion lies within fingers' reach, palpation for tenderness is most helpful. Such palpation is not indiscriminate; it is confined to the tissue at fault. It must never be undertaken until every movement bearing on the functional assessment has been studied. Palpation too early on in the examination of a patient has been practised on a large scale, and until recently was probably the commonest cause of mistaken diagnosis in the whole of medicine. One has only to consider the former universality of 'fibrositis' to realize how widespread was the adoption of this approach.

The farther down the limb a lesion lies, the more precision in diagnosis palpation affords. At the trunk, shoulder and hip areas, it is seldom of value and often misleading. At the knee and elbow, palpation is helpful, and at the wrist and hand, ankle and foot, it has great importance. Sometimes there is no tenderness over the site of a proximal lesion. The examiner must not let himself be dismayed in such a case since, for example, in supraspinatus tendinitis the tendon is no more tender than its fellow on the other side; and in subdeltoid bursitis the part of the bursa involved may lie under the acromion, inaccessible to the investigating finger. Only when the decision has been reached that the lesion lies quite superficially can absence of tenderness be regarded as showing the diagnosis to be wrong. By contrast, he must be on his guard against the phenomena of referred and associated tenderness already discussed.

The presence or not of pulsation in the arteries is often important diagnostically. In intermittent claudication the popliteal pulse can seldom be felt. In thrombosis or coarctation of the aorta, of which an early sign may be vague pains in the lower limbs on walking, the femoral pulses are absent. Thrombosis of the external iliac artery leads to claudication and a cold foot after walking; again the femoral pulse is absent. Sometimes in the thoracic outlet syndrome, and in many normal people, approximation of the scapulae abolishes the radial pulse.

Palpation may also reveal the presence of deformity, e.g. a Paget tibia, warmth, swelling, fluid or crepitus. Fluctuation may identify a haematoma or fluid in a joint or bursa. (Any muscle appears to fluctuate when tested transversely; hence the examiner's fingers must lie at different levels along the length of the belly.) Bony tenderness may provide the sign suggesting a fracture. In rupture of a muscle or tendon the gap may prove palpable.

Palpation can detect a difference in mobility at one spinal joint as compared with its fellows; lay manipulators lay great stress on this examination. But the question arises whether it is the hypomobile joint that should be considered pathological. In fact, laymen often find lesions at the upper two lumbar joints by palpation, whereas these are the very levels where trouble is so rare; hence I am not convinced of its diagnostic value. Laymen also allege that they can single out sublaxations of one vertebra on another by this means; however, different exponents' findings show marked discrepancy.

In my view, the best criterion is to move each spinal joint in turn and find out at which level symptoms are most strongly evoked.

LOCAL ANAESTHESIA

When an anatomical localization has been arrived at by correlation of the patient's symptoms with the deductions based on a series of responses to many diagnostic movements, followed or not by palpation, there is still room for error. Whenever possible, therefore, confirmation or disproof should be sought from the induction of local anaesthesia, at any rate for the first few years of the clinical work of the future orthopaedic physician. Otherwise he may erroneously ascribe some particular pattern to a certain disorder and never find out his mistake. If 2 to 10 c.c. (depending on the size of the lesion) of a 1:200 solution of procaine in saline is injected into the point of origin of the pain, the symptoms disappear for the duration of anaesthesia—about 90 minutes. A stronger solution affords no better anaesthesia and the after-pain is more severe.

In the limbs, if the wrong spot is chosen, the pain, being merely referred thither, fortunately does not disappear. Hence, the criterion in these parts of the body is good. Unhappily, the same does not apply to the trunk, especially its posterior aspect. *Pain due to unilateral disc-protrusion in the neck, thorax or lumbar region can sometimes be abolished for the time being by a local anaesthetic injection into the tender paraspinal areas.* This phenomenon is difficult to account for, but a possible explanation has been put forward by Whitty and Willison (1958). They suggest that *any* reduction in the impulses which pass to the centre of summation may modify the referred sensation by diminishing the total sensory inflow.

Five minutes after the infiltration, the patient is requested to repeat whichever movement was found on examination to be the most painful, and is asked if it still hurts. It is by no means enough to ask the patient as he lies on the couch if his pain has gone. In addition, if limitation of some movement existed, its range should be estimated again, e.g. straight-leg raising in sciatic root-pressure after epidural infiltration or active elevation of the arm in patients with a painful arc. If the pain has nearly or quite disappeared, the right spot has clearly been chosen. If it remains, and the solution has been injected into the intended spot, the diagnosis has been shown to be mistaken; hence the patient must be examined again to see where the error in deduction lies. If he says that the pain is only slightly eased, no attention should be paid, since many patients like to avoid discomfiting the doctor, especially if students are present.

Local anaesthesia is a most valuable method of confirming localizations arrived at in soft tissue lesions. There is no other criterion comparably effective. By using it in every suitable case, the physician makes the patient the judge of the correctness of the diagnosis. It is very easy to fall into the habit of assuming that a certain set of symptoms and signs designate some lesion, and it is only when local anaesthesia has conspicuously failed in several consecutive cases that the physician is brought to realize that he has misconceptions on this particular point. In those numerous soft tissue lesions which lie deeply and in which the radiograph cannot help, it is the patient who, with the help of local anaesthesia, assists the physician to confirm where the lesion lies.

FAILURE TO ARRIVE AT A DIAGNOSIS

Patients in whom a thorough examination on the lines suggested in this chapter fails to disclose the source of the pain fall into five main categories.

1. Slight Pains

When the degree of pain is small, the diagnostic movements may not elicit it in the expected way. If such patients are examined again a week or two later, some of them will be found to have recovered spontaneously. Others will have got worse, and the lesion becomes clearly definable. This applies particularly to some cases of neuritis or of herpes zoster in which the first symptom may be severe pain unaccompanied by any physical signs. The characteristic signs may not appear for several days; until then no certain diagnosis is possible.

2. Very Severe Pain

During the first day or two after an injury of any severity, the pain may be such that the patient cannot state accurately which movements hurt and which do not. Moreover, especially at the shoulder and ankle, every passive and resisted movement may be found to cause pain, no clear pattern emerging at all. When localized tenderness is sought, widespread swelling may obscure it by making all spots painful on pressure. When real doubt exists, re-examination at the end of a few days suffices.

In the presence of severe pain, clinical examination may prove extremely difficult on account of an excess of physical signs, For example, in severe lumbago or sciatica the patient may be found lying very still, the smallest movement of any part of his trunk or lower limbs causing intense exacerbation. In such a degree of pain, the patient cannot allow the range of movement at unaffected joints (e.g. the hip) to be tested, nor can he cooperate when the power in his muscles is to be ascertained. Justifiable fear of pain rightly prevents him from moving.

In these cases the history must be given its full weight; gross signs such as muscle wasting or absence of tendon-reflexes must be noted and considered in the light of the fact that only a limited number of lesions cause agonizing pain. A radiograph may not be obtainable at first because of the difficulties of moving the patient. One must not forget to take such a patient's temperature; for a septic process of slow onset may give rise to pain starting in much the same way as disc lesions or secondary malignant deposits.

3. Lesions Outside the Sphere of Orthopaedic Medicine

The diffuse pains that characterize some diseases of the nervous system and viscera may be difficult to distinguish from the equally diffuse pains so often set up by lesions of the moving parts. Thus the absence of signs of disease of the bones, joints, muscles, etc., of a limb should lead to a neurological and arterial examination. X-ray of the lungs should be included. Inquiry about general health and visceral function must be made and, if necessary, followed up.

4. Genuinely Difficult Cases

Most of these are patients with obscure pain in the trunk, especially when the symptoms are felt anteriorly only. The distinction between visceral pain and that caused by lesions of the vertebral column may be most difficult. Moreover, not only may thoracic disc lesions give rise to purely anterior thoracic or abdominal pain, but both cervical and lumbar disc lesions may set up dural pain felt in the trunk far outside the relevant dermatome. Hence the search must be wide and areas examined from which, in theory, symptoms of such distribution cannot arise.

Another source of difficulty is a minor lesion obscured by psychogenic overlay, the patient putting forward a reasonable story but alleging a number of inconsistent responses on examination. It is then often advisable to have the patient treated for a week or two by the physiotherapist, even without a definite diagnosis, and to ask the almoner for a domestic inquiry. The handling to which the patient becomes accustomed, together with contact with two sensible and dispassionate persons, improves his capacity as a witness when he is next seen. Such treatment is less an evasion of responsibility than preparation for further examination after a clearer picture has developed.

Yet another difficulty is a double lesion. When two lesions lie close together, especially when a major lesion overshadows a minor one in its vicinity, or two adjacent tissues appear both affected, a decision on what action to take is not easy. For example, both the supraspinatus and the infraspinatus tendons may appear at fault, or a neck and a shoulder lesion to co-exist. In determining the best approach, the following criteria are useful:

(a) The most tractable

If, say, a patient has a minor cervical disc-displacement causing scapular pain and appears to have some disorder at the shoulder too, it is a matter of only a few minutes to carry out manipulative reduction at the neck and, when the pain derived from the neck has ceased, re-examine the shoulder.

(b) The commoner

Since supraspinatus tendinitis is twice as frequent as infraspinatus tendinitis, the statistical approach is reasonable in such cases.

(c) The most obvious

If one disorder is identified with certainty, it is either anaesthetized or treated until it no longer causes symptoms. This allows the second lesion to emerge during clinical examination later.

(d) *The most painful*

Severe pain from one lesion overshadows discomfort emanating from a lesser disorder. This will declare itself only after cure of, or anaesthesia induced at, the greater trouble.

(e) *The articular*

Vague aches apparently arising from extra-articular sources may be elicited when in fact only the joint is affected. The joint should be treated first and, when it has recovered, the patient is examined again.

5. Pain Devoid of Organic Basis

Patients with assumed or purely psychogenic symptoms constitute a real problem in orthopaedic medical clinics, to which are properly sent all cases of obscure pain for which an adequate physical explanation seems lacking. For the sake of the practitioner of orthopaedic medicine himself, no less than that of the staff of the department, such cases *must* be sorted out. Otherwise he may be led to adopt unwarranted opinions on the efficacy of some form of treatment, since dramatic (though usually ephemeral) cure may follow any therapeutic measure, merely as a result of suggestion. Moreover, it is most disheartening to the staff of a department to have to give treatment endlessly to patients who have no organic lesion.

Detection is seldom difficult. The patient's story may arouse suspicion as a most uncommon sequence of events is described and the pain found to spread more and more distantly as the narrative continues. The circumstances attending the onset of pain may be curious and tendentiously put forward and the patient emphasizes suffering rather than symptoms throughout. There may be reference that grossly transgresses the segmental boundaries. The pain may come and go in a most unlikely manner, and may not obey the generalization that referred pains do not cross the midline. The degree of disablement may vary from day to day, and be much in excess of the patient's complaints and of what examination reveals later.

A great number of active, passive and resisted movements should be performed, the examination beginning at joints as distant as possible from the site of alleged pain. Thus, if the upper limb is stated to hurt, the trunk movements may well be tried first. The examiner may find that the painfulness or not of a movement depends on variations in his tone of voice when asking if pain is elicited, or on the care and expectant attitude with which he attempts some passive movement. The same movement tested in different ways may elicit different answers, as may even the identical movement repeated a few minutes later.

The most striking finding in patients with pain devoid of organic basis is that no coherent pattern emerges, the patient appearing to answer at random and often contradicting himself. Alternatively, every movement at every joint may be stated to cause pain. Again, movements may be said to hurt in areas that they cannot affect. No patient, not even a doctor, when asked to perform a series of movements at several joints, can work out quickly in his mind which should and which should not cause pain. Diffuse tenderness is to be expected, and has led to the erroneous idea of 'diffuse fibrositis', 'generalized muscular rheumatism', and 'myalgia'.

It is less, however, on the failure to make a pattern out of the patient's responses than in the discovery of clear inconsistencies that a diagnosis of psychogenic pain may be confidently made. The response to the same movements may alter when performed with the patient standing and lying or on lying prone and lying supine. The range of movement at a joint may be found much limited in one direction and full in all the others in a manner that does not occur at that joint. Or the patient may be unable voluntarily to move a joint at which the passive range is full and muscle power, as tested by resisted movement, normal. If real doubt still exists, the patient may be put on to some indifferent treatment for a fortnight and then examined again. The examiner has recorded the findings, but the patient cannot remember his previous responses (unless they were all positive or all negative) and differences found on the two occasions afford a clear pointer.

The examiner should be on his guard against considering the symptoms of hypersensitive patients as psychogenic. Mere exaggeration does not prove that there is no lesion, for many patients endeavour to impress the examiner by too great a show of pain. In such cases there are no errors of quality but only of quantity. It is both unfair to patients and a hindrance to advancement in diagnosis to label every obscure pain as psychogenic or of little account. On the contrary, if difficult cases are examined repeatedly, some patients will be found ultimately to be suffering from a condition with which the examiner was previously unfamiliar. In others, the increasing disparity between the findings at different times confirms the lack of organic basis for the complaint.

Unfortunately, no test has yet been devised to distinguish between pain deliberately assumed (e.g. for financial purposes or to evoke domestic sympathy) and psychoneurosis, in which the disorder is unconsciously motivated.

THE NEED FOR ACCURACY

The question may be asked whether the time and trouble necessary to arrive at a correct diagnosis in soft tissue lesions is well spent. When methods of treatment with a wide effect are employed alone, the answer is in the negative. Clearly heat, exercises, diffuse massage and electrotherapy affect a large area rather than one spot; hence these measures can be ordered without a precise diagnosis, the more so as they do not afford appreciable benefit in any soft tissue lesion.

In orthopaedic medicine proper, however, great diagnostic accuracy is required. The question of when to manipulate and when not, may hinge on accurate localization of a lesion to within a quarter of an inch (e.g. in tennis-elbow), or an exact knowledge of its size and consistency (e.g. in a disc lesion). If 1 c.c. of hydrocortisone is to be injected, very little diagnostic latitude is allowable. Deep massage is a valuable remedy only when applied to the affected spot; therefore it can profitably be used only when a diagnosis correct to within a finger's breadth has been made.

The time saved by exact diagnosis is a great virtue. The lesion is singled out, the patient accurately treated; recovery is swift. He may be seen for a moment once or twice after the first occasion; then attendance ceases. By contrast, patients with vague disorders receiving vague treatment continue to attend, often for years, not only wasting the hospital's time and money and exasperating the physiotherapist, but in the aggregate taking up more of the doctor's time than if he had spent a reasonable period examining the patient at the first attendance. Again, by the time a doctor has driven half a dozen times to and from the house of a patient with lumbago in the course of some weeks, he has expended more time than he would by manipulative reduction at the first attendance. Humanitarian considerations and enlightened self-interest point the same way.

The Avoidance of Accurate Treatment

Accurate treatment of the types described in this book should be reserved for cases with an exact diagnosis. Nothing is more damaging to the cause of rational physiotherapy (and nothing is more disheartening for the physiotherapist herself) than to exert her best skill, time and strength on patients with ill-defined disorders. If adequate examination does not result in a clear diagnosis, the patient should receive palliative treatment (e.g. analgesics) or, if a more stimulating effect appears indicated, be put into an exercise class or given faradism. If such indifferent methods alleviate the symptoms, it is obvious that there was nothing much wrong

F

and the doctor is spared a mistaken supposition that a correct diagnosis was made and that accurate treatment was remarkably successful. If no benefit accures from such 'treatment', a second opportunity for examining the patient is afforded. Since precise treatment is adapted to each individual lesion, and has real effect on the tissues treated, it follows that harm can result when the wrong type of disorder is thus treated. Consider, for example, the damaging effect of massage to the area about the greater tuberosity of the humerus in a patient thought to have a supraspinatus tendinitis and in fact suffering from subdeltoid bursitis. Or the result of manipulating a supposed tennis-elbow if the true lesion is a traumatic arthritis of, or a loose body displaced within, the elbow joint. Such errors are by no means unknown and unjustly bring precise methods into disrepute.

Effective treatment by massage or manipulation nearly always hurts. Hence the individual as well as his lesion must be considered. Will the patient, though the nature of his disorder has been ascertained, be able to stand the requisite treatment? Alternatively, is the patient's frame of mind such that, if anything uncomfortable is done, he will wrongly allege that treatment has caused him lasting harm? A highly neurotic patient with, say, lumbago or a tennis-elbow may be quite unable to allow the proper manipulations. It is most unwise, in that case, to advise such treatment; for the physiotherapist will not be able to give it, and the patient feels that the medical man shows callousness and (after all, correctly) lack of understanding in ordering it. Again, patients anxious to prolong their disability welcome stern measures; for they can then claim that lasting harm has resulted. Even if such patients have some minor lesion on which the exaggerated complaint and excessive disablement are based, it is dangerous to treat that lesion without due regard for the patient's mental attitude. In pain largely psychogenic, removal of its minor organic basis is often very successful; in wilful exaggeration this endeavour is sure to fail.

Accurate physiotherapy will lapse into undeserved disregard if both lesions and patients are not selected with adequate care. Patients who cannot tolerate a painful measure, patients who are anxious not to get well and patients in whom an adequate diagnosis has not been made—in all these, exact treatment should be avoided.

Note

The matter set out in this chapter in successive editions of this book over the last twenty years has been in part repeated and confirmed by Beetham, Polley, Slocumb and Weaver (1965). The interested reader is referred to their book *Physical Examination of the Joints* (W. B. Saunders, Philadelphia).

7

The Head, Neck and Scapular Area

The chief difficulties when investigating pain in the head, neck and scapular area are these: (1) the misleading way in which pain and tenderness are referred; (2) belief in cervical spondylosis as a cause of pain and as a contra-indication to manipulation; (3) uncertainty about 'fibrositis'.

THEORETICAL CONSIDERATIONS

Pain of ligamentous origin appears to occur at the joints between occiput and atlas, and atlas and axis; it results in the old man's matutinal headache. This arises spontaneously in the elderly and is connected with the degeneration and limited movement that designate osteoarthritis, although equal degrees of osteophytosis can exist radiographically in those who do, and do not, have discomfort. At the remainder of the cervical joints osteoarthritis of itself causes no symptoms; there is no pain, merely a painless limitation of movement that makes the patient complain of stiffness and inability to turn the head properly when backing a car. An intra-articular displacement, i.e. pressure from a protruded fragment of disc, causes pain at a cervical joint no less than at a thoracic or lumbar level, whether or not osteoarthritis is present. The fact that attrition of the disc and osteophyte formation are symptomless becomes clear after manipulative reduction has been carried out on an allegedly 'osteoarthritic' neck. Moreover, in most cases the history, even taken by itself—rules out 'osteoarthritis' patients complaining of intermittent pain, unilateral pain, pain on coughing, sudden twinges on some movements; in such cases examination reveals the partial articular pattern of internal derangement. During manipulation the end-feel is not the bone-to-bone of osteophytes engaging but the softer resistance that is overcome with the production of the small click that heralds cessation of symptoms. Understanding of disc lesions in middle-aged and elderly patients will remain clouded until the idea of osteoarthritis or osteophyte formation as a cause of pain at any level between the third cervical and the fifth lumbar is laid at rest. Osteophytosis is the result, not the cause, of the disc lesions, and it is the latter which cause all the intermittent pain.

Osteophytes do at least exist. By contrast, cervical, scapular or pectoral 'fibrositis' is a purely imaginary concept based on palpation without previous assessment of the function of the relevant tissues. The secondary nature of what used to be called 'fibrositis' can be shown by clinical examination. This discloses that some of the active and passive neck movements evoke or increase the scapular pain, whereas the resisted neck, scapular and arm movements do not. The lesion ascribed to 'fibrositis' is thus shown to have a cervical articular origin, devoid of muscular component. An even more convincing proof lies in manipulation. Before this begins, the patient and examiner identify the very spot. As manipulative reduction at the neck progresses, the spot shifts from, let us say, the infraspinatus muscle to the supraspinatus, then to the rhomboid, then to the trapezius and, finally, when a full range of painless movement has been restored to the affected cervical joint, it has disappeared. In no circumstances could an area of real inflammation in a muscle be made to shift to another muscle and then to yet another in the course of seconds by manipulating a near-by joint.

Cervical Spondylosis

Spondylosis is a general term for the many different results of degeneration of the intervertebral discs. It is not a diagnosis, since the results of degeneration are so varied. A blunderbuss name of this sort is useful as an indication of aetiology, but is not exact enough a description for any decision on treatment; for no indication is afforded whether the pressure is due to an osteophyte or a protruded disc.

Spondylosis is in part a beneficient phenomenon. The osteophytes that form limit movement and ultimately serve to stabilize a joint containing a fragmented disc. They also increase the area of the weight-bearing surfaces, thus distributing the load over a larger area. Since clinical differentiation is not difficult if the instructions in this chapter are followed, the word should be dropped and replaced by the appropriate diagnosis.

'Spondylosis' at the neck includes:

(1) Symptomless osteophyte formation, seen radiologically, at vertebral body or foramen

(2) Symptomless narrowing of one or more joint spaces, indicating wear on the disc

(3) Osteoarthritis causing upper cervical pain or headache

(4) Osteophytic compression of one or more nerve-roots

(5) Osteophytic compression of the spinal cord, causing paraesthesia in hands and feet

(6) Osteophytic compression of the anterior spinal artery, causing paraplegia

(7) Osteophytic kinking of the vertebral artery by an outcrop on the superior articular process, affecting the basilar circulation

(8) Cervical disc lesion with unilateral or alternating scapular pain.

(9) Cervical disc lesion with bilateral pain in the neck

(10) Cervical disc lesion causing headache by extra-segmental dural reference

(11) Cervical disc lesion with unilateral scapulo-brachial pain without root-palsy

(12) Cervical disc lesion with unilateral scapulo-brachial pain with root-palsy

(13) Cervical disc lesion with bilateral aching in the upper limbs and paraesthetic hands as the result of bilateral protrusion

(14) Cervical disc lesion causing paraesthesia in hands and feet, as the result of central protrusion

(15) Cervical disc lesion compressing the spinal cord with one or more root-palsies in one or both upper limbs and spastic paresis in the lower limbs.

(16) The mushroom phenomenon at a cervical level.

Clearly, many of the conditions that are lumped together as 'cervical spondylosis' cannot be anything of the sort, since they get well after a time. Any disorder that was genuinely caused by a narrowed disc and osteophyte formation could never improve, since cartilage is avascular and cannot regenerate and osteophytes cannot become smaller.

REFERRED PAIN

Headache

Much doubt exists concerning the circumstances in which pain in the head can spring from the neck. Some disbelieve in the possibility altogether, ignoring the way pain may be made to radiate experimentally from the neck to the head (Cyriax, 1938). This was confirmed by Campbell and Parsons (1944) and by Brain (1963) who supported the concept of what he terms 'spondylotic' headache. Others point out that no nerve runs from the occiput to the forehead; but this anatomical objection is invalid, since referred pain does not travel down any nerve, being an error in cortical perception. In fact, reference of pain from neck to head is a commonplace, and has been described in succeeding editions of this book since 1947 but, as the symptoms do not correspond with the known headaches and may go on for years without altering or giving rise to signs of overt disease, these are often mistakenly dismissed as due to neurosis or, at least, as possibly organic but incurable. At times, differentiation is indeed difficult, but the distinction is important; for headache arising from the neck is among those most easily and lastingly relievable. It is therefore a great pity when the diagnosis is missed, since a situation arises in which lay-manipulators receive a gratuitous advertisement from medical men. A not uncommon sequence is: An elderly man is told that his headaches are caused by high blood pressure, whereas they are in fact unconnected and result from upper cervical osteoarthritis so apt to occur coincidentally at this age. He goes to a bonesetter; his neck is manipulated; his headache ceases. The patient, and doubtless the lay-manipulator too, are misled into supposing that manipulation of the neck alters autonomic tone and is the cure for hyperpiesis. Since these laymen assert their ability to cure a number of disorders that manipulation does not in fact alter, unhappy verisimilitude is given to these claims, and patients who really do suffer from arteriosclerosis are induced to waste time and money on fruitless visits.

Referred Headache

There are two ways in which headache arises from the neck: by segmental or extra-segmental reference (Cyriax, 1938, 1962).

Segmental Reference

The head is formed from the first and second cervical segments (the mandible from the third). The first and second cervical vertebrae are also derived from these two segments. Hence, on anatomical grounds, lesions of the occipito-atlantoid-axial joints give rise to pain felt to spread to any part of the head. Painful capsular contracture occurs some time after an injury—traumatic osteoarthritis leading to post-traumatic headache—or as age advances. The pain is usually felt to start at the centre of the upper neck, spreading to both sides, to the vertex (C1) and/or to the temples and forehead (C2). As happens elsewhere, local pain may be wholly absent, the patient then complaining only of the referred headache.

In this type of headache, the cardinal symptom is pain on waking every morning, felt in the occiput and head, or head only. This begins to ease after some hours, and it has gone by midday. The patient is then free till the next morning. There is nothing periodic about this headache; it appears on waking every day without fail, tending to last longer into the day as the years go by.

Extra-segmental reference

As has already been stated, the dura mater is the only tissue related to the locomotor system from which pain is referred extra-segmentally. Patients often describe pain felt to radiate from the mid-neck down to the scapular area and up to the temple, the forehead and behind one or both eyes, rarely to the bridge of the nose. This description of a pain occupying the territory of the upper thoracic to the second cervical dermatomes (i.e. traversing twelve segments) naturally directs attention to the dura mater, and therefore to the common cause for pressure on it: a disc protrusion.

A central disc lesion at a mid or lower cervical level may give rise to bilateral pain extending from the scapulae to the occipital area. Such widespread symptoms may suggest a multiple origin, and the cause is often thought to be cervical osteoarthritis at several levels, a notion to which the radiographic appearances in any elderly patient will lend spurious colour. An important diagnostic feature in these cases is provocation of dural pain by coughing, a symptom that is, of course, absent in pain of articular origin. Realization that osteoarthritis at the cervical joints other than the two uppermost of itself causes no discomfort should prevent this misdiagnosis. It is an important error; for such patients can often be fully relieved of their symptoms, but the manipulative technique required is different from that suited to matutinal headaches resulting from segmental reference.

Pain in the face

Local. There are a number of well-recognized local lesions that cause pain in the face. This may stem from an infected tooth or sinus, from the tempero-mandibular joint or from the facial bones themselves as the result of fracture, neoplasm, abscess or osteitis deformans. Then there is postherpetic neuralgia, trigeminal neuralgia (sometimes bilateral in disseminated sclerosis) and arteritis, which may set up intermittent claudication in the tongue or masseter muscles. Just as intracranial arterial dilatation gives rise to migraine, so may a similar affection of the arteries of the face give rise to periodic attacks of pain there.

Referred. It must be remembered that the face forms part of the second cervical segment; hence pain in the face may originate from the neck. There are two mechanisms: (*a*) segmental reference from a disc-lesion at the axial-third-cervical joint; (*b*) extra segmental reference from pressure on the dura mater exerted at any part of its cervical course. It is important, therefore, to examine the joints of the neck in any patient with obscure or long-lasting pain in the face. This also applies to patients with vertigo, tinnitus and positional nystagmus (Cope and Ryan, 1959).

Thoracic Reference

Pain can be referred extra-segmentally upwards to the head from a lesion causing pressure on the dura mater at an upper thoracic or any cervical level. Pain at one or both aspects of the upper posterior thorax may originate locally, but it is far more often referred from the lower cervical extent of the dura mater. Indeed, the probable cause of scapular pain is a cervical disc protrusion in the early (reducible) stage. Uncommonly, the pain may be pectoral, but felt within the body, less superficially than the scapular aching which appears to the patient to lie close under the surface. Anterior extra-segmental referred pain is no more a transgression of the boundaries of the dermatomes than posterior pain, but is rare, and may well be misdiagnosed as angina. Equally unanatomical is the interscapular pain, without any neckache, that may result from a cervical disc lesion protruding centrally and compressing the dura mater. Since it is accompanied by the same referred tenderness, this time centrally, as occurs unilaterally with scapular pain, the central thoracic pain and tenderness may well be ascribed to an upper thoracic spinal lesion. Compression of the eighth cervical or first or second thoracic nerve-roots by a disc-protrusion causes lower scapular pain, often felt at the fifth to seventh thoracic dermatome area. Diagnosis may prove difficult before the pain in the upper limb appears and outlines the relevant dermatome there. When the root-pain is absent, it can be extremely difficult to know whether such thoracic pains start from the neck or the upper thoracic part of the spine.

This diagnostic difficulty is enhanced by the fact that the neck-flexion stretches the dura mater in both the cervical and the thoracic regions; pain elicited by this movement is therefore ambiguous. If the other cervical and not the thoracic, or the other thoracic and not the cervical, movements hurt, the diagnosis is established, but there are cases with rather mixed signs which are anything but clear. Pain on scapular approximation strongly suggests a thoracic lesion, but is not a certainty. Yet, one must at least know beforehand whether manipulative reduction is to be attempted at a cervical or an upper thoracic joint.

Paraesthesia

Which fingers are involved and how far proximally the pins and needles extend should always be ascertained. If the inner one and a half, or one aspect of the outer three and a half digits, are involved, the relevant nerve-trunk must be examined from the base of the neck as far as the hand; no indication of the level of the impingement is afforded, except that it is not at the intervertebral foramen itself. If pins and needles are felt running from the hand to, say, the forearm, the source of pressure cannot lie at the wrist, since the lesion is always proximal to the upper level of the paraesthesia. If, by contrast, all the digits are affected, or any combination other than those mentioned, the level of pressure must lie above the final differentiation of the nerves forming the brachial plexus. Hence a complaint of pins and needles in fingers not supplied by *one* peripheral nerve affords a good indication that the pressure is exerted above the level of the shoulder. In such cases, a dermatomic distribution is to be expected and affords great diagnostic help. If pins and needles are felt in the feet as well, a cervical disc or osteophyte may be projecting centrally and transfixing the spinal cord, but diseases like a spinal neuroma, pernicious anaemia, diabetes and peripheral neuritis must then be excluded.

Misleading Tenderness

When the dura mater is compressed, tenderness of the muscles at the site of the pain thus caused is a constant and most misleading phenomenon. This is a genuine, deep, localized muscular tenderness, and digital pressure here is stated by the patient not only to have established the exact site of his trouble, but also may evoke the pain referred to the limb. Palpation without previous examination of function in such cases has led to the ascription of such pains to a disorder—regarded as imaginary (Cyriax, 1948)—called 'fibrositis', and various authorities have described myalgic spots and trigger-areas. These exist; but they are the result, not the cause, of the lesion, as reasoned evaluation of the physical signs present will quickly demonstrate.

The suggestion has been made that such tender areas are the result of small areas of fasciculation, secondary to the lower motor neurone lesion. This is not so; for the tender areas are commonly found at the trapezius, rhomboid or spinatus muscle in, for example, seventh cervical root-palsies: muscles belonging to quite other segments, at which the electromyograph can in any case be employed to prove that fibrillation is absent. This phenomenon must be recognized; otherwise minor subluxations in the cervical joints will continue to be misdiagnosed as muscle lesions until root pain supervenes ('fibrositis of the trapezius leading to neuritis'), and the best moment lost for performing manipulative reduction. Palpation for tenderness must be avoided in cervical disc lesions, for it is positively fallacious. It is only in the rare event of the pattern for a muscle lesion appearing when the diagnostic movements are interpreted that the muscles at the base of the neck and scapula should be palpated.

TEMPORAL ARTERITIS

Giant-cell arteritis scarcely occurs before the age of sixty and the main incidence is over seventy. It is a self-limiting disorder, seldom lasting longer than a year. As elderly patients usually have evidence of osteo-arthritis in X-rays of the neck, the pain of arteritis is often mistaken for 'cervical spondylosis'. Years of matutinal headache should not be confused with the short history of increasing pain in scalp, face and neck of arteritis. The scalp may become so tender that the pressure of the pillow at night hurts.

Examination shows the temporal arteries not to pulsate, to be tender and, often, nodular. The pterygoid muscles may claudicate, and if the lingual arteries are affected the tongue cannot be protruded fully.

Energetic treatment with high doses of cortisone is an urgent necessity; for thrombosis of the ophthalmic artery with irretrievable blindness may occur and must be prevented at all costs.

THE BASILAR SYNDROME

Vertigo may be dependent on the position of the neck.

The basilar artery is formed by the junction of the two vertebral arteries. Blood is supplied to the temporal lobes and visual cortex by the two posterior cerebral arteries that spring from the basilar artery. If the circle of Willis is atheromatous and cannot quickly supply extra blood, temporary ischaemia (without thrombosis) of these areas of the brain can be caused by pressure on the vertebral arteries. Vertigo on neck extension is the common complaint; or the patient may have to change from sitting to lying very slowly for fear of severe giddiness. Vision may be momentarily blurred as posture alters.

Rotation about the odontoid process accounts for at least 45 degrees, the remaining movement up to 90 degrees being distributed between the other cervical joints and de Kleyn (1939) noted that rotation and extension of the neck to one side obstructed the vertebral artery on the stretched side at the level of the atlas. Young (1967) showed by angiography that the vertebral artery is also compressed at the second to sixth levels by rotation towards that side. Hence the vertebral artery may be menaced by osteophytes: both those projecting anteriorly from a facet joint and those projecting laterally from the intervertebral joint. It is also endangered by each inferior articular facet if the vertebra moves backwards during movement towards extension. When, therefore, an elderly patient complains of non-progressive symptoms of this kind related to posture and neck-movement without deafness, tinnitus or evidence of neurological disease, it is highly probable that osteophytosis is compressing the vertebral arteries, thus reducing the basilar flow momentarily.

A test has been devised to detect deficient circulation through the vertebral artery. The patient stands with his eyes closed and his arms stretched out horizontally in front of him, keeping quite still. He is then asked to rotate his head fully to one side and stay so for a minute, then to turn his head the other way. His outstretched arms are observed and any straying of the arm away from the parallel suggests cerebral ischaemia caused by the cervical rotation. If the test is positive and careful manipulation during strong traction has no effect, decompression of the vertebral artery at the point of impact as demonstrated by arteriography may be indicated.

MIGRAINE

The vascular origin of migraine is not in doubt; for angiography has demonstrated the vascular spasm in the cerebral arteries. By contrast, the extracranial blood vessels dilate, and may be felt throbbing not only by the patient but by the examiner. The factors that trigger off an attack in susceptible subjects are unknown, nor do we know whether, in different individuals, the attacks are provoked by a common mechanism.

The history is particularly valuable in distinguishing migraine. In clear cases, a long history—often starting in adolescence—of sudden onset of unilateral throbbing headache is characteristic. It may change sides; it spreads to the whole neck; photophobia, visual hallucinations, tunnel-vision and prostration occur; vomiting brings relief. Sometimes, however, the headache is bilateral and not accompanied by typical symptoms; then the diagnostic feature is recurrent severe headache of unprovoked onset, without stiffness of the neck, followed by sudden complete subsidence of all pain until the next attack. Occipital migrainous neuralgia also behaves in this way.

An attack of migraine can sometimes be instantly aborted by strong traction on the neck. Half a minute's traction in some cases is regularly successful, in others not. The mechanism is obscure (it may be connected with the stretching of the carotid artery) and the phenomenon would clearly repay further study, since it affords one criterion whereby two different types of migraine can be differentiated.

For many years, I supposed, on what appeared to me logical grounds, that manipulation of the neck could have no preventive effect on migraine, but only on those headaches mistaken for migraine. But a minority of patients have reported, some years after the reduction by manipulation of a cervical disc-displacement, that ever since then attacks of obvious migraine have ceased. Since this happy result is obtained only in the middle-aged or elderly, it may well be that an occasional factor in periodic headache is that described by A. Kovass (1955). His careful radiological studies showed that the superior articular process of a cervical vertebra can develop an osteophyte that presses on the vertebral artery and the sympathetic fibres running with it. Were pressure at this point exerted by a small displaced fragment of exfoliated articular cartilage within the lateral joint, manipulative reduction could prove lastingly successful.

HISTORY IN NECKACHE

In the case of cervical disc protrusion the history is usually characteristic. There are eight recognizable stages. *First*, the young patient is apt to suffer attacks, once a year perhaps, of waking with severe unilateral pain in the neck, which is fixed in visible deformity: acute torticollis. The pain is constant and severe for two or three days, spontaneous recovery taking seven to ten days. Recurrence is to be expected. Acute torticollis is the analogue of lumbago: a sudden large displacement of a fragment of disc. *Secondly*, attacks of intermittent scapular aching begin during the patient's late twenties or thirties. They last several weeks and again are unilateral, but not always on the same side of the neck. *Thirdly*, during the fifties or later the ache becomes constant, the loose fragment of disc no longer spontaneously returning to its bed. *Fourthly*, at any time after the age of thirty-five, the scapular ache may become much worse and progress to unilateral severe root-pain, much worse at night with or without pins and needles in the hand. The brachial pain gets worse for a fortnight, remains severe for four to eight weeks and then subsides gradually. Patients with a root-paresis usually lose their pain in three months; those without, in four months. *Fifthly*, a bilateral protrusion may set up discomfort in both upper limbs with pins and needles in all the digits of both hands. *Sixthly*, a central protrusion may bulge out the posterior ligament and compress the dura mater, which becomes adherent. At this stage, constant bilateral aching from occiput to scapulae is to be expected in a patient aged sixty or more. *Seventhly*, the spinal cord becomes compressed and pins and needles appear in hands and/or feet, with bilateral aching in the upper limbs. *Lastly*, an osteophyte obliterates the anterior spinal artery and paraplegia results.

The common site for pain arising from a cervical disc lesion is the scapular area, often with upward reference towards the ear. Rarely the pain is pectoral or felt in one axilla only. Cough seldom hurts, whereas in a thoracic disc lesion both cough and a deep breath usually increase the pain. Swallowing may be uncomfortable in cervical disc protrusion. Scapular pain also occurs in neuralgic amyotrophy and suprascapular and long thoracic neuritis. Rarely, pain may be referred from the shoulder joint or the sterno-clavicular joint to the base of the neck. There is nothing very characteristic about the head- and neckache of temporo-occipital arteritis. It should be suspected if the headache is severe and comes on without previous attacks of neckache in an elderly patient, whose neck on examination reveals no articular signs sufficient to cause more than minor discomfort.

In elderly patients, headache or bilateral occipito-cervical pain can arise from the ligaments of the upper two cervical joints. This is the elderly patient's matutinal headache, easing after some hours. Though the pain is not severe, it is very trying since the ordinary analgesics have little or no effect on it. Unilateral cervical pain in the elderly is usually caused by a disc lesion with displacement of a fragment of cartilage within the osteo-arthritic joint; it is *not* due to osteoarthritis as such. It is the displacement that hurts, whether or not osteoarthritis is present, as manipulative reduction quickly demonstrates. In younger patients, ankylosing spondylitis gives rise, of course, to pain and stiffness at the neck radiating to the head; as a rule the history of lumbo-sacral pain finally reaching the neck gives the clue; but the lumbo-thoracic condition may evolve painlessly, and difficulty in turning the neck be noticed as the first symptom.

Secondary deposits give rise to central pain and marked limitation of movement coming on much more quickly than the slow onset of osteo-arthritic stiffness. This speed of onset is characteristic. Movement becomes rapidly limited and the pain more severe week by week rather than year by year.

Inspection of the Neck

The neck may be held in an asymmetrical posture; if so, note should be taken whether the deformity is a pure lateral list or contains an element of rotation as well; if there is pain, the deviation may be towards or away from the painful side. The existence of a compensating thoracic curve is determined. If this is present, adolescent scoliosis, unilateral cervical rib, Klippel-Feil deformity or a past thoracoplasty is probably the cause of the asymmetry.

Congenital Torticollis

Painless congenital contracture of one sterno-mastoid muscle results in the neck being fixed in side-flexion towards the affected side and rotation away from it. In babies there may be a swelling on the muscle, but usually there is not.

Neglected cases are seen in which the contracture has resulted in permanent postural deformity of the neck and facial asymmetry. Treatment should have been instituted by stretching out the sterno-mastoid muscle and subsequent maintenance of the overcorrected position as soon as the baby was born. If this was not done, division of the muscle is required in adolescence, followed by vigorous after-treatment.

Acute Torticollis in Children

This is an interesting condition. Children between the ages of five and ten, usually after a sore throat, suddenly develop a stiff neck, with little or no pain. Inspection shows the neck to be held in flexion towards one side and rotation in the opposite direction. The resisted neck movements are not weak but may be slightly painful. There may be glands in the neck, particularly on the contracted side, suggesting recent tonsillitis. The radiograph reveals the postural deformity, of course, but no other lesion.

I feel sure that this condition is not caused by a cervical intervertebral disc lesion, nor by acute myositis or anterior poliomyelitis. It resolves spontaneously in about a fortnight, and probably results from a swollen gland lying under and irritating the sterno-mastoid muscle, thereby causing reflex spasm. This seems to be a minor form of the well-known fixation of the neck from glandular enlargement that characterizes the anginal variety of glandular fever. At all events, cure appears to be hastened by short-wave diathermy to the mid-cervical area; manipulation and exercises are useless and unkind.

In children occasional cases of afebrile otitis media occur. The presenting symptom may then be merely pain in the neck, and the only sign, for the first week or two, asymmetrical fixation. The neck is held immobile by muscle spasm and the slightest attempt at any passive movement provokes pain and is resented and strongly resisted. This is a greater degree of limitation of movement than occurs in the transient torticollis described above, moreover, movement is equally limited in every direction. Such signs, in the absence of X-ray evidence of disease of the cervical spine, should lead to aural examination. Retropharyngeal abscess may also start in this way.

Acute Torticollis in Adults and Adolescents

Acute torticollis is rare before the age of twelve but begins to be quite common at about fifteen. Whereas disc lesions at thoracic and lumbar levels causing root pain are not infrequent in adolescence, cervical disc lesions, though a common cause of scapular aching, appear not to cause other than ephemeral brachial pain before the age of thirty-five. Exceptionally, patients who have suffered a severe accident to the neck may develop root pain some years younger.

The patient, usually aged fifteen to thirty, wakes with a 'crick in his neck', i.e. the neck fixed in side-flexion sometimes towards, sometimes away from, the painful side, but without rotation deformity. Marked limitation of only one lateral and only one rotation movement is found on examination, and the pain is unilateral. In other words, part of the joint is blocked by displacement of a fragment of disc. The patient has lain with the neck held sideways and rotated for hours and the constant angulation of the joint has led to a slow shift of the loose fragment. This becomes suddenly and very painfully apparent when the patient sits up and applies weight-bearing to the joint at the same moment as he tries to move it to the neutral position. The pain is constant and severe for a few days and then eases; all symptoms have gone by seven to ten days after the onset.

Lumbago may cause lateral deviation of the lumbar spine, but more often fixation in flexion. In acute torticollis, the frequency is reversed and a list to one side is common, but a neck fixed in flexion is rare. But it does occur in early postero-central displacement in youngish persons, and such cases must be treated with great care to avoid further retropulsion towards the spinal cord or stretching of the posterior longitudinal ligament.

Spasmodic Torticollis

The diagnosis is made on inspection. The patient is seen suddenly to twist his head, always in the same direction, by an apparently irresistible active movement. The complaint is of social inconvenience, not pain. The movement can be prevented by the patient's or the examiner's manual pressure, which can also be used to overcome the muscles and rotate the head back into the neutral position. The muscles give way in the manner suggesting neurological hypertonus; there is strong resistance at first, but when the muscles begin to give, all resistance ceases. Apart from the repeated movement, nothing abnormal is found when the neck is examined. In organic disease, associated movements may relax the spasm. For example, the patient's head may be fixed in extreme rotation from which position he cannot move it except by bringing his hand to his mouth, whereupon the head automatically turns forward.

Spasmodic torticollis had always been regarded as a tic, hysterically produced. Critchley (1938), however, distinguishes four types: (1) purely psychogenic; (2) following epidemic encephalitis (often transitory); (3) forming part of a more widespread extrapyramidal lesion; and (4) a gradually progressive tonic-clonic spasm not confined to the neck muscles. By performing an intracerebral injection, Russell (1938) produced spasmodic torticollis accidentally in a monkey. Post-mortem examination showed a subthalamic infarct.

In early mild cases, it is worth while trying to teach a co-operative patient to move the head in the opposite direction at the moment when he feels the involuntary movement about to begin; this may keep the head still. Other physiotherapy is useless; hypnotism has an occasional success. If the symptoms warrant, assessment of which muscles are causing the movement should be attempted; denervation by means of root-section and/or division of the spinal accessory nerve may then bring about marked improvement.Sorensen and Hamby (1966) describe excellent results in half of all cases. Since sterotaxic surgery has proved a success in dealing with the torsion spasm of muscular dystonia deformans. Cooper (1965) has reported on this approach in spasmodic torticollis.

Hysterical Torticollis

These cases are easy to detect; for the patient contracts his vertebro-scapular muscles, thus keeping the scapula hunched, as well as flexing the neck towards that side. Elevation of the scapula can play no part in the organic lesion resulting in the head being held fixed in side-flexion. Moreover, no disorder exists in which an adult's neck becomes suddenly so painfully fixed that no movement is possible in any direction. This is also hysterical, the muscle contraction being easily overcome by passive movement during persuasion.

In Parkinsonism, the neck may become gradually stiff and painful, owing to muscle rigidity, and in such elderly patients the radiograph is sure to show 'osteoarthritis', thus obscuring the true diagnosis. Inspection of the facies affords the clue.

Inspection of the Scapular Area

The level at which the scapulae lie is noted; a downward and outward displacement suggests trapezial weakness secondary to accidental division of the spinal accessory nerve during an operation for glands in the neck.

A localized neuritis of this nerve is a rarity. Prominence of the vertebral border of one scapula suggests a long thoracic neuritis with paralysis of one serratus anterior muscle: this may be called 'winged scapula' but should not; for it draws attention to the result and not the cause. If both scapulae are affected thus, and both muscles found weak, myopathy is highly probable. A thoracic kyphosis in children and thin adults makes the lower angles of the scapulae stand out prominently. The appearance results from a flat bone being held against a convex surface. As the scapula is applied to the thorax superiorly by muscular tension, it is the lower part of the bone that projects. (Such patients should be treated for the causative kyphosis; exercises to strengthen the thoraco-scapular muscles naturally have no good effect.) Occasionally inspection of the scapula reveals isolated wasting of the infraspinatus muscle; rupture, myopathy, traumatic or suprascapular neuritis or severe arthritis of the shoulder then have to be considered. The contour of the thorax itself and of the arm is also noted.

Fixation of one scapula at a higher level than the other characterizes congenital elevation of the scapula (Sprengel's shoulder). The levator scapulae muscle is then replaced by abnormal bone—the suprascapula.

Enlargement of the clavicle provides an occasional manifestation of osteitis deformans; subluxation at the sterno-clavicular joint gives rise to false appearance of enlargement by making the bone prominent. Congenital absence of the clavicle, nearly always bilateral, and with such undue mobility of the scapulae that the shoulders can be made to meet in the front of the sternum, characterizes cleido-cranial dysostosis.

Examination of Neck Movements

To examine the active, resisted and passive movements of the neck, the patient sits on a couch or stands. The former is preferred as he is then prevented from moving his trunk as well when asked to move his neck, and the examiner is well placed for resisting the neck and scapular movements. Neck movements are: flexion, extension, flexion to each side, rotation to each side. Their range is noted, whether or not each sets up pain, and if a movement hurts, where the pain is felt. The painfulness of the resisted movements is assessed; weakness is a rarity. The passive movements show whether or not a full range at the cervical joints exists and provide useful data for correlation with the findings on active movement. If the passive movements are tested with the patient lying supine, it must be remembered that a greater range exists in this position than when the patient sits up, on account of the postural tone present in the muscles during the erect position. Hence, minor discrepancies in the range of movement have no significance and provide no evidence that a psychogenic disorder is present.

Since testing the resisted movements so seldom causes pain (except in fracture of the first rib, anginal glandular fever or acute adult torticollis), it becomes clear that at the neck articular lesions predominate and muscle lesions hardly occur. Therefore, the chief virtue in examination of the muscles against resistance is the information afforded in cases of suspected psychogenic disorder.

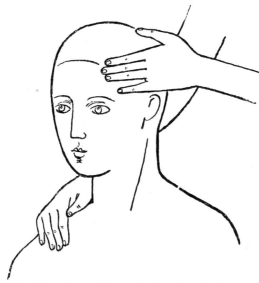

FIG. 23. Resisted side-flexion of neck. The examiner's one hand steadies the patient's shoulder while the other resists the movement of the head.

Gross wasting of both trapezius muscles and of the erector muscles of the neck occurs in myopathy. The patient has difficulty in holding the head up for long, and the muscle wasting on each side results in great prominence of the spinous processes of the cervical vertebrae. Scleroderma of face and hands may coexist in these cases. On account of the flexion deformity and muscle wasting, these signs may be mistaken for arthritis at the cervical joints: an error that the radiograph, if the patient is middle-aged, appears to confirm. Myasthenia gravis occasionally first shows itself as an inability to hold the head up for long, e.g. at the theatre. In paralysis agitans, pain and limitation of active neck movements are sometimes the presenting symptoms, but the passive range is not limited. This discrepancy leads to immediate realization that voluntary control is at fault. A sudden extension strain to the neck muscles may overstretch the longus colli muscles; if so, the patient cannot lift his head from the pillow in bed and resisted flexion remains weak for about a fortnight.

Examination of Scapular Movements

The patient is asked to shrug his shoulders; this demonstrates whether or not the scapula possesses normal mobility in relation to the thorax.

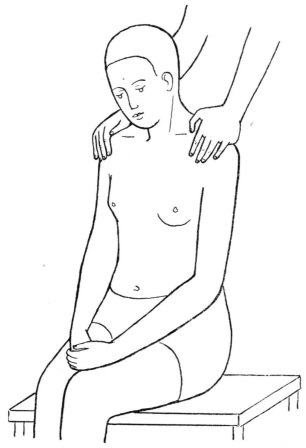

FIG. 24. Resisted elevation of scapulae. The examiner's hands press downwards as the patient shrugs his shoulders.

Crepitus on this movement is noted. Pulmonary neoplasm, contracture of the costocoracoid fascia, arthritis at the sterno-clavicular joint and secondary malignant deposits in the scapula limit passive mobility. In advanced spondylitis ankylopoetica the acromio-clavicular joint may suffer ankylosis; scapular movement is then grossly limited and the arm cannot be raised beyond the horizontal. If paraesthesia appears in the hands after the scapulae have been kept elevated for a minute or so, the thoracic outlet syndrome is present. Bringing the scapulae strongly backwards may abolish the radial pulse when the space between the clavicle and the first rib is unduly small. This occurs in some normal persons, but also suggests the thoracic outlet syndrome.

The resisted scapular movements are tested next: (1) elevation (trapezius and levator scapulae muscles), (2) forward movement (pectoralis minor and serratus anterior), (3) backward movement (rhomboids and lower trapezius), and (4) pressing against a wall with the arms held forward horizontally (serratus anterior). It must be remembered that the active scapular movements also affect the joints at each end of the clavicle. Scapular approximation stretches the dura mater via the uppermost thoracic nerve-roots, thus causing pain in the chest in thoracic disc lesions.

Although the neck, thorax and scapulae have now been tested, it is quite unsafe to stop the examination at this point, even if the patient has purely scapular or cervical pain. The upper limb must be examined next for evidence of a neurological lesion. Unless muscular weakness is carefully sought, a lesion of a nerve-root or a nerve-trunk may escape detection. Moreover, pulmonary sulcus tumour or neoplasm in the cervical spine cannot be excluded in the earliest stage merely by relying on the radiograph. This may reveal nothing at a time when examination of the forearm and hand reveals marked muscle weakness. Finally, evidence of an upper motor neurone lesion should be sought; for a central posterior protrusion at a cervical or thoracic joint may compress the spinal cord.

Summary

Full examination for scapular pain of somatic origin thus consists of:

(1) Inspection

(2) Testing the joints of the neck, scapula and thorax by active and passive movements

(3) Testing the muscles of the neck, scapula and arm by resisted movements

(4) Neurological examination of the upper limb for lower motor neurone lesion

(5) Neurological examination of the lower limb for upper motor neurone lesion.

Interpretation

Neck Movements

Neck-flexion stretches both the cervical and the thoracic extent of the dura mater; hence this movement will elicit the pain in both a cervical and a thoracic disc lesion; at either level central or unilateral pain at any scapular level may result. The diagnosis rests on which *other* movements prove painful—cervical or thoracic. Pain on scapular approximation nearly always indicates that the thoracic spine is affected, since this movement draws up the thoracic but not the cervical extent of the dura mater.

The *capsular pattern* at the cervical joints is: no limitation of flexion, equal degree of limitation of side-flexion and rotation, some or great limitation of extension. Painless restriction in an elderly patient signifies osteoarthritis, i.e. painless stiffness. If any passive movement other than flexion causes pain, and especially if this is unilateral, a disc lesion is present at the symptomless osteoarthritic joint. Gross limitation of passive movement in a young person, coming on slowly, characterizes ankylosing spondylitis. If so the lumbo-thoracic spine is already fixed and the sensation of bone-to-bone is evoked early at the extremes of passive rotation and side-flexion at the neck. Marked limitation of movement in the capsular pattern, coming on quickly (i.e. in the course of weeks or at most a few months), accompanied by pain steadily increasing in severity, strongly suggests secondary neoplasm. Invasion at the fourth to seventh levels is easily identified by the neurological signs when the upper limbs are examined, even though no particular discomfort has yet reached the arm. But at the upper three levels muscle weakness is seldom found; hence detection is more difficult. However, in secondary neoplasm the muscles are invaded too, with the result that the resisted rotation also proves painful, so painful sometimes that the patient is unwilling to press hard. If doubt still exists, and the radiograph is uninformative, gentle passive movements carried out with the patient supine elicit the twang of muscle spasm, when metastases are present. If this sensation is elicited, the radiograph taken a few weeks later discloses the osseous rarefaction.

In myeloma, however, the onset is more gradual and the restriction of movement less obvious, even when the subsequent radiograph shows considerable erosion of bone; in such a case, a root-palsy in the upper limb that is too extreme or bilateral or has lasted too long provides the diagnostic hint.

Arthritis

Limited movement in the capsular pattern at the cervical joints may be caused by (1) osteoarthritis, (2) spondylitic arthritis, (3) rheumatoid arthritis, (4) recent fracture, (5) post-concussional adhesions, and (6) disease of bone.

Osteoarthritis at the upper two cervical joints leads to a ligamentous contracture, causing pain in the occiput and forehead, worst in the morning. The patient also finds, for example, that he is embarrassed in trying to reverse a car by inability fully to turn his head. Osteoarthritis at the lower cervical joints causes no symptoms, merely painless stiffness. If a disc lesion occurs at an osteoarthritic joint, pain results identical with the pain caused by a displacement at a joint devoid of osteoarthritis.

Since osteophyte formation is the result of degeneration of the disc leading to ligamentous pull and consequent raising up of periosteum at the articular margins, disc lesions are particularly common at osteoarthritic joints, not as the result but the cause of the osteophytes visible on the radiograph. This has led to the idea that osteoarthritis at the neck is painful. It is important theoretically for, if osteoarthritis were the cause of patients' symptoms, no treatment could avail. In fact, if the displacement can be corrected, the allegedly osteoarthritic pain ceases. The demonstration of osteophytes and diminished joint spaces by radiography in no way contra-indicates manipulation by the methods employed by the orthopaedic physician, whereas forcing movement by the methods of osteopathy or chiropraxy is apt to aggravate the condition, as does manipulation under anaesthesia. The elderly patient's tolerance of discomfort is diminished and the amount of distraction possible at his joint is reduced by osteophytes and capsular contracture. Hence, the orthopaedic physician's technique involving strong traction is the method of choice in such cases.

Ankylosing spondylitis results in increasing fixation and finally ankylosis in flexion; stiffness in the joints in this disorder precedes local radiographic evidence of the disease by many years. If lumbo-thoracic involvement has progressed painlessly—as may happen—the diagnosis may remain obscure unless the whole back is inspected. The radiographic appearance, not of the cervical spine, but of the sacro-iliac joints, is diagnostic.

Wedge-fracture of a cervical vertebral body, left untreated, usually becomes symptomless after a month. It is often first discovered years later when the neck is X-rayed on account of a disc lesion. Radiographic signs of osteophyte formation at the cervical spinal joints is compatible with full painless function; by contrast, in some elderly patients with capsular contracture causing marked limitation of all cervical movement, the radiograph does not show a single osteophyte.

Rheumatoid arthritis may affect the spinal joints, usually after many years of chronic disease, causing bone atrophy and even such inflammatory destruction of ligament that the bones subluxate. Conlon, Isdale and Rose (1966) studied 658 patients' necks, half with osteo- and half with rheumatoid arthritis. They found disc-degeneration equally in both groups more often at the fifth–sixth joint, but multiple disc-narrowing without osteophytosis and atlanto-axial subluxation was confined to the rheumatoid cases. Rheumatoid arthritis of the cervical joints occurring in the early stage of the disease or as an isolated phenomenon is rare. The diagnosis is made when the patient lies down and the feel of the joint on passive movement is ascertained. In spondylitis the end is reached abruptly by bony block; in osteoarthritis the movement comes to a fairly hard stop, but in early rheumatoid arthritis the joint has the characteristic 'empty' feeling, i.e. the movement ends without any contact of bone, ceasing at a point which the examiner can tell is far short of how far the joint will go structurally. Manipulation is strongly contra-indicated; indeed, no treatment helps appreciably.

There is one disorder that may give rise to combined articular and muscular pain: post-concussional syndrome. The patient lies in bed for some months after a head injury, often fracture of the skull. During this time it is not feasible to give neck exercises. Hence healing in the absence of adequate movement occurs both at the damaged upper cervical joints and at the muscular attachments at the occiput. Such patients are often suspected of psychoneurotic pain; yet massage to the muscle origin together with manipulation of the joints often affords lasting relief.

Disc lesions

In disc lesions the partial articular pattern is found. In acute torticollis, the pain is unilateral and though the extremes of five, rarely all six, passive and active movements provoke considerable pain, the pattern of limitation is diagnostic. Gross limitation is present of one side-flexion movement, and of the rotation movement towards the same side; often no movement at all in either of these directions is possible. By contrast the other four movements are of full range, most extremes hurting. In minor more chronic displacement, four, three or two movements prove painful at the extreme, and two, three or four do not. The examiner should beware if only one passive movement hurts, the other five not, especially if the painful movement is side-flexion away from the painful side. Any costo-scapulo-clavicular lesion, or one at the apex of the lung, may cause pain when it is passively stretched. If resisted side-flexion towards the painful side also hurts, a lesion at the first rib, e.g. stress fracture, is the

probability. A painful arc, usually on extension or on rotation is pathognomonic of a disc lesion. When root-pain is present, some of the neck
movements increase the scapular pain in exactly the same way as if root-
pain were not present. Occasionally, one, two or three of the six movements provoke brachial pain, or paraesthesia in the hand, or both. If so,
the likelihood of possible reduction is very small. When a patient has
nearly recovered from an attack of root-pain, the neck movements may
no longer hurt in the scapular area, the diagnostic clue (apart from the
history) being the characteristic pattern of root-weakness on examination
of the upper limb. In chronic central posterior disc protrusion, the neck
movements, surprisingly enough, may be merely uncomfortable in a
vague general sort of way; alternatively a full (for his age) and painless
range may be present. Sometimes the extreme of neck-flexion may elicit
the pins and needles in hands or feet or both—a sign that is shared with
disseminated sclerosis, when an active plaque is present at a lower cervical
or upper thoracic level of the cord.

Subacute Arthritis of the Atlanto-axial Joint

This is a rare condition, encountered in my experience only in men
aged twenty-five to forty years old. The patient complains of several
weeks' increasing stiffness and discomfort in the centre of the upper neck.
There has been no previous neck trouble, and, if the patient has had osteopathy, it has merely caused some hours' added pain.

Examination shows a full range of flexion, extension and side-flexion at
the joints of the neck, but gross limitation of rotation, which may be
restricted to 10 degrees or 20 degrees in both directions. This unusual
finding naturally engenders caution, but fever is absent, the X-ray picture
and the E.S.R. are normal; there has been no sore throat; no glands or
mastoid tenderness is present, and examination of the limbo-thoracic spine
shows no evidence of ankylosing spondylitis.

The patient is asked to lie down and the end-feel of rotation is assessed.
The movement comes to a soft stop, quite unlike the bone-hard end-feel of
spondylitis or advanced osteoarthritis (neither of which could come on in
a few weeks), the crisp end-feel of a disc lesion, or the twang of the muscle
spasm that characterizes secondary malignant deposits.

The cause of this condition is not clear, but it is presumably caused by
non-specific inflammation since a few days' indomethacin (25 mg. t.d.s)
restores full painless range. The fact that this disorder is treated by lay-
manipulators makes me very sceptical of the alleged sensitivity of their
hands, since I should have said that anyone could feel the unsuitability of
the end-feel.

Other Disorders

Limitation of movement in the capsular pattern appearing at once after injury suggests fracture. The same limitation of movement coming on gradually after a severe injury suggests 'traumatic osteoarthritis'. This lesion, if organic lesion it is, appears confined to patients who are claiming compensation for an injury, and though the limitation of passive range is perfectly genuine, and can be felt to be so when the joint is moved during manipulation, I am in two minds whether it really causes symptoms. Limitation of active, but not passive movement at the neck occurs in paralysis agitans. Annoyingly enough, in the early stage of neuralgic amyotrophy, although there is no articular lesion, the neck movements often hurt in the cervico-scapular area in an uncharacteristic manner. The nature of the disorder is ascertained when the upper limbs are examined and muscles found paralysed at random, not according to the pattern of one root.

Pain on resisted movement occurs in neoplasm, occipital arteritis, when resisted extension and side-flexion compress the tender artery. After concussion, a patient may have lain unconscious or uncooperative for days after the accident and adhesions may have formed both about his cervical joints and at the muscle insertions at the occiput.

No lesion exists that causes sudden complete inability to move the head in an otherwise healthy patient. This event characterizes hysteria, when active movement may suddenly become impossible in all directions. Examination shows the exaggeration, and when passive movement is attempted, much resistance is encountered at first. It gradually gives, and finally a full range of passive movement is disclosed, with no pain at extremes but a gush of tears instead.

Scapular Movements

If scapular pain is brought on by the scapular movements, the following seven patterns occur.

(1) The active and passive scapular movements all hurt; the resisted do not. A first or second thoracic root-lesion. Some radiation will soon appear to the ulnar border of the forearm and palm (T1) or along the medial aspect of the arm to the inner side of the elbow (T2).

(2) Active, and full passive, elevation of the scapula hurts; the forward and backward movements do not. The resisted movements are painless. (a) Arthritis at the sterno-clavicular joint. When its posterior ligaments are affected, the pain may be felt only at the back of one side of the neck. (b) Strain of the costo-coracoid fascia. If so, full elevation

of the arm also hurts at the pectoro-scapular area. (c) Healed apical phthisis. Dense scarring here also limits the mobility of the costo-coracoid fascia.

(3) Active and passive elevation of the scapula are painful and limited but the resisted movements painless. History of trauma and no damage to bone: (a) haematoma lying in contact with the costo-coracoid fascia. No history of trauma: apical pulmonary neoplasm should be suspected and the small muscles of the hand examined. The radiograph soon becomes diagnostic.

(4) Active and passive approximation of the scapulae hurt; the resisted movement does not. An upper thoracic intraspinal lesion is compressing the dura mater: almost certainly a thoracic disc-protrusion.

(5) Moving the scapula up and down may elicit discomfort and crepitus, sometimes marked enough to be audible across the room.

(6) If pain is present at one side of the base of the neck and it is brought on by neck-flexion and side-flexion towards the painless side, by active and passive scapular elevation and by full elevation of the arm, the lesion almost certainly lies at the joint between the first rib and the transverse process of the first thoracic vertebra.

(7) If active and passive elevation of the scapulae hurt at the pectoral area, in combination with pain elicited also by resisted depression of the bone, the subclavius muscle is at fault.

Scapular pain unaffected by neck or thoracic movements, taken together with normal X-ray appearances of the lungs and ribs, suggests herpes zoster or infectious neuritis. The vesicles appear after four days, and the pain of infectious neuritis lasts only three weeks. In neuralgic amyotrophy the brachial pain comes on within a few days. Hence pain that has continued without spreading for more than a month suggests visceral disease such as atypical angina.

X-RAY EXAMINATION

This yields mostly negative information, showing the absence of tuberculous disease, fracture or neoplastic erosion. But secondary deposits can be detected clinically before enough erosion takes place to show by X-rays. Minor wedge-fracture of the body of a vertebra does not set up symptoms after the first few weeks unless the disc was damaged at the same time.

Diminution of one or more joint spaces is a commonplace in painless necks. Some osteophyte formation is all but universal in other than young patients, and is compatible with a full and painless range of movement.

Gross osteoarthritis leads to limitation of movement, not necessarily to any discomfort. Ossification in the anterior longitudinal ligament leads to painless stiffness at the affected joint. Congenital fusion of two vertebrae limits movement slightly and is symptomless in itself but leads to overuse of the joints above and below. Disc lesions occur at joints whose space is not visibly diminished; and a narrowed joint space, though it shows the disc to be thin, cannot be taken as evidence of protrusion. If a disc lesion is known to be present, the fact of narrowing does not prove that that joint contains the lesion. For example, a diminished space at the fifth cervical level is often found in cases of seventh or eighth cervical root-palsy, i.e. a sixth or seventh cervical disc lesion. Lateral angulation at one joint only (as is occasionally seen at the lumbar spine) can never be detected, even when the neck is recently fixed in gross deformity. In normal individuals spondylolisthesis may be seen at the third or fourth cervical joint; this has no pathological import and is no bar to manipulation, but the secondary spondylolisthesis of advanced rheumatoid disease is of course significant, and would provide a contra-indication to manipulation except for the fact that manipulation is already contra-indicated in rheumatoid arthritis without spondylolisthesis. The radiograph serves merely to exclude unsuspected disease of other kinds, but in early cases of vertebral malignant invasion, it cannot even be relied upon always to do that. It is, of course, patients with secondary deposits not yet visible by X-rays who reach the orthopaedic physician.

A common source of error today is attempted diagnosis by radiography. A patient aged, say, fifty develops an arthritis in his shoulder, or supraspinatus tendinitis or a tennis-elbow. The radiograph at that age is sure to show some narrowing of a disc or two with osteophytosis. The radiographic appearances of the shoulder and elbow are normal, since the capsule of a joint and a tendon are both radiotranslucent structures. The patient's pain is now attributed to his neck on radiographic grounds. Things have gone so far that articles have even been published stating that cervical spondylosis *causes* tennis-elbow. It would be equally easy to prove, since both occur at the same age, that it causes angina or intermittent claudication.

The posterior osteophyte that compresses the spinal cord is not visible on a plain radiograph, though it is disclosed by myelography. When the anterior spinal artery is, or is in danger of becoming, compressed, radiography with contrast medium is indicated, since decompression or removal of the osteophyte offers the patient the best hope of recovery. Such osteophytes are often multiple. Naturally, a suspected neuroma requires myelography at once.

SECONDARY MALIGNANT DISEASE

Upper Three Cervical Vertebrae

Secondary deposits at the upper three cervical levels are difficult to detect; for the nervous involvement that makes the situation so clear at lower cervical levels is absent. The patient complains of rapidly increasing stiffness and pain in the neck coming on in the course of two or three months. Examination shows gross limitation of active movement in every direction, and when the passive movements are tested, muscle spasm is felt to spring into action to prevent movement; the bone-to-bone feel at the extreme of range of an osteophytic joint is noticeably absent. The resisted movements are then found also to hurt—evidence of a gross lesion. Since the patient is usually elderly, and the radiograph may at first show just osteophytes, a mistaken diagnosis of osteoarthritis is often made. Any patient whose 'osteoarthritis' has caused grossly restricted movements and increasingly severe pain at the neck in the course of weeks or a very few months should be regarded as suffering from malignant invasion, and X-rayed at intervals until the deposit shows or time shows the ascription to be incorrect.

Lower Four Cervical Vertebrae

Diagnosis is easy. Suspicion is aroused when marked articular signs (as above) are found in conjunction with a short history. But, when the upper limbs are examined, neurological signs are detected far in excess of anything a disc lesion can produce. In disc lesions there is severe pain and some muscle paresis; in malignant disease the root-pain is far less severe, but the paresis much more complete and extensive. Discrepancies are of several sorts. In disc lesions, one root only is affected; in cancer often two or three. Disc lesions set up unilateral weakness; in cancer the paresis is often bilateral, and perhaps at different levels. Some muscles always escape in disc lesions; e.g. radial deviation of the wrist and flexion of the thumb are never found to be weak however severe a discogenic palsy is present. Discovery that wrong muscles are affected thus puts the examiner on his guard.

Upper Thoracic Vertebrae

A first thoracic root-palsy is, in my experience, never the result of a disc lesion. This causes lower scapular pain with radiation of root pain to the ulnar aspect of the hand, but I have never yet detected any root weakness. If the small muscles of the hand are weak, there is often a Horner's syndrome present as well; if so, a pulmonary sulcus neoplasm must be sought radiologically. If the apex of the lung is clear, the vertebrae must be X-rayed at intervals.

Difficulty arises with the upper thoracic vertebrae below the first. Malignant invasion, as happens also at the upper three cervical vertebrae, causes no detectable root-palsy. But at the upper cervical joints marked limitation of movement can be detected, whereas at upper thoracic levels limitation of movement, however gross, cannot be detected. Unless the root-pain is bilateral, only a past history of operation for cancer puts the physician on his guard. In difficult cases (as they all are) one can manipulate if patient, family doctor and previous surgeon agree; or wait several months and only then, if the radiograph remains clear, manipulate.

FRACTURE

A recent fracture of a vertebral body leads to marked limitation of movement in each direction, especially of extension. The pain is bilateral or central, and the patient has had to hold his neck quite stiff ever since the accident. The patient is not often of the age for malignant deposits, although a pathological fracture occurring, e.g. at tennis, may afford a misleading history. The radiograph is confirmatory, but the appearances are often difficult to interpret.

CERVICAL NEUROFIBROMATA

These are rare and diagnosis may be anything from very easy to impossible. Any patient who appears to have a cervical disc lesion causing root-pain in the upper limb for more than six months should be suspected of a neurofibroma and the case reviewed with this possibility in mind. Naturally enough, articular signs are absent, for there is nothing wrong with the joint. Unhappily, when a cervical disc lesion with brachial pain has been present for some months and spontaneous cure is well advanced, the articular signs often disappear; however, this coincides with relief from pain, whereas the pain of a neuroma goes on increasing.

Neurofibromata have lately appeared in my department at the rate of three or four a year, and the possibility must always be considered. Warning points are:

(1) The patient's age. A cervical disc lesion causing considerable root-pain does not occur under the age of thirty-five; even after a severe accident to the neck it does not appear before thirty. Any patient, therefore, in his twenties suffering from what might otherwise be thought to be persistent root-pain caused by disc protrusion should be regarded as suffering from a neuroma.

(2) Cough hurts. The pain of a cervical disc lesion is seldom aggravated by coughing, and if it is, it is nearly always felt in the scapular area, not down the arm.

(3) Primary postero-lateral onset. Though it is true that a disc lesion in the neck may start in the reverse fashion (i.e. paraesthetic hand, aching forearm then arm, finally scapular pain), this is uncommon. By contrast neuromata usually start this way.

(4) Length of history. Unilateral root-pain, especially if a root-palsy supervenes, very rarely lasts more than three or four months, and does not get worse after the first month. A neuroma causes pain increasing indefinitely.

(5) Extent of weakness. The experienced clinician knows what is the maximum amount of root-palsy that a disc protrusion will cause. Weakness too great in degree, or affecting muscles that are not usually involved, or a paresis that extends to two or more roots, is strongly suspicious.

(6) Bilateral development. If a disc protrusion shifts to one side, it moves away from the other side; hence the pain is strictly unilateral. Elderly patients, it is true, may suffer minor bilateral protrusion, and thus get pins and needles in both hands, but they have scarcely any root-pain. Hence any young or middle-aged patient, whose unilateral root-pain becomes bilateral, probably has a neuroma.

(7) Cord symptoms. Pins and needles felt all over the body and evoked by neck-flexion are characteristic of a neuroma. Elderly patients with cord pressure from a disc or an osteophyte may have intermittent paraesthesia in one or both hands and feet, but scarcely ever in the entire trunk as well. · Moreover, the pins and needles often come and go causelessly, and are only seldom brought on by neck-flexion.

(8) Cord signs. If pressure on the pyramidal tracts is displayed by a spastic gait, incoordination or an extensor plantar response, myelography will be considered whatever the lesion is thought to be.

In neuroma, the straight radiograph reveals nothing relevant at first, but may show misleading narrowing of one or more joint spaces if the patient is no longer young.

If suspicion arises but no convincing signs are detectable, the patient should be kept under observation for as long as is necessary—not less than a year. He should not be referred to a neurological department. Here, when nothing much is found, a patient may be discharged. I have had to wait as long as eighteen months for acceptable neurological signs to appear; hence the patient should be encouraged to continue attending.

OSTEOPHYTIC ROOT-PALSY

The symptoms and signs are quite different from those of a cervical disc lesion. The bony outcrop enlarges very slowly, thus causing very little aching, as it gradually grows to transfix the nerve-root in the course of years. There is not much neckache; the upper limb may not hurt at all, the patient complaining merely that it is weak. Alternatively, some root-pain may be present, changing little in the course of months. Scapular pain is often slight or absent.

Naturally the patient is elderly, fifty or over. Examination shows a neck stiff from osteoarthritis but often the movements of the neck do not alter such symptoms as are present. When the upper limb is examined, a severe root-palsy at one level only is discovered, most often at the fifth level, since inability to abduct the arm draws attention to itself much more forcibly than a sixth or seventh paresis.

An oblique radiograph of the relevant foramen shows the projection, but the converse does not hold; for many patients with such intra-foraminal osteophytosis have no symptoms and no weakness.

If the palsy is severe, the foramen should be explored and the osteo-phyte drilled away with a dental burr. If it is not severe, the patient should be reviewed at three-monthly intervals for assessment of the degree of root-weakness. If it increases, as is to be expected, operation should not be deferred, especially if the abductor muscles of the shoulder are wasting, since inability to raise the arm from the side is a severe disablement. If the paresis remains stationary, it is safe to wait. Only once have I encountered a patient whose palsy had recovered spon-taneously by a year later, and it is scarcely worth waiting for this slim chance. Lay manipulation has often been carried out on these patients, and as far as I can see no real harm has resulted. Nevertheless, it can only drive the osteophyte harder against the nerve, and I regard manipulation as contra-indicated in these cases.

NEURALGIC AMYOTROPHY

This is an uncommon disorder, often mistaken for a cervical disc lesion with root-pain. However, the history is different and examination shows the disorder to have picked out muscles regardless of root derivation, or the muscles of several roots.

History

Violent pain starts suddenly at the centre or both sides of the neck. There is no trauma nor causative strain and the patient remembers that, despite the pain, he could move his head quite well, thus contrasting strongly with the marked restriction of movement that accompanies the early stages of internal derangement. Moreover, the pain is central, whereas in a non-traumatic stiff neck the symptoms are nearly always unilateral. After a few days, the pain spreads down both arms often to the hands, but there are rarely pins and needles. It then leaves one upper limb, but remains in the other, which aches very severely for about two months, and it takes another two or three months for the pain gradually to subside completely.

Signs

Examination reveals a full range of movement at the neck, but some of the cervical movements may provoke local discomfort, which may also be aggravated by a cough or a deep breath. Examination of the one painless upper limb occasionally reveals that one muscle, usually the infraspinatus, is paralysed, all the other muscles being of full strength. Examination of the painful limb shows that several muscles are paralysed, the others belonging to the same segment retaining full power. A common pattern is paralysis of the infraspinatus with the triceps, or with the extensors of the fingers, or with the extensors of the thumb. It is rare, whatever other muscles are affected, for the infraspinatus muscle on the painful side to escape. The affected muscles are paralysed, not just weak, as in a disc lesion.

Severe cases occur, but do not reach the orthopaedic physician. When a complete palsy of most of the muscles in both upper limbs results from a sudden attack of neuralgic amyotrophy, the patient is bedridden and requires strong analgesics for several months.

POST-CONCUSSIONAL HEADACHE

Much confusion exists about this syndrome. Sympathetic doctors regard it as organically determined; the more objectively-inclined, as due to neurosis. There being no objective criteria for evaluating headache, the diagnosis is apt to reflect individual doctors' attitude to disorders that do not set up detectable physical signs. Headache—an undisprovable symptom—is, of course, often alleged by patients wishing to strengthen their claim for compensation after injury to the head and neck.

Clearly organic headache complicates concussion; so does neurotic headache; so does assumed headache. But the only rapidly relievable headache of these three is that arising from the neck. Naturally, any force severe enough to cause concussion must expend some of its impact on the neck as well. The joints, less often the muscles, are damaged at the moment of the blow, and the immobility imposed by the damage to the brain prevents early movement. Adhesions form about the occipito-atlantoid-axial ligaments, and scars may also form at the occipital insertion of the semi-spinalis muscles. The former are easily rupturable by manipulation, and the latter by deep friction.

The only difficulty is diagnosis. The headache caused by cerebral commotion is not, of course, alterable by manipulating the neck. Nor will the traumatic neurasthenic be persuaded thus to drop his law-suit. In either case, the neck is not at fault, and treating it is fruitless.

Diagnosis is made first by careful assessment of the history—the lack of tendentious statements, the correspondence between symptoms and disablement, the absence of additional symptoms such as giddiness and inability to concentrate. A straightforward account given in an objective manner inspires confidence. When this is supported by an examination devoid of inconsistencies or exaggeration, the patient must be regarded as sincere. Such patients should receive manipulation of the upper two cervical joints and deep friction to the occipital insertion of the muscles. Success results even in cases where the neck-signs are so slight that little benefit is anticipated. Hence one treatment should be given as soon as the patient is seen, and repeated if necessary. Only two or three treatments are required; if the patient is not well by then, it is useless to go on.

Bechgaard (1966) in a review of over three hundred cases of injury to the cervical spine found that in 64 per cent there was a dramatic initial improvement in symptoms after manipulation. Of these, twenty-three were patients with late post-traumatic headache. Three-quarters of these patients improved after one to three manipulations. Follow-up showed that two patients relapsed after a fortnight, six experienced partial relief only, two remained symptom free six months later and eight were still well after a year. Since it is in this type of case that orthopaedic medical manipulation during traction is considerably more successful than manipulation by other techniques, these results represent a minimum.

8

Cervical Intervertebral Disc Lesions

From the clinical point of view the cervical spine includes the upper two thoracic vertebrae, which are examined with the other segments forming the upper limb. Hence the two uppermost thoracic joints are tested with the neck, the thoracic type of examination becoming relevant from the third to the twelfth thoracic levels.

ANATOMY

The intervertebral discs lie between the opposing surfaces of the bodies of the vertebrae, except at the joints between occiput and atlas, and atlas and axis. Here no discs exist; hence the first disc lies between the axis and the third cervical vertebra. There is a curious anatomical abnormality at the first and second cervical levels. The uppermost two cervical nerves emerge in front of the articular masses, whereas at the whole of the rest of the spine the nerve-roots emerge posteriorly. The first and second roots are thus very seldom pinched. The disc compresses the nerve-root one greater in number than itself; i.e. a protrusion at the fourth level compresses the fifth root and so on. The discs are adherent to the cartilaginous end-plates that cover the articular surface of the adjacent vertebral bodies and blend with the anterior and posterior longitudinal ligaments. They are somewhat thicker anteriorly, thus contributing to the cervical lordosis. As elsewhere, the disc consists of annulus fibrosus and nucleus pulposus, but from the clinical point of view nuclear protrusions form only a small minority of cervical disc protrusions. Wolf (1956) found the average antero-posterior diameter of the neural canal to be 1·7 cm., and considers that a protrusion that diminishes the canal to less than 1 cm. will compress the spinal cord, but before this has happened adherence of the dura mater to the posterior longitudinal ligament may lead to damage to the cord on neck-flexion. In the normal adult, the root-foramen is four times the size of the nerve-root; hence encroachment must be considerable before conduction is interfered with and in fact quite large foraminal osteophytes may be visible radiographically that cause no pain and no interference with root conduction. Each nerve-root possesses a dural sleeve, pressure on which sets up pain felt in any part, or the whole of the relevant dermatome. Pressure on the nerve-trunk just beyond its exit from the foramen is painless, distal paraesthesia and a lower motor neurone lesion resulting.

Wilkinson (1964) points out that pressure from disc-material may compress the nerve-root in two ways:

(1) Postero-lateral protrusion that does not invade the foramen, but compresses the root against the lamina.

(2) Postero-lateral protrusion lying a little farther laterally which compresses the nerve-root against the articular process.

In her series of seventeen patients, all of whom came to autopsy (most of them with multiple protrusions,) the frequency was:

Joint	Number of protrusions
C2	4
C3	11
C4	12
C5	16
C6	9
C7	2

This is quite different from the frequency in the cases of less advanced disease seen by the orthopaedic physician. The root-signs indicate that protrusion is very rare at C2 and 3, uncommon at C4 and 5 and 7, and very common at C6. In nine patients out of ten with a root-palsy, it lies at the seventh level, i.e. a C6 disc lesion. Todd and Pyle (1928) measured the thickness of adults' cervical discs and found the spaces: C2, 3·7 mm.; C3, 4 mm.; C4, 4·4 mm.; C5, 4·8 mm.; C6, 5·6 mm.; C7, 4·4 mm. Clearly the instability is likely to be greatest where the intervertebral ligaments are longest, and this may well be the cause for the great preponderance of seventh cervical root-palsies.

Naturally, a bulging disc exercises ligamentous traction and lifts up periosteum; bone grows to reach its lining membrane and an osteophyte forms. Spondylitic myelopathy is 'one of the commonest diseases of the spinal cord found in middle-aged and elderly people' (Wilkinson, 1964) and 'It has become increasingly apparent in recent years that cervical spondylosis is the commonest cause of disease of the spinal cord over the age of fifty.' (Leading article in British Medical Journal, 1963.)

These two quotations are cited to emphasize that many neurologists now regard cervical protrusions (of disc-material and of bone) as the main cause of disease at the cervical extent of the spinal cord. Once gross osteophyte formation or adherence of the dura mater to a bulging posterior ligament has taken place, obviously nothing can be done by conservative treatment to remedy, let alone reverse, this process. But it stresses the importance of the view that I have expressed for so many years, viz. that reduction at a time when this is still possible is the only effective prophylaxis against irremediable damage to the spinal cord years later. This is contrary to current treatment of a protruding disc, which is to leave it where it is, apply a collar and hope for the best. Judging by the neurological opinion recorded above, this attitude does not get the spinal cord very far in the long run.

During full flexion, the neck is 3 cm. longer than in full extension. Patients with dural adhesion to the posterior ligament may well damage the cord when they stretch it by neck-flexion; now wearing a collar is a rational precaution. This increase in length provides the reason why neck-flexion so often aggravates the pain of a thoracic or lumbar disc protrusion: the dura is pulled upwards along its whole extent, engaging or tautening the relevant nerve-root against the intraspinal projection. Though the cervical nerve-roots also angulate as the dura mater is drawn upwards during neck-flexion, it is remarkable how seldom this movement sets up increase of the brachial pain in root-compression whether from an osteophyte or a disc protrusion.

Examination

The principles underlying the examination are four. First, examination of neck, by active, resisted and passive movements to decide if an articular lesion is present. Secondly, examination of the upper limb for root-paresis. Thirdly, examination of conduction along the spinal cord. Fourthly, if complaint is made of what suggests root-pain, examination of the upper limb for an alternative cause for the pain in the arm. Cervical disc lesions are so common that patients often develop a painful disorder of the upper limb at a time when they happen to have scapular pain caused by a cervical disc lesion, and the brachial pain is then apt to be mistakenly attributed to root-pressure: an error to which the radiographic appearances of a middle-aged patient's neck misleadingly afford apparent confirmation.

Articular signs

The patient performs six active movements: flexion, extension, side-flexion each way, rotation each way. He states whether or not each movement hurts, and if so where; the examiner notes the range of movement. The same six movements may then be tested again passively and against resistance, the patient reporting the result. These findings are then collated.

The articular signs are the same whatever the level of the lesion; this can be deduced with certainty only if root-signs appear. In recent cases, Maitland's vibratory technique can be used to detect the joint that resents passive movement. The patient lies prone and the thumbs are applied at either side of each cervical spinous process in turn. When a vibratory movement is applied, the examiner feels the muscles spring into contraction to protect the joint when he reaches the affected level. In internal derangement, the pain is usually unilateral and felt all over or anywhere in the neck and scapular area. The symptoms are provoked in the manner of a blocked joint, some active movements hurting unilaterally, others not. Common patterns are two, three or four movements out of the six hurting and four, three or two proving painless. Active rotation towards the painful side nearly always hurts at the extreme; this movement is sometimes unilaterally limited. The passive movements reproduce the same pattern, and hurt more than the active. The resisted movements prove painless, except that resisted flexion is sometimes uncomfortable, presumably as result of the consequent compression strain on the affected joint.

In acute torticollis in young people (fifteen to thirty), the articular signs are gross and obvious: the onset is sudden, usually on waking; the neck deviates, often away from the painful side; side-flexion and rotation in one direction cannot be performed actively or passively; yet movement in the other directions remains little affected.

Since cervical disc lesions often give rise to upper posterior thoracic pain, as do also upper thoracic disc lesions, it is important to realize that neck-flexion is an articular movement as regards the cervical joints, but pulls the dura mater upwards at its thoracic extent. Hence upper thoracic pain provoked by neck-flexion is an ambiguous finding; diagnosis depends on what other movements of the neck, scapula and thorax do and do not reproduce the symptoms.

When a patient is recovering from severe root-pain, there is often a moment when the neck movements become full range and painless but the upper limb still hurts considerably. The history, the presence of the root-palsy and the fact that he states that his neck was very stiff originally provide the clue.

The articular signs in central posterior protrusion vary a great deal. In a recent case in a young or middle-aged patient the neck may be fixed in flexion: the analogue of lumbago. Long-standing gradual protrusion in the elderly may leave the neck movements entirely painless even in the presence of a large projection squeezing the spinal cord, and the limitation of movement may be no more than is usual at that age in trouble-free patients.

Bilateral postero-lateral protrusion also sets up little in the way of articular signs. The patient is elderly, complains of an ache in both upper limbs and paraesthetic hands. Examination shows some discomfort at each side of the neck on the cervical movements; there is often considerable limitation, but often not more than can exist in patients without symptoms.

Root-signs

The symptoms are three-fold; scapular pain caused by unilateral compression of the dura mater; root-pain due to pressure on the dural sleeve of the nerve-root; weakness and tingling due to parenchymatous involvement. The signs are three-fold; for there is no way of testing the mobility of a cervical nerve-root at the intervertebral foramen in a manner analogous to stretching the lower three lumbar nerve-roots. They are thus:

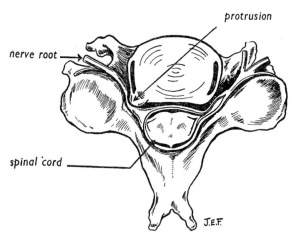

FIG. 25. Protrusion of disc substance at a lower cervical joint causing root-pressure

(1) articular signs; (2) ascertaining if a cervical movement increases the pain in the arm or brings on the pins and needles in the hand; (3) estimating conduction along the root. However, the examiner must not expect the neck movements to hurt down the arm; this is uncommon. Nor must he await the appearance of a clear root-palsy before diagnosing cervical disc lesion; this must be done on the articular signs alone. By the time a root-paresis makes the diagnosis obvious, the time for effective treatment has passed. If this were realized, root-pain would become a rarity, manipulative reduction having been carried out at the stage of scapular pain only.

The upper limb is examined for root-paresis; if present, this indicates the level of the protrusion. The following movements are tested against resistance.

Rotation of neck: C1
Shrugging shoulders: C2, 3, 4
Abduction and lateral rotation at shoulder: C5

Flexion at elbow: C5, 6
Extension at wrist: C6
Extension at elbow: C7
Flexion at wrist: C7
Ulnar deviation at wrist: C8
Extension and abduction of thumb: C8
Approximation of fourth and fifth fingers: T1

Cutaneous analgesia is sought at the fingers: it is absent in fifth-root lesions, often present at the thumb and index in sixth-root lesions, the index, long and ring fingers in seventh-root lesions; the middle and two ulnar fingers in eighth-root lesions. In first-thoracic-root lesions the fingers retain sensation.

The tendon jerks are elicited, the biceps jerk (C5, 6), the brachio-radialis jerk (C5, 6) and the triceps jerk (C7).

Cord Signs

A spastic gait, incoordination of the lower limbs and an extensor plantar response indicate pressure on the spinal cord.

Upper Limb Signs

An alternative cause for the ache in the arm becomes apparent during examination of the upper limb for root-paresis. If e.g. limitation of passive movement at the shoulder or, say, a tennis-elbow is found, the patient with articular signs at his neck as well must have two lesions. Difficulty arises when a patient has a cervical disc lesion and also presents rather vague signs at the shoulder joint—a full range of movement but a suggestion perhaps of subdeltoid bursitis or a tendinitis as well. These secondary signs may prove false. The situation is clarified when manipulative reduction is carried out at the neck at once, and the shoulder is then examined again. In at least half the cases, the shoulder 'signs' will be found to have disappeared.

Pressure on Individual Roots

The first intervertebral disc lies between the second and third cervical vertebrae. The first cervical root emerges between the occiput and the atlas, and the eighth cervical root between the seventh cervical and the first thoracic vertebrae. It follows that a cervical intervertebral disc, when it protrudes, compresses the root one greater in number: e.g. the disc at the sixth joint affects the seventh root. In the list appended here, the maximum root-signs are set out, but partial palsies do occur, though not so often as in the lower limb.

First and Second Cervical Roots

False Reference

Cases are not infrequently encountered of pain in the neck, spreading to the vertex of the skull (C1) or to one temple, the forehead and behind one or both eyes (C2). Examination shows the pain to originate in the joints of the neck. In young patients there is no question yet of occipito-atlanto-axial osteoarthritis leading to bilateral capsular pain felt in the head; moreover, the pain may be unilateral. The cause cannot be a disc lesion at the upper two joints, since they do not contain a disc. Pain in the head associated with a cervical disc lesion is only another example of extra-segmental reference from the dura mater; it has nothing to do with the first and second cervical nerve-roots. In fact it is no more unreasonable for a disc lesion at the sixth or seventh level to set up pain in the upper neck (C3) and occiput (C2) than in the forehead, which is also part of the second cervical dermatome. The degree of extra-segmental reference is the same.

Root-pressure

Unilateral pain felt at the upper neck accompanied by *tingling* in the occipito-parietal region on the same side is a rare complaint in elderly patients; this appears to be a true localizing sign. Examination of movements shows the articular pattern accompanied by marked limitation of movement in every direction. Rotation may be reduced to 10 degrees range. Gross osteoarthritis at one side of the atlanto-axial joint is presumably responsible, with an osteophyte engaging against the second cervical root.

Third Cervical Root

This is rarely affected. Possible symptoms in addition to the unilateral pain in the neck are: pins and needles and numbness felt at the pinna, the posterior part of the cheek, the temporal area and the whole lateral aspect of the neck, with a forward projection under the body of the mandible. I have met with two cases in which the paraesthesia extended to half the tongue. Clinically I have never detected muscular weakness. Occasionally unilateral analgesia of the skin of some part of the neck is present. Rarely, paraesthesia in one cheek is the only symptom; naturally this draws immediate attention to the trigeminal nerve. When repeated expert neurological examination reveals no lesion of this nerve, and time shows that the trouble is not progressive, the patient is usually regarded as imaginative or, at best, as suffering from an undiagnosable disorder.

Fourth Cervical Root

These cases are rare. The pain spreads outwards from the mid-neck and is concentrated at the shoulder. This distribution is slightly different from that caused by pressure on the side of the dura mater at any cervical level; for in the latter event scapular pain is felt posteriorly, seldom at the point of the shoulder, and it does not end abruptly at the deltoid area. Pins and needles are absent, but a horizontal band of cutaneous analgesia, 2 to 4 cm. wide, may be found along the spine of the scapula, the mid-deltoid area and the clavicle, like a half-hoop. No muscle weakness is detectable.

Fifth Cervical Root

The pain extends from the scapular area to the front of the arm and forearm as far as the radial side of the hand; it does not extend to the thumb; pins and needles are, in my experience, absent. *The weak muscles are:* the two spinati, the deltoid and the biceps. The biceps-jerk may be sluggish or absent; the brachio-radialis jerk sluggish, absent or inverted.

Differential Diagnosis

The most difficult finding, leading to frequent errors, especially in elderly patients, is a combination of cervical disc lesion causing scapular pain, and some other lesion (e.g. supraspinatus tendinitis or osteoarthritis of the shoulder) giving rise to pain felt in the arm. Since at this age, radiological alterations are always visible at the cervical vertebrae, and the radiograph in most painful shoulders reveals no local abnormality, X-ray examination can be most misleading.

The other conditions to be kept in mind are enumerated below:

(1) Traction palsy of the fifth cervical root

(2) Palsy of the axillary nerve after dislocation of the humerus at the shoulder

(3) Infectious neuritis of the long thoracic or suprascapular nerve

(4) Traumatic palsy of the suprascapular nerve

(5) Herpes zoster

(6) Myopathy affecting the deltoid and spinatus muscles, complicated by capsular pain (due to disuse contracture) emanating from the shoulder joint

(7) Rupture of the supraspinatus tendon

(8) Rupture of the infraspinatus tendon

(9) Secondary malignant deposits at the scapula

(10) Diaphragmatic pleurisy.

Sixth Cervical Root

The pain spreads down the front of the arm and forearm to the radial side of the hand, and pins and needles felt in the thumb and index finger are often a conspicuous feature; cutaneous analgesia may be detectable at the tips of these digits. *The weak muscles are:* biceps, supinator brevis and the extensores carpi radialis. Wasting of the brachio-radialis muscle may be visible. Occasionally the subscapularis muscle is weak too. The biceps jerk is sluggish or absent, sometimes as an isolated finding.

Differential Diagnosis

At this level, the difficulty lies in the fact that the muscular weakness is often slight. Electromyography may assist, but paresis detectable clinically often appears before electrical testing reveals any abnormality. The conditions that give rise to similar symptoms are:

(1) Pressure on the median nerve in the carpal tunnel

(2) Pressure of the first rib or of a cervical rib on the lower trunk of the brachial plexus

(3) Tendinitis or partial rupture of the biceps muscle

(4) Rheumatoid perineuritis, especially if it complicates monarticular rheumatoid arthritis of the shoulder joint

(5) Tennis-elbow.

Seventh Cervical Root

This is by far the commonest root affected; at least nine out of ten cervical disc lesions occur at this level. The pain extends from the scapular area down the back of the arm, via the outer forearm, to the finger-tips; pins and needles are usually felt in the index, long and ring fingers. Rarely the pain is pectoral instead of scapular; indeed, a few patients with weakness due to a seventh-root-palsy never develop any brachial discomfort at all, but only unilateral anterior upper thoracic pain. Some of the neck movements provoke the pectoral pain; the thoracic movements and resisted adduction of the arm do not, and it is examination of the symptom-free upper limb that clarifies the diagnosis. *The outstandingly weak muscle is* the triceps; the radial flexor, much less often the extensors (or both), of the wrist may be weakened too. The triceps-jerk is seldom affected even when the triceps muscle is extremely weak. Cutaneous analgesia is often found at the dorsum of the long and index fingers. After severe and prolonged pressure, complete wasting of the mid-fibres of the pectoralis major muscle may appear as a triangular depression lying between the parts of the muscle developed from the sixth and eighth myotomes. Rarely, a larger part than usual of the serratus anterior is developed from the seventh myotome and partial winging of the scapula results. Though the seventh root cannot be painfully stretched, the patient finds relief from putting his hand on his head: a posture that relieves tension on the root. Patients should be told to adopt this position when trying to fall asleep.

Differential Diagnosis
  (1) Radial palsy from pressure—e.g. of a crutch, the edge of a chair or bed or fracture of the shaft of the humerus
  (2) Lead poisoning (always bilateral)
  (3) Carcinoma of the bronchus
  (4) Tennis-elbow; golfer's elbow
  (5) Tricipital tendinitis
  (6) Fracture of the olecranon

Eighth Cervical Root

The pain occupies the *lower* scapular area, the back or inner side of the arm and the inner forearm; pins and needles are usually felt at the third, fourth and fifth fingers. *The weak muscles are:* the extensor and adductor muscles of the thumb, the flexor and extensor muscles of the fingers. The triceps muscle is sometimes a little weak too. Cutaneous analgesia may be detected at the fifth finger.

Differential Diagnosis
  (1) Cervical rib. The muscles derived from the first thoracic myotome are affected.
  (2) Pressure on the lower trunk of the brachial plexus by the first rib.
  (3) Secondary deposits at the seventh cervical or first thoracic vertebra. This is their usual site at the cervical spine and the condition is easy to detect; for the pain is not severe in proportion to the weakness, which is extreme. Moreover, the seventh and eighth, alternatively the eighth cervical and first thoracic, roots are *both* involved, with the result that the whole hand and forearm are virtually paralysed. Disc lesions in the neck very rarely give rise to multiple palsies; hence evidence of involvement of two roots immediately suggests secondary neoplasm, whether or not the radiograph shows bone erosion.

(4) Pancoast's tumour. The neck movements are usually of full range and painless, although side-flexion away from the painful side may prove uncomfortable. Full elevation of the scapula may be painful; if so, full passive elevation of the arm is too. Horner's syndrome and a first thoracic palsy are present; X-ray examination of the apex of the lung reveals an opacity.

(5) Angina. Although cervical disc lesions usually give rise to scapular pain spreading to the upper limb, cases are occasionally encountered of unilateral reference to the front of the chest. Pain in the neck and the left pectoral area spreading down the upper limb to the ulnar aspect of the hand naturally suggest a myocardial disorder, especially if the patient is no longer young.

(6) Traction palsy of the lower two roots of the brachial plexus.

(7) Frictional ulnar neuritis at the elbow.

(8) Pressure on the ulnar nerve at the wrist. Occupational; or a ganglion connected with the flexor carpi ulnaris tendon.

(9) Thrombosis of the subclavian artery. The upper-limb pain is claudicational and the radial pulse is lost.

First Thoracic Root

Disc lesions at the first thoracic level are very rare. Most patients with symptoms attributable to this root are, in fact, suffering from some other disorder, e.g. cervical rib, pulmonary sulcus tumour, secondary neoplasm, or pressure on the median or ulnar nerve-trunk.

The pain is felt diffusely in the lower pectoro-scapular area and spreads down the inner aspect of the arm to the ulnar border of the hand, where pins and needles and slight numbness may be noted. The fingers are un-affected. In first thoracic disc lesions, *there is no weakness of the hand*; if this is found, neoplasm or a cervical rib is the likely cause.

The first thoracic root can be painfully stretched by:

(1) Forward movement of the scapula during elevation.

(2) Abduction of the arm to the horizontal and then stretching the ulnar nerve by flexing the elbow.

Both these movements should aggravate the thoracic pain, as do coughing and neck-flexion. Reduction by manipulation is difficult; if it fails, spontaneous recovery is not to be expected in less than six to twelve months.

Second Thoracic Root

I have met with two cases. A man of forty lifted a heavy weight while crouching and felt a click in one scapular area. Within some hours he had unilateral pain in the pectoro-scapular region, spreading to the inner side of the elbow. He had had constant pain for six weeks, aggravated by a deep breath or cough. The movements found to increase the brachial pain were: (1) neck-flexion during full elevation of the painful limb, (2) neck-flexion during scapular approximation, (3) elbow-flexion with the arm horizontal, i.e. touching the back of his neck.

In one case a fortnight's treatment by head-suspension, and in the other two sessions of manipulation afforded full relief.

Cervical Disc Lesions Causing Pressure on the Spinal Cord

Nowadays it is generally agreed that a common, probably the commonest, cause of upper motor neurone disease in elderly patients is central posterior protrusion of disc-substance, or the development of an osteophyte in this situation. In either case the spinal cord suffers compression.

1. Sudden Onset with Pain in the Neck

These cases used to be called transverse myelitis if the onset was unprovoked, and contusion of the spinal cord if the cause was severe trauma to the neck. Severe pain in the neck is followed by pain, weakness and tingling in both upper limbs, or in all four limbs. A central posterior protrusion or a fold of ligament has squeezed the spinal cord.

2. Pain in Both Upper Limbs

The patient develops pain in both scapular areas, soon radiating to the arms and forearms. The hands tingle, rarely the pain in the arms alternates; if it is more severe on one side, it is correspondingly less on the other. Then pins and needles appear at the soles of the feet, often increased or brought on by neck-flexion.

In these cases, since the displacement is central and interferes little with the joint from which it protrudes, the articular signs at the neck may be quite inconspicuous, the commonest being considerable limitation of extension. The symptoms often suggest the thoracic outlet syndrome or, less often, a sensory stroke, and differential diagnosis is not easy. The protrusion being central, there is no tendency to spontaneous cure such as characterizes unilateral pain caused by a postero-lateral protrusion. The brachial pain may thus last for years; by corollary, manipulative reduction may prove possible also after years of pain and paraesthesia.

3. Painless Slow Onset

The patient finds difficulty in walking and on examination is found to have an upper motor neurone lesion affecting both legs. Hands and feet tingle; a common complaint is pins and needles from the front of both knees to all the toes. Investigation by radiography with a contrast medium shows the protrusions, which are often multiple. They may be the result of osteophyte formation or of disc-herniation; the two are distinguishable only at laminectomy. Later on pressure may be exerted on the anterior spinal artery causing widespread local degeneration of the cord with paraplegia. The posterior longitudinal ligament forms adhesions to the dura mater, which becomes thickened. Neck-flexion may then over-stretch and damage the spinal cord further; hence wearing a collar may well prevent aggravation and even bring about some improvement in the course of months.

In patients who have had, say, a severe car accident considerable damage without fracture at the neck is a commonplace. These patients may develop disc lesions at any time during middle-age; the resemblance then to disseminated sclerosis is considerable. The patient starts limping and drags one leg; there is not necessarily any neckache. Examination shows the upper motor neurone disturbance. In cases of doubt a myelogram must be performed.

4. Paraesthetic Fingers: Acroparaesthesia

In elderly patients advanced degeneration with protrusion of disc-substance at one or more lower cervical levels may give rise merely to pins and needles in both hands. This may continue for years unchanged. Minor bilateral postero-lateral protrusion has taken place. In due course, pins and needles usually appear in the lower limbs as well—sometimes in the feet only, sometimes including the thighs and legs as well. This denotes a central protrusion, giving rise to a triple bulge.

The Mushroom Phenomenon

This is a rarity at the neck. The patient is elderly and states that, lying down, he is perfectly comfortable and with his head supported on a pillow he can move it painlessly. After sitting or standing for some time, he

SUMMARY

Disorder (traditional name)	History	Articular Signs	Neurological Signs	X-ray Signs	Treatment
Acute 'rheumatic' torticollis	Sudden onset, often on waking, of unilateral pain in neck; young patients	Obvious. Often postural deformity. Marked limitation of movement in at least two directions	None	None	Manipulative reduction
'Scapular fibrositis'	Unilateral scapular aching of unexplained onset in middle age	Full range. Extreme of several neck movements evokes scapular pain	None	None	Manipulative reduction
'Brachial neuritis'	35 years old and over. Unilateral scapular pain spreading to upper limb. Often paraesthetic digits	Same as in 'scapular fibrositis' unless neck movements also elicit pain in arm (seldom)	Some progress to root-palsy, others not	None	Palsy: await spontaneous recovery in 3–4 months. No palsy: attempt reduction
'Acroparaesthesia' (caused by bilateral cervical disc protrusion)	Vague aching in neck or both scapular areas; paraesthesia in hands and or feet	Very slight, even absent. Traction on neck may abolish symptoms during the pull	None. Extensor plantar response only after years	Elderly changes	Plantar response flexor: attempt reduction. Response extensor: collar or laminectomy
Amyotrophic lateral sclerosis. Progressive muscular atrophy	Nothing to attract attention to neck	No more discomfort and limitation of movements at cervical joints than is expected at that age	Lower motor neurone lesion in upper limbs; upper ditto in lower limbs. Plantar response often extensor	Elderly changes	Laminectomy
Osteophytic root palsy	Painless weakness of upper limb	Ditto	Gross weakness of muscles supplied by one root only	Large osteophyte seen on oblique view occluding osteophyte foramen	Removal of osteophyte
Rheumatic headache	Matutinal headache of elderly men	Limited movement, especially rotation, which may evoke headache	None	Elderly changes	Stretch out upper two cervical joints by manipulation

feels neckache, i.e., after the affected joint has borne the weight of the head. If this compression is maintained for long, discomfort in both arms and pins and needles in the hands begin. The patient has found that lifting his head upwards with his hands stops all symptoms.

Examination reveals an osteoarthritic neck with limited movement, not necessarily with much aching at the extremes of the possible range. Neurological signs attributable to the root-pressure are absent and conduction along the spinal cord is unaffected.

The diagnosis rests on the typical history and the negative examination. A weight-relieving collar or arthrodesis provide the only effective alternatives.

Whiplash Injury

There exists a tendency to regard this accident as causing a disease *sui generis* and to suppose that the use of the term 'whiplash' indicates that a diagnosis has been made. This is not so; 'whiplash' is merely a statement on how the injury was caused. In severe cases, the anterior longitudinal ligament may rupture; the upper facets then slide down wards on to the lower facets. This causes marked anterior folding of the now relaxed ligamentum flavum. This fold compresses and damages the spinal cord, even causing death. In such cases the radiograph shows neither fracture nor dislocation and post-mortem examination reveals no disc protrusion.

More often an ordinary cervical disc lesion results, no different from that acquired without a memorable accident. In the end precocious degenerative change at the affected joint develops. This can be kept to a minimum by immediate manipulative reduction carried out as for a similar displacement occurring without an accident, but medico-legal questions usually bar effective treatment.

Typically, the patient is seated in a stationary car which is run into from behind. He has no warning and cannot brace his muscles as he would when seeing a car about to collide with him head on. His body is shot forwards, leaving the head behind and the cervical joints are forcibly hyperextended. The head recoils now into excessive flexion, unless the forehead hits the windscreen, which is just as damaging, owing to the severe articular jarring. The patient is stunned for a moment and taken to hospital complaining of pain in head and neck. The X-rays are negative, and the patient sent home where he spends a few days in bed. The neckache may abate somewhat but continues; more radiographs are taken, physiotherapy given, collars worn, all to no avail. Finally, the question of traumatic neurasthenia is raised, the more so since there is nearly always a compensation claim pending.

Some doctors are incurably sanguine in their prognoses in this disorder; they find evidence merely of muscle and ligamentous strain which they report will soon repair itself. Naturally, those concerned with compensation do not relish the idea of damage to an intervertebral disc—an avascular structure which can never repair itself.

Unfair attitudes abound on both sides. Considerable damage to a disc without concomitant fracture may cause genuine severe symptoms which are apt to be disbelieved; by contrast, a fracture without concomitant injury to the disc unites and usually causes no further trouble. But the deformity is visible radiologically and a 'fractured spine' is very acceptable legally. The patient is in a cleft stick; if he is sincere and alleges minor aching, he gets little compensation; if he exaggerates his symptoms considerably, he is apt to receive a larger sum, even if the traumatic neurasthenia is recognized. If he overdoes his symptoms blatantly he may be regarded as a malingerer and lose his case. A properly designed clinical examination alone can decide what is the true position, and ensure a report based on observed facts and not on opinion.

It is my habit to explain the position to those patients who are sincere. I offer them an immediate attempt at manipulative reduction, if their main interest is relief from symptoms; but point out that, if this proves successful, the amount of compensation will be much reduced. If they are uncertain, I advise them to consult their solicitor before receiving treatment, and emphasize that, although the lesion is most probably reducible today, there is no certainty that this situation will continue until the suit has been concluded several years hence. Patients with responsible work to do seldom hesitate; they merely wish their pain relieved so that they become effective again. Those with an uninteresting job are naturally more concerned with the benefits of compensation; they often decide to take their chance with reducibility when the case is settled.

TREATMENT OF CERVICAL DISC LESIONS

Prophylaxis

Young patients wake up with a stiff neck, having gone to bed comfortable the night before, obviously as the result of lying for several hours with their head twisted on their shoulders. Intra-articular displacement comes on gradually during this time and, on waking, they think they 'have been sleeping in a draught'. Hence posture at night is an important point in prophylaxis. The patient, if he sleeps supine, should have one thin pillow; if he lies on his side, the thickness of the pillow should be so adjusted that his cervical and thoracic vertebrae form a horizontal line. The habit of lying prone in bed, so useful for patients with lumbar disc lesions, results in the head being kept fully rotated for hours during sleep. Patients should be warned that this otherwise beneficial position must be avoided once stiff neck has begun to show itself. A bath towel twisted into a rope four to six inches in diameter and wound round the neck provides an effective stabilizer at night for those who keep getting attacks.

A head rest on the car-seat prevents the sudden extension movement of the neck on impact from behind, but a safety belt increases the force of the flexion rebound by limiting it to the cervical spinal joints.

By day, the cervical lordosis should be maintained. Patients liable to stiff necks, or who have just had a displacement reduced, must avoid keeping the neck bent for a long period: they should extend the neck every so often for a second or two when reading, writing, sewing, knitting, etc. Alternatively, during reading they should raise a book, for example, to the level of their eyes.

Prophylaxis of Root and Cord Pressure

If a damaged cervical disc protrudes repeatedly, sooner or later the displacement, instead of undergoing spontaneous reduction again, will increase in size, and any time after the age of thirty-five an attack of severe root-pain may incapacitate the patient for several months. Alternatively, a posterior central bulge may form and increase slowly in size; it may draw out an osteophyte by ligamentous traction lifting up the periosteum. Both these processes are encouraged by today's normal attitude towards even an obvious disc-displacement—passive resignation. There are various ways of doing nothing that do not make this negative attitude obvious to the patient: e.g. the prescription of analgesic drugs, or heat, or massage, or exercises, or the provision of a collar. If the displacement is left where it is to get larger or smaller as fortune dictates, it will sometimes take the latter course. Even so, the longer the protrusion lasts, the more time it has to stretch the posterior longitudinal ligament, perhaps irretrievably, thus enhancing the likelihood of further attacks. The prevention of eventual pressure on a root or the spinal cord is clearly the reduction of the displacement when it first appears. In other words, reduction now, repeated as the years go by as often as proves necessary, affords the best—indeed the only—hope of preventing attacks of severe pain and eventual crippling in old age.

Reduction by Manipulation

In his book on 'Cervical Spondylosis' (1967) no less an authority than Lord Brain maintains that the chief use of manipulation of the neck is 'to reduce an intra-articular displacement . . .' Since cervical spondylosis is secondary to changes in the disc, and the symptoms, especially in the early stages, stem from minor degrees of disc protrusion, we have here clear confirmation that the prophylaxis and treatment of choice in cases not too advanced is manipulative reduction. It is the first treatment to be considered, no less so at the neck than at, say, the knee. Unless some contra-indication exists, manipulative reduction should be attempted within the hour. It is my habit to carry this out as soon as the diagnosis is established; for, in the early case, waiting some hours or a day may make a great difference to the reducibility of the protrusion. This should be pointed out to patients who, usually because of some important engagement, wish to defer treatment.

Contra-indications

Evidence of an upper motor neurone lesion shows that (a) manipulation is unsafe; (b) it will fail. I have tried on two patients, at the request of the doctor and the orthopaedic surgeon looking after them. They were made no worse but certainly no better, and cases have been reported of tetraplegia after manipulation in disc lesions of this type. However, a central posterior protrusion may exist not yet large enough to interfere with conduction along the pyramidal tracts. In such a case, the symptom is usually pins and needles in hands or feet, or both. A patient with a cervical disc lesion with this *symptom*, but no *sign* as yet of pressure on the spinal cord, may be treated by an attempt at manipulative reduction. It must then be most carefully carried out with *a maximum of manual traction and a minimum of articular movement*. In particular, rotation must be avoided during the manipulation. It is in this type of case that manipulation under anaesthesia is apt to make the condition worse, since the common manœuvre is rotation. Chiropraxy is also dangerous; osteopathic methods are unsuccessful but less harmful. Maitland's oscillating manipulation may help a little, but the best hope of reduction lies in really strong manual traction. Since this method of treatment is the one least practised, those who regard manipulation as unsuited to this type of case are, in general, right, the more so since disc lesions that have been aggravated by unsuitable techniques often prove very difficult to reduce afterwards.

In basilar ischaemia (see p. 140) manipulation is dangerous.

Criteria of Reducibility or Not by Manipulation

Four questions must be answered: (1) How large is the protrusion? (2) Is it central, unilateral or bilateral? (3) Do the articular movements affect it? (4) How long has it been present?

Central and bilateral displacements require strong traction and slight articular movement for their reduction; these cases are unsuited to osteopathy and chiropraxy, but Maitland's mobilizations may help. Unilateral displacement requires strong movement during traction and, if there is no root-pain, osteopathy and chiropraxy may succeed.

The larger the protrusion the more marked the neurological signs. Evidence of pressure on the spinal cord shows manipulation to be dangerous. A root-palsy shows the herniation to be larger than the aperture whence it emerged. Therefore, it cannot be put back, but the vain endeavour is not dangerous. Pins and needles as an isolated phenomenon can be ignored.

If several of the neck movements set up or markedly increase the scapular aching, the displacement clearly lies where the articular movements influence it. Such 'good' neck signs suggest reducibility. If the neck movements set up pain in the upper limb, reduction is always difficult and often impossible. Pain felt at one side of the upper neck and caused by a cervical disc lesion at the second and third level nearly always proves more difficult to abolish than when an apparently identical displacement exists at the fourth to seventh levels, setting up pain in the lower neck and scapular area. If the ordinary manipulations do not secure reduction, the technique suitable for a central displacement may succeed.

The time factor also comes into play, but only from the moment that unilateral root-pain has become established. As long as the pain is cervico-scapular only, there is no time limit to successful manipulative reduction. After two months of unilateral root-pain reduction can seldom be secured by manipulation, but this limitation does not apply when the root-pain is bilateral.

Osteophyte formation and attrition of one or more discs do not contra-indicate an attempt at manipulative reduction. It is true that ligamentous contracture makes traction less effective, the patient's age makes him less tolerant of discomfort; but the endeavour is perfectly safe. Less is done at one sitting and post-manipulative soreness is apt to last a couple of days instead of some hours; moreover, it cannot, at really stiff cervical joints, be abolished by a lateral glide. Hence it is best to see the patient two or three times in all at weekly intervals. But the treatment of a cartilaginous displacement within an osteoarthritic cervical joint is identical with the same condition in a joint devoid of osteophytosis. In fact, reduction has been successfully achieved in patients over eighty years old.

It should be noted that none of these criteria relates to the presence or not of diminished joint spaces or osteophyte formation on the radiograph.

The possibilities are:

(1) Scapular pain without root-pain. Good or bad neck signs without neurological weakness. Reducible in one or two sessions.

(2) Unilateral scapular pain with root-pain. Good neck signs; no neurological signs. Almost certainly reducible.

(3) Unilateral scapular pain with root-pain. Neck movements hurt down the upper limb as well as in the scapular area. No neurological weakness. Probably irreducible.

(4) Bilateral scapulo-brachial discomfort with paraesthetic hands and/or feet. Fair neck signs, no neurological signs. About half are reducible in four to eight sessions.

(5) Unilateral root-pain followed by scapular pain. Symptoms begin at the hand and slowly progress upwards to the scapular area. Such primary postero-lateral protrusions, as at the lumbar spine, are irreducible. N.B. Cervical neuromata often begin this way.

(6) Unilateral scapular pain with root-pain. Good neck signs and minor paraesthesia only. Sometimes reducible, especially if the brachial pain has lasted less than a month.

(7) Unilateral scapular pain with root-pain. Poor neck signs and major root-palsy. Certainly irreducible.

(8) Unilateral scapular pain and root-pain of more than six months' standing. Fair neck signs and a recovering root-palsy. One manipulation will often restore full and painless movement to neck, abolishing the scapular ache. The root-pain is unaltered there and then, but slowly begins to ease some days after the manipulation. Two or three sessions at fortnightly intervals are required. In these cases, the manipulation appears to restart the mechanism of spontaneous cure which normally would have become complete in four months.

(9) Unilateral scapular pain persisting for months after a root-pain has ceased. Only one neck movement elicits the discomfort. Irreducible.

(10) Paraesthetic hands and/or feet. Neck-flexion evokes the symptoms. Gait not spastic. Plantar response: flexor. Usually reducible.

(11) Swift progression. Scapular pain one day followed by root-pain and paraesthesia the next day. Good neck signs and no neurological weakness yet. Very seldom reducible.

(12) Elastic recoil. Rarely manipulation is confidently started in a patient with signs suggesting that reduction by manipulation will prove simple. When this is attempted a rubbery rebound is felt when the

extreme of passive rotation is reached. No matter how often this movement is forced, apparent full range being achieved each time, no increase in the active movement is found when the patient sits up. When manipulation fails in this rare type of primary nuclear displacement, it is wise to pass on at once to sustained traction in bed.

(13) Paraesthetic hands and/or feet with extensor plantar response. Irreducible.

Gross Deformity

Torticollis

Acute torticollis in patients aged under thirty should be treated differently from other disc lesions. On examination one side-flexion and the rotation movement towards the same side are grossly limited. Manipulation consists in carrying out, during strong traction, the movements of rotation and side-flexion *only* in the painless direction. If this is repeated several times, the patient's pain will be much diminished, he can sit up and hold his head in the neutral position, but the range of movement in the two very restricted directions will not have increased. He is then lain on a couch and the head is gradually pushed more and more over towards the unobtainable side-flexion. It may take an hour of repeated small shiftings by the physiotherapist to achieve this end. The same has then to be done for rotation. Hence it may well be three hours in all before a full and painless range of movement is restored to the affected cervical joint. An alternative in these acute cases is vibratory treatment to the affected joint while the patient lies prone. My father, Edgar Cyriax, used to use his finger-tips, Maitland uses his thumbs, for the manual vibration. In either case the patient should be seen the next day, since some degree of relapse is common.

Curiously enough, acute torticollis in patients aged over thirty can be treated in the ordinary way; indeed the disorder is not, at that age, so severe. The deformity is less pronounced; the limitation of movement in the two directions is less extreme; there is no particular tendency to recurrence the next day.

In Side-flexion

Gross side-flexion deformity with scapular pain calls for manipulation repeatedly in the line of the deformity until the neck can be held painlessly in the mid-position. A most dangerous treatment—far worse than doing nothing—is to push the head over the other way during anaesthesia. Gross intractable fragmentation of disc substance, severe root-pain or pressure on the spinal cord often results.

In Flexion

Patients who are forced to hold their chin on their chest, hardly able to extend the neck at all, have a herniation lying posteriorly and centrally. Manipulation in such cases must be very gradual, involving a great deal of traction without, at first, any attempt being made to extend the neck; otherwise the manipulation carries with it the risk of increased posterior protrusion with damage to the spinal cord.

Anaesthesia

Manipulation of the neck is widely regarded as dangerous. This is correct when laymen's techniques are used, since little or no traction is employed. Indeed, Maigne insists that it is safe only to manipulate the neck osteopathically in the direction that does not hurt. He is right, particularly when one remembers that only a local examination by palpation of the neck is considered sufficient by lay manipulators. This view also applies when manipulation is carried out under anaesthesia. But the fact that manipulation with little or no traction and without the benefit of the patient's co-operation may well have unfortunate results is no reason for avoiding manipulation carried out with proper safeguards on suitable cases. Manipulating the cervical joints under anaesthesia is equivalent to crossing the street with the eyes shut: no argument at all against crossing the street.

General anaesthesia is strongly contra-indicated; for a set manipulation is not performed. What to do next, whether to repeat a manœuvre or avoid it, whether to stop or go on, depends on re-examination after each manœuvre. When it appears to be required, i.e. because the displacement proved irreducible in its absence, it will be found that those protrusions that could not be reduced without anaesthesia cannot be reduced with anaesthesia either. Anaesthesia leaves the manipulator wholly in the dark, depriving him of that most essential adjuvant—the patient's co-operation. In fact, adequate relaxation can be readily secured without anaesthesia, for as soon as adequate traction is applied, the patient's pain ceases. Hence he automatically relaxes.

Manipulative Technique During Traction

All cervical manipulation is carried out during traction (see Vol. II). This has a fourfold effect: (1) The cessation of compression on the displacement stops the pain and the patient is happy to relax his neck muscles. (2) The posterior longitudinal ligament is rendered taut. (3) The loose fragment becomes free to move. (4) The sub-atmospheric pressure produced at the joint induces suction. If, then, anything moves, centripetal force ensures that it moves towards the centre of the joint and away from its posterior edge. The fact that manipulation is carried out in slight extension—never in flexion—ensures that more space exists at the front than the back of the joint; this too encourages the intra-articular fragment to move forwards thus ensuring that the spinal cord is not touched as the fragment shifts. Extension also prevents overstretching of the posterior longitudinal ligament during the traction.

Strong traction is applied and maintained for a second or two until the manipulator feels that he has taken up all the slack in the joints of the neck. Traction is maintained and the required movement is pressed home until a small click is felt. This may occur long before full range is reached, particularly during rotation. The patient sits up and the result on the pain is reported by the patient and on the range of movement noted by the manipulator. If this manoeuvre has helped, it is repeated; if it has not, another technique is tried, and so on, the result being evaluated after each attempt. Cervical reduction does not take place with one resounding thud, as at the lower lumbar spine; it involves a series of small clicks. If no click is felt, nothing has been achieved; but a click does not mean that any benefit has necessarily resulted. It is only when it is followed by improved symptoms and signs that it has any significance. After each manoeuvre, the conscious patient sits up and moves his neck; the manipulator assesses the effect on the range of movement and the patient on the degree of pain.

If the pain and tender spot have shifted, the patient is asked to point out their new situation. It is a good sign when a pain felt in the upper thorax moves upwards and medially. With this knowledge of the effect of each step, the manipulator can see at once if any particular manoeuvre has done good, has had no effect, or has done harm. Decision on the next step depends on this knowledge. It is quite possible in difficult cases to spend the whole of the first session in finding out what particular manoeuvre helps—and there may be only one. At the patient's next attendance, this particular technique may be repeated, say, a dozen times. It is my view that only the patient's active co-operation renders manipulation in cervical disc lesions simple, effective and really safe. When the manipulator feels that, at the extreme of rotation, bone meets bone, it is no use continuing forcing in that direction. During side-flexion, the feeling of coming up against a leathery block also indicates that no more can be expected from that manoeuvre.

No exercises 'to maintain range' follow manipulative reduction; for the same movements as the manipulator carried out during traction have the opposite effect of that intended when repeated with centrifugal force acting on the joint.

True failure of manipulation in what appears a thoroughly suitable case raises the question of an error in diagnosis. Since nuclear protrusions are rare, pulmonary neoplasm, occipital arteritis, myeloma, chordoma, or an intra-spinal neuroma must be reconsidered.

Amount of Traction

An experiment was made to find out how much pull I exerted when reducing a cervical disc-displacement. The maximum was found to be 300 lb. Miss Moffatt, then my senior physiotherapist at St. Thomas's, reached 220 lb.

Radiography was carried out before and during fairly strong traction on the neck. It showed that traction increased each joint space by 2·5 mm.—in other words, almost doubled the distance between the bones. No wonder cervical disc lesions are not difficult to reduce so long as the traction is adequate.

Dr. P. Flood's report was:

'Two antero-posterior films were taken. The first before pull was applied and the second while you pulled on the head. In the preliminary film the distance between the upper surface of the first dorsal vertebra and the upper surface of the fourth cervical vertebra is on measurement 7 cms.; during pull this distance is increased to 8 cms. In order to avoid magnification the position of the spine relative to the film was, as far as was possible, similar in both cases. This is confirmed on measurement of the transverse width of the spine which does not vary by more than a millimetre.

'The increase of 1 cm. over the distance of the bodies of the lower four cervical vertebrae must therefore be due to opening of the intra-vertebral spaces' (see Plates 7 & 8).

Novice's Routine

A suitable routine for the novice would be as follows, evaluation following each step. The neck is never manipulated in flexion.

(1) Rotation half the way towards the painless side
(2) Full rotation towards the painless side
(3) Rotation three-quarters of the way towards the painful side
(4) Full rotation towards the painful side
(5) Side-flexion towards the painless side
(6) Lateral gliding

Many variations are imposed by what happens at each manœuvre, and greater and lesser degrees of extension can be used during the preliminary traction. Obviously, if one technique is found to help, it is repeated, perhaps many times at slightly different angles. If a manœuvre does harm, or shoots pain down the patient's arm, it is avoided. If two or three manœuvres are without effect, or increase symptoms, manipulation is abandoned.

Osteopathy

The main school of manipulation in France is headed by Dr. R. Maigne, who manipulates only in the 'direction indolore'. As far as this applies to osteopathic manipulation, of which he is a past master, this is doubtless excellent teaching. However, this restriction does not apply to the orthopaedic medical type of manipulation during traction, since a centri-petal force is now acting on the joint during each manœuvre. Indeed, it is very often rotation during traction in the painful direction that proves the most effective. Nor does the converse hold; for, even if Maigne's restric-tion is observed, harm may nevertheless result if manipulation is attempted in really unsuitable cases.

Patients are often met with who have received manipulation for months even years, from a layman. Though it is true that osteopathic or chiro-practic manipulation, without adequate traction, takes more sessions of treatment to achieve its effect than the orthopaedic physician's methods, the fact remains that what can be shifted by manipulation does so almost at once. What has not begun to move after two orthopaedic medical or six of layman's attempts clearly cannot be benefited thus, and alternative methods of treatment must be considered. Four sessions of treatment for postero-lateral, and eight for postero-central, protrusions are my maxi-mum to date, even in cases where osteopathy or chiropraxy had already failed.

Maintenance of Reduction

If a loose body in a joint has moved once, it can move again. Patients with only cervico-scapular pain often describe a number of previous attacks, and others are to be expected unless the patient is careful about the posture of his neck, especially at night. A recurrent displacement should be reduced again at once. The patient must be warned that the longer a protrusion is left unreduced, the more ligamentous stretching results and the greater the likelihood of recurrence and the eventual supervention of root or cord pressure. Even if previous attacks were self-limiting, there is no guarantee that this will be so again in the present attack. Hence, immediate complete reduction is the first line of defence.

Recurrence is not to be expected after root-pressure that is allowed to run its full course untreated. By contrast, if reduction succeeds in cases of root-pain, the position is the same as in scapular pain—namely, the protrusion has gone back to its original bed and what has shifted once can obviously shift again.

1. A Moulded Collar

It occasionally happens that reduction, though fully achieved, proves very unstable. This is most apt to occur in protrusions of some years' standing and after ill-advised manipulation under anaesthesia.

A moulded plastic collar is made; being transparent, it is remarkably inconspicuous. It must support the mandible well, and the occipital piece must not tend to push the head forwards. When careful trying-on shows that the collar fits, the patient's disc lesion is reduced again and the collar applied while he remains lying on the couch. It must be worn by day for three or four months. Then it should become possible gradually to discard it. It would naturally be an advantage if it were also worn at night for the first few weeks, but it is rare to meet a patient who can sleep in it. If the displacement recurs during the night, reduction by manipulation must be repeated.

A patient with recurrent trouble may find that daily suspension keeps him comfortable. The apparatus is installed at his home and he gives himself ten minutes traction every day (see Vol. II). Others find that they can restore movement caused by a recent and minor subluxation by active movement while the head is floating. The patient lies supine in a warm bath, only his nostrils projecting above the surface of the water. The weight of the head is now borne by the water; hence compression strain on the joint ceases. The head is now moved voluntarily into the position previously unattainable, and held there for some time. If this manœuvre is carried out early enough, reduction often ensues.

2. Operative Fixation

Arthrodesis is, of course, successful in the maintenance of reduction, so long as it is done when no displacement sufficient to cause symptoms is present. It is the only really effective treatment for the mushroom phenomenon, avoiding compression of the joint during the time the neck bears the weight of the head.

3. The Avoidance of Exercises

Movement of the neck during the time that the weight of the head is borne on the cervical spine may well have the opposite effect of the same movement carried out during traction. In the one case centrifugal, in the other centripetal, force is acting on the joint. Most patients after manipulative reduction are advised, even by osteopaths, to perform exercises. The effect is the opposite of that intended. Many patients, particularly those attending hospitals, are given exercises (often after heat or massage) without reduction. This is most unkind; for the symptoms can only increase if, during weight-bearing, the edge of the joint is forced by muscular action against the displacement that blocks movement. No one advises exercises before reduction of a torn meniscus at the knee. The same applies at a spinal joint.

Dangers of Cervical Manipulation

The dangers of medical treatment are usually assessed in relation to the harmful effects likely to accrue when the work is carried out under the best auspices. No one warns against the dangers of appendicectomy when carried out in a cottage by candle-light. The important results are those of competent surgeons working under ideal conditions. A great deal is heard about the dangers of manipulating the joints of the neck, without any reference to the operator or the cases selected. This is quite unrealistic; the dangers and successes must be assessed by the results obtained at an efficient hospital properly staffed, not what happens when any comers are manipulated cheerfully by laymen or when anaesthesia is used.

In the U.S.A. five cases have been described, three by Pratt-Thomas and Berger (1947), and two by Ford and Clark (1956), in which manipulation of the neck proved fatal owing to thrombosis of the basilar artery. Four of these manipulations were carried out by chiropractors, one by the patient's own wife. All patients were in the age group thirty-two to forty-one. A further fatal case of infarction of the brain stem has been described by Smith and Estridge (1962). The patient, aged thirty-three, died three days after chiropraxy to the neck. The authors ascribe the extreme softening of stem and cerebellum found post-mortem to ischaemia consequent upon arterial spasm. Since the vertebral artery on one side is compressed on full rotation of the neck to the other side, bruising can occur at the atlanto-axial level.

Thrombosis of the internal carotid artery, twenty-four cases of which have been described by Boldrey, Maass and Miller (1956), can be caused by compression where the artery crosses in front of the lateral process of the atlas. In six of these patients, rotation of the head away from the side on which the affected artery lay appeared a causative factor, especially when adhesions bound the artery down to bone. Manipulation is not mentioned in this series.

I have encountered one such case. A man of sixty-five with a disc lesion causing pain in the scapular area and upper limb was manipulated with due care as regards rotation. Then side-flexion away from the painful side was carried out and his leg on that side became spastic with extensor plantar response. He recovered fully in a week. The fact that we have had no lasting trouble after manipulation may be because our technique is different from laymen's, or merely to the misfortune being such a rarity. There are estimated to be 16,000 manipulators in the U.S.A. who must be regarded as likely to manipulate not less than one neck each day. If five cases have occurred in ten years, this risk works out at about one in ten million manipulations, and is no argument against manipulative reduction in suitable cases. As a safety measure, Smith and Estridge recommend that, before the neck is manipulated, the head should be rotated and extended. If vertigo or sensory disturbances appear, the attempt should be abandoned.

The Danger of Not Manipulating

Manipulation of the neck is usually done by laymen with little or no training and no knowledge of what lesion they are proposing to affect, or by surgeons under anaesthesia. It is rightly regarded by most doctors, in these two sets of circumstances, as dangerous. I wholeheartedly agree. But this applies to all effective manœuvres; they are dangerous when wrongly performed or when unsuitable cases are chosen. These facts must not be allowed to discredit manipulation of the cervical joints by trained persons, in suitable cases, during traction and without anaesthesia. Bad results in poor circumstances do not preclude good results when due care is taken. When the indications for treatment are considered, it is usual to weigh the dangers of action against the dangers of inaction. Contemporary medical literature is littered with warnings against manipulation of the cervical spinal joints, particularly when X-rays show osteophytosis, without due attention to other aspects of the question: what is likely to happen if manipulation is withheld? Manipulation can relieve pain, perhaps of years' standing, that might well have continued for a lifetime, and it can reduce a disc lesion that is slowly enlarging, or by ligamentous traction is drawing out an osteophyte. In either case, the spinal cord is menaced and eventually pressure may lead to thrombosis of the anterior spinal artery, whereupon not even laminectomy can help. Left where it is (the standard procedure in Britain) such a cervical protrusion can lead not only to pain but to crippledom. Since paraplegia from cervical disc lesion and consequent osteophytosis is by no means rare, it is worth contemplating an even greater danger—leaving the early minor displacement unreduced. The time for quick and simple reduction is missed, and the displacement left to get larger or smaller, to raise osteophytes by ligamentous pull or not as fortune dictates. There comes a time when manipulation is no longer any use; later still, it may become dangerous. When the patient has died, post-mortem studies show that the pressure on the spinal cord could not *then* have been relieved by manipulation. To argue from this that manipulation should not have been used early on involves casuistry unworthy of our profession. The harm caused by not manipulating may not show for some or many years, but if the right moment has been missed the harm done may be irretrievable. This delay obscures the connection between the missed opportunity and the later disablement, but this does not make the situation any less real, nor any more excusable.

Prolonged Traction

There are three ways of doing this.

1. Head Suspension

This measure is used far too often. Numerous cases with neck symptoms receive endless traction, either with no result or with some benefit after ten or twenty sessions, whereas one or two manipulations would have given full relief.

Suspension has its indications, but they are few and infrequently encountered.

(a) *For stability*. Manipulative reduction has succeeded but by next morning the case has relapsed. Manipulative reduction is repeated, but with the same relapse next day. After the third reduction, the patient is treated by suspension, say, daily for a week, in order to attempt to secure a more stable position of the loose fragment.

(b) *For reduction*. An extremely nervous patient may be unable to bear the idea of manipulation. If a genuine slight disc-displacement is present, daily suspension for two or three weeks may achieve what could have been done in a few minutes by manipulation.

Small postero-central displacements in patients not too elderly, presenting with a minimum of articular signs, may also benefit in the long run.

(c) *Prophylaxis*. Patients with a very unstable fragment of disc can often be kept free from trouble by head-suspension for ten minutes daily, usually for years on end.

Contra-indications

Suspension is unsuited to the elderly or to patients so heavy that the neck cannot stand such weight, or when the dura mater is adherent to the cervical spine. However, the real contra-indication is trying in vain to reduce a cervical disc lesion by traction alone, when this can be effected quickly and easily by manipulation during traction. My advice to a physiotherapist who has been asked to give neck-suspension to an obviously reducible cervical disc lesion is to carry out 'passive movements during suspension' and do her best that way.

2. Long Traction

This is seldom indicated. It can be used for patients with severe pain in the arm, not controllable by drugs, and preventing sleep. The patient lies on a sloping couch; a collar is placed round his neck and a 15 to 20 lb. weight attached over a pulley. After a few minutes' traction, the brachial pain ceases and the patient falls asleep. He can then stay so for as many hours as is convenient. When he walks out of the hospital, his pain returns to its former pitch, but he is rested. This method can therefore be used in severe root-pain while awaiting spontaneous resolution; it does not alter the displacement nor expedite cure but, by affording sleep, makes the patient's condition, pending recovery, much more bearable.

3. Traction in Recumbency

This is the method of choice in patients with:

(a) *A nuclear protrusion.* This is rare, but is encountered between the ages of twenty and thirty. Scapular pain results, reproduced by rotation of the neck towards the painful side; the active movement is 45 degrees limited, whereas all the other movements are of full range and either quite or nearly painless. When rotation is carried out passively during traction, full range is easily achieved, but when the patient sits up, the limitation of active movement is unaltered. The neck is then manipulated in the same direction again, rather harder, and the elastic recoil characteristic of a nuclear protrusion is felt. Such a displacement can go on for many years unchanged, and the only remedy is sustained traction in bed.

(b) *A disc-displacement with root-pain but no root-palsy.* Though neurological signs are absent, the displacement has proved irreducible by manipulation. The patient is then told that he must await spontaneous recovery, due four months after the onset of the brachial pain. He avers very reasonably that he cannot endure such severe pain for so long. Continuous traction in bed is then the alternative, but should not be initiated without warning the patient that it is quite an ordeal. It should not be prescribed for root-pain with a root-palsy, nor for ordinary cartilaginous disc lesions; it is very seldom successful. Traction, however prolonged, fails to reduce many cartilaginous displacements and I have on a number of occasions easily reduced a displaced fragment of annulus causing severe root-pain in patients who had had up to a fortnight's fruitless traction in bed elsewhere.

Method. Traction in bed is best carried out in hospital, because the patient requires full nursing day and night. He cannot feed himself or move his head appreciably. The principles of treatment are: (1) to give the patient enough drugs to prevent his feeling the mandibulo-occipital pain of the collar and that down his upper limb; (2) never to allow the traction to abate for one moment. The well-intentioned nurse who tries repeatedly to adjust the collar, meanwhile relieving the traction, ruins the success of this method. No one may touch the harness or weights. So long as the severe brachial pain continues, it overshadows all else and the patient is kept well drugged. Heroin is much preferable to morphia unless cyclizine (50 mg.) is added; otherwise vomiting may make removal of traction imperative. Dipipanone (Diconal) is useful since it contains cyclizine.

Ten or twelve pounds traction day and night is maintained during heavy sedation until the brachial pain ceases—usually in twenty to forty hours. Traction is then diminished in force, and after two days the patient is allowed to lie without weights. At the end of three or four days he sits up for short periods. Hence, even in the most satisfactory case in which all pain ceases at the end of twenty-four hours, five days in bed are the least that can be hoped for; more often seven days elapse before the patient is fit to go home. As soon as the pain ceases and the stronger analgesics are no longer required, the patient makes every sort of complaint about the collar and indeed every aspect of his treatment; he becomes difficult and may need several visits a day. Not being in any way ill, he has plenty of will-power; hence traction in bed, although often effective, should be undertaken with great reluctance. (For details of apparatus, etc., see Vol. II.)

Awaiting Spontaneous Recovery

It is curious that, however long a disc protrusion exerts pressure at or near the mid-line, no tendency to spontaneous recovery is manifest at any spinal level. A disc lesion causing central or unilateral neckache or scapular pain can continue indefinitely. If the bulge is wide enough to give rise to bilateral scapular or bilateral brachial pain, there is the same likelihood of continuance. If the bulge moves a little to one side, giving rise to unilateral scapular pain, there is still no tendency to recovery. It is quite useless, therefore, to predict that unilateral or bilateral neckache or scapular pain of some months' standing will ever cease; it may or it may not. Once the displacement has moved postero-laterally, compressing the dural investment of the nerve-root with consequent brachial pain, spontaneous cure in three to four months becomes extremely probable. The more marked the palsy, the more quickly the pain abates. Full strength will almost certainly have returned to the muscles by, say, three to six months after the symptoms ceased. The only exception is an eighth root-palsy which may take up to six months to disappear and may occasionally leave a patient with a permanently weak thumb.

The normal course of unilateral root-pain due to a cervical disc lesion is intermittent scapular pain for some or many years. Then increasing scapular pain comes on followed by pain in the upper limb. This becomes severe in the course of a week and pins and needles are apt to begin in the fingers corresponding to the dermatome. The pain remains severe, much worse at night, for four to six weeks, then begins to ease. In severe root-palsy, the pain has often eased after two months, and very seldom lasts longer than three months. When the protrusion is smaller, and unilateral root-pain without muscle paresis results, cessation of pain may well take the full four months. (The time must be reckoned from the onset of brachial pain, not of scapular aching.) As stated above, when the root-pain is bilateral, with merely some aching in the arms and pins and needles in the hands as the important symptom (acroparaesthesia), there is no limit to the duration of symptoms.

During the period of unavoidable root-pain pending spontaneous cessation, not much can be done. The possibilities are:

1. Explanation

The patient who is told he has a displacement that cannot be put back naturally expects that he will suffer his present pain for life. Hence, learning that the symptoms subside in the end affords considerable reassurance, and the time when relief may be expected to begin can be foretold with considerable accuracy by merely assessing the severity of the root-palsy.

The ordinary course of events is quite different, and has unfortunate repercussions against the medical profession. The patient starts his

H

brachial pain; he sees his doctor and is given analgesics with only temporary benefit. After a month he goes to hospital where he is told he has a
'slipped disc', he is given either physiotherapy, traction or a collar; the
pain continues unchanged. After a month of this 'treatment' (i.e. two
months in all), he presumes that the medical profession cannot help him
and he goes to a lay-manipulator who treats him two or three times a
week for another month. During this (the third) month, his symptoms
slowly abate spontaneously, but both he and the layman ascribe the relief
to the manipulative treatment. This series of events must not be allowed
to continue for it gives futile manipulation and laymen a gratuitous and
undeserved advertisement.

The prognosis should be explained to the patient, he should be prescribed a strong analgesic to enable him to sleep, and he should be seen
fortnightly until the forecast has been fulfilled. This continued interest in
the patient by the physician prevents him from going elsewhere to waste
his time and money. Moreover, watching to see what the degree of root-
palsy demands in length of time needed for the pain to stop increases the
physician's prognostic accuracy. It is this unrealized spontaneous recovery
that has led to belief in the efficacy of every sort of treatment for what
used to be called 'brachial neuritis'. Massage, electrotherapy, salicylates,
vitamin B, etc.—all appear successful if persisted in for long enough. It is
the fashion nowadays to put patients into a collar while they are awaiting
spontaneous recovery from a cervical disc lesion causing root palsy. This
measure neither diminishes immediate symptoms nor hastens eventual
cure, and it entails the patient enduring the additional and pointless discomfort of the collar.

This view of the uselessness of all treatment in established root-palsy has
been emphasized in succeeding editions of this book since 1954. It was
confirmed by Nichols (1965) who reported a trial on 493 patients divided
into five groups and treated respectively by (a) traction, (b) a collar,
(c) advice on posture, (d) physiotherapy, and (e) placebo tablets. At the
end of a month, 80 per cent of the members of group (c) were relieved,
75 per cent of those on traction, wearing a collar or receiving physiotherapy, whereas only 56 per cent of group (e) were better. Clearly,
treatment has no effect on established unilateral root-paresis, which ceases
spontaneously whatever is or is not done. Nichols draws the modest
conclusion that physiotherapy does not materially affect the eventual
course of cervical spondylosis. He is right, but that does not imply that
logical treatment in cases without root-paresis is without value. St.
Thomas's offered to join in this investigation, but my suggestion was
declined by his committee.

2. Analgesics and Posture

The pain at night is severe and minor analgesics like aspirin are useless. Pethedine, Physeptone or one of the stronger drugs of this sort are required. There is one posture that considerably eases the nocturnal pain: sleeping with the affected arm elevated. This relaxes the nerve-root and many patients can get off to sleep with their hand on their head.

3. Manipulation

This helps in two sets of circumstances, even when a root-palsy is present.

(a) *Marked articular signs.* Usually, by the time that root-pain has continued for two or three months, the articular signs become inconspicuous. An occasional case is encountered of marked limitation of movement in some directions persisting with considerable scapular pain evoked at the extreme of range. In this event, one reason for the patient's broken sleep is scapular pain waking him each time he turns in bed. One session of manipulation, even in the presence of a root-palsy, can be relied on to restore a full and almost painless range of movement to the neck without, unfortunately, affecting the root-pain. Much better nights often follow.

(b) *Overdue root-pain.* A patient may have had an attack of unilateral root-pain which has not resolved in the proper time. It is rare for an attack of brachial pain due to a cervical disc protrusion not to subside spontaneously, but such a case may be encountered, lasting, say, a year or two. The articular signs do not amount to much and, had the root-pain been of a month or two's standing, manipulation would be quite useless. In fact, after the lapse of six months it is often effective, but in a different way. It appears to afford no benefit then and there; yet a few days later brachial pain, of say a year's duration, begins to ease. A second manipulation a fortnight later leads to disappearance of the pain in the upper limb. It is difficult to understand exactly what has happened, but the aborted mechanism of spontaneous recovery has clearly been restarted.

4. Epidural Local Anaesthesia

Root-pain that has lasted say a year and has shown no tendency to resolve spontaneously, and is not helped by manipulation, is a rarity. Epidural local anaesthesia is then called for. Ten c.c. of 1:200 procaine are injected at the required level, and the root-pain ceases within a few minutes. It does not return to its previous intensity, and should disappear after two to four inductions at say fortnightly intervals.

Laminectomy

Cervical laminectomy is a dangerous operation and is to be avoided as far as possible. The situation is quite different from lumbar laminectomy which, in competent hands, is regularly successful and cannot make the patient worse. During the operation, the fall in blood pressure together with the flexion of the neck may provoke thrombosis of the anterior spinal artery, and the reported results mostly claim not more than 50 per cent success. The indications are: (1) Advancing spastic paresis. If the myelogram shows one large indentation, the result of laminectomy is usually better than in cases with smaller protrusions at several levels. (2) Advancing weakness of the hand—i.e. progressive muscular atrophy. (3) Sudden bilateral advance of paralysis of the brachial nerve-roots, such that root-conduction is being lost at the rate of, say, a level a day. In such emergencies in elderly patients, whose general condition is poor, decompression without any attempt to deal with the lesion lying in front of the spinal cord may prove the only practicable measure.

Osteophytic root-palsy demands removal of part of the facet or grinding away the bony outcrop with a dental burr.

TREATMENT OF CAPSULAR DISORDERS

The degree of osteoarthritis must be assessed clinically, not by radiography.

Post-traumatic stiffness of the cervical joints comes on after immobilization, especially if the patient has lain unconscious for some days, unable to move his neck. The manipulation consists of a quick jerk at the extreme of the possible range, rupturing adhesions (see Vol. II). Traction is not required.

Traumatic osteoarthritis in middle-aged patients often appears uninfluenced by treatment, but since many of these patients are claiming compensation it is difficult to be sure if this condition really causes symptoms or not.

In *osteoarthritis* of the upper two cervical joints, capsular contracture is present and leads to considerable limitation of movement. Rotation and side-flexion manipulations are performed, but now they are carried out during traction with the slow strong pressure calculated to stretch out a tough structure. As a result, not only is the pain in the upper neck abolished, but the matutinal occipito-frontal headache also disappears. There is no upper age limit to manipulation, which can be safely carried out after the age of eighty. However it is often best to force only one movement at a session; hence the really elderly patient may have to come two or three times for as much treatment as, had he been ten years younger, could have been carried out at one session. General anaesthesia is occasionally requested by sensitive or apprehensive patients, and makes the manipulator's task somewhat easier.

The stiffness of *spondylitis ankylopoetica* can be temporarily offset by the same gradual stretch. Sooner or later, the manipulator feels bone hitting bone when forcing is attempted; if so, the contracture is too advanced to benefit. *Rheumatoid arthritis* of the cervical joints is best treated by a collar and indomethacin. Manipulative stretching is contra-indicated. Subluxation requires arthrodesis.

TREATMENT OF MUSCLES

Painful scarring at the occipital insertion of the semispinalis capitis muscle may follow the prolonged rest in bed necessitated by concussion. This results in headache, elicited by the resisted neck movements. The treatment is deep massage there (see Vol. II); permanent relief is obtained in two to six sessions of proper friction.

It is a curious fact that a patient who receives deep massage to the muscles overlying a joint which is the site of internal derangement may temporarily recover a full range of active movement, though nothing else has been done. As a result, massage to the semispinalis capitis muscle at the requisite level may also be ordered as a means of securing localized relaxation of muscle before manipulative reduction is attempted.

TREATMENT OF LIGAMENTS

I am not at all sure in what circumstances ligamentous disorders occur at the neck. The following are the views of my colleague, R. Barbor:

The ligamentum nuchae becomes affected in three circumstances:
   (i) As the ligamentous component of a 'whiplash injury'.
  (ii) As a chronic strain following repeated internal derangement at a cervical intervertebral joint.
 (iii) As an occupational stress when the patient has to hold his neck in a flexed position for long periods.

In all these cases, stretching the ligament causes discomfort or pain, and there is abnormal tenderness to palpation usually between C5 and C6, or C6 and C7 spinous processes.

The treatment consists of intraligamentous injection of dextrose sclerosant solution mixed with a local anaesthetic agent on one to three occasions.

This should be followed by the patient maintaining a full range of movement at the cervical joints twice a day until all discomfort has ceased.

Technique of Injection

The patient sits on a chair and leans forward to rest the forehead on a table. In this position the cervical spine is flexed so as to facilitate palpation of the ligamentum nuchae at the lower two cervical levels.

A 2-ml. syringe is used and a flexible type 2-in. medium fine needle, filled with 1 ml. of 2 per cent procaine and 1 ml. of P.25G., dextrose sclerosant solution.

The skin is sterilized and the needle inserted just above the seventh cervical spinous process and is injected at, and to either side of, the spinous process. The needle is partly withdrawn: skin and needle are then pulled upwards and the process repeated about the sixth spinous process. The ligamento-periosteal attachments are infiltrated at both levels through one skin puncture.

9

The Jaw, the Thoracic Outlet, the Sterno-clavicular Area

THE TEMPORO-MANDIBULAR JOINT

When this joint is affected, the patient himself nearly always supplies the diagnosis. It should not be forgotten that a painless stiffness of the joint may be the first symptom of tetanus.

Anatomy

The temporo-mandibular joint is essentially one in which both the bone and the socket move.

The joint space is divided horizontally into two compartments by the meniscus. At the upper, the meniscus glides to and fro on the temporal bone; at the lower the mandibular condyle hinges on the meniscus. On opening the mouth fully the condyle and meniscus move forward together, i.e., the mandible and its socket move as one on the temporal bone.

Examination

The patient is asked to open and close the mouth, to deviate the mandible to right and left and to protrude it forwards. He then clenches his teeth and attempts to open the mouth against the examiner's resistance under his chin. The joint is then palpated while the patient opens and shuts his mouth and deviates each way. The examiner's finger should be placed just below the zygomatic process when opening is examined, and in the external auditory meatus when the jaw closes.

Whether or not each condyle of the mandible moves forwards or not on to the articular tubercle can be felt, together with any click or crepitus.

I. Clicking Jaw

This is due to a momentary luxation of the intra-articular meniscus. It can usually be relieved by so strengthening the muscles of mastication that they hold the jaw steady. To this end, resisted exercises are practised, i.e. opening the mouth, protrusion and lateral deviation. There is seldom any need to give a resisted exercise to the muscles that close the jaw; for these the patient maintains for himself by chewing. If dislocation of the meniscus takes place during the exercises, this must be prevented by the physiotherapist's finger pressing against the side of the jaw while the movements are resisted with the other hand.

2. Fixed Dislocation of the Meniscus

When this occurs the patient finds himself suddenly unable to open his mouth more than one centimetre. Full closing of the jaw is painless. Lateral deviation towards the affected side is usually painless and may be the position of ease.

Manipulative reduction without anaesthesia usually succeeds. The operator inserts his thumb and presses downwards on the molar teeth on the affected side. The point of the patient's chin is cupped between the operator's fingers and palm. During strong disengagement of the temporal bone and the mandible, this is rocked backwards and forwards, in alternate deviation laterally. The click is felt (see Vol. II). If the endeavour fails, under general anaesthesia, the patient's jaws are merely forced apart with a dental gag until the meniscus slips home (Fig. 26). Reduction by this means presented no difficulty even in a case of two years' standing.

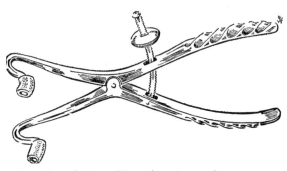

FIG. 26. Dental gag, for reducing a dislocated meniscus at the temporo-mandibular joint

3. Osteoarthritis

If this causes symptoms, there is pain on, seldom limitation of, the extreme of each movement. Crepitus is felt. Treatment consists of deep friction to the capsule of the joint followed by forcing movement (see Vol. II).

4. Sympathetic Arthritis

A day or two after the extraction of molar teeth, the patient may notice increasing difficulty in opening his mouth. On examination, movement is limited in every direction and the bone in the region of the tooth-socket is tender. This type of sympathetic irritation of the joint appears analogous to that occurring in connection with any abscess near the extremity of a bone.

Spontaneous cure of the arthritis may take two or three weeks. Treatment is seldom required, but must be directed to the dental sepsis, not the joint.

5. Non-specific Arthritis

Occasional cases are seen of arthritis of one temporo-mandibular joint for no apparent reason.

In the course of some weeks the patient develops increasing pain in the cheek and inability to open the mouth. This may remain slight, but may also progress to the point where opening beyond one centimetre is impossible; it may go on for months unchanged. Eating is painful and if much limitation is present the patient has to live on slops.

No clear cause is discernible. Gonorrhoeal ankylosis is a disease of the past, and neither Still's disease nor ankylosing spondylitis is present. In some cases, monarticular rheumatoid arthritis is apparently responsible, since hydrocortisone injection once or twice into the joint is curative. It should always be tried, even if the sedimentation rate and other tests are negative (as they so often are when only one large joint is affected).

Technique of Injection

The patient lies on his side, with the affected joint uppermost. The zygoma is identified and just below, level with the tragus, the physician can feel the condyle of the mandible moving as the mouth is opened as much as possible and then closed. A thin needle attached to a syringe containing 0·5 cc. of hydrocortisone suspension is inserted at the base of the tragus and pointed slightly forwards, aiming at the space left behind when the condyle has shifted anteriorly as far as possible by the patient opening his mouth as wide as he can. The needle becomes intra-articular at about 1·5 cm.

Stretching

If hydrocortisone has no effect, the only alternative is stretching the joint first with a Hallam's gag, then with a dental gag. It is remarkable that this treatment should be effective, but it is. Within a couple of months, full, painless movement is often restored, without tendency to recurrence.

6. Ankylosis

This is apt to follow a rheumatoid, septic or, in times past, a gonorrhoeal infection.

If the ankylosis is unsound, Hallam's gag may be used so long as enough space exists between the teeth for the introduction of the steel plate. It is opened by turning a screw and bears on all the front teeth (Fig. 27). He

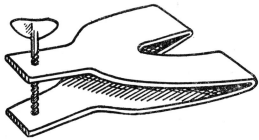

FIG. 27. Hallam's gag, for forcing movement slowly at the temporo-mandibular joint

suggests that pressure should be exerted in this way for twenty minutes every three hours. Arthroplasty is a most satisfactory operation for intractable limitation of movement. It should not be performed too late in cases of Still's disease, for lack of growth of the mandible from disuse leads to unsightly facial deformity.

7. Pain Arising in the Pterygoid Muscles

Rarely, the track of a local anaesthetic injection for dental purposes in this area becomes secondarily infected. Seward (1966), in hospital practice, estimates this occurrence as only two or three times in 100,000 injections. A day or two after the visit to the dental surgeon, pain in the cheek and stiffness set in. The history of a local anaesthetic injection is clear, and examination shows limitation of jaw opening. But clenching the teeth hurts, as does resisted deviation towards the painful side. If these resisted movements hurt, the patient's temperature should be taken and treatment by antibiotics is called for at once.

Intermittent claudication of the pterygoid muscles occurs in giant-cell arteritis. Cortisone must be started without delay for fear of blindness from involvement of the ophthalmic artery.

8. Loss of Molar Teeth

The patient complains of a constant deep burning pain inside the temple and the upper part of the cheek, not necessarily made worse by eating. Examination reveals pain at the extremes of all movements at the temporo-mandibular joint, and loss of all the molar teeth, on the same side as the painful joint, on the opposite side, or on both sides.

The arthritis is caused by excessive upward pressure of the mandible against the articular fossa of the temporal bone, due to loss of the distance-maintaining apposition between the molar teeth of mandible and maxilla. Dentures restoring the proper distance between the jaws lead to the disappearance of the pain in a few weeks.

9. Hysteria

Obviously, patients, especially adolescents, wishing to draw attention to themselves by a reluctance to eat or speak, readily develop difficulty in opening the mouth. They are apt, however, to describe too diffuse a pain, extending perhaps all over the head and face, and to hold the neck stiffly as well. The circumstances attending the onset may ring false.

Examination of the jaw in an uncooperative patient is difficult, for he may merely hold his jaw closed and allege such pain that he cannot open his mouth. It is wise, therefore, to test the resisted movements of the neck first and to palpate indifferent spots (e.g. the maxilla) for tenderness in suspicious cases. Except in tetanus, gross limitation of movement does not come on suddenly on both sides at once; moreover, in subluxation of the meniscus at least 1 cm. of opening range is always retained.

The result of treatment often proves conclusive, persuasion aided by gentle forcing restoring range in a few minutes.

THE THORACIC OUTLET SYNDROME

It has long been recognized that pressure on a nerve, if sustained or severe, sooner or later interferes with the parenchyma; the signs of loss of conduction characterizing a lower motor neurone lesion then appear. If, however, the pressure is slight or intermittent, conduction may not become impaired, even after many years of symptoms. Hence intermittent pressure on a nerve-trunk may never result in the development of the neurological deficit that would be expected sooner or later to clarify the diagnosis. Yet the patient's sensations, particularly his complaint of pins and needles, indicate that a nerve is affected. This is often the situation at the thoracic outlet in middle-aged women. The nerve recovers by night as fast as it is compressed by day, no loss of conduction ever supervening.

The thoracic outlet syndrome is an affection of the brachial plexus, not

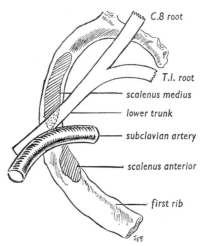

FIG. 28. Anatomy of thoracic outlet
(after Rogers)

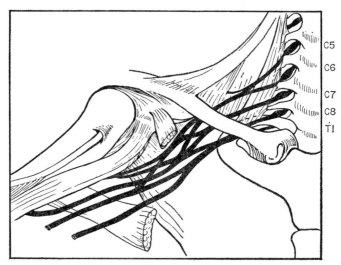

FIG. 29. The relations of the brachial plexus
Note the proximity of the lower trunk to the first rib.

the nerve-roots. The patient, therefore, experiences no symptoms at the base of the neck where the lesion lies, but only those referred to the distal part of the upper limb. The nerves derived from the eighth cervical and first thoracic roots, i.e. the lower trunk, are affected alone. The mere discovery, therefore, of neurological signs at or above the seventh cervical level, excludes pressure at the thoracic outlet as the cause.

There are two main types of pressure at the thoracic outlet: (1) that associated with a cervical rib, and (2) that associated with the first rib. Cervical ribs show, of course, by X-rays, but it must be remembered that patients with every gradation of bony abnormality, from unusually long transverse processes at the seventh cervical vertebra to large cervical ribs, may have no relevant symptoms at all. By contrast, a strong fibrous band in the position of a cervical rib but without ossification does not show radiologically, but can cause just as much trouble as a bony rib.

Cervical Rib

The symptoms are wholly distal and more often related to pressure on nerves than on the subclavian artery or vein. Pins and needles and numbness of median or ulnar distribution, more often the latter, are commonly the first symptoms. The complaint is usually bilateral, but often more severe on one side than the other. The patient, who is usually in his twenties or thirties, notices that carrying anything heavy or even wearing a winter overcoat brings on the paraesthesia in the hands. Sometimes he states that dependence of the arm for any length of time is followed by aching in the hand, which remains white and cold for some hours. This can be confirmed objectively, and indicates pressure on the subclavian artery. If the pressure is exerted on the subclavian vein, the hand may become oedematous and, less often, cyanosed for hours or days. Occasionally, he is concerned to see that, albeit painlessly, bilateral wasting of the abductor pollicis brevis muscle has slowly become complete over a period of years; the patient then attends merely to find out the cause of the alteration in the contour of his thenar eminence.

On examination, scapular elevation, and holding the arms up for a while, bring on the pins and needles but alleviate the vascular signs. Approximation of the scapulae draws the clavicles backwards and often stops the radial pulse, but this is not uncommon in normal individuals. Passive depression of the scapulae by the examiner seldom has any effect, but making the patient carry a weight for some time may increase or bring on the symptoms. Palpation at the root of the neck anteriorly may reveal a unilateral increase in the ease with which subclavian pulsation is felt. By contrast with these scapular findings, the movements of the neck are free and painless; and examination of the upper limb usually reveals no abnormality until the hand is reached, when ulnar or median weakness sooner or later becomes detectable. In early cases no abnormality is necessarily found.

Radiography shows the cervical ribs. It must be borne in mind that supernumerary ribs, visible by X-rays, do not necessarily cause symptoms.

In due course, in cases of median development, wasting of the abductor pollicis brevis muscle begins to show itself. In cases of ulnar development, the hypothenar and interosseous muscles weaken. Cutaneous analgesia is seldom a prominent feature. After some years, all the small muscles of the hand and the flexor digitorum profundus to the fourth and fifth fingers may become very weak.

Pressure exerted by the First Rib

Acute Onset

Rare cases occur of pressure at the thoracic outlet arising suddenly. A young person, after carrying a heavy weight for some distance—usually a suitcase on a journey—suddenly feels faint and develops pain in the chest and upper limb. Within a few minutes the hand and forearm blanch, but, since breathing usually hurts, consequent shallow respiration often leads to the patient's immediate admission with a provisional diagnosis of spontaneous pneumothorax. The radial pulse and warmth and colour return to the upper limb within a few hours.

Even more uncommon are attacks of severe, momentary pectoral pain caused by sudden impingement of the clavicle against a prominent costochondral junction of the first rib. If the diagnosis is confirmed by local anaesthesia and the attacks are severe and frequent, osteotomy of the clavicle is warranted.

Slow Onset

When the pectoral girdle droops during middle-age and subjects the lower trunk of the brachial plexus to pressure from the first rib by day, the symptoms are altogether different and the radiograph is normal.

The patient, nearly always a middle-aged woman, complains that each night she is woken two or three hours after falling asleep (i.e. between 1 and 3 a.m.) by severe pins and needles in both hands. She soon learns that if she lets her arms hang over the edge of the bed, or if she sits or stands up, the symptoms quickly subside. She falls asleep again, and the same thing may happen some hours later, or she may then sleep uninterrupted until the morning. Often the hands feel numb on waking; if so, the patient has difficulty for the first half-hour with small actions such as turning on the light; for she cannot feel the switch between her fingers.

By day, she is little troubled unless she carries a heavy weight on one arm, e.g. a shopping-basket, which soon brings on the pins and needles. These are seldom confined to any one part of the hand; they usually affect all five digits equally, on both aspects or within the palm. After some months or years, nocturnal pain begins in the hands and forearms, later still reaching to the shoulders. The patient sometimes comes to realize that the more she exerts herself by day, the more pain she will have that night; she may also notice that after a few days in bed with, say, influenza or while on a lazy holiday, her nocturnal symptoms disappear. The hands do not change colour. Sometimes the paraesthesia is purely unilateral. Rarely, patients present themselves with pain in the arm and forearm without pins and needles in the hand. If so, psychogenic pain is closely simulated, but the absence of exaggeration when the patient is examined makes the organic nature of the pain obvious and suggests the thoracic outlet as a possible source of pain.

The paraesthesia is a release phenomenon; it comes on only when the day's constant downward strain is taken off the pectoral girdle, i.e. at night, when the relief from the weight of the upper limb on lying down allows the lower trunk of the brachial plexus to move upwards out of contact with the first rib. Recovery takes some time after a whole day's compression, and it is therefore some hours before the paraesthesia appears and reaches an intensity that wakens the sleeping patient. Since the nerves recover each night, no signs of a lower motor neurone lesion may ever become manifest, even in those patients who have had severe nocturnal symptoms for several years.

Examination of all the movements of the neck and upper limb reveals full power and full painless range, except that sustained (1) elevation of the scapula and (2) elevation of the arms bring on the symptoms. If a patient appears to be suffering from compression at the outlet, these two postures should be maintained for several minutes, since the pins and needles and/or pain never come on instantly. If these two tests fail, the patient should lie supine with the arms above her head for five or ten minutes. Throughout the examination, it is the negative response to all the diagnostic tests, combined with a positive response to one or other of these ways of lifting the lower trunk of the brachial plexus off the first rib that, together with a suggestive history, enables a firm diagnosis to be made.

Differential Diagnosis

(1) Bilateral protrusion of the seventh cervical intervertebral disc: acroparaesthesia. The symptoms nearly always begin at the scapulae; there is pain on moving the neck, and the muscles affected are different. (2) Central cervical disc lesion. Pressure on the spinal cord may give rise

to pins and needles in the hands only, but they usually appear in the feet as well quite soon. The paraesthesia comes and goes in a wholly irregular way, most marked by day. Movement of the cervical spine is limited and bilaterally painful. Neck flexion may bring on the pins and needles in the hands. (3) Pulmonary sulcus tumour (Pancoast). Horner's syndrome is present: severe weakness of the small muscles of the hand (they are all affected) comes on rapidly. The radiograph of the apex of the lung is diagnostic. In advanced cases, erosion of the first and second ribs is also visible, and the patient may be hoarse owing to paralysis of one vocal cord. (4) Friction on the ulnar nerve at the elbow. (5) Compression of the median nerve in the carpal tunnel. (6) Compression of the ulnar nerve at the wrist.

Treatment
Operation

When cervical ribs set up marked signs of pressure on the brachial plexus or the subclavian artery, operation is usually indicated, especially in younger patients. If the obstruction is fibrous, not bony, the radiograph is misleadingly negative. Nevertheless, exploration of the outlet is warranted, especially in cases with vascular symptoms, in order to avoid the development of thrombosis, or later of a subclavian aneurysm. Unless operation is done early in vascular cases, gangrene of the fingers or ischaemic contracture may supervene (Rob and Standeven, 1958). Many different mechanical abnormalities exist. Hence the surgeon exposes the outlet and examines the relationship of the first rib and its muscles to the artery and the lower trunk of the brachial plexus, planning any subsequent operation according to what is found at the time.

Conservative Treatment

In the middle-aged patients who provide the majority of sufferers from pressure at the thoracic outlet, conservative treatment is usually very effective. Within two or three weeks the patient loses her longstanding symptoms and, as long as she keeps to her regimen, remains well. After a time, the nerves lose the heightened sensitiveness resulting from repeated bruising; some months later the patient finds that she can relax her precautions a good deal. If she suffers relapse, she knows its cause and its remedy.

Treatment requires the patient's co-operation and comprises:

(1) *Explanation*
It is important to make the patient understand the mechanism by which

her pain is produced. If she takes it as a release phenomenon, she bears with it until it ceases, realizing that the presence of pins and needles characterizes recovery and implies that she has adopted an eventually beneficial position. In the absence of such guidance, she unwittingly makes herself worse by, logically enough, avoiding such postures as bring on her unpleasant symptoms. Once she realizes that her pain is abolished by renewed compression of the nerve, she can appreciate why she must reverse her attitude. Otherwise she merely postpones her symptoms voluntarily, and has to suffer the more each night in consequence.

(2) *Elevating the Scapulae*

It is quite useless merely to give exercises to the trapezius muscles. In the first place, these muscles are extremely strong in all healthy individuals. In the second place, strengthening a muscle in no way hinders it from fully relaxing when not in use. The patient must learn to keep her shoulders very slightly shrugged all the time, in other words, to maintain a slight constant postural tone in the trapezii. This habit can be inculcated; exercises to make the muscles contract and then relax misses the point altogether. Before lifting anything heavy she must shrug her scapula right up and maintain it so all the time that she is carrying the weight. So far as possible, she must avoid wearing an overcoat. A basket on wheels is a great help to the housewife. Provision of domestic help fully relieves some patients, as study of the history may indicate.

(3) *The Armchair*

Each evening, after supper, she must sit in an armchair with her arms adducted to her sides and the forearms so supported on the arms of the chair that the scapulae are held well up without effort on her part. After a while, this posture results in the appearance of the familiar symptoms. She remains seated thus until the paraesthesia has ceased, however long this may take—at first often twenty to thirty minutes, later only a few minutes. The nerve-trunk having now recovered, she can go to bed, free from fear of being woken.

(4) *Support*

Occasionally, it is wise to take the downward strain off the thoracic outlet. In unilateral cases, a sling can be worn bearing on the other shoulder only. In bilateral cases, it is necessary to provide a belt with adjustable gutters supporting the upper forearm (Fig. 30). The patient rests her elbow on the gutter all the time that the arm is not in active use.

(5) *Raising the Trapezius Muscles*

The operation devised by Cockett should be employed in resistant cases. The trapezius muscles are detached from the spinous processes of the cervical vertebrae and then sutured back again higher up, thus providing the scapulae with a permanent brace.

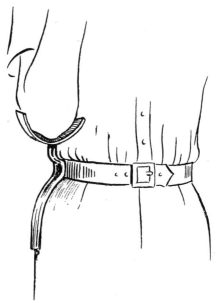

FIG. 30. Gutter-belt. The patient rests her elbow on the gutter whenever the arm is not being used, thus relieving the pectoral girdle of the weight of the upper limb.

SUBCLAVIAN OCCLUSION

The chief symptom is intermittent claudication in the arm, i.e. pain after continuing hard work for a while. Hence, the patient complains of an increasing ache in whatever muscles he has been using most strongly, whereas the examiner finds no lesion when he makes the patient contract each muscle momentarily. It is the pain brought on by persistent exertion that suggests thrombosis of the subclavian artery, and a negative examination makes it the more probable. The diagnosis is made when the radial pulse is found absent. The aortogram reveals the exact state of affairs.

If, as the result of vigorous use of the arm, the brachial demand for arterial blood becomes so great that the pressure in the circle of Willis falls below that in the subclavian artery, blood is drawn to the arm from the cerebrum. Reversal of blood flow in the vertebral artery occurs when the subclavian stenosis lies proximal to the origin of the vertebral artery. In these cases, in addition to the increasing discomfort, exertion of the arm makes the patient feel faint from diminution in the blood-flow to the brain.

RARE CAUSES OF SCAPULO-CLAVICULAR PAIN

A number of conditions exist in which the movements of the neck and scapula both hurt, sometimes of the arm too. Such a multiplicity of painful movements suggests psychoneurosis, but the following conditions must be eliminated before such an attribution can be confidently made.

Cervical Disc Lesion

The pain is in the upper scapular area, and is brought on in the usual way by some but not other of the active and passive neck movements. However, in acute cases, testing the scapular and arm movements against resistance may hurt too, since the scapula must be fixed by contraction of the scapulo-vertebral muscles before the arm can be pushed hard in any direction, thus compressing the spinal joint. But the pain is felt at the base of the neck, not the arm. There is occasionally a painful arc. A patient with really acute torticollis may be unable to get his arm up voluntarily above the horizontal. Resisted lateral rotation at the shoulder and resisted flexion at the elbow may also cause pain, but again in the scapular area.

The diagnosis is immediately clarified by reducing the cervical displacement by manipulation; then the same arm and scapular movements are tested again. If, as often happens, they no longer hurt, the cervical displacement is shown to be responsible for the whole syndrome. All patients, therefore, who clearly possess a cervical disc lesion, and perhaps also trouble in the scapular area or arm, should be treated thus. After manipulative reduction, it becomes clear if they arose from transmitted stress or because two lesions are present.

Fractured First Rib

Since this is usually a stress fracture, there is no history of trauma; merely the unprovoked appearance of pain at the root of the neck. The neck movements hurt, especially side-flexion away from the painful side, when the scalenes pull on the rib adjacent to the fracture. Resisted side-flexion towards the painful side is also painful for the same reason. Raising the arm is painful and often cannot be carried out beyond the horizontal, but full passive elevation is seldom more than uncomfortable. Since a fractured rib unites in two months, this disorder need be considered only when the history is short—a few weeks. The radiograph is diagnostic.

Clay-shoveller's Fracture

This is a stress fracture, caused by unaccustomed exertion, usually digging, by an unfit person. The pain is central at the base of the neck and active and passive flexion and extension of the neck prove painful. However, elevation of each scapula also hurts and again the arms cannot be actively elevated beyond a small amount of abduction.

This time the pain is central and the inability bilateral, and again spontaneous recovery takes two months; hence this diagnosis need be considered only in short-lived cases. The seventh cervical or first thoracic spinous process is tender. The radiograph is diagnostic.

The Costo-coracoid Fasciitis

Idiopathic Contracture

This is a very uncommon cause of limited elevation of the arm. The symptom is gradually increasing, upper pectoro-scapular pain on one side only. It is provoked at first only by full elevation of the arm. After a year or two elevation becomes slightly limited, and any prolonged reaching upwards leads to some hours' or days' increased aching.

The syndrome is difficult to recognize, because the symptoms suggest a cervical disc lesion and the signs, unless carefully studied, suggest a psychogenic disorder. The key to the condition is the discovery of slight painful limitation of elevation of the scapula.

Examination of the neck-movements reveals that active side-flexion away from, and resisted side-flexion towards, the painful side hurt at the root of the neck. Upward movement of the scapula, active or passive, is painful at its extreme and slightly limited. Resisted elevation is painless. Forward movement of the scapula is usually full and painful; backward, full and painless. Since the patient seldom asks advice for the first year or so, by the time he is seen, active and passive elevation of the arm has become about 10 degrees limited by pectoro-scapular pain; but passive movements at the gleno-humeral joint are neither restricted nor painful. All the resisted shoulder movements hurt a little at the base of the neck.

This curious pattern occurs only in contracture of the costo-coracoid fascia. When inspection of the range of elevation of both scapulae together discloses limitation on the painful side, this rare condition is brought to mind. One cause is dense adhesions at the apex of one lung such as occurs in long-standing tuberculosis. However, not all cases show such a shadow. Follow-up for several years reveals no ultimate cause, nor any tendency to spontaneous recovery; indeed the contracture tends to become very slowly worse. My youngest patient had had it for a year when she was first seen aged twenty-three. It does not appear to start after the age of fifty.

Traumatic Fasciitis

Occasionally, these symptoms and signs come on after trauma. If so, a deep breath also hurts and pneumothorax is suspected, but the radiograph excludes this disorder. I regard these cases as caused by a small haematoma lying beneath the costo-coracoid fascia. No treatment avails, and spontaneous resolution takes about three months.

Treatment

Conservative treatment is vain. Forcing elevation of the arm brings on increasing aching for several days; no benefit follows. If the cause is tuberculous fibrosis at the apex of the lung, forcing is contra-indicated since it might well disturb the healed area. The patient must just accept that he cannot lift his arm right up.

So far only one patient has accepted operation. She was a secretary and typing made her upper pectoral area ache so severely that she could not go on. In 1967, my surgical colleague D. R. Urquhart exposed the fascia, which appeared quite normal and divided it and the pectoralis minor muscle. She retains some 5 degree limitation of elevation a year later, but is symptom-free and works well.

Pulmonary Neoplasm

Some early cases can be mistaken for a shoulder lesion. The neoplasm interferes with the diaphragm and pain at the point of the shoulder results. When it begins to erode the chest wall, the pectoralis major protects the ribs by going into spasm when the arm is elevated. Hence, pain at the point of the shoulder and limitation of elevation of the arm beyond the horizontal result. The neck and scapular movements may cause slight discomfort, but the range of both is full. The passive range of movement at the shoulder joint is full and painless, thus forming a strong contrast with the fact that the arm cannot be lifted even passively above the horizontal, in the presence of a fully mobile scapula. When the agent responsible for this restriction is sought, the pectoralis major can be seen to contract and prevent further movement.

The radiograph of the lung reveals a large shadow.

Subclavian Muscle

This muscle is occasionally strained, expecially in patients with a lax sterno-clavicular joint. The pain is felt accurately at mid-clavicle, and may be brought on slightly by passive elevation of the scapula, but is severe when the patient presses his pectoral girdle downwards against the examiner's resistance applied to the elbow, while the arm is approximated to the patient's trunk.

However long the symptoms have continued, deep massage to the muscle affords permanent relief.

STERNO-LAVICULAR JOINT

This joint allows some 60 degrees range of elevation, 60 degrees of rotation and 30 degrees of forward movement, the range being limited by the fact that the scapula has reached its extreme of range.

The joint may be sprained as the result of a fall and any capsular stretching that occurs there is permanent. The weight of the upper limb makes the medial end of the clavicle ride upwards, after capsular rupture, as far as the costo-clavicular ligament permits. A permanent prominence is then visible. Subluxation is common also in osteoarthritis and after a bacterial infection.

The patient himself supplies the diagnosis; for the pain is felt exactly at the joint and does not radiate. Movement at the joint produced by the active scapular movements usually evokes slight discomfort, but the main discomfort appears at the extreme of each movement of the humerus at the shoulder: a more powerful way of straining the joint. Adduction of the arm across the chest hurts most and in recent sprains may prove painful enough to be limited. On palpation, the joint is prominent and tender. In osteoarthritis, the joint may appear swollen and feel soft in a manner more suggestive of rheumatoid arthritis, but this finding need not arouse alarm. Syphilis is said to have a special predilection for the inner end of the clavicle, but this appears no longer so.

Treatment

Recent Sprain

A sling should be worn for a couple of days to relieve the joint of the weight of the upper limb and hydrocortisone injected as soon as the patient is seen. Recent and chronic cases respond equally well. Subsequent instability, provided that it is painless, is of no inconvenience to the patient. Exercises are contra-indicated since the sterno-clavicular joint is dependent for stability on ligaments alone; hence movements only cause further stretching. Moreover, no adhesions can form in a joint about which no muscle exists that could hold it too still.

Chronic Cases

Pain follows exertion (the joint is already osteoarthritic or subluxated), and may continue indefinitely in spite of the avoidance of exertion. One injection of hydrocortisone into the joint abolishes the symptoms, but the patient must permanently restrict exercise thereafter, otherwise pain will return and a further intra-articular injection will be required.

Posterior Sterno-clavicular Syndrome

This is a rare condition. For no apparent reason, a middle-aged patient develops unilateral pain at the *posterior* aspect of the neck, which continues unchanged for years. The pain is not severe, but constant, worse on using the arm. There is no discomfort anteriorly in the region of the sterno-clavicular joint.

On examination, the neck movements, passive and resisted, do not hurt, but scapular elevation is painful at its extreme, passively as well as actively. There is no scapulo-thoracic crepitus. No weakness or pain is revealed when scapular elevation is tested against resistance. Full elevation of the arm is difficult to achieve because of pain felt at the base of the neck, whereas full abduction at the gleno-humeral joint is painless. Examination of the rest of the upper limb reveals no abnormality. The anterior sterno-clavicular ligaments are not tender. Thus nothing draws attention to the sterno-clavicular joint. Patients are apt to receive treatment intended to restore full elevation to the arm, but this increases the symptoms. Yet 1 cc. of hydrocortisone injected into the posterior sterno-clavicular ligament, either through the joint or by approaching the back of the joint from above, relieves the condition, apparently permanently.

SCAPULO-THORACIC CREPITUS

When one or other scapula—sometimes both—is actively moved up and down against the thorax, painless crepitus may be palpable. Occasionally, a loud creaking audible across the room is provoked. If the scapulae are abducted, the crepitus on movement ceases. The condition is clearly due to roughening of the posterior thoracic wall just beyond the lateral edge of the ilio-costalis muscle.

When the crepitus occurs in young people, there may be concern lest the crepitus prove the precursor to 'rheumatism'. Explanation that the crepitus is permanent and insignificant is usually all that is necessary.

Occasionally the patient complains of considerable scapular aching after exercise. Typists, gymnasts and physiotherapists may become scarcely able to work. In such cases, the area whence the crepitus originates must be outlined by discovering just how far the scapula need be abducted for the crepitus on movement to cease. The roughened area now lies just medial to where the vertebral border of the upper scapula lay. Deep massage must be given to this spot. The patient feels no special tenderness here; the physiotherapist cannot feel any crepitus as she gives the massage; hence the spot must be found mathematically. The crepitus on scapular movement does not cease; yet say twenty such treatments largely or wholly abolish the ache, even when it is of many years' standing.

The patient may begin to develop a tic, moving his scapula repeatedly so as to elicit the crepitus; this naturally increases the ache, though he imagines that the action provides temporary relief. Advice to resist this habit suffices.

Should massage fail and the symptoms warrant, excision of the upper inner angle of the scapula affords permanent cure, but I have only once met sufficient disability to warrant this.

10

The Shoulder: Examination

PART I: LIMITED RANGE

The problems discussed in these three chapters concern the nature and site of the numerous painful processes that occur in the shoulder region, and the factors governing the choice of treatment.

Special difficulties attend identification of the many possible lesions, since the pain is in much the same place whatever its source, and the physical signs that render differentiation possible are slight and wearisome to evaluate. Moreover, double lesions are encountered quite often, thus increasing the complexity of the problem. Therefore, many doctors regard disorders at the shoulder as uninteresting, undiagnosable and incurable, but tending to recover in the end. Nothing could be further from the truth; for many shoulder lesions persist unchanged for years and nearly every one is fully, often permanently, relievable. The many separate lesions are all distinguishable, and with a clear-cut diagnosis, they are nearly all curable. Purely clinical testing suffices and is indeed merely an exercise in applied anatomy. Auxiliary methods such as radiography and blood tests seldom add any information and may prove misleading.

Pain

Symptoms arising from the tissues at the shoulder are seldom felt at the shoulder itself. The exception is the acromio-clavicular joint. This is developed within the fourth cervical segment and cannot, therefore, refer pain to the arm. All the other common lesions at the shoulder affect structures derived largely from the fifth cervical segment. Hence, wherever the actual source lies, the pain is often felt to start at the lower deltoid area and to spread along the relevant dermatome, which ends at the radial side of the wrist, the pain radiates as far as the base of the neck.

How far the pain is referred depends on the severity of the lesion. For example, in slight arthritis or tendinitis, the pain is usually felt at the upper arm only, whereas the same lesion, if more intense, leads to radiation of pain as far as the wrist. This extended reference is an error of perception occurring in the sensory cortex. Precise delineation of the extent of the pain has two values: (a) it outlines the dermatome and thus shows within which segment to look for the lesion; (b) it indicates the severity of the pathological process.

Whatever the disorder at the shoulder may be, the pain is apt to be felt in the same place except for the ache at the point of the shoulder that suggests a lesion of the acromio-clavicular joint. For example, whether arthritis, bursitis or tendinitis is present, the lesion lies in a structure of largely fifth cervical derivation; hence fifth cervical reference is common to each. Furthermore, the same lesion, when its severity alters, may at different times give rise to pain at different sites; for the symptoms are confined only by the segmental boundaries.

No matter what the position of an articular or para-articular lesion at the shoulder, if it is severe, the patient feels a deep burning ache running down the antero-lateral aspect of the arm and the radial side of the forearm. He has little idea of its source; if he indicates an exact point, he is usually wrong. Whenever such diffuse pains are met with in the upper limb, examination of the entire forequarter is always required. Nor must the examiner stop when one disorder has been identified; for combined lesions are fairly common in this area.

PRESENT-DAY MISCONCEPTIONS

There are a number of important errors in current medical thought on the shoulder leading to difficulty in correctly interpreting the clinical findings. The most important error is to ascribe capsular lesions to disorder of the tendons about the joint. This is considered below.

Tendinous Lesions Thought to Cause Limitation of Movement

There is a widespread belief that limitation of movement at the shoulder can result from tendinous lesions. Limitation of *active* movement can, of course, be due to, say, supraspinatus tendinitis, when so painful an arc exists that the patient cannot by his own efforts get the arm beyond the horizontal. But full passive elevation relaxes the supraspinatus muscle and can always be obtained. Hence, tendinous lesions do not limit the *passive* range of movement, and it is the passive movement, not the active, that informs the examiner what is the true range. Tendinitis leading to capsulitis is a neat idea, but bears no relation to what is found on clinical examination of painful shoulders. Another notion is that degenerative change in the biceps and supraspinatus tendons leads to subsequent arthritis; this theory creates a pleasant unity, but is without justification. Tendinous and capsular lesions at the shoulder are quite separate, and each may be present for years without affecting the other; they do not merge, however long the patient is kept under observation.

Bicipital tendinitis is held by many authorities to be the forerunner of a 'frozen shoulder'. In fact, the tendon of the long head of biceps does not move during abduction of the humerus, the bone gliding under the stationary tendon. Were the tendon to become inflamed or fixed to bone, it is conceivable that limitation of adduction of the humerus might in theory result; but passive abduction could not become restricted. If the tendon is frayed, degenerated or chronically inflamed, the only symptom would be pain on resisted flexion and supination of the forearm.

More recently orthopaedic surgical opinion has accused the rotator cuff as the primary lesion in a frozen shoulder. This alternative is equally mistaken. In fact, the muscles about any joint do not go into spasm spontaneously. They do so to protect the joint, and it is here that the primary lesion lies. In any case, no lesion (short of ossification) of any tendon can give rise to limitation of passive movement; the characteristic finding in arthritis of the shoulder. Were the rotator cuff to contract, the pull of the subscapularis and infraspinatus muscles would cancel each other out, but no tendon lies inferiorly to counterbalance the pull of the supraspinatus tendon. Hence, did the 'rotator cuff syndrome' exist, it would lead to fixation of the shoulder in full abduction—the exact contrary of what actually happens.

The idea that tendinous disorders can limit movement at the shoulder has arisen in three ways, as follows:

(1) Because limitation of active movement, in spite of its ambiguity, is taken at its face value. If active movement is limited, either joint range is restricted or the muscle will not move the arm properly. Hence, if the examiner does not then test the passive movement, he is misled. No one denies that tendinous lesions can lead to limitation of the voluntary range, but they cannot restrict the range on passive testing.

(2) Because of the difficulty often experienced in distinguishing between the earliest stage of an arthritic shoulder and a tendinous lesion.

(3) Because injury to both the capsule of the shoulder joint and the supraspinatus tendon is fairly common. As a result of the tendinous lesion, the patient has considerable pain on attempting active abduction. He therefore avoids this movement and the damaged shoulder joint develops post-traumatic adhesions. Thus a traumatic supraspinatus

tendinitis, accompanied initially by a full range of movement at the shoulder joint, may later lead to a joint at which true limitation of movement from disuse has supervened.

'Periarthritis'

Presumably 'periarthritis' can only mean that some tissue about a joint, rather than those forming it, is at fault. This word is unhelpful; for it fails to answer the vital question—which of the periarticular structures is affected? At the shoulder, the condition to which the term 'periarthritis' is least ill-suited is subdeltoid bursitis, which should be described as such.

The false concept of 'periarthritis' has arisen from a mistaken belief in the diagnostic value of radiography. Limitation of movement at the shoulder associated with normal X-ray appearances has been thought to exclude a diagnosis of arthritis. This is not true. Many types of arthritis at other joints continue for a long time without showing any radiological changes and yet are unhesitatingly and correctly ascribed as arthritis; e.g. traumatic or rheumatoid arthritis of the fingers; traumatic, gonorrhoeal or infective arthritis at the knee; gouty arthritis of the foot. The fact that what had, on negative radiological grounds, been called 'periarthritis' was a capsular lesion meriting the term arthritis, was finally proved by Neviaser (1945). He dissected post mortem, or inspected at operation, sixty-three shoulders with limited movement on clinical examination. He found that the capsule of the joint, instead of showing the normal laxity, was tight, closely applied to the head of the humerus and under such tension that it gaped widely when incised anteriorly. He found the densest adhesions between the two capsular surfaces (see Fig. 31) inferiorly, thereby limiting abduction. His conclusions were that the lesion was not a 'periarthritis', but thickening and contracture of the capsule which microscopy showed to be the site of reparative inflammatory change. He suggested 'adhesive capsulitis' as a suitable term. These findings provide clear pathological confirmation of the views, then based on clinical considerations only, expressed in the original edition of this book. Viessel (1949) carried out arthrography with pyelosil on three cases of frozen shoulder and also found 'a degree of obliteration of the inferior joint recess'.

J. H. Young confirmed this finding (1952) by postmortem dissection. Capsular contracture was the only lesion in six cases of blocked shoulder opened by de Sèze et al. (1959). Reeves (1966) found a marked reduction of the volume of fluid that was injectable at constant pressure in arthritic shoulders, less so when the lesion followed trauma.

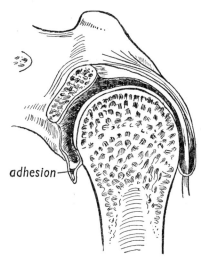

adhesion—

FIG. 31. Coronary section of the shoulder. A dense adhesion has formed at the inferior aspect of the joint, binding together the capsular fold (after Neviaser).

Possible Sources of Shoulder–Arm Pain

The preliminary examination singles out pain referred to the shoulder from elsewhere, e.g. diaphragm. Radiography identifies lesions of the bones. When these two possibilities have been excluded, pain felt in the shoulder and upper limb should be sought at the following twelve sites.

1.	Capsule of the shoulder joint	C_5
2.	Subdeltoid bursa	C_5
3.	Subcoracoid bursa	C_5
4.	Acromio-clavicular joint	C_4
5.	Costo-coracoid fascia	?
6.	Subclavian artery	?
7.	Supraspinatus tendon	C_5
8.	Infraspinatus tendon	C_{5-6}
9.	Subscapular tendon	C_{5-6}
10.	Subclavius muscle	C_5
11.	Biceps tendon	C_{5-6}
12.	Triceps muscle	C_7

EXAMINATION OF THE SHOULDER

History

The object of taking a history is twofold. First, to help decide whether or not the source of pain is likely to be in the shoulder region. Second, to assist further in assessment when the conditions that cause limitation of movement at the shoulder are encountered. In these cases, the answers to the questions set out below help to determine the stage that the lesion has reached. By contrast, if a tendon is found at fault, none of the points raised in the history is relevant.

Ten questions are enough:

(1) Where is your pain?

If the patient indicates the point of his shoulder, a lesion of the acromio-clavicular joint is suggested; pain felt anywhere in the arm is common to all the other possible lesions.

(2) Was there any injury?

If later examination shows the capsular pattern, this suggests traumatic arthritis.

(3) What is your age?

Age is relevant to the distinction between the different types of arthritis at the shoulder.

(4) How long have you had it?

If the capsular pattern is present, the stage that a freezing arthritis should have reached follows a chronological sequence. Too much or too little limitation of movement for the time that has elapsed since the onset suggests monarticular rheumatoid arthritis. Acute subdeltoid bursitis leads to gross limitation of movement in a few days; the non-capsular pattern is present, and spontaneous recovery takes six weeks. In palindromic rheumatism, the capsular pattern is present and the pain and limitation last only three days.

(5) Have any other joints been affected?

An affirmative answer suggests rheumatoid, psoriatic or lupus erythematosus arthritis or that complicating ankylosing spondylitis.

Gout is rare at the shoulder and in most gouty patients with shoulder trouble the lesion there is unconnected.

(6) Has your pain spread?

The farther down the upper limb the pain goes, the more severe the lesion. Radiation to the arm excludes the acromio-clavicular ligaments.

(7) When did the pain reach your elbow and your wrist respectively?

When freezing arthritis begins, pain is felt at the deltoid area, on movement only, for the first month. It reaches the elbow during the second month, and the wrist at the end of the third month, by which time it has become continuous. Two or three months later the pain diminishes and shortens, so that at the end of eight months the discomfort is once more evoked only by movement and has returned to the deltoid area. In freezing arthritis, aggravation and spontaneous cure follow a chronological pattern, scarcely varying from case to case. Hence, the length of time since the onset and the behaviour of the pain can be correlated; this sequence often distinguishes freezing from monarticular rheumatoid arthritis.

(8) Can you lie on that side at night?

If not, and the capsular pattern is present, treatment by forcing movement is inappropriate.

(9) Is there pain by day even when your arm is kept still?

If there is, forcing is contra-indicated.

(10) Have you ever had an operation?

This and questions about visceral function are relevant only if the pattern for malignant invasion at the shoulder emerges.

Examination: First Part

The first question is: does the pain felt at the shoulder arise from the tissues about the shoulder? The second is: if the shoulder is at fault, which of the structures there contains the lesion? The first part of the examination decides the former point, and since any patient with armache is complaining of pain felt within a dermatome between the fourth cervical and the second thoracic, these segments must be fully examined. The first stage of the examination, therefore, consists of a quick survey from neck to hand. If the lesion is found to lie within the shoulder area, this is then examined more carefully. If the pain is found to be referred to the shoulder from some other moving part, examination is concentrated there. If no abnormality, i.e. neither limited movement, pain nor weakness is found at all, the lesion clearly lies outside the moving parts, and conditions like angina or diaphragmatic pleurisy are brought to mind. If all the movements, or a number of contradictory movements, are stated to hurt, the question of a psychogenic disorder arises.

The examination proceeds as follows, the patient being asked, as he performs each movement, if it hurts and, if so, where, while the examiner notes if weakness is apparent on any of the resisted movements.

Neck	active flexion, extension,
	both side-flexions,
	both rotations;
	resisted rotation (C1)
Scapula	resisted elevation (C2, 3, 4)
Shoulder	active elevation (C5)
Elbow	passive flexion and extension,
	resisted flexion (C5 and C6) and extension (C7)

Wrist   resisted flexion (C7) and extension (C6)
Thumb   resisted extension (C8)
Finger   resisted adduction of fourth and fifth fingers (T1)

If this examination shows that the lesion lies about the shoulder, this is examined in detail. However, if abnormality is detected on movements other than those of the shoulder, the lesion is shown to lie elsewhere.

Examination: Second Part

The Twelve Movements

It is just as important to carry out not more than twelve movements as to test not less than twelve. Too few movements means incomplete examination, but too many muddle the examiner, especially if he attributes significance to impure movements that test two structures simultaneously. When the arm is brought away from the side in the coronal plane, the amount of movement of which the arm is capable is referred to as *elevation*. This is possible through 180 degrees. The amount of movement existing in this direction between the scapula and the humerus is called *abduction*. This is possible through 90 degrees.

Since combined lesions are not uncommon at the shoulder, the fact that there is limitation in every direction must not lead the examiner to omit trial of the resisted movements. A fall on the shoulder may, for example, damage the fifth cervical nerve-root as well as the joint; partial rupture of the supraspinatus tendon may set up a secondary subdeltoid bursitis; myopathy may result in capsular contracture from disuse; neoplasm may invade both joint and tendons, and so on. Hence, the *resisted movements must be examined even in cases in which the discovery of limitation of range makes the diagnosis appear obvious.*

Normally, however, capsular lesions are uncomplicated and trial of the resisted movements does not set up pain or show weakness. This fact provides clear evidence that, as at other joints, there is no primary lesion of the muscles in arthritis at the shoulder.

The twelve movements are:

1. *Active Elevation*
The patient is asked to bring his arm up as high as he can and is asked what he feels. His active range of movement and statement on pain are noted for correlation later.

Patients do not know how the arm gets up to full elevation; most imagine that 180 degrees of movement are present at the shoulder joint.

In fact, the first 90 degrees of elevation take place at the scapulo-humeral joint. The next 60 degrees result from rotation of the scapula. The last 30 degrees involve adduction of the humerus, the surgical neck crossing in front of the coracoid and acromion processes which rotation of the scapula has now made to point upwards instead of forwards. This knowledge is important in detecting psychogenic limitation of active elevation. If the scapula is mobile and its muscles intact, even if the shoulder is ankylosed, 60 degrees of active abduction must be attainable by scapular movement alone.

2. *Passive Elevation*

The examiner pushes the patient's arm up as high as possible and notes (a) whether full elevation is obtainable; (b) if it hurts; and (c) if active and passive elevation correspond in range or not. During passive elevation and the two passive rotations, there is an opportunity to note the end-feel. This may be important both in diagnosis and deciding treatment. If pain comes on well before the extreme of range is reached, and the end-feel is soft, subdeltoid bursitis is suggested. If full range is present, all extremes hurting, a hard end-feel characterizes a capsular lesion. If the point when pain comes on and the extreme of the possible range lie very close together, the capsule is probably at fault. By contrast, when chronic bursitis, tendinitis or an affection of the acromio-clavicular joint causes pain at the extremes of full range, the hard capsular end-feel is absent and over-pressure results in increased pain but no more resistance than that of the normal joint. There is a characteristic free feel to the extreme of full elevation of the normal joint which has a strong positive significance and is easily identified after a little experience.

3. *Painful Arc*

This applies only when 90 degrees of abduction range at the shoulder joint is present, passively or actively. The patient is asked to bring his arm up outwards and to state if, at any point in the upward movement, he feels an ache, and if so, if it disappears again. Pain starting at the horizontal and continuing until full elevation is reached is not an arc. If the pain disappears above the horizontal but returns at full elevation, an arc is present. It is pain abating on either side of the painful point that has diagnostic significance. Since the abductor muscles draw the head of the humerus upwards and medially, an arc is usually best elicited on voluntary movement. However, an arc is an arc, whether felt on the way up only, down only, or both, active or passive.

A painful arc can often be seen, the arm faltering momentarily in its upward movement at about the horizontal. Alternatively, the patient

I

may have learnt how to avoid it by bringing his arm forwards into the sagittal plane before the horizontal is reached. So severe an arc, that active elevation stops at the horizontal and the patient uses his other hand to push the arm up farther, suggests calcification in bursa or tendon.

4. *Scapulo-humeral Range of Abduction*

The examiner fixes the lower angle of the scapula with his thumb, applying the heel of his hand to the patient's mid-thorax, and lifts the elbow outwards with his other hand until he feels the scapula start to move. He notes the amplitude of this angle (normal 85 degrees to 100 degrees).

5. *Passive Lateral Rotation*

The patient bends his elbow to a right angle and the examiner holds the forearm pointing straight forwards. The humerus is now rotated outwards, first on the good, then on the affected side. The range is usually 90 degrees, occasionally a little more in the young, and often 10 degrees to 20 degrees less in the elderly. If the restriction is due merely to age, it is painless and bilateral.

If lateral rotation is limited, the angle by which this falls short when the two sides are compared is estimated, and the examiner tests for the capsular end-feel. Whether the pain appears before or at the extreme of range, and whether or not over-pressure increases the pain, are all noted.

6. *Passive Medial Rotation*

The normal range, starting from the forward position of the forearm (as above) is 90 degrees. The examiner rotates the patient's humerus inwards and notes if full painless, full painful, or limited range is present, and in the latter case assesses the amplitude of this limitation.

Rarely a painful arc exists on medial rotation (never on lateral); if so, a tender structure is being pinched. It is important that the physician should not be too tender-hearted when medial rotation is tested, or he will stop at the arc and suppose that medial rotation is limited. If so, misdiagnosis is inevitable.

7. *Resisted Adduction*

The patient's elbow is brought a few inches from his thorax and he is then asked to pull his arm to his side as hard as he can. The examiner prevents all movement by placing one hand on the inner side of the patient's elbow, and the other on the patient's flank. The patient says whether pain is evoked or not, and, if so, where. The examiner notes the strength of the muscles.

8. *Resisted Abduction*

The patient pushes his elbow laterally as hard as he can; the examiner holds the elbow so strongly that the shoulder joint does not move. Pain is reported; strength noted.

9. *Resisted Lateral Rotation*

The patient bends his elbow to a right angle, the forearm pointing forwards. Keeping his elbow well into his side actively, he tries to rotate the arm outwards against the examiner's pressure, applied to the patient's lower forearm (not his hand), so strongly that the shoulder joint does not move. Pain is reported; strength noted.

10. *Resisted Medial Rotation*

The same as for lateral rotation, except that the resisted movement takes place towards the trunk.

11. *Resisted Extension of the Elbow*

The patient's elbow is bent to a right angle; he then presses his forearm down against the examiner's resistance applied to his lower forearm (not the hand). Pain is reported; strength assessed.

12. *Resisted Flexion to the Elbow*

The same as for resisted extension, except that the patient flexes his elbow.

MOVEMENT AT THE SHOULDER

The normal range of movement at the shoulder-joint is a matter of dispute. Clearly, the general belief—90 degrees at the shoulder joint and 90 degrees at the scapula—when the arm is moved from its dependent position to full elevation, is incorrect; for inspection shows that the vertebral border of the scapula never lies horizontally when the patient's arm is held vertically upright. The actual mechanism is as follows: from the adducted position to the horizontal position the arm moves at the scapulo-humeral joint. At 70 degrees, the greater tuberosity of the humerus is approaching the acromion, at 80 degrees it lies immediately beneath and the head of the humerus moves slightly downwards as the tuberosity passes under the coraco-acromial ligament. At 90 degrees, the tuberosity has moved beyond the arch and engages against the upper edge of the glenoid labrum. This is how a painful arc comes about (Fig. 32).

The next 60 degrees of elevation are performed by rotation of the scapula by the serratus anterior muscle. In doing so, the lower angle of the scapula moves well forward, and the whole bone now lies tilted so that the coracoid and acromion processes lie pointing vertically (see Fig. 34). At the same time the clavicle, being attached to the acromion, has to rotate also. It possesses about 60 degrees range of rotation at the sterno-clavicular joint. The last 30 degrees of elevation now take place as a result of adduction of the humerus (Fig. 35), largely owing to contraction by the pectoralis major muscle. The coraco-acromial ligament no longer hinders the movement when the scapula has rotated fully, for the surgical neck of the humerus can now glide along it anteriorly.

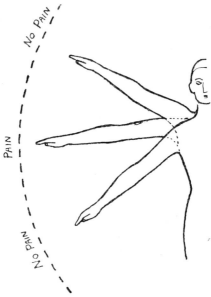

FIG. 32. Painful arc at shoulder. As the arm passes the horizontal, pain is elicited, disappearing as this point is passed in either direction.

The range of rotation at the shoulder joint is 180 degrees. It is best measured from the mid-position (i.e. the forearm pointing straight forwards) and the humerus is then normally capable of being turned 90 degrees medially and laterally.

Psychogenic Disorders at the Shoulder

The outstretched arm affords somatic evidence of welcome; by contrast, revulsion is evinced by withdrawal, characterized by the arm held close to the side. Since the position of the arm is closely connected with the emotions, patients with a distaste for their circumstances or their company readily develop inability to abduct the arm, holding it rigidly adducted.

In the detection of limited movement at the shoulder joint of hysterical origin, exact knowledge of the sequence described above is essential.

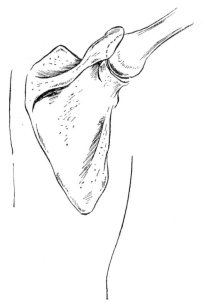

FIG. 33. Abduction at the shoulder joint. The scapula does not move appreciably. The humerus moves through 90 degrees, until the abduction movement is stopped by engagement of the greater tuberosity against the rim of the glenoid fossa.

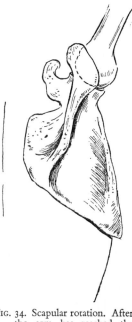

FIG. 34. Scapular rotation. After the arm has reached the horizontal, the next 60 degrees of elevation are brought about by active rotation of the scapula. This rotation brings the lower angle of the scapula antero-laterally with the result that the acromion and coracoid processes point vertically.

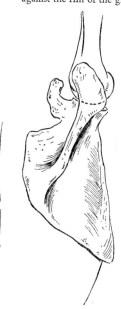

FIG. 35. Final stage of elevation of arm. During the last 30 degrees of elevation the scapula does not move. The neck of the humerus glides past the coraco-acromial arch by a movement of adduction, which can now be carried out in the vertical instead of the horizontal plane on account of the rotation of the scapula.

Moreover, even if the shoulder joint is completely fixed, 60 degrees of abduction can always be obtained by scapular rotation. If the scapula was found normally mobile during the preliminary examination, this is the minimum range of abduction possible. The patient has no idea of these facts. Hence, gross inconsistencies are quickly detected.

A common self-contradictory situation is as follows: The patient can raise his arm voluntarily only to the horizontal. Since 60 degrees of this movement is scapular, he can possess only 30 degrees range of abduction at the shoulder joint. But passive abduction may reveal 90 degrees scapulo-humeral range. Further examination may show the serratus anterior and supraspinatus-deltoid muscles to be perfectly strong when tested against resistance. The patient's limitation of elevation can result only from unwillingness, due to either psychoneurosis or malingering.

A malingerer, if middle-aged, who keeps his arm firmly to his side or wears a sling for some weeks, soon develops genuine limitation of movement at the shoulder. This should be remembered when gross inconsistencies are found in conjunction with an immobilizational arthritis at the shoulder joint.

INTERPRETATION

When the patterns that emerge on clinical examination come to be interpreted, there are four main divisions:

1. Limited passive movement; capsular pattern.
2. Limited passive movement; non-capsular pattern.
3. Full passive range; one resisted movement hurts.
4. Full passive range; one or more muscles are weak.

The Capsular Pattern

The presence of the capsular pattern indicates arthritis. At the shoulder there exist 90 degrees range of abduction, 90 degrees range of medial rotation and 90 degrees range of lateral rotation. The capsular pattern is: so much limitation of abduction, more limitation of lateral rotation, less limitation of medial rotation. Probable proportions are:

Arthritis	Abduction limited by	Lateral rotation limited by	Medial rotation limited by
Slight	10°	30°	Full and painful
Medium	45°	60°–70°	10°–15°
Gross	70°–80°	90°–100°	30°

An interesting confirmation of this pattern was provided by Reeves (1966) who illustrates an arthrogram of an arthritic shoulder which shows 'less restriction of posterior distribution of dye than anterior'. Clearly, if the anterior aspect of the capsule is more contracted than the posterior, lateral rotation will be more limited than medial rotation. The pattern is the same whatever the cause of the arthritis, which has to be decided on the criteria set out below. Moreover, the stage that a capsular pattern has reached is often as important as its nature, in particular when treatment is considered; the end-feel is very informative in this respect.

There are twelve separate disorders characterized by limitation of movement at the shoulder joint in the capsular pattern.

1. Traumatic Arthritis

A minor injury is reported by a middle-aged or elderly patient. After the immediate pain has ceased, he feels little or nothing for some days, then the upper arm begins to hurt, first on certain movements only; later, a constant ache sets in, soon spreading down to the elbow. Untreated, the pain and limitation of movement continue to get worse for four months. Then the pain begins to ease and at the end of a year full painless movement has returned spontaneously to the joint.

This is an avoidable condition, but is rarely prevented. Since it occurs so seldom before the age of forty-five, and never before the age of forty, except with fractures, prophylaxis is not necessary under that age. What is so often apt to happen is that, when the radiograph of the sprained shoulder shows no bony injury, the patient is merely reassured. No instructions on movement are given. In consequence, a traumatic arthritis leading to increasing pain and limitation of movement is allowed to develop. There comes a moment after three to five weeks when the joint has become so irritable that an attempt to treat it by stretching the capsule out aggravates the disorder, whereas, in the early stage, maintenance of mobility would have prevented the onset of the arthritis.

No muscular wasting occurs in traumatic arthritis, and in the common uncomplicated case, the resisted movements show that the muscles are not involved.

2. Immobilizational Arthritis

When an elderly patient's arm is put in a sling for any reason, e.g. Colles's fracture, limitation of movement of the capsular pattern is apt to come on quite quickly and lead to a painful arthritis indistinguishable from a traumatic arthritis, except by the history. A patient with early hemi-plegia is very prone to the same disorder, since he cannot move the paralysed arm himself and passive movement is not always ordered at once.

The maintenance of the range from the first, actively in immobilization, passively in hemiplegia, is all that is required in prophylaxis.

3. Freezing Arthritis: Type A

This is a rare phenomenon, without parallel at any other joint. Freezing arthritis usually comes on between the ages of forty-five and sixty. It follows, with only slight variations, a fixed course. Freezing arthritis is a good descriptive label; for, after freezing, the joint then thaws.

For no apparent reason, a middle-aged patient begins to feel an ache at the shoulder on moving the arm. There is no pain when the arm is kept still. Examination reveals almost a full range of movement at the shoulder joint, each extreme hurting when tested passively; the resisted movements are painless. After a month or two, the pain on movement becomes more severe and spreads as far as the elbow; a constant aching sets in, worse at night and worse still if the patient lies on that side in bed. Limitation of movement at the shoulder joint of the capsular type is now apparent. At the end of two or three months the pain has become constant and severe, reaching to the wrist. Severe pain on the slightest jarring of the joint may compel the patient to wear a sling. Examination now shows an abduction range of only 30 degrees to 45 degrees with corresponding limitation of rotation. The shoulder, however, never becomes, strictly speaking, 'frozen'; for complete fixation of the scapulo-humeral joint (such may occur in rheumatoid arthritis) is absent. No further diminution in the range of movement takes place after four months.

At the end of four months the pain is at its worst, but during the fifth month the symptoms begin to abate. At the end of the sixth month the constant ache has largely ceased. Once more pain is felt only when the shoulder is moved, and it leaves the forearm, remaining only in the arm. He begins to be able to lie on that side again at night. Later still, the pain produced by movement becomes confined to the deltoid area, and after eight months from the onset the range of movement begins to return to the joint. At the end of about a year the patient is well; the ache has ceased and full range of movement has been restored. It will be noted that the pain and limitation come on together during the first four months; the pain ceases during the next four months but the limitation of movement remains. Range returns during the last four months. There is little deviation from this course. Clearly freezing arthritis is not a degenerative condition since it recovers spontaneously and does not come on after the age of sixty.

Examination throughout shows the capsular pattern in its various degrees; the resisted movements remain strong and painless.

4. Freezing Arthritis: Type B

The existence of this rare variety came to light only when hydro-cortisone could be relied upon to differentiate between freezing and monarticular rheumatoid arthritis. I had previously confused this type of lesion with monarticular rheumatoid arthritis.

The patient is aged forty-five to sixty and gives the ordinary history of arthritis at the shoulder: pain in the deltoid area increasing and spreading down the upper limb as movement becomes increasingly restricted. How-ever, the pain goes on getting worse for nine months. At six or nine months, 30 degrees of abduction range exist but, by about the ninth month, this range has fallen to 5 degrees or 10 degrees and at the same time the pain eases greatly. Spontaneous return of full movement to the shoulder may then take a further year.

Examination reveals the capsular pattern and some wasting of the deltoid muscle. This finding, together with the wrong chronology for a freezing arthritis, naturally leads to a diagnosis of monarticular rheuma-toid arthritis, and indeed this usually proves correct. However, in this condition hydrocortisone injected intra-articularly affords no benefit, and the disorder runs its course unaffected by treatment.

This does not appear to be an example of a particularly severe freezing arthritis, since the course is so much longer and the pain eases when the limitation of movement is at its greatest: the reverse of the state of affairs in freezing arthritis.

5. Monarticular Rheumatoid Arthritis

Traumatic arthritis and monarticular rheumatoid arthritis are, in civilian practice, about equally common, whereas freezing arthritis is responsible for less than a tenth of all cases of limited movement in the capsular pattern.

Rheumatoid arthritis at the shoulder starts in the same way as a freezing arthritis, and at first they can scarcely be distinguished clinically. The radiograph affords no assistance and the sedimentation rate is seldom raised. However, *rheumatoid arthritis of this sort is much commoner than a freeze*, and, in cases of doubt, all patients should be tested therapeutically by the response to intra-articular hydrocortisone. Differentiation is most important since monarticular rheumatoid arthritis at the shoulder responds dramatically to hydrocortisone injected into the joint, whereas steroids have no effect on freezing arthritis.

In either case, for no apparent reason, pain begins in the deltoid area, spreading down the upper limb as far as the wrist, as the arthritis advances. Examination shows limited movement in the capsular pattern. Certain points arise that help to distinguish the two disorders.

(a) *Age*

Rheumatoid arthritis can come on at any age, whereas freezing arthritis is to be expected only between the ages of forty-five and sixty.

(b) *Paraesthesia*

Rheumatoid perineuritis may complicate the arthritis, and pins and needles in the hand of the affected side are apt to occur at, or just before, the onset of the arthritis. Perineuritis must be distinguished from ulnar paraesthesia appearing on waking only, caused by pressure on the nerve at the elbow owing to the unusual position which the arthritis compels the patient to adopt at night.

(c) *Timing*

The predictable four, four and four months' progress of freezing arthritis has been described above. Even at its height, 30 degrees of abduction range are always retained, and the speed with which movement lessens and returns follows a standard. Hence, if the timing is wrong for a freezing arthritis, the lesion is almost certainly rheumatoid. For example, if the pain is still getting worse after six months, if less than 30 degrees abduction range exists, if 60 degrees of abduction range have been lost after only a month's pain, if only 10 degrees of movement have been lost after four months, the chronology is wrong for a freeze.

Rheumatoid arthritis may recover spontaneously, seldom in under two years, or it may rarely proceed to fibrous ankylosis, or it may flare and subside at intervals for decades.

The arthritis at the shoulder that complicates psoriasis also responds well to intra-articular hydrocortisone, but is apt to go on for several years if not treated in this way.

The arthritis that is caused by osteitis deformans is apt to go on indefinitely, and in monarticular cases arthrodesis is warranted.

(d) *Other Joints*

If other joints are found affected by rheumatoid arthritis, or the patient has ankylosing spondylitis, psoriasis, Reiter's disease, lupus erythematosus or gout, the suggestion is clear.

Freezing arthritis in my experience, never attacks the same shoulder twice, though it may, within two to five years, attack the other shoulder. Hence recurrent attacks naturally suggest a rheumatoid type of lesion. Palindromic rheumatism has a predilection for the shoulders, but the attacks, however severe at the time, last only a few days, and eventually signs of rheumatoid arthritis at other joints are apt to appear.

(e) *Muscle Wasting*

Freezing arthritis is not a severe lesion and no muscle wasting ever becomes apparent. In rheumatoid arthritis of any severity, wasting is detectable.

(f) *Both Shoulders*

Freezing arthritis in both shoulders at the same time is a great rarity, whereas, especially in the elderly, it is often bilateral in rheumatoid cases. It is then apt to be mistaken for 'cervical spondylosis', since the limitation of movement may not be extreme and thus escape detection. The radiograph of the shoulders reveals no abnormality, and that of the cervical joints will almost certainly, at that age, show osteophytosis and narrowing of one or more disc spaces. Though freezing arthritis does not attack the same shoulder twice, rheumatoid arthritis may flare again at any time, at the same shoulder, the other one, or at joints elsewhere.

(g) *Confirmation*

If these points are all considered, diagnosis seldom presents difficulty. If doubt exists, the therapeutic test of injecting 50 mg. hydrocortisone into the joint settles the matter. If monarticular rheumatoid arthritis or one of its variants is present, the spontaneously appearing pain ceases in two days and a week later the patient reports continuation of the marked relief.

6. Osteoarthritis

Osteoarthritis at the shoulder joint is usually symptomless. The patient is aware of crepitus on movement of years' standing and a tendency to minor ephemeral aching after considerable exertion. Primary osteoarthritis causing symptoms is uncommon, but the presence of this degeneration makes the joint very apt to develop a superimposed traumatic arthritis after quite a slight, often indirect, strain on the joint or merely some overuse. Alternatively, quite a brief period of immobility, e.g. rest in bed after a coronary thrombosis, may set up a similar condition.

Myopathy and hemiplegia have the same effect. Hence, it is open to argument whether what is called osteoarthritis of the shoulder in these circumstances often merits the term; for the arthritis is usually brought to light by the injury or the immobilization. Osteoarthritis at the shoulder is not necessarily connected with osteophyte formation visible on the radiograph. Many shoulders affording such X-ray evidence possess a full and painless range of movement; others with pain, capsular contracture and marked crepitus on movement, are found normal on X-ray examination. Moreover, the presence of an osteophyte does not protect a patient against tendinitis or bursitis. It is thus a clinical diagnosis only.

The first pointer to osteoarthritis, other than the patient's age, is gained on examination of the painless shoulder which is found to be the site of symptomless osteoarthritis. The characteristic finding is slight limitation of elevation, such that the patient's arm, instead of reaching his ear, lies forward of this line, level more with his nose. Rotation is of full range and painless. Crepitus is palpable on movement, showing articular cartilage at the glenoid fossa to be fragmented.

Examination of the passive movements at the affected shoulder reveals the capsular pattern, combined with palpable crepitus. The resisted movements are painless.

7. Shoulder–Hand Syndrome

This is a variety of monarticular rheumatoid arthritis occurring in an elderly patient. After the age of sixty, pain in the arm and marked limitation of movement at the shoulder joint sets in. At the same time, the hand on the same side becomes stiff and the skin of the fingers undergoes trophic change. The ordinary capsular pattern is present at the shoulder joint; in addition, movement at the wrist, metacarpophalangeal and interphalangeal joints becomes markedly limited. Often the stiffness is such that it prevents the patient from gripping things in his hand at all. The fingers are shiny and red, and the skin atrophic; the nails may cease to grow. Recovery is uncertain. J. H. Young's postmortem dissection (1952) of a shoulder showing this syndrome revealed the same inferior capsular adherence as Neviaser described in freezing arthritis.

It has been suggested that the shoulder–hand syndrome is in some way connected with taking large doses of phenobarbitone, but cases certainly occur without any such drug having been ingested.

8. Bacterial Arthritis

Bacterial arthritis is uncommon whether septic, gonorrhoeal or tuberculous; in tuberculosis, by the time the patient is first seen, destruction of part of the articular surface of the humerus is already established, and permanent ankylosis unavoidable.

9. Bony Block

Patients with tertiary syphilis or syringomyelia may develop painless limitation of movement at the shoulder. When the joint is forced, a bony block is felt, but no pain is evoked. The radiograph shows huge osteophytic outcrops, engagement of which clearly restricts range. Examination of the nervous system reveals the cause of the neuropathic arthropathy, usually syringomyelia.

Displacement of a fractured tuberosity under the acromion also leads to a bony block, but there is a history of severe injury. Again, the radiograph is diagnostic.

10. Secondary Neoplasm

Invasion of the upper humerus and glenoid area by secondary malignant desposits affects the joint and the adjacent muscles. Hence the signs are dual: marked limitation of movement at the shoulder joint, accompanied by severe muscular weakness and pain when the resisted movement is attempted. The muscle wasting is greatly in excess of any attributable to the arthritis, and follows a bizarre pattern, not conforming to any one neurological lesion nor being confined to any one muscle. X-ray examination is confirmative.

Localized warmth felt at part of the scapular area may prove the first sign of a malignant deposit eroding bone. Within at most a week or two of this observation, a palpable tumour will have appeared and erosion of bone will be visible on the radiograph.

11. Primary Neoplasm

This occurs chiefly in young patients, in whom the slightest causeless limitation of movement at the shoulder should lead at once to study of the radiographic appearances. If the tumour originates from the shaft of the humerus, the first symptom may be pins and needles in the hand associated with fixation of the biceps and triceps muscles, leading to limitation of movement at the elbow. Chronic afebrile osteomyelitis and sarcoma are sometimes indistinguishable radiologically; biopsy or the response to penicillin may then be required to establish the diagnosis.

12. Haemarthrosis

After a slight injury the joint becomes painful quickly and the capsular pattern is found present on examination. When this happens in a young man, the cause is always haemophilia.

THE RADIOGRAPH

There are few joints where the radiographic appearances afford so little assistance as at the shoulder. Usually nothing abnormal is seen, even after the shoulder has been the site of severe arthritis for months. Traumatic capsulitis, no matter how long-standing, does not give rise to radiographic change.

Monarticular rheumatoid arthritis is often associated, at first, with a normal picture; later, slight general decalcification may be seen. Osteophyte formation may be seen but may be symptomless. Huge osteophytes limit movement, of course, at times all but painlessly. It should not be forgotten that osteophyte formation at the shoulder does not protect a patient against other lesions, to which all the symptoms may be attributable.

Calcification may appear in the subdeltoid bursa, but even a large area of calcification of the bursa is consistent with full and painless function at the shoulder joint; by contrast, many cases of bursitis display no calcification. Often, only one shoulder has been hurting, but the calcification is bilateral. Small calcified nodes may be seen at various places, most often in the supraspinatus tendon, but do not usually cause symptoms; on the other hand, large deposits in the tendon do cause pain, both at the arc and on active abduction. *Deposits should be regarded as significant only when they correspond in situation with the lesion already determined by clinical examination.*

Tuberculosis, neuropathic arthropathy, primary and secondary neoplasm, dislocation, fracture, osteoma, bone abscess, chondromatosis, osteitis deformans—it is conditions like these that show on the radiograph, whereas all the common causes of pain arising at the shoulder fail to show. Hence, radiography provides no short cut to diagnosis.

CLINICAL STAGES OF CAPSULAR LESIONS

The division of capsular lesions at the shoulder into acute, subacute and chronic has proved unsatisfactory, in so far as these words can be used equally well to describe how recent or how severe the lesion is. It so happens that, soon after an injury, the capsulitis is acute in the sense that it is recent, but chronic in the sense that the lesion is not yet severe and responds well to active treatment. Equally, after some months, the inflammation may become acute, i.e. severe, when the passage of time clearly warrants the designation chronic. This nomenclature has, therefore, been abandoned and the stages merely numbered. Severe, moderate and mild are not satisfactory alternative qualifications; for a lesion leading to little pain but marked limitation of movement at the shoulder clearly cannot be termed 'mild' even though, like a recent capsulitis associated with little restriction of range, it responds well to active treatment.

First Stage of Capsular Lesions

But, as occasionally happens, should these criteria be satisfied only in part, the capsulitis in in the second stage. For example, a patient may have pain confined to the shoulder and yet be unable to lie on the affected side at night.

1. When the pain is confined to the deltoid area or at least does not extend beyond the elbow
2. When the patient can lie on the affected side at night
3. When there is no pain except on movement
4. When the end-feel is elastic.

But, as occasionally happens, should these criteria be satisfied only in part, the capsulitis is in the second stage. For example, a patient may have pain confined to the shoulder and yet be unable to lie on the affected side at night.

Third Stage of Capsular Lesions

When the following criteria are satisfied, the arthritis is in the stage when all active measures directed to the joint are harmful. It is at this stage that intra-articular hydrocortisone is so valuable.

1. Severe pain extends from the shoulder to the forearm and wrist
2. The patient cannot lie on the affected side at night
3. The pain is greatest at night, and persists even when the arm is kept still
4. The end-feel is abrupt.

As stated above, the *second stage* of capsular lesions comprises those cases in which a mixture of these two sets of criteria exists. When the cause of the capsular lesion is clearly traumatic, an arthritis in the second stage can often be cautiously treated as if in the first stage; when the onset is unprovoked, the opposite holds.

THE NON-CAPSULAR PATTERN

The presence of limitation of passive movement in other than the capsular proportions shows that a lesion other than arthritis is present. This cannot be a tendinous lesion, since it is anatomically impossible for a tendinous lesion of itself to limit passive range, although pain on voluntary movement may deceptively restrict the active range. Those who test the range of passive, as well as active, movement cannot be deceived by this reluctance. The causes of limited movement in the non-capsular pattern are:

    Acute subdeltoid bursitis
    Pulmonary neoplasm
    Capsular adhesion
    Subcoracoid bursitis
    Contracture of the costo-coracoid fascia
    Fracture of the first rib
    Clay-shoveller's fracture
    Psychogenic limitation

Acute Subdeltoid Bursitis

The bursa exists to provide two gliding surfaces that enable the greater tuberosity to slip smoothly under the acromion; otherwise the two projections would catch against each other. It has two parts: subacromial and subdeltoid. The subacromial part covers the superior aspect of the supraspinatus and infraspinatus tendons, extending medially as far as the acromio-clavicular joint line. The subdeltoid part reaches about an inch below the greater tuberosity, covering the entire outer aspect of the uppermost part of the humerus.

1. Swift Onset
A distinguishing feature is the speed of onset. A patient who, without injury, in the course of two or three days, loses almost all capacity to abduct the arm is almost certainly suffering from acute subdeltoid bursitis. Since it is apt to recur at two to five year intervals, on the same or the other side, there is often a history of previous attacks, subsiding in about six weeks. The only other disorders are septic arthritis, which is a febrile disease, and palindromic arthritis which lasts only three days.

2. Age
There is scarcely any limit. My youngest patient was a girl aged

seventeen who had three previous attacks during two years. Acute bursitis is very uncommon after sixty-five.

3. Non-capsular Pattern

In acute bursitis, 60 degrees limitation of abduction is usually associated with little limitation of either rotation. This is very different from arthritis when 60 degrees limitation of abduction would correspond to some 90 degrees limitation of lateral rotation. When so much limitation of abduction is present, the characteristic painful arc cannot be elicited; hence lack of the normal articular proportions provides a physical sign of the first importance.

4. No Muscle Spasm

The second distinguishing feature is that, the joint not being involved, the range is limited by the patient's declaring that he cannot, because of increasing pain, allow further movement; there is no involuntary muscle spasm at all. Finally, if the examiner continues to move the joint farther, the patient voluntarily brings his arm down again by using his own muscles; this takes place at a variable point, depending upon how much he will let himself be hurt at any particular moment. By contrast, in a capsular lesion, however often the movement is attempted, muscle spasm occurs at the same point and no amount of forcing without anaesthesia increases the range.

5. Disproportionately Limited Active Abduction

A fourth feature is the fact that the range of active abduction may be limited to, say 10 degrees at a time when the passive range in this direction is, say, 30 degrees or even 45 degrees. Apparently the abductor muscles, on account of their intimate relationship to the bursa, are inhibited from any but slight contraction in the acute stage. Unless this fact is kept in mind, severe bursitis may be mistaken for a psychogenic disorder.

6. Palpation

Palpation for tenderness follows. In acute subdeltoid bursitis, the tenderness is very obvious when the two sides are compared. Exceptionally, unilateral thickening of the bursal wall may be felt, and even less often fluctuation may be detected. If so, aspiration shows whether blood or clear fluid is present.

7. Painful Arc

In acute bursitis, this valuable sign is lacking, but, as the patient recovers his range of abduction, the painful arc eventually appears, thus confirming the diagnosis retrospectively.

Pulmonary Neoplasm

This may cause pain felt at the shoulder with limitation of elevation at the shoulder joint—a very deceptive pair of facts. Muscles have only one pattern of response; any serious lesion is apt to produce spasm in near-by muscles. For example, a Brodie's abscess at the upper tibia sets up muscle spasm limiting movement at the knee joint; appendicitis causes rigidity of the abdominal muscles, and so on.

If the neoplasm interferes with the diaphragm, pain will be felt at the fourth cervical dermatome, i.e. at the deltoid area. If it encroaches on the ribs, stretching the muscle attached to the ribs leads to sympathetic spasm of the pectoralis major. When the shoulder is examined, the patient is unable to lift his arm beyond the horizontal, and passive elevation beyond this level is impossible because of pain and spasm. By contrast, the scapula is mobile, and a full range of passive movement is present at the shoulder joint without muscle weakness. This may at first glance suggest psychogenic limitation, but further examination shows otherwise. The reason for inability to elevate the arm is spasm of the pectoralis major muscle.

The diagnosis of pulmonary neoplasm is now obvious and confirmed radiologically. The patient is apt to come with a radiograph of the shoulder and the apex of his lung, just missing the lower lung field.

The same signs are also found in contracture of the pectoral scar after radical mastectomy.

Capsular Adhesion

It is surprising how seldom injury to part of the capsule of the shoulder joint results in one localized patch of capsular scarring. Although this does occur, subsequent traumatic arthritis with increasing limitation of movement in *every* direction is much the commoner result.

The history of injury is clear; often it is of a reduced dislocation. The patient's immediate post-traumatic pain ceases, but the deltoid area goes on aching during exertion for months or years afterwards. The condition persists, tending to get neither better nor worse.

Examination of the passive movements reveals a non-capsular pattern. Elevation is of full range and painful; medial rotation is of full range and painless; lateral rotation is limited in range and painful. Such a finding might suggest a lesion of the subdeltoid bursa, but for the absence of the painful arc. After a dislocation, the scarring in the capsule lies anteriorly, hence it is lateral rotation that is then limited in range. Examination of the resisted movements shows that the muscles are not involved.

A similar pattern emerges many months after complete rupture of the infraspinatus tendon. Since the patient has lost the capacity voluntarily to rotate his arm laterally, he finally loses part of this movement, even when attempted passively, from localized capsular contracture. The range of abduction and medial rotation is not affected. When resisted lateral rotation shows the infraspinatus muscle to be powerless, the cause of the localized contracture becomes obvious.

Lateral rotation is also limited alone in subcoracoid bursitis, but in such a case passive adduction is painful at its extreme and, when the arm is elevated to the horizontal, the limitation of lateral rotation disappears.

Subcoracoid Bursitis

This is also rare, and confusingly enough gives rise to isolated limitation of lateral rotation, as does the anterior capsular contracture (p. 244) due to trauma, or after rupture of the infraspinatus muscle.

Differential diagnosis rests on: 1. The absence of a history of a severe injury to the front of the joint. 2. The absence of the capsular feel and of spasm limiting the amount of lateral rotation range. In consequence, the patient can, by disregarding the pain, allow rather more movement. 3. If the humerus is abducted to the horizontal, a full range of lateral rotation can be achieved in bursitis, but not, of course, without pain. In capsular contracture, it is unattainable whatever the position of the arm. 4. Passive adduction hurts at the extreme of range.

Contracture of the Costo-coracoid Fascia

This is a very uncommon cause of limited elevation of the arm. The symptom is gradually increasing upper pectoro-scapular pain on one side only. It is provoked at first only by full elevation of the arm. After a year or two, elevation becomes slightly limited and any prolonged reaching upwards leads to increased aching for some hours or days.

The syndrome is difficult to recognize; for the symptoms suggest a cervical disc lesion and the signs, unless carefully studied, suggest a psychogenic disorder. The key to the condition is the discovery of slight limitation of elevation of the scapula (p. 214).

Fracture of the First Rib

This may be a stress fracture, without history of trauma. The pain is at one side of the base of the neck and is brought on by the neck and scapular movements. Voluntary elevation of the arm stops at the horizontal, but a full passive range exists at the shoulder. The radiograph is diagnostic.

Clay-Shoveller's Fracture

This is usually a traction fracture. The pain is at the centre of the lower neck. Though the neck movements scarcely hurt, the patient can hardly abduct either arm actively at all. The passive range is full. The radiograph shows avulsion of the tip of the spinous process of the seventh cervical or first thoracic vertebra.

Acromio-clavicular Joint

At the extreme of each passive movement at the shoulder, the acromio-clavicular joint is stretched, more than on scapular movements. Hence, these may well prove painless, but the extreme of every shoulder movement may hurt, usually passive adduction the most. Patients with a lesion at the shoulder joint complain of pain in the arm, whereas disorders of the acromio-clavicular joint give rise to purely local symptoms. Thus pain confined to the point of the shoulder elicited by the passive shoulder movements, associated with a full range of movement at the shoulder joint, draws attention to the acromio-clavicular joint even if the scapular movements are painless. None of the resisted movements hurts.

Psychogenic Limitation

The shoulder joint is closely connected with emotional tone. The outstretched arm is a symbol of pleasure and welcome; the arm held into the side expresses repugnance. Hence, those who feel withdrawn from the world or view it with disgust readily develop an inability to abduct the arm. This is therefore common in endogenous depression or conversion hysteria. But the patient does not realize that, even if the shoulder joint is ankylosed, mobility of the scapula permits 60 degrees of abduction and that the arm must be capable of this amount of abduction unless the scapula has also become fixed. Hence, detection of psychogenesis is simple if the range of voluntary and passive elevation is contrasted with the range of passive abduction at the scapulo-humeral joint. In organic disability, the range of passive elevation equals the passive scapulo-humeral range plus 60 degrees.

The large number of patients who have carried off this psychogenic conversion undetected, and have in consequence enjoyed years of treatment, confirms the diagnostic importance of comparing the responses to active, passive and resisted movements.

11

The Shoulder

PART II: FULL RANGE

The causes of limitation of movement at the shoulder have been dealt with in Chapter 10. The presence of a full range of movement at the shoulder excludes arthritis and acute bursitis, and concentrates attention on the tendons and on chronic bursitis.

For the diagnosis of a tendinous lesion, it is essential that *a full range of passive movement should exist at the joint.* Some discomfort may be elicited at one or more extremes of range, but the range is *full.* Hence there is all the difference in the world between 1 degree of limitation of movement and full range, and no effort must be spared to be sure, even at the expense of hurting the patient. There is not necessarily a full range of active movement, since a patient may be prevented by severe pain on using an injured muscle, or by a painful arc on abduction or medial rotation, from achieving more than partial movement. It is then *passive* testing that demonstrates that the range is full. This is the basis of the divergence of opinion between orthopaedic surgeons and myself; for they often make a diagnosis of a tendinous lesion in the presence of limited range. Agreement on the different significance of the active and passive ranges of movement would quickly resolve this situation.

During the first part of the examination (outlined in the previous chapter) lesions of the moving parts referring pain to the shoulder will have been detected. Visceral pain must also be considered if the examination from neck to fingers is negative. For example, diaphragmatic pleurisy may set up pain felt at the shoulder on deep breathing and coughing, and myocardial pain may be felt in one or both upper limbs, without any pain in the chest. In such a case, exertion unconnected with use of the arm (e.g. walking upstairs) brings on the symptoms and examination of the upper limb reveals no abnormality. If continued exertion of the arm sets up claudicational pain in the arm and shoulder, subclavian occlusion should be suspected. If so, the radial pulse is absent.

It is when the movements of the shoulder prove painful, but a full range of passive movement is present, that attention is paid to pain evoked by a resisted movement. These are tested one by one—abduction, adduction, lateral rotation, medial rotation at the shoulder, followed by flexion and extension of the elbow. Care should be taken to have the patient's arm near the mid-position and to resist the contraction so strongly that no movement of the joint takes place.

Lesions simultaneously affecting every muscle about the shoulder joint do not, in my experience, occur except in neoplasm; if so, the passive range is also very limited. If every resisted movement hurts in the presence of full passive range then there is nothing wrong with the muscles being tested. The scapula has to be fixed by contraction of the vertebro-scapular muscles before any strong movement of the arm can be begun; hence, pain on all resisted movements suggests a severe lesion in the cervico-scapular area; alternatively, psychoneurosis. When pain on every resisted movement accompanies pain on every passive movement, the question of psychogenic or assumed disability comes very much to the fore. Alternatively, there may be constant pain to which the patient refers each time, since he fails to realize that the question is one of *aggravation* by movement. Renewed explanation is therefore required.

In the first place, resisted abduction, adduction, medial and lateral rotation are tested. If one movement proves painful, each of the others should still be tried for the reason adduced above—that the response to pain produced by one resisted movement can be regarded as significant only if others are stated not to hurt. Alternatively if one movement is found weak, it is by discovering what other movements are or are not weak that a diagnosis is reached. If one resisted movement hurts, a group of muscles is thereby incriminated; various subsidiary movements are then tested to show which individual of that group is at fault. The movements may be tried in any order, but they must *all* be tried.

EXAMINATION

Resisted Abduction Movement

The term 'abduction' cannot be properly applied to positions of the arm after it has passed the horizontal and, to avoid ambiguity, will be reserved for movement away from the body *below* the horizontal. The movement is resisted by the examiner's hand placed at the outer aspect of the patient's elbow (see Fig. 36).

In theory, pain on a resisted abduction movement can arise from the supraspinatus or the deltoid muscle. Apart from direct injury, complete recovery from which is usually swift, lesions of the deltoid muscle do not

occur. Hence, pain on the resisted movement towards abduction incriminates the supraspinatus muscle. To be quite sure, the patient's arm is held
passively at the horizontal by the examiner, who resists a forward and
backward movement; this elicits pain from the anterior and posterior

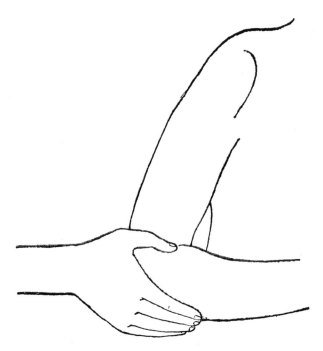

FIG. 36. Resisted abduction of arm. The patient pushes his elbow away from his side while
the examiner's hand resists the movement so strongly that none takes place.

fibres of the deltoid muscle in turn. If, as expected, neither of these movements hurts, the fault lies with the supraspinatus muscle.

The position of the lesion within the supraspinatus muscle is then identified as follows (Fig. 37):

(1) A painful arc exists. This shows the lesion to lie superficially near
the teno-periosteal junction, just medial to the greater tuberosity of the
humerus.

If the painful arc is more marked when the abduction movement is
carried out in medial rather than lateral rotation of the arm (i.e. palm
down or palm up), additional information is afforded. If the arc is more
marked when the arm is brought up palm-upwards, the lesion lies at the
anterior aspect of the teno-periosteal junction; if palm-downwards hurts
more, the posterior part of the tendinous insertion is singled out. These

accessory localizing signs are particularly useful when hydrocortisone is to be injected.

The mere presence of a painful arc exculpates the deltoid muscle; it does not lie between tuberosity and acromion and thus cannot be pinched.

(2) Full *passive* elevation of the arm hurts. This implies tenderness of that part of the tendon which is pinched between the greater tuberosity and the glenoid rim: i.e. the deep aspect of the teno-periosteal junction. If

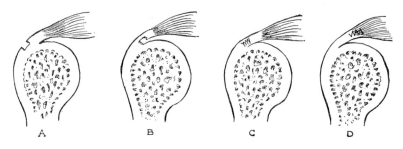

    A   B   C   D

Fig. 37. Supraspinatus tendinitis. Accessory signs indicate the exact position of the lesion.

A. Painful arc. The lesion lies superficially at the teno-periosteal junction. B. Pain on full passive elevation. The lesion lies deeply at the teno-periosteal junction. C. Both a painful arc and pain on full passive elevation. The lesion traverses the distal end of the tendon. D. Neither an arc nor pain on full passive elevation. The lesion lies at the musculo-tendinous junction.

this sign is found together with a painful arc, the lesion clearly traverses the distal end of the whole tendon. The fact that full *active* elevation hurts has no localizing significance; for during this movement the supraspinatus muscle is contracting and pain will be elicited wherever the lesion in the muscle happens to lie.

3. The absence of a painful arc and of pain elicited on full passive elevation suggests a lesion of the supraspinatus at the musculo-tendinous junction, since the belly itself is very rarely affected. Tenderness of the musculo-tendinous junction may be sought, and the two sides compared, deeply within the angle formed by the clavicle and the spine of the scapula while the arm is passively supported horizontally. However, local anaesthesia should always be used to verify this diagnosis; for an occasional case of tendinitis at the teno-periosteal junction unexpectedly fails to show either of the two appropriate localizing signs.

In spite of the intimate relation of the supraspinatus tendon to the sub-deltoid bursa, a resisted abduction movement, when properly tested, is painless in even acute bursitis.

Weakness of abduction occurs in: (a) rupture of the supraspinatus tendon; if so, a painful arc is present: (b) suprascapular palsy: (c) a lesion of the fifth cervical root: (d) partial rupture of the supraspinatus tendon.

This is uncommon and leads to pain *and* weakness when resisted abduction is tested. (e) A secondary deposit in the acromion.

Resisted Adduction Movement

The arm is brought a short distance away from the body and the adduction movement resisted by pressure against the inner side of the elbow (see Fig. 38). The muscles responsible are the pectoralis major, latissimus dorsi and the two teres. Pain, except when it arises from the axillary portions of the pectoralis major or latissimus dorsi muscles, is usually correctly appreciated by the patient at the anterior or postero-lateral aspects of the thorax respectively. When the patient's sensations are no guide and an adduction movement hurts, the next part of the examination is to ask him to bring his arm first forwards then backwards against resistance. If the former hurts, the pectoral muscle is at fault and confirmation may be sought by asking him to press his hands together as in Fig. 39. If the backward movement hurts, the fault lies in one of the other three muscles. The teres muscles may be differentiated by the fact that the major is a medial, the minor a lateral, rotator of the humerus. The latissimus dorsi and teres major muscles, being identical in function, cannot be distinguished by any test. In fracture of an upper rib anteriorly, testing the pectoralis major muscle hurts at the upper part of the thorax, and full elevation of the arm also pulls painfully on the broken bone.

Palpation follows when the pectoralis major muscle is affected. The fibres just below the lateral half of the clavicle or those at the lower extent of the outer edge are the probable sites.

If the lesion lies at the pectoral insertion at the bicipital groove the pain evoked by resisted adduction is felt at the shoulder and upper arm. The latissimus dorsi muscle is usually affected at the upper part of the outer edge.

Resisted Lateral Rotation Movement

The patient's arm must be kept at his side with the elbow held at a right-angle and the movement resisted by pressure applied just above the wrist (Fig. 40). If the pressure is applied at the hand, the response to resisted wrist extension complicates the picture, and the examiner, who may think he is testing the infraspinatus muscle alone, may, in fact, be eliciting pain from a tennis-elbow.

Patients are very apt to abduct the arm when asked to rotate it outwards; this must be avoided, otherwise a supraspinatus tendinitis may be mistaken for an infraspinatus tendinitis. If resisted lateral rotation hurts

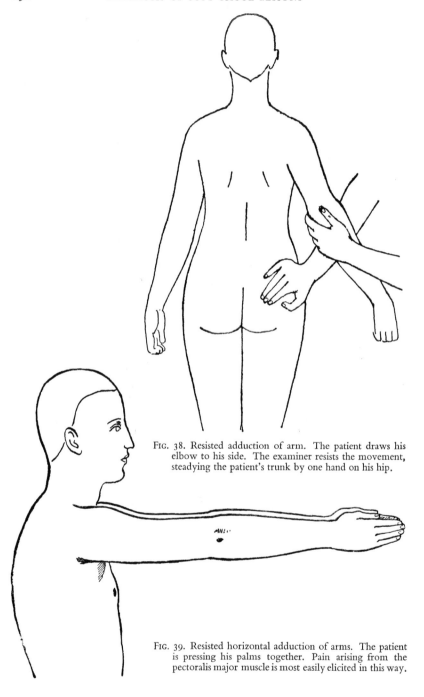

FIG. 38. Resisted adduction of arm. The patient draws his elbow to his side. The examiner resists the movement, steadying the patient's trunk by one hand on his hip.

FIG. 39. Resisted horizontal adduction of arms. The patient is pressing his palms together. Pain arising from the pectoralis major muscle is most easily elicited in this way.

alone, infraspinatus tendinitis is present. If a resisted adduction movement also hurts—which is very uncommon—the teres minor muscle is inculpated. A painful arc on elevation occurs with infraspinatus tendinitis, when the lesion lies at the distal and superficial fibres of the tendon, i.e. where it can be pinched between tuberosity and acromion. In the absence of a painful arc, there is no way of telling which part of the tendon is

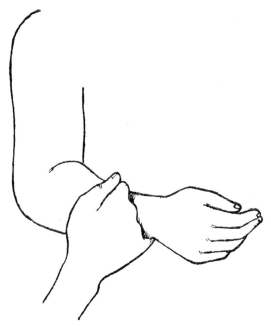

FIG. 40. Resisted lateral rotation of arm. Keeping his elbow at his side, the patient pushes his wrist away from his body. Note that the examiner's hand is placed at the lower forearm avoiding pressure on the patient's hand. The patient's forearm is supported by the examiner's fifth finger. No outward movement is allowed to occur

affected except by palpation for tenderness supplemented by local anaesthesia. Palpation is carried out in the position for massage of the tendon (see Vol. II).

It is not uncommon for pain to be evoked both by resisted abduction and resisted lateral rotation, even when correctly carried out. In such cases, a double lesion is usually present, and both tendons require treatment. Occasionally, however, this combination characterizes chronic subdeltoid bursitis. (I call it 'Skillern's bursitis', after the physiotherapist who first pointed this out to me.) Before a confident diagnosis of two tendinous lesions is made, therefore, it is well to palpate the subdeltoid bursa for a tender spot and, if one is found, induce local anaesthesia there diagnostically. A painful arc is common to all three lesions; hence this finding is no help. Intendinitis, since the supraspinatus is affected twice as often as infraspinatus, the former should be infiltrated with hydrocortisone first. In some cases, both movements become painless after this injection.

In rupture of the infraspinatus tendon, painless weakness with a painful arc at first is very noticeable. After a year or two, the arc ceases but some 30 degrees of the range of lateral rotation at the shoulder becomes lost. The infraspinatus muscle is weak and wasted in suprascapular palsy and in some cases of neuralgic amyotrophy.

Resisted Medial Rotation Movement

This movement (Fig. 41) provides information about pain arising from the subscapularis, pectoralis major, latissimus dorsi and teres major muscles. The last-named three muscles are all adductors, whereas the subscapularis muscle is a weak abductor. It suffices, therefore, to show the

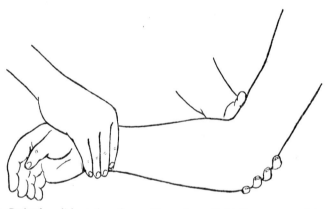

FIG. 41. Resisted medial rotation of arm. The patient pulls his forearm towards his trunk. The examiner steadies his elbow and resists the movement by pressure against his wrist.

absence of pain on a resisted adduction movement to demonstrate that the subscapularis is the muscle affected. If a lesion of this muscle has thus been shown to exist, two further localizing signs should be sought. (1) A painful arc. If this is present, the lesion is at the uppermost part of the teno-periosteal junction, since only the top of the lesser tuberosity can engage against the coraco-acromial arch. The presence of a painful arc also serves to exculpate the adductor muscles. (2) Pain on passive adduction across the front of the chest. At the extreme of this movement the lower part of the lesser tuberosity is squeezed against the coracoid process. This shows the lesion in the tendon to lie at the humeral insertion at its lower extent. Lesions in the subscapular belly appear not to occur. Complete rupture of the tendon is rare and leads to great weakness on resisted medial rotation.

Resisted Forward Movement

When pain is elicited by this movement alone, the lesion has on each occasion been found to lie at the upper extremity of the coraco-brachialis muscle. In theory, resisted adduction should also hurt; in practice, it does not do so.

Resisted Flexion and Supination at the Elbow

Though part of the biceps and triceps muscles exist at the shoulder, they control the elbow. Hence no examination of the shoulder muscles is complete until the resisted elbow movements have been tested. If pain is felt at the shoulder and examination of the passive and resisted shoulder movements is negative, the resisted elbow movements must be tested. Pain brought on at the shoulder by resisted flexion and supination at the elbow arises from the biceps muscle, probably the tendon of the long head; trouble at the short head is very uncommon indeed. Unless, as is rare, a painful arc exists, there is no way of finding out which part of the long tendon is affected except by palpation for local tenderness.

A snapping long head of biceps seldom causes clinical tendinitis.

Resisted Extension at the Elbow

When this hurts in the upper arm, it should not be assumed that the lesion necessarily lies in the triceps muscle; for it may well arise when a tender structure lies between the acromion and the head of the humerus. Strong contraction of the triceps muscle forces the humerus upwards, and thus pinches painfully any lesion lying between these two bones. It is then another way of eliciting the pain when a painful arc is present.

If no painful arc is found, the upper part of the belly of the triceps is palpated for tenderness. A lesion here is a real rarity and requires confirmation by local anaesthesia before it can be accepted.

Local Anaesthesia

Whenever possible, all diagnoses based on the indirect evidence afforded by which movements prove painful should be confirmed by local anaesthesia.

Indeed, it is by trial and error over the past twenty-five years that I have taught myself the proper interpretation of these similar but not identical patterns, and have been able to evolve methods of effective treatment.

PAINFUL ARC OF MOVEMENT

Since the acromion itself is very seldom at fault, this finding implies that there is tenderness of a structure lying between the humerus and the acromion. The lesion is pinched when the prominent tuberosity passes under the arch, i.e. at 80 degrees of abduction (Fig. 42).

The pain is elicited better on active than on passive movement and is usually greater on the way upwards than downwards. Since the pain is due to pressure of one or other tuberosity towards the coraco-acromial

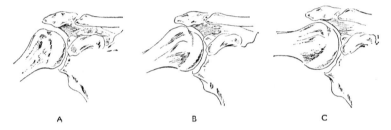

  A   B   C

FIG. 42. The mechanism of a painful arc at the shoulder

A. *No pain.* At 70° of abduction the humeral tuberosity is approaching the acromion. As yet no pain is felt. B. *Pain.* At 80° of abduction the tuberosity lies under the acromion. If a tender structure lies between two bones, it is now painfully squeezed. C. *No pain.* At 90° of abduction the tuberosity has passed the acromion and the painful pinching ceases

arch, it is greatest when the abductor muscles are contracting and the head of the humerus is held well-lodged against the arch. Once the arm has passed beyond the horizontal in either direction, the pain ceases abruptly. A painful arc can sometimes be obviated by bringing the arm up forwards instead of outwards. Many patients have learned this for themselves and may be seen, as the proposed movement reaches the horizontal, to bring the arm forwards and rotate it outwards so as to minimize the painful pressure. Sometimes the painful arc appears solely on the upwards, less often only on the downwards, passage of the arm. Rarely, there is a painful arc on medial rotation of the arm; if so, it can happen that the patient stops medially rotating his arm when he reaches the arc, and apparent limitation of range results. The examiner who, when testing passing range, stops too soon because of the strong ache, is also misled. Since limited range has so different a significance from a painful arc, firm pressure, even if it does hurt the patient, must be used in such an instance to make sure.

A painful arc nearly always indicates tenderness of a structure lying between the acromion and one or other humeral tuberosity. It is only rarely that the arch itself is tender, as the result of a severe sprain at the deep fibres of the acromio-clavicular joint, or rarely, malignant invasion of the acromion. The possible causes of a painful arc are thus as follows:

1. Supraspinatus Tendinitis

This is by far the commonest cause and implies tenderness at or very near the greater tuberosity, either from strain of, scarring in, calcification in, or rupture of, the supraspinatus tendon. In the first three instances, the power of abduction is full and this movement is painful when resisted. The radiograph reveals nothing. In the last, the power of initiating abduction is lost and the presence of a painful arc discoverable only on a passive elevation movement; the radiograph is normal. Calcification is of course clearly visible radiographically (Plate 12), and is suggested clinically by a *very* painful arc.

2. Subdeltoid Bursitis

If this causes a painful arc, the bursitis is localized; for in acute bursitis pain prevents movement long before the arc is reached. The affected part of the bursa can remain tender for years. In such cases there is a painful arc, with or without pain at the extreme of each passive movement; none of the resisted movements hurts. Often there is *only* an arc. This finding differentiates chronic bursitis from lesions of the supraspinatus, infraspinatus or subscapular tendon, all of which are characterized by pain elicited by the appropriate resisted movement. Many authorities regard bursitis and tendinitis at the shoulder as identical or, at least, indistinguishable. This is by no means so, if the examiner tests the function of the tendons by resisted movement.

Calcification may be visible lying in the bursa at a point below the insertion of the tendons. A deposit lying higher up cannot be ascribed to any one structure by examination of the X-ray picture; clinical examination is required.

3. Infraspinatus Tendinitis

A painful arc is often associated with pain on resisted lateral rotation. If so, the lesion in the infraspinatus tendon lies at the uppermost part of the tendinous insertion at the humeral tuberosity.

4. Subscapular Tendinitis

In this case, the painful arc is associated with pain on a resisted medial rotation movement. The presence of the painful arc singles out the upper extremity of the tendinous insertion at the lesser tuberosity.

5. Biceps Tendinitis

The intra-articular extent of the long head of biceps is very seldom affected, the tendon being usually at fault where it lies in the bicipital groove. Here it cannot be pinched. However, intracapsular bicipital tendinitis is identified when the arc is associated with pain elicited by resisted supination of the forearm and resisted flexion at the elbow. The passive and resisted movements of the shoulder are all painless.

6. Sprain of the Inferior Acromio-clavicular Ligament

This is also rare. The painful arc is associated with the pattern suggesting that the acromio-clavicular joint is at fault. It is not easy to differentiate chronic strain of the inferior acromio-clavicular ligament from long-standing subdeltoid bursitis, since, both are lesions of adjacent inert tissues. The fact that the scapular movements set up localized aching and that the extreme of passive adduction at the shoulder joint hurts, suggests the acromio-clavicular joint, but only local anaesthesia settles the matter.

7. Metastases in the Acromion

Secondary neoplasm of the acromion alone is rare. It causes tenderness of the bone itself, demonstrated indirectly by the existence of a painful arc and detectable superficially by palpation. Localized warmth is found when erosion of bone is proceeding rapidly.

The action of the supraspinatus muscle is grossly impeded. Hence, pain and marked weakness on testing abduction, associated with bony tenderness, leads to immediate radiography.

8. Capsular Laxity at the Shoulder

After a dislocation or sprain, residual capsular laxity at the gleno-humeral joint may give rise to momentary subluxation of the head of the humerus as the arm moves upwards towards the horizontal position. At about 80 degrees, it clicks back into place, perhaps with some discomfort. The examiner can see the momentary arrest of the movement and feel the

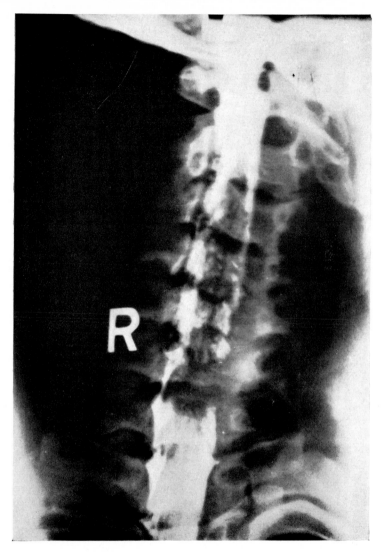

PLATE 9

Cervical myelogram. Contrast radiograph of a sixth cervical disc lesion, taken four months after the onset of the brachial symptoms, when the root-pain had almost ceased. Note the unilateral arrest of contrast medium at the sixth level.

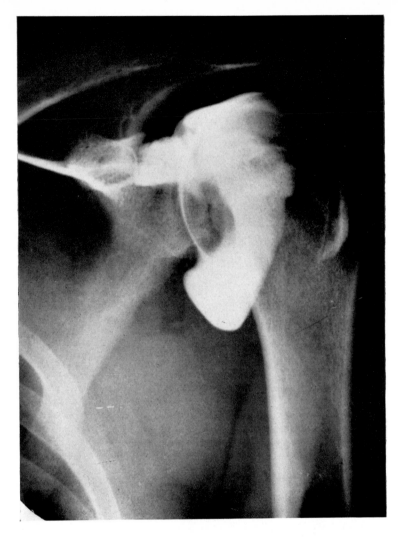

PLATE 10

Arthrogram of shoulder. Normal appearances. The articular cavity is outlined, together with the subcoracoid and bicipital bursae. (By courtesy of Professor J. Debeyre,
Paris.)

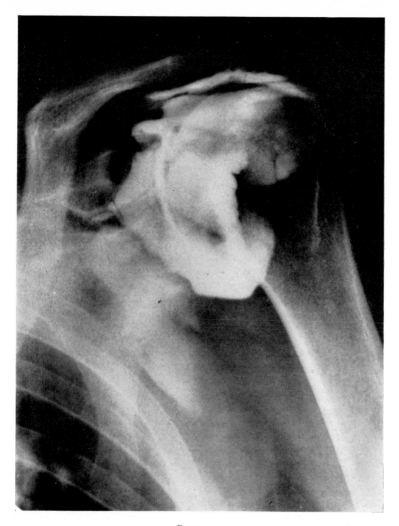

Arthrogram. The supraspinatus tendon is ruptured and the contrast medium, injected into the joint, has passed through the gap, outlining the subdeltoid bursa. (By courtesy of Professor J. Debeyre, Paris.)

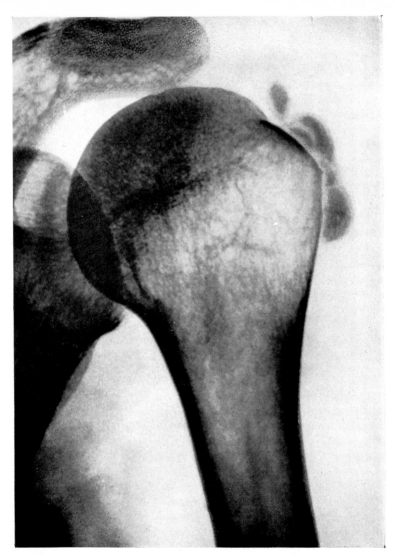

PLATE 12

Calcification in the subdeltoid bursa. Radiograph of the shoulder of a woman aged 33 who had suddenly developed severe brachial pain four days previously. Marked limitation of movement of the non-capsular pattern was present.

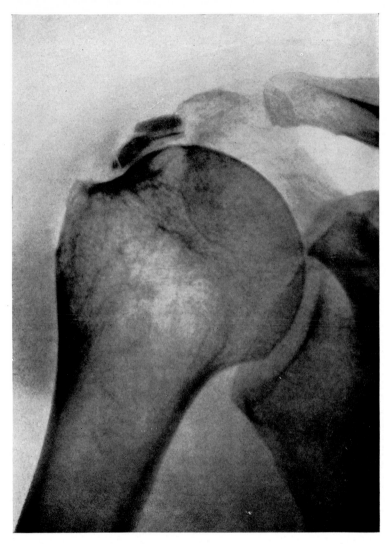

PLATE 13

Calcification in the supraspinatus tendon. The clinical signs of tendinitis were present.

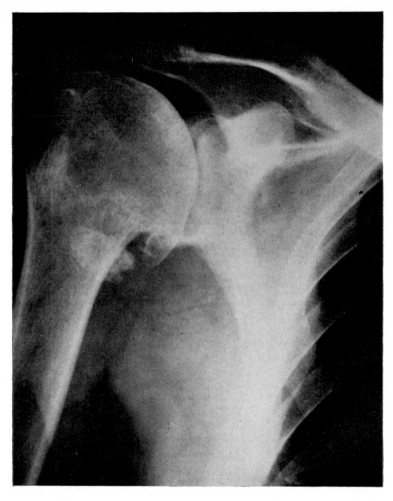

PLATE 14

Osteo-arthritis of shoulder with loose body. Man of 68 had had repeated twinges in his upper arm for three years.

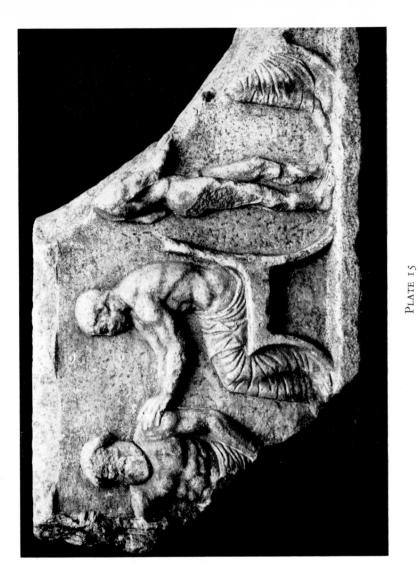

PLATE 15

Massage to shoulder. A relief two thousand years old at the museum in Cyrene, Libya. (By courtesy of the Curator of the Department of Antiquities.)

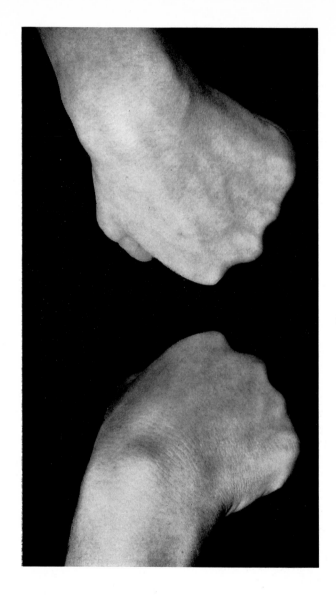

PLATE 16

Subluxation of capitate bone. The radiograph showed no displacement.

click. This is not a true painful arc, but the resemblance may be close, and its spurious nature must be realized.

9. A Cervical Disc Lesion

An extraordinary occasional finding in disc lesions with pain in the scapulo-humeral area is the presence of a painful arc as the affected arm is elevated. Patients with pain in the region of the shoulder often believe that they cannot move the arm away from the side; this is merely another manifestation of the common, deep-rooted idea that function is necessarily impaired at a painful member. Most can be gradually persuaded fully to elevate the arm actively, but when the arm passes the horizontal, the muscular effort is at its greatest and some secondary tautening of the cervical muscles takes place, leading to such pain that the arm falters, and a false localizing sign appears. This phenomenon has created the mistaken idea that certain neck conditions give rise to disorders occurring at—not just pain felt in—the shoulder. Osteopaths even claim cure of various types of shoulder trouble by manipulating the neck. Since differential diagnosis is sometimes difficult, it is easy to see how this error arose. In a case of this sort, showing indefinite signs at both the neck and the shoulder, manipulative reduction at the neck should be performed at once until a full and painless range has been restored. The shoulder should then be examined again and, in many instances, the previous signs at the shoulder will have disappeared.

Subclavian Occlusion

In this disorder, claudicational pain comes on after the arm has been powerfully used for some time, accompanied by a feeling of weakness. If the brachial artery dilates enough, and the thrombosis lies proximal to the root of the vertebral artery, the direction of flow through this artery becomes reversed and after strong exertion the patient feels faint.

Examination of the muscles and joints of the upper limb reveals no disorder, since exertion has to be continued for some while before a concentration of the products of muscular metabolism is reached enough to cause pain. But the history of pain coming on in the arm after a time, accompanied by weakness, in a patient with normal joints and muscles, should lead to palpation of the radial pulse. This is absent and arteriography reveals the state of affairs.

Subdeltoid Bursitis

Six types of bursitis occur:

K

1. Acute Bursitis

If an afebrile patient, because of increasing pain, loses all capacity to abduct his arm actively in the course of a few days, much the likeliest cause is acute subdeltoid bursitis. In dislocation, there is a history of trauma and the deformity is obvious. In pathological fracture the limitation of movement is immediate. Palindromic rheumatism recovers in three days.

Acute bursitis is an uncommon condition, occurring equally in men and women. It is self-limiting within six weeks, and apt to recur at intervals of two to five years. The cause is unknown and injury plays no part in the aetiology. At the earliest stage, which lasts only a day, a painful arc can be elicited; after that the range of abduction becomes too restricted for this point to be reached. It is then limitation of movement of the non-capsular pattern that draws attention to the bursa. The usual finding is marked limitation of abduction with very little restriction of lateral rotation: the reverse of the findings in arthritis; moreover, the capsular feel is absent. This pattern leads to palpation of the bursa, the whole of which is exquisitely tender.

The bursitis takes two or three days to become really acute. First an ache sets in at the shoulder; pain soon spreads down the arm to the wrist; after three days it becomes severe and constant. The patient's sleep is now disturbed, and he soon finds that he can barely move his arm at all. After seven to ten days of severe pain, the symptoms abate somewhat; at the end of two or three weeks there remains only an ache, and active abduction may have reached half-range. At the end of four to six weeks the patient has fully recovered. When he is nearly well the painful arc reappears again for the last week.

2. Chronic Localized Bursitis

Chronic localized bursitis does not result from an acute bursitis that has not resolved completely; it is a separate entity. It is quite a common cause of painful shoulder.

The onset is gradual and apparently causeless; the pain may continue for years. Sometimes the radiograph shows a calcified deposit; more often no abnormality is revealed. Men and women are attacked at ages ranging from fifteen to sixty-five. Rarely, localized bursitis is the result of direct contusion. If so, thickening of the bursal wall is visible and palpable and there may be a small effusion.

The pain is felt in the lower deltoid area and examination discloses a painful arc and often nothing else. Sometimes, in addition, though the

passive range is full, every extreme is uncomfortable. No resisted movement hurts. This finding implies that of the four tissues tenderness of
which can give rise to a painful arc—the supraspinatus, infraspinatus, and
subscapular tendons, the subdeltoid bursa—it is not any of the tendons,
since the resisted movements are painless. There remains only the
bursa.

The question is now which part of the bursa is affected. Half of it lies
under the acromion and out of finger's reach. The subdeltoid moiety is
palpated for tenderness and, if such an area is found, it is anaesthetized
with 10 ml. 0·5 per cent procaine. After five minutes, the patient is asked
to elevate his arm again and to state whether the arc has been abolished or
not. All diagnoses of subdeltoid bursitis are tentative, until confirmed by
this test.

If none of the mional accessible part of the bursa proves tender, the
lesion must lie subacromiconally. Again local anaesthesia must be used to
decide the diagnosis (especially in incomprehensible bursitis, p. 262). The
same amount of solution as before is introduced with a 5-cm. needle
deeply between the acromion and the tendons, and the patient declares the
result.

Spontaneous painless effusion into the bursa may, as happens at other
joints, complicate severe rheumatoid arthritis; doubtless it would give rise
to a painful arc if the arthritis at the shoulder did not prevent movement
to that point.

3. Bursitis with Calcified Deposit

Judging by the literature, calcification of the bursa occurs less often in
England than in the U.S.A. and, when it is met with in this country, the
patient is often of mid-European descent.

The onset is sudden and unprovoked. Within a few days the patient
finds himself unable to move the arm appreciably because of severe pain
spreading from the shoulder to forearm and wrist. The pattern of limitation is non-capsular; the capsular end-feel is absent; the bursa is very
tender and the radiograph reveals quite a large area of calcification. There
is often a smaller similar shadow at the other (symptomless) shoulder. The
disorder recovers rather more quickly than acute bursitis without a deposit,
usually in a month. There is some tendency to recurrence. After recovery
the calcification remains, sometimes disappearing spontaneously after
several years. The sequence of events is so similar to that in gout, that
blood uric acid estimations were carried out in a small series of cases.
However, the highest figure obtained was 4·0 mg. and some were low
normal levels (under 2·0 mg.).

4. Haemorrhage into the Subdeltoid Bursa

In my experience this occurs only in old age. The haemorrhage is apparently spontaneous in all cases except one in which the bleeding was secondary to rupture of the supraspinatus tendon. The complaint is of swelling and pain. Visible bruising is occasionally present. The bursa is prominent and tense; fluctuation is easily detectable. Aspiration reveals blood. In long-standing cases, fibrous clots can be felt to move about inside the bursa.

The range of movement is limited more by the bulk of the fluid than by the bursitis; it is slight, but after a period of immobilization owing to pain, greater limitation due to capsular contracture may well supervene. Recurrent haemorrhage into the bursa after aspiration suggests haemangioma.

5. Crepitating Bursitis

Patients are seen, usually a year or two after a subdeltoid bursitis with effusion has subsided, complaining of creaking at the bursa on moving the arm and some aching in the deltoid area after exertion. (No treatment appears to make any difference, but the disability is very minor.)

6. 'Adhesive Bursitis'

This is an alleged entity copied from one textbook to another. In my experience, it does not occur and inquiry from surgeons who operate on shoulders shows that they do not encounter bursal adhesions either.

7. Incomprehensible Bursitis

Patients are rarely encountered who have pain felt at the shoulder arising only during, and for some hours after, considerable exertion. They can carry on in spite of the pain, which is disagreeable but not disabling, and persists for years.

Examination shows one of four patterns:

(1) Full range; both passive rotations hurt; full elevation is painless; there is no arc; the resisted movements do not hurt.

(2) Full range with discomfort at extremes; painful arc; resisted abduction and lateral rotation both hurt.

(3) A changing pattern of pain on resisted movement. Full painful range of passive movement. The resisted movements hurt in an erratic

way, the response being pain, then not, when the test is repeated. Slight arc.

(4) Slight limitation of passive abduction alone or passive medial rotation alone. The resisted movements are painless or all equally painful. No arc.

It cannot be explained how these signs signify bursitis, but infiltration of the affected area of the subdeltoid bursa is immediately curative after every other known treatment has failed. If no part of the subdeltoid bursa is found tender, local anaesthesia has to be induced under the acromion repeatedly until the right spot is found.

Interpretation of Pattern

Summary of Significant Findings

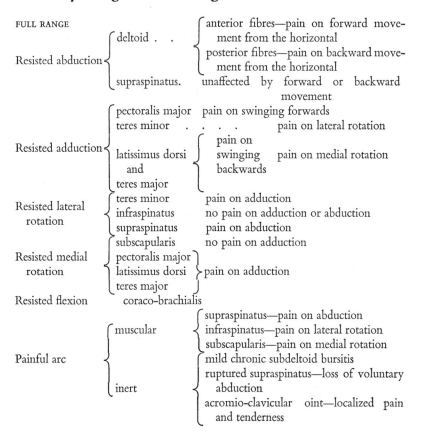

FULL RANGE

Resisted abduction
- deltoid
  - anterior fibres—pain on forward movement from the horizontal
  - posterior fibres—pain on backward movement from the horizontal
- supraspinatus. unaffected by forward or backward movement

Resisted adduction
- pectoralis major   pain on swinging forwards
- teres minor . . . .   pain on lateral rotation
- latissimus dorsi and teres major   pain on swinging backwards   pain on medial rotation

Resisted lateral rotation
- teres minor   pain on adduction
- infraspinatus   no pain on adduction or abduction
- supraspinatus   pain on abduction
- subscapularis   no pain on adduction

Resisted medial rotation
- pectoralis major
- latissimus dorsi   pain on adduction
- teres major

Resisted flexion   coraco-brachialis

Painful arc
- muscular
  - supraspinatus—pain on abduction
  - infraspinatus—pain on lateral rotation
  - subscapularis—pain on medial rotation
- inert
  - mild chronic subdeltoid bursitis
  - ruptured supraspinatus—loss of voluntary abduction
  - acromio-clavicular oint—localized pain and tenderness

LIMITED RANGE

Capsular pattern
- traumatic capsulitis—history—no radiographic change
- osteoarthritis—age, crepitus, other shoulder too
- freezing arthritis—unprovoked onset, characteristic three-phase course, no muscular wasting, age 45 to 60
- monaticular rheumatoid arthritis—sedimentation rate, muscular wasting, wrong chronology
- bacterial arthritis—great wasting, radiographic change

Noncapsular pattern
- acute subdeltoid bursitis—site of tenderness, disproportionate limitation of abduction, calcification
- subcoracoid bursitis—disproportionate limitation of lateral rotation ceasing when arm horizontal
- anterior capsular adhesion—disproportionate limitation of lateral rotation persisting when arm horizontal
- secondary neoplasm—bizarre pattern, radiographic change
- neoplasm of lung—radiographic change, Horner's syndrome, weak fingers

Bony block
- neuropathic arthropathy—no pain, radiographic change, W.R., syringomyelia
- displacement of fractured tuberosity under acromion—pain, recent injury, radiographic change

MUSCULAR WEAKNESS IN SHOULDER AND ARM

If a patient cannot reproduce actively a movement of which his joint can be shown by passive testing to be capable, one or more muscles must be out of action, either from intrinsic or nervous defect. Alternatively, the disorder may be psychogenic. In many cases, although the voluntary movements are not limited in range, trial of the resisted movements displays weakness. On the whole, weakness is much easier to detect than wasting; for inspection of the serratus anterior and spinatus muscles, except in thin subjects, is difficult; even at the deltoid muscle a minor degree of wasting is surprisingly difficult to see. Naturally, the examination for weakness must continue from scapula to hand; for if the lowest cervical or first thoracic root or the lower trunk of the brachial plexus is involved, it is only examination of the hand that affords the clue. The test for winging of the scapula must not be forgotten.

Eleven possible findings are:

1. Painless Weakness of the Deltoid Muscle

This may result from traumatic compression of the axillary nerve, usually by the head of the humerus when it dislocates. The bony displacement may have been momentary only; hence, there may not be clear history of dislocation. A patient with a powerless deltoid but with a strong supraspinatus muscle possesses a full range of active elevation, but he cannot bring his arm backwards from the horizontal position. Gross wasting of the deltoid is usually obvious and a patch of cutaneous analgesia is found at the mid-deltoid area. An interesting sign in the early case is involuntary spasm of the trapezius muscle, lasting a week or two. The scapula is thus kept elevated, relieving tension on the axillary nerve. In such a case, full side-flexion of the neck away from the weak side is apt to hurt in the area of cutaneous analgesia at the upper arm.

Treatment consists merely of making sure that the patient uses his supraspinatus muscle so as to maintain a full range of movement at the shoulder joint pending recovery of the deltoid muscle. This often takes six months.

2. Pain Weakness of Deltoid, Biceps and Both Spinatus Muscles

This combination characterizes a lesion of the fifth cervical nerve-root. It may result from a *fourth cervical disc lesion*. If so, some of the cervical movements give rise to scapular pain. If the cause is a *traction palsy*, there is a history of an accident depressing the shoulder-girdle and the cervical movements are of full range and painless.

Myeloma may result in monoradicular weakness, but secondary neoplasm sets up widespread weakness. In neuroma, the weakness may be too great for a mere disc lesion or it may affect the muscles relevant to more than one root. In gradual osteophytic compression of the root, pain is slight or absent.

No treatment avails in a disc lesion that has already caused a root-palsy. Spontaneous recovery must be awaited; this takes three to four months for the root pain and six to eight months for the return of muscle power, from the onset of the pain in the upper limb, not from when the scapular ache began. In traction palsy there is little discomfort, and the muscles recover in about six months. If necessary, the patient is taught meanwhile to maintain a full range of movement at the shoulder joint. Residual weakness is rare. A fifth cervical root-palsy caused by encroachment on the fourth intervertebral foramen is best treated surgically by drilling away the osteophyte.

3. Painless Weakness of the Supraspinatus Muscle Alone

This results from rupture of the supraspinatus tendon. The disorder may come on insidiously without a history of trauma, since the tendon can slowly degenerate, parting gradually until it finally gives way altogether. Alternatively, a strain or a fall on the shoulder may be responsible. The diagnosis suggests itself when a middle-aged patient suddenly loses all power to abduct his arm. In this circumstance, the deltoid is powerless to act as an abductor; for its contraction merely moves the head of the humerus upwards into the hiatus left superiorly by the gap in the supraspinatus tendon. As the head of the humerus must move downwards as abduction proceeds, the deltoid cannot work alone and all power of active abduction below the horizontal is lost. When he tries, rotation and elevation of the scapula, combined with lateral flexion of the trunk away from the affected side, give rise to an apparent range of at most 20 degrees. On inspection, the deltoid muscle is not wasted. Passive elevation is full—except in neglected cases—and a very pronounced painful arc is discovered as the examiner lifts the patient's arm past the horizontal. After the arm has been passively raised just above the horizontal, past the arc, voluntary elevation once more becomes possible and the patient now has no difficulty in bringing his arm right up by using his deltoid and serratus muscles.

Radiography is often confirmative, since the gap between acromion and head of the humerus can be seen to be much narrowed, the bone having subluxated upwards into the gap left by the parted tendon.

The above description applies to cases seen within the first month or so of the occurrence of the rupture. Since the condition is almost confined to the middle-aged or elderly, capsular contracture from disuse soon sets in. In such cases the picture is complicated by the addition of limitation of movement in the capsular proportions from immobilizational arthritis.

Wasting of the supraspinatus muscle belly is detectable at the end of some weeks, and is permanent.

4. Painful Weakness of the Supraspinatus Muscle Alone

This implies a partial rupture of the supraspinatus tendon and is difficult to differentiate from uncomplicated tendinitis. Supraspinatus tendinitis is clearly present, but marked weakness as well as pain becomes apparent when the abduction movement is attempted against resistance. If, in such a case, local anaesthesia destroys the pain but leaves the weakness unaltered, mere unwillingness to perform a painful movement can be ruled out. There is no particular tendency for a painful partial rupture to become complete, at any rate within some years. Malignant invasion of the acromion also leads to pain and weakness of abduction of the arm.

5. Painless Weakness of the Supraspinatus and Infraspinatus Muscles

This is likely to come to light only if the power of resisted lateral rotation movement of the two arms is compared. Pain constantly day and night lasting three weeks is felt in the scapular area and upper arm. No movement of the neck, scapula or upper limb affects it. Voluntary movement of the arm is not lost because the deltoid and teres minor muscles remain in action. Except in fat subjects, wasting of the supra- and infraspinatus muscles can be detected on inspection and palpation. The cause is neuritis involving the suprascapular nerve alone. No treatment is required; recovery is spontaneous and seldom takes more than four to six months.

The lesion is occasionally traumatic. If an injury results in severe traction on the arm pulling it away from the trunk, the suprascapular nerve may be caught against the edge of the bony notch it traverses at the upper border of the scapula. Rarely, the nerve is ruptured completely and permanent palsy results.

Bilateral painless disappearance of the spinatus muscles suggests myopathy. If so, the serratus anterior muscles are often also affected. Since the cases of myopathy usually seen by an orthopaedic physician occur in middle-aged patients, secondary limitation of movement may have occurred at the shoulders as a result of capsular contracture from disuse. The wasting, if perceived at all, is then ascribed to arthritis. The great wasting and weakness contrast strangely with the small degree of limitation of movement; moreover, in uncomplicated arthritis the muscles are not clinically weak.

6. Painless Weakness of the Serratus Anterior Muscle

This weakness is detected when the patient is asked to elevate his arm actively, when 45 degrees limitation of elevation is found, whereas passive elevation is full and painless. This means that there is a full range of voluntary movement at the shoulder joint but that active rotation of the scapula is defective. When the patient is asked to lean forward with his arms stretched out in front of him and to push against a wall, winging of one scapula at once becomes apparent. The cause is a long thoracic nerve-palsy—another manifestation of neuritis. Most patients suffer two or three weeks' constant aching in the scapular region and upper arm unaffected by movement, but the neuritis sometimes comes on painlessly. Spontaneous recovery is the rule, and takes four to eight months. No treatment is necessary.

Occasionally the palsy follows direct or indirect trauma to the nerve. In one case a horse had trodden on the patient's scapula (and a year later no recovery had begun), and in another the scapula had been wrenched away from the body laterally and recovery began six months later.

Partial weakness of the serratus anterior muscle is occasionally detectable (with some difficulty) in a cervical disc lesion resulting in a sixth cervical root-palsy. A suggestion of winging is perceptible; voluntary elevation of the arm is lacking in only the final 5 degrees.

Bilateral painless disappearance of the serratus anterior muscles charac-terizes myopathy.

7. Painless Weakness of the Infraspinatus Muscle Alone

The cause is rupture of the infraspinatus tendon; it is rare. The patient is middle-aged or elderly, and has suffered some accident or overstrain involving the shoulder. In the early case, examination reveals a painful arc accompanied by great weakness of lateral rotation of the arm; if the teres minor muscle escapes, the movement can just be performed actively; if not, the active movement is completely lost. After many months, the remnants of the tendon still attached to the tuberosity lose their tenderness and the painful arc ceases. The weakness is permanent, and leads to painless capsular contracture anteriorly; as a result, after a year or two 30 degrees to 45 degrees of lateral rotation range have been lost, abduction and medial rotation remaining of full range.

Treatment consists of infiltrating the remnants of the infraspinatus tendon with hydrocortisone to abolish the arc, and showing the patient how to maintain the range of lateral rotation by using his other hand daily to rotate the arm outwards.

8. Painless Weakness of the Subscapular Muscle Alone

This too is rare and results from rupture of the subscapular tendon. The history is of trauma followed by weakness at the shoulder. Examination shows a painful arc and great weakness of medial rotation of the arm. It is remarkable, considering the strength of the pectoralis major, latissimus dorsi and teres major muscles, how little power remains when medial rotation is tested. The weakness is permanent, but the painful arc on elevating the arm usually disappears within a month or two. The patient should be shown an exercise to strengthen the intact medial rotator muscles and how to maintain a full range of movement at the shoulder. Hydrocortisone injected at the lesser tuberosity desensitizes the tender tendinous remnants and should be carried out at once in all cases with a painful arc.

9. Weakness of the Triceps and Forearm Muscles

This is nearly always due to protrusion of the sixth cervical intervertebral disc, setting up a seventh cervical root-palsy. The pain may be concentrated at the scapula and arm, rarely it is confined to the pectoral area, but on examination the scapular muscles, the shoulder joint and the muscles controlling it are all normal. By contrast the neck movements set up the thoracic pain. The triceps muscle may be weak alone, or in conjunction with the flexors of the wrist. The triceps jerk is seldom affected.

10. Weakness of the Biceps and Forearm Muscles

This finding characterizes a sixth cervical root-palsy. The loss of power of flexion and supination at the elbow is often minor but is accompanied by clear weakness of the extensor muscles of the wrist. The biceps and brachio-radialis jerks are usually sluggish or absent. The only common cause is a fifth cervical disc lesion.

Examination shows that the neck, but not the shoulder, movements cause the pain felt in the scapular area.

11. Neuralgic Amyotrophy

The first symptom is central neckache, then pain in both arms, then concentrating in one upper limb only. The pain is severe and takes from four to six months to cease completely. Pins and needles are seldom experienced; if they are, they occupy the fingers relevant to the muscles most severely affected.

The affected muscles are completely paralysed from the outset and the weakness is of individual muscles, irrespective of segmental origin. The infraspinatus muscle is often involved, whatever other muscles are found weak, sometimes bilaterally.

Snapping Shoulder

This is nearly always the result of subluxation of the long head of biceps. As the result of rupture of the transverse humeral ligament, the tendon slips in and out of the upper end of its groove. It is almost invariably painless, and in most snapping shoulders the cause of pain and the snapping are unrelated, although the patient naturally associates the two.

STATISTICAL ANALYSIS

The frequency of lesions at the shoulder was determined by analysing 150 consecutive cases:

Traumatic arthritis	40 cases
Monarticular rheumatoid arthritis	36
Supraspinatus tendinitis	29
Subdeltoid bursitis	23
Infraspinatus tendinitis	8
Acromio-clavicular strain	6
Subscapular tendinitis	6
Freezing arthritis A and B	5
Bicipital tendinitis	2

Recapitulation

A few unusual patterns are listed here for speedy reference:
(a) *Passive elevation is full, but active elevation is limited.*
Ruptured supraspinatus
Fifth cervical root-palsy
Suprascapular neuritis
Long thoracic neuritis
Clay-shoveller's fracture
Fractured first rib
(b) *Passive elevation is limited but there is 90 degree abduction range at the scapulo-humeral joint.*
Contracture after radical mastectomy
Pulmonary neoplasm
Posterior sterno-clavicular syndrome
Contracture of the costo-coracoid fascia
Ankylosis of the acromio-clavicular joint
(c) *Passive lateral rotation is limited alone.*
Anterior capsular scar (old dislocation).

Subcoracoid bursitis.
Ruptured infraspinatus tendon.
(d) *Full range with incomprehensible pattern.*
Probably localized subdeltoid bursitis.

Chronology of Limited Movement

Only approximate periods can be given

Three Days

Limited movement of capsular pattern. Frequent recurrence. Spontaneous recovery in three days.
Palindromic rheumatism

One Month

Limited movement of capsular pattern. Spontaneous recovery in one month.
Chondrocalcinosis (pseudo-gout)

Six Weeks

Limited movement of noncapsular pattern. Recurrence each two to five years at either shoulder. Spontaneous recovery in six weeks.
Acute subdeltoid bursitis

One Year

Limited movement of capsular pattern. Spontaneous recovery in one year.
Freezing or traumatic arthritis

Two Years

Limited movement of capsular pattern. Spontaneous recovery in two years.
Monarticular rheumatoid arthritis

Indefinite Limitation

Limited movement of capsular pattern. Spontaneous cessation of pain in two years, with, often permanent, residual limitation of movement.

Arthritis complicating ankylosing spondylitis
Psoriasis or lupus erythematosus

ACROMIO-CLAVICULAR JOINT

When this joint is affected, usually after a fall on the shoulder, the patient complains of pain exactly at the site of the joint. There may be a slight aching also in the upper deltoid area, but such reference is uncommon and does not deceive; for when asked to indicate whence the pain springs, the patient places one finger on, or very close to, the joint. Rarely, the inferior aspect of the capsule bears the brunt of an injury. If so, the pain at the joint is sometimes felt to travel as far as the mid-arm and a painful arc may then occur on abduction at the shoulder. Hence a puzzling picture emerges, very similar to that of localized subdeltoid bursitis. Local anaesthesia has to be employed to clarify the diagnosis; for tenderness cannot be elicited either at the deep aspect of the joint or at the subacromial part of the bursa. Since they are both inert structures lying in contact and beyond reach of the examiner's finger, differentiation is difficult.

If any movement at the acromio-clavicular joint hurts at the point of the shoulder, diagnosis is simple. But it often happens that no scapular movement hurts; it is only when the extremes of passive movement at the shoulder are tested that pain is evoked. These, surprisingly enough, appear to strain the joint more effectively than do the scapular movements. A useful distinction is to test full passive adduction of the arm across the front of the upper thorax. This is often the most painful movement when the acromio-clavicular joint is affected, but causes little discomfort in chronic subdeltoid bursitis. If the posterior acromio-clavicular ligament is severely strained, passive adduction of the arm may become so painful as to appear limited. Another difficulty is the very earliest stage of arthritis at the shoulder, when full range at this joint is still retained with merely pain at extremes. The site of the pain helps, for gleno-humeral capsular pain is rarely felt at the point of the shoulder. The end-feel is also useful diagnostically; it is normal at the shoulder when the acromio-clavicular joint is at fault. Moreover, in arthritis at the shoulder, passive testing discloses that it is the extreme of lateral rotation, not of adduction, that hurts most.

Severe stretching of the acromio-clavicular joint leads to laxity and a tendency to subluxation, which may be visible and is usually easily palpable. Recurrent subluxation soon becomes a painless clicking; its degree is limited by the length of the conoid and trapezoid ligaments. It does not constitute an appreciable disability in itself, and in any case the capsular laxity is permanent. Osteophyte formation at the acromio-clavicular joint leads to prominence of the ends of the bones; these may be slightly tender. Such osteoarthritis seldom causes more than some temporary aching after exertion, but is a common radiographic finding in elderly patients. It is thus usual to find patients credited with a lesion of the acromio-clavicular joint on the strength of misapplied X-ray findings, although the most cursory examination would have revealed, for example, limitation of movement at the shoulder joint. No degree of arthritis at the acromio-clavicular joint can affect the range of movement at the shoulder joint. In advanced ankylosing spondylitis fixation of the acromio-clavicular joint occasionally becomes complete. The arm can then be raised only to the horizontal, but a full range of passive movement is found at the scapulo-humeral joint. Examination of the scapular movements then shows that rotation and elevation are not possible, i.e. that the limitation of elevation of the arm is dependent on fixation of the scapula.

Treatment

Since no muscle effectively spans the acromio-clavicular joint, the patient cannot voluntarily stabilize it after a sprain. Even less can he hold it too still, in such a way as to lead to the formation of post-traumatic adhesions. Hence this joint is always treated by rest rather than movement.

Recent Case without Subluxation

All that is required is to get rid of the post-traumatic inflammatory reaction. Hydrocortisone is therefore injected, care being taken to deal with the inferior aspect of the joint no less than the rest. The patient should be symptom-free after two days and fit then to return to full activity.

Technique of Injection
The area of tenderness lying superiorly and anteriorly is mapped out and infiltrated all over, using 2 ml. of hydrocortisone suspension.

Although the bones lie so superficially, the joint-line is tiny and difficult to palpate except in thin subjects. The right spot is thus difficult to identify, and it assists to have the patient's arm, his elbow by his side, held in full lateral rotation by an assistant, so as to distract the clavicle from the acromion as far as possible.

The inferior acromio-clavicular ligament is now injected by putting a

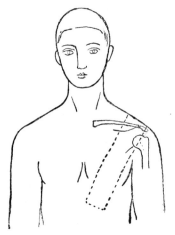

2·5 cm. needle vertically into the joint and pushing it on until the resistance of the ligament is encountered on the far side. A drop is injected at half a dozen different places along the ligament, by altering the angle of the needle at each little withdrawal and reinsertion.

Occasionally, a wider infiltration of the inferior surface of the joint is required than can be achieved from this approach. If so, the anterior joint-line is identified and approached from 2 cm. below this point with a needle 4 cm. long. When the tip of the needle is felt to reach bone, 2 ml. of hydrocortisone suspension are now used to infiltrate the ligamentous attachments at each side of the joint-line.

FIG. 43. Strapping for acromio-clavicular joint. The strapping passes from the lower ribs, over the joint, to the lower scapular area.

Recent Case with Subluxation

In addition to hydrocortisone injection, relief from tension is required. The arm should, therefore, be supported in a sling for a few days, so that its weight does not pull the clavicle and acromion apart. Strapping should be applied from the lower sternum, passing over the joint and reaching the lower ribs behind (Fig. 43) and kept on for ten days. Exercises are contra-indicated except that, as always, a full range of movement is maintained daily at the shoulder joint if the patient is over forty.

Naturally enough, the laxity of the ligaments persists indefinitely, but so long as there is no pain, there is no appreciable disability.

Osteoarthritis

The shoulder is apt to ache after overwork, e.g. digging, and sometimes after a spell of overuse goes on aching. Such a persistent ache can be dispelled by an injection of hydrocortisone, but the condition of the joint has not been altered and the patient must be warned that further exertion will lead to relapse.

12

The Shoulder

PART III: TREATMENT

The shoulder is a most rewarding joint when accurate diagnosis is followed by accurate treatment, since an effective remedy exists for nearly every disorder. In the past, many conditions at the shoulder were considered incurable. This was, and in part remains today, a justified view; for how to arrive at an accurate diagnosis at the shoulder was not known, and the diagnostic methods set out in the previous two chapters are still not practised widely enough. In consequence, even today, many easily curable conditions remain uncured. Patients are told they will recover without treatment in a year, which often proves a most inaccurate prognosis in arthritis, and even more so in tendinitis which may go on for years. Further difficulty arises from the general but erroneous belief that tendinous lesions cause, or by extension to adjacent structures result in, limitation of movement. Clearly, if the earliest stage of arthritis is mistaken for tendinitis, it is logically assumed that the later supervention of marked limitation of movement results from extension of the alleged tendinitis. This notion, unfortunately, is widespread, undisputed and based on excellent authority . . . yet false. Clinical perseverance and an open mind are the first essentials; adequate injection techniques and a properly trained physiotherapist provide the next requirement.

GENERAL PRINCIPLES

Treatment at the shoulder is a pleasure. The abiding problem is diagnosis. Once the right lesion has been singled out, almost every disorder is quickly relievable.

The objects of treatment are:

1. To Restore a Full Range of Painless Mobility at the Joint

There are three different approaches:

(a) *Intra-articular hydrocortisone.* In recent traumatic arthritis, the injection may of itself suffice, the range returning spontaneously as the injections allay the synovial inflammation. If not, once the joint enters the stage when active treatment is indicated, stretching out should begin. In mon-articular rheumatoid arthritis, the injections are enough in themselves. Stretching out is contra-indicated.

(b) *Stretching out the joint.* This entails gradual and repeated forcing by the physiotherapist. The capsule is first rendered analgesic by the increased local circulation that follows short-wave diathermy. It is then stretched out two or three times a week until the range has been restored.

(c) *Manipulation under anaesthesia.* This is rarely required. When real indications exist, it is made much more quickly effective by injecting hydro-cortisone into the joint the day before. The post-manipulative reaction is thus largely avoided and after-treatment shortened and simplified.

2. To Restore Painless Function of a Tendon

There are two approaches. One is to break down unwanted scar-tissue, by deep friction given across the fibres of the tendon. The other is to leave the scar-tissue in being, but to remove the traumatic inflammation from it by infiltrating the lesion with hydrocortisone suspension.

3. To Abolish Tenderness of a Bursa

Procaine and hydrocortisone can both be used for this purpose.

4. To get rid of Calcified Material

Repeated infiltration with procaine dissolves a deposit; alternatively, it can be removed at operation.

CAPSULE OF SHOULDER-JOINT

Prophylaxis of Stiffness

This is most important; for stiffness at the shoulder is often as easy to prevent at the time as it is troublesome to put right afterwards. For example, when a middle-aged or elderly patient's upper limb is kept in a sling for some time for any reason, and no instructions are given about moving unaffected joints, the immobilization imposed on the shoulder joint is purely wanton. The same applies after hemiplegia.

Post-traumatic adhesions are very apt to form at the inferior aspect of the joint (Fig. 31, p. 223) where damaged folds of lax capsule lie in contact so long as the patient keeps his arm to his side. Since this is what he naturally does in order to avoid pain, treatment by early movement is essential after any sprain of the capsule of the shoulder joint in any patient over forty. The joint movement is maintained passively; active repetition follows.

Fracture

Examination of the shoulder in cases of united fracture of the surgical neck of the humerus shows that, when treatment by movement is not instituted at once, stiffness supervenes rapidly from traumatic arthritis. Hence, in this type of fracture it is not the broken bone that governs treatment, but the damage done to the joint by a force sufficient to break bone. Any bruised shoulder, whether associated with a simple fracture or not, should be taken seriously and treated by immediate movement. In fracture of the surgical neck, movement must of necessity by given passively for the first week. Since it is movement at a joint, however induced, that prevents stiffness, passive movements are strongly indicated. During the first few days after an injury, the passive movement may be possible over quite an ample range at a time when no amount of encouragement induces much active movement. For the first fortnight after fracture of the surgical neck of the humerus, abduction is the principal movement to maintain. Rotation is more likely to occur at the site of the fracture than at the shoulder joint, and should therefore be avoided. When the abduction movement is carried out, the physiotherapist must place one hand on the shoulder and the other under the elbow (Fig. 44) and press the fractured ends together. In this way the humerus is made to move in one piece as the physiotherapist abducts it; there is very little pain, and movement at the joint, not at the fracture line, is secured.

Treatment of Arthritis

Treatment depends on the type and stage of arthritis present.

When two disorders co-exist at the shoulder, the capsular lesion always takes precedence. Until full movement has been restored, little advantage accrues from treating, e.g. a tendinous lesion.

Immobilizational Arthritis

If the arm is put in a sling for any reason, stiffness of the shoulder must be prevented from the outset. The older the patient, the sooner does immobility lead to an arthritis. In recent hemiplegia, the patient cannot use his muscles to move the shoulder and the range has to be maintained passively until voluntary movement returns.

From the first, the patient must take the arm out of the sling night and

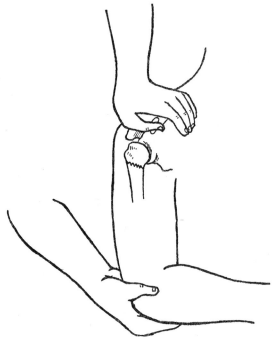

Fig. 44. Passive movement at the shoulder in recent fracture of surgical neck of humerus. The bone-ends are kept opposed by pressure exerted upwards from the elbow while the shoulder is held down. In this way a good range of movement can be maintained at the shoulder joint pending the return of active movement.

morning and move the shoulder joint through its full range. If stiffness has already set in, the shoulder must be stretched out daily by the physiotherapist until the full range is restored. If the arthritis has got to the stage when such stretching is no longer effective, hydrocortisone must be injected into the joint. Unsuitability for stretching is signalled by three criteria—namely, the patient cannot lie on that side at night; he is in pain even when the arm is kept still; the ache spreads to the forearm.

After fracture the same stiffness results unless the shoulder joint is stretched out by the physiotherapist a little more each day until the full range has been regained.

Traumatic Arthritis

This can be avoided by early gentle forcing of the joint, which leads to rapid restoration of the full range of movement. Once limitation has set in, stretching by the physiotherapist remains successful if the signs of activity are absent, i.e. there is no pain when the arm is kept still, no reference of pain below the elbow and the patient can lie on that side at night. If these signs point to a degree of activity contra-indicating active treatment, hydrocortisone is the only alternative. Injected into the joint, it allays the inflammatory reaction at the synovial membrane. If the first injection relieves, the second is given as soon as its effect is passing off—usually one to two weeks later. Others are given at whatever intervals prove necessary. More than three or four injections are seldom required. The pain subsides, and the joint enters the first stage again. If the range has increased spontaneously as the result of the intra-articular hydrocortisone injections, they are kept up until it is clear that recovery will continue spontaneously. If the joint reaches the first stage but no increase in range results from the injections, stretching is cautiously begun by the physiotherapist. If the joint tends to flare, hydrocortisone is repeated and the forcing postponed for a few weeks. If all goes well, treatment can usually cease before full range has been quite restored, final resolution occurring spontaneously.

Technique of Injection

There are several ways of entering the shoulder joint, but the method described has the advantage that the patient cannot easily move his arm, since he is lying on it; thus he cannot perform the sort of abrupt movement that may break the needle. The patient lies prone on a couch with his forearm under his upper abdomen. This keeps the arm still in considerable medial rotation and, however arthritic the shoulder, the posture is not painful. The articular surface of the humeral head now faces posteriorly, and provides a large target for the needle. The operator identifies the posterior bony projection where the acromion and the spine of the scapula meet at right-angles. He selects a spot 1 cm. below this point and thrusts in a thin needle 5 cm. long. He identifies the tip of the coracoid process anteriorly and aims the needle directly at it. He feels nothing as the needle traverses the infraspinatus tendon, but the capsule of the joint offers clear resistance. Once the capsule of the joint is pierced, the needle engages against articular cartilage—another characteristic sensation, quite unlike the impenetrable surface offered by bone. The needle is now withdrawn half a millimetre and 50 mg. of hydrocortisone are run into the joint cavity. No appreciable pressure is needed, and care is taken that the needle remains intracapsular, just touching cartilage.

Freezing Arthritis

In the recent case, stretching is no help and increasing pain and limitation of movement develop whatever is or is not done. At this point, say three or four months after the onset, a common error is to manipulate under anaesthesia. This discredits manipulation at the shoulder. Ill-timed manipulation further diminishes range of movement at the shoulder by the next morning, and causes an extra one or two months' severe pain.

Freezing arthritis of six or more months' duration re-enters the first stage and responds very well to stretching. This hastens cure; a full range of movement may be regained in, say, six weeks when spontaneous recovery would have taken another four months. Manipulation under anaesthesia is also successful at this stage, but several weeks' after-treatment is required. Hence little time is saved and there is little advantage in this more forcible treatment.

Hydrocortisone injected intra-articularly is without effect, and confirms the distinction between freezing and rheumatoid arthritis.

Osteoarthritis

The presence of osteophytes and the crepitus indicating roughening of the surface of cartilage cannot be altered by any treatment. But the cause of pain is capsular contracture which may come on as the result of the degenerative process itself, but much more often results from minor injury or even mere overuse, e.g. sawing wood for some hours. Osteoarthritis makes the joint very susceptible to outside influences, which easily evoke a traumatic arthritis superimposed on the symptomless osteoarthritis.

Hydrocortisone has no effect on osteoarthritis without a secondary traumatic arthritis. The only effective treatment is gradual stretching of the joint. But the joint may not be in the first stage, in which case little can be done except wait until time has brought the joint into a treatable condition. Alternatively, the patient may be, as so many old people are, intolerant of any uncomfortable treatment; the disorder is then also intractable. However, the results are good in those cases that can be treated actively.

Monarticular Rheumatoid and Spondylitic Arthritis

Even when fully within the first stage, this condition provides a permanent contra-indication to forcing movement at the joint whether by the physiotherapist after heat or, even worse, under anaesthesia. It is the existence of this condition that is the major reason for the gradual abandonment of mobilization under anaesthesia for what is almost always misdiagnosed as a 'frozen shoulder'. No one would force movement, still less under anaesthesia, at a hot and swollen rheumatoid knee or wrist; neither should this be performed at the shoulder, even though the capsule lies too deep for the heat and swelling to be detectable.

Steroid therapy is strongly indicated. All other measures are harmful, as no one knows better than I from the futile attempts that I made to help before hydrocortisone became available in 1952. The relief of monarticular rheumatoid arthritis at the shoulder affords one of the most dramatic results in all orthopaedic medicine. The patient, pale, miserable and worn-out by months of constant pain and lack of sleep finds that, twenty-four hours after the first injection, his pain when the arm is kept motionless has ceased, and that he can turn and lie on that side at night and sleep without difficulty. He comes again some days later, scarcely recognizable as the wan creature of the previous week. The joint is injected again. The principle is to repeat the injection just *before* it begins to relapse. A likely sequence is seven, seven, ten, fourteen, twenty-one days' interval between injections. Six to ten will probably be required in all and, when the patient is doing well on monthly or six-weekly injections, they can be stopped. Though pain ceases, except when the joint is stretched, as from the first injection, increase in range is seldom noted for the first month or two, and is apt to begin only after, say, the fourth injection. The patient is asked to return at once if the interval between injections has been misjudged, the pain beginning to reappear before the allotted period has elapsed. Since monarticular rheumatoid arthritis tends eventually to recur at the same or the other shoulder, the patient is warned—though he scarcely needs the advice—to come at once if either shoulder troubles him again.

Psoriatic arthritis at the shoulder responds well and quickly to intraarticular hydrocortisone; the arthritis complicating lupus erythematosus takes a larger number of infections and the range may not be fully restored even though pain ceases.

When an arthritis judged rheumatoid proves unexpectedly to be refractory to hydrocortisone—this is rare—the presence of freezing arthritis, type B, should be considered. If so, no treatment avails, and spontaneous recovery takes two years.

STRETCHING THE SHOULDER

This is not so simple as it sounds. If the physiotherapist does too much, she provokes a reaction that leads to a diminished range of movement, whereas if she is too gentle, she achieves nothing. Considerable judgement and care are required.

Heating the joint capsule by short-wave diathermy is a useful preliminary to forcing, since the temporary increase in circulation acts as an analgesic. The patient lies on the couch and the physiotherapist notes the range of passive movement, paying great attention to the end-feel. Discomfort is, of course, evoked when the arm is pushed towards the extreme of the restricted range. If sustained pressure can be felt to coax a little further movement from the joint, without increasing this pain or provoking the abrupt onset of muscle spasm, the joint should respond well to stretching. Again, this is likely to succeed if the resistance to movement begins before any pain is elicited. If, by contrast, pain and spasm come on sharply together, or pain stops the movement before the extreme of the possible range has been reached, the experienced physiotherapist will refuse to force the joint, probably stating merely that it does not 'feel right'; for these sensations imparted to the hand are difficult to put into words. Assuming that she finds the end-feel satisfactory, she next forces the arm up for a few moments, then brings it down again. If the pain ceases at once it is clear that treatment can be reasonably strenuous; if it continues, a cautious start must be made. The physiotherapist puts one hand on his sternum (to keep the thorax on the couch) and the other on his elbow and pushes this upwards. Increasing pressure is exerted for, say, a minute. There is no jerk; it is a sustained movement. She then relaxes gradually, pauses, and repeats the manipulation. Her first treatment is fairly gentle, and at the patient's next visit she asks him for how long he was sore afterwards and assesses anew the range of passive movement. He should experience increased aching for one or two hours after the forcing, the symptoms then returning to their previous level. This period of exacerbation is her criterion, and she adjusts the vigour of her treatment to secure this result. This rule is a great safeguard; for not all shoulders respond well to forcing, even when fully within the first stage. If she finds the patient is still suffering from increased pain a day or two after his first treatment, it is clear that forcing has been ordered in error and that an injection of hydrocortisone into the joint should be substituted. By contrast, if she provoked no lasting reaction at all, she must press harder, at times with great strength and persistence, to get her result.

This applies as much to the physiotherapist's after-treatment of mobilization under anaesthesia as to the gradual stretching out that is required in: (1) recent traumatic or immobilizational arthritis (to prevent adhesions forming); (2) long-standing traumatic or immobilizational arthritis (to break adhesions); (3) the second six months of freezing arthritis; (4) osteoarthritis.

Long-standing Cases

After many days' vigorous forcing of movement by the physiotherapist without apparent effect, a loud crack may be heard as a discrete band parts. Thereupon, the range of movement increases and the pain diminishes. After an interval the same happens again. Thus, in these cases, the shoulder recovers by a series of sudden improvements punctuating stationary periods.

Manipulation under Anaesthesia

This should be undertaken with caution, forethought and unwillingness. Occasionally in long-standing traumatic arthritis or osteoarthritis *in the first stage*, it becomes immediately clear that fractional mobilization under general anaesthesia is required. In others the physiotherapist reports at the end of two or three weeks that even strenuous treatment is without effect on the range of movement or the pain. If so, forcing under anaesthesia should be carried out at once. The day before the manipulation, 50 mg. of hydrocortisone are injected into the joint, to diminish the otherwise severe reaction. A small amount of pentothal given quickly suffices, since only half a minute's relaxation is necessary. The patient lies supine on the couch. The operator brings the patient's arm up as far as it will go without forcing, allowing it to rotate so that his hand is pressing on the medial aspect of the elbow (see Vol. II). Quite gentle sustained pressure suffices, the operator continuing his pressure until one large band of adhesions is heard to part; *no more should be attempted, and no endeavour is made to force either rotation*. This was an empirical finding, but now that Reeves has shown that stretching out rotation is apt to rupture the stretched tendon, the inadvisability of forcing this movement rests on a sound theoretical basis.

Reeves (1966) exposed two shoulders at operation and watched the effect of manipulation. Abduction was obtained when the inferior aspect of the capsule of the joint ruptured close to the glenoid attachment. He then forced lateral rotation and saw the subscapular tendon and the front of the capsule rupturing together. Curiously enough, there was no bleeding. A post-manipulative arthrogram showed the contrast material leaking out from the tear and tracking down the shaft of the humerus.

The physiotherapist's after-treatment is vigorous and lasts several weeks, i.e. until the full active range is retained between treatments.

Comment

It should be clear from the above remarks that *nothing is easier than to force movement at the shoulder joint under anaesthesia, whereas to know when to carry this out and, in particular, when to abstain requires great judgement.*

Manipulation has no effect in acute or chronic subdeltoid bursitis; a full range is found to exist under anaesthesia but the symptoms and limitation of movement remain unaltered when the patient regains consciousness.

Arthrodesis

Intractable continuing arthritis at the shoulder is very uncommon. If all treatment fails and time brings no relief, arthrodesis affords a satisfactory solution. The patient retains 60 degrees of abduction by rotating his scapula and becomes fit for quite heavy work once more.

THE SUBDELTOID BURSA

Localized Bursitis

Every diagnosis of localized subdeltoid bursitis is tentative, since the signs are so often closely mimicked by minor degrees of tendinitis. Hence, confirmatory local anaesthesia is always required. The accessible portion of the bursa is palpated for tenderness, and the chosen spot infiltrated with 5 or 10 cc. 0·5 per cent procaine solution, the amount depending on the size of the tender area. If no tender spot can be found, and the signs indicate that subdeltoid bursitis is undoubtedly present, the conclusion must be drawn that the affected area lies in the half of the bursa beyond fingers' reach, i.e. under the acromion. A longer needle is now used to infiltrate the bursa here. In either case, after waiting five minutes for the local anaesthesia to take effect, the patient is examined again to determine if the signs, in particular the painful arc, have ceased. If the right spot has been chosen, no movement now causes pain; if the diagnosis of bursitis is mistaken, or if it is correct but the wrong spot has been infiltrated, the symptoms persist. The procedure must be tried again.

The diagnostic injection also provides the treatment. A couple of infiltrations at the correct spot with procaine solution is usually curative. If it fails, 5 cc. hydrocortisone suspension is used, and, as the result of the previous diagnostic local anaesthesia, the exact spot to inject is known in advance. One, at most two, such infiltrations are always curative.

No physiotherapy has the slightest effect on subdeltoid bursitis. Manipulation is likewise futile, for there is already a full range of movement at the shoulder joint.

Contusion of the bursal wall by a direct blow requires no treatment; recovery is spontaneous.

Acute Bursitis

The severe pain lasts seven to ten days; hence the treatment described below is called for only if the bursitis has lasted less than a week. Since it is a recurrent condition, patients soon learn when an attack is beginning and should attend at once for repetition of treatment.

In acute subdeltoid bursitis the whole accessible bursal wall is very tender; it may even be somewhat swollen. The patient lies in bed, the entire area is mapped out and the skin marked to define the edge. He is now given a strong analgesic, e.g. morphia. The entire area is now infiltrated, a drop at each point, with 5 cc. of hydrocortisone suspension. Another 5 cc. are then injected all over the subacromial extent of the bursa, and the morphia repeated two or three hours later. The next morning the patient wakes with rather a sore shoulder but with virtually no pain. Most of the movement has returned and he is able to go about his business. A few days later, if any aching persists, some small point missed during the diffuse infiltration may need injecting with, say, another 2 cc. of the suspension.

This treatment aborts an attack but does not, of course, diminish the tendency to further bouts, which are apt to recur at two- to five-yearly intervals. If the patient is seen after ten days, a sling for a week and butazolidine are indicated by day. By night, the patient is repeatedly woken because in bursitis involuntary muscle spasm is absent (unlike arthritis). Hence each time he moves in bed, his arm is shifted into the painful range. A figure of eight bandage round the thorax and the arm avoids this phenomenon and should be worn for a week or two. Butazolidine mg. 200 three times a day is particularly suited to bursitis and may be continued for a week.

Bursitis with Calcification

Acute Episodes

Although symptomless for years at a time, calcification renders a patient liable to attacks of acute bursitis; if so, severe pain accompanied by little or no movement at the shoulder joint results from a subdeltoid bursitis of sudden onset which, within a few days, has already reached the third stage. The treatment is the same steroid infiltration as for acute bursitis without calcification.

Persistent Pain

If calcification gives rise to persistent symptoms—and a small shadow on the radiograph is no guarantee that it causes whatever symptoms attributable to the shoulder the patient may have—local anaesthesia is the treatment of choice. Whether the acid solution dissolves the deposit or acupuncture liberates it—indeed, the two actions may be combined—is uncertain, but the results are usually good. However, six to eight weekly injections may be required before the radiograph shows that the deposit has faded. Radiotherapy is said to abolish pain and to lead to disappearance of the deposit, but did so in only one of a trial series of ten cases thus treated. Spontaneous disappearance of the deposit and of the symptoms may take place in the course of two or three years. This is not invariable, and deposits have persisted for up to seven years. Removal of the deposit at open operation is not often required, but is very successful.

Rheumatoid Bursitis

This causes a prominent swelling at one or both shoulders and fluctuation is easily detectable. Bursae may also be swollen elsewhere. The symptoms are rarely due to the bursitis, but to associated rheumatoid arthritis at the shoulder joint. Aspiration can be performed and hydrocortisone injected, but little benefit accrues.

Haemorrhagic Bursitis

Aspiration, perhaps more than once, is all that is required. Immediate return of the blood after aspiration occurs in angioma.

SUBCORACOID BURSITIS

Hydrocortisone should be injected in the region of the bursa. Three or four infiltrations are often required, since great accuracy in the placing of the injection is unattainable. Nevertheless, they must be continued until the patient is well; for the condition may last many months, showing little tendency to spontaneous cure within the first year.

Technique of Injection

The tip of the coracoid process is identified. A spot 2 in. below this point is chosen and a needle 5 cm. long inserted backwards and medially, tangentially to the curve of the process and aiming at its base. When it strikes bone at the neck of the scapula, it is pulled back 1 cm. The area hereabouts is infiltrated with 2 ml. hydrocortisone suspension by a series of withdrawals and reinsertions at a slightly different angle.

TENDONS AND MUSCLES

General principles apply at the shoulder. Tendinous lesions respond to hydrocortisone, which disinflames the painful scar; massage breaks up the scar tissue itself and is also effective, but is more painful and takes longer. The lesions of a muscle belly are rare at the shoulder, but when they do occur, deep transverse massage is quickly curative.

Supraspinatus Tendon

Tendinitis

This common lesion often shows no tendency to spontaneous recovery, and cases of many years' standing are encountered. Hence this otherwise trivial lesion may permanently make a man unfit for heavy work or unable to follow his favourite sport. Yet, cure is simple.

The tendon may be affected at:

1. The superficial aspect of the teno-periosteal junction anteriorly/ posteriorly
2. The deep aspect of the teno-periosteal junction
3. The musculo-tendinous junction.

At the tendon, hydrocortisone is the treatment of choice; the alternative is deep massage which is naturally more effective when the superficial rather than the deep fibres of the tendon are affected. At the musculo-tendinous junction, only massage avails (see Vol. II). Local anaesthesia is required in diagnosis, since only a few supraspinatus lesions lie at this point, but it affords no lasting benefit. Surgical removal of the acromion used to be carried out for supraspinatus tendinitis, but is now out of date; for it abolishes the painful arc leaving the tendinitis unaltered. It thus helps only a little. It also has the unintentional merit of improving access for the physiotherapist's finger, and has thus facilitated cure both of infraspinatus and of supraspinatus tendinitis with greater ease than in unoperated cases.

Technique of Injection

The position of the arm is the same as for massage (see Vol. II) since the tendon must be clearly palpated before any injection can be given. To this end the patient sits leaning against his forearm behind his back. The tendon has now a forward course, emerging from the anterior edge of the acromion and running anteriorly to the tuberosity of the humerus. Both these bony points can be felt and a 1 cm. stretch of tendon identified in the groove between them. The anterior edge of the tendon, now running sagittally, can be felt. A 1 cc. tuberculin syringe fitted with a fine needle 2·5 cm. long is filled with hydrocortisone suspension and inserted vertically downwards towards the tendon. The resistance afforded by dense fibrous tissue identifies the superficial surface of the tendon. By a series of little withdrawals and reinsertions a drop of hydrocortisone suspension is injected at a dozen different adjacent points, deeply or superficially, anteriorly or posteriorly, according to where the accessory signs show the lesion to lie.

Calcification in the Tendon

The first approach is to ignore the calcification and merely inject the tendon itself in the ordinary way, since the lesion may be adjacent to the area of calcification and not due to the deposit at all. But a large deposit may cause symptoms; if so, an endeavour must be made to get rid of it. No notice need be taken of tiny nodes visible radiographically; they have no significance.

Local anaesthesia should be induced at the deposit once every week or two until the symptoms cease; six to eight injections of 10 cc. are usually required. Whether the acid solution of procaine hydrochloride dissolves the deposit, or the acupuncture releases it—or both—is uncertain.

In the event of the injections failing, removal of the deposit at open operation is curative.

Complete Rupture

The immediate objective is to get rid of the painful arc. To this end hydrocortisone is injected into the tendinous remnants at the humeral tuberosity to destroy their sensitivity. As soon as the arc ceases, the patient should be shown how to initiate the abduction movement of the arm by placing his hand against the outer side of his thigh and then giving a twitch to his hip and simultaneously bending his trunk over to the opposite side. The supraspinatus muscle alone initiates abduction; this manœuvre swings the arm outwards to the point where the action of the deltoid muscle becomes effective and, since a painful arc no longer halts the movement, he can elevate his arm fully. If the rupture is of some standing, secondary capsular contracture from disuse may supervene. If so, the physiotherapist must stretch the joint out until the full range is restored. Permanent loss of power abduction is inevitable, but return to all but heavy work is possible within a few weeks. A patient with a light job need not take time off from work at all.

Operation

Since supraspinatus rupture affects chiefly the elderly, surgery is seldom indicated.

If it is decided upon, exposure of the belly usually shows that contracture prevents direct suture of the tendinous remnants. If so, the belly is freed and slid along the fossa until the proximal end of the torn tendon can be fixed into a cavity prepared for it in the humeral tuberosity. Debeyre (personal communication, 1968) followed up his cases for six years and reported 45 per cent cures, 25 per cent improvement and 30 per cent failures.

Infraspinatus Tendon

Hydrocortisone should be injected into the affected part of the tendon, or deep massage given at that point.

Technique of Injection

The patient lies prone, propped up on his elbows (see Vol. II). The bodyweight now forces the scapula to a right-angle with the humerus, thus uncovering the tuberosity. The tendon is identified below the lateral aspect of the spine of the scapula and followed along to the humeral head. If a painful arc exists, the lesion lies distally and superficially; if there is no such localizing sign, the tendon is palpated for tenderness. If no part of the tendon is more sensitive than another, the first point to try is the deep aspect of the teno-periosteal junction.

A 1-ml. tuberculin syringe is fitted with a fine needle 3 to 4 cm. long, the length depending on the thickness of the patient's subcutaneous tissues. The needle can be felt to enter the substance of the tendon and a dozen little injections are given close together in the region of the lesion.

Subscapular Tendon

Massage at the subscapular tendon is more painful and less successful than at the spinatus tendons. It is thus a fortunate circumstance that hydrocortisone is particularly effective here. Indeed, investigating the results of hydrocortisone in tendinitis in eighteen consecutive cases, one single infiltration of hydrocortisone gave relief in every instance, whereas at the other tendons the first injection cured only half of all cases.

The decision on which part of the teno-periosteal junction to aim at depends on finding a painful arc (uppermost extent) or pain on full passive adduction of the arm (lower extent), or both.

Technique of Injection

The patient lies face upwards, his hand resting on the front of his thigh. In this position the bicipital groove lies directly anteriorly and is palpable. Just medial to its upper end, the lesser tuberosity can be felt with ease through the deltoid muscle. This point is marked with a skin pencil.

A 2-cm. needle is thrust straight backwards until at about 1 cm. it reaches the tendon. A dozen small infiltrations are made in the region of the lesion, using a total of 25 mg.

Bicipital and Pectoral Tendon

Tendinitis of the long head of biceps, even of years' standing, recovers with two to four sessions of transverse friction. Therefore, no alternative treatment seems worth considering. Strain of the tendinous insertion of the pectoralis major at the edge of the bicipital groove is also best treated by deep friction, but recovers more slowly. However, infiltration with hydrocortisone all along the edge would clearly prove very difficult technically.

Pectoralis Major and Latissimus Dorsi Bellies

Local anaesthesia usually has a good lasting therapeutic effect on lesions of the belly of these two muscles; should it fail, deep massage is quickly effective.

Contracture of the Costo-coracoid Fascia

This is a disorder for which no conservative treatment exists. Stretching the arm into elevation causes several days' increased pain, but does no permanent good or harm. In one case, operative division of the costo-coracoid fascia and the tendon of the pectoralis minor, kindly carried out by my surgical colleague D. R. Urquhart, proved curative.

If the contracture is secondary to apical fibrosis of the lung, it is best left alone.

Subluxation of the Humeral Head

When a false painful arc occurs at the shoulder as the result of sub-luxation upwards of the head of the humerus during abduction, the patient must be taught how to depress the bone as the arm goes up. He can avoid the upward movement by using his pectoralis major and latis-simus dorsi muscles; the physiotherapist teaches him how to do this.

13

The Elbow

There is no line of demarcation between the shoulder and elbow regions. Pain in the arm may originate at the shoulder with reference downwards, or less often at the elbow with reference upwards. Most pains indicated by the patient at the elbow or forearm have a local origin, since at the more distal part of the upper limb the capacity for correct localization is good. If he describes the pain as occupying an ill-defined area, it is almost certain that a pain referred from above is present. If the slightest doubt exists, the patient is examined from neck to fingers.

Once it is clear that the elbow region is at fault, the joint and the muscles about it are tested by ten movements.

(a) Four. Passive extension, flexion, pronation, supination—full range, limited range, painful, painless.

(b) Four. Resisted extension, flexion, pronation, supination—strong, weak, painful, painless.

(c) Two. Resisted flexion and extension at the wrist—painful, painless. The muscles that perform these two movements arise from the humeral epicondyles and a lesion in either often causes pain felt at the elbow although the tissue affected is not functionally a part of the elbow (i.e. tennis- and golfer's elbow).

PAIN ON PASSIVE MOVEMENTS

The passive range of flexion, extension and rotation is ascertained and the end-feel noted. When extension is tested, the hard end-feel of the normal joint or of arthritis contrasts with the soft end-feel of an impacted loose body. If the passive, but not the resisted, movements hurt, the joint is affected. If the passive movements are painless, but one, or two compatible, resisted movements hurt, the trouble lies in the muscle thus singled out.

Early arthritis at the elbow shows itself as an isolated affection of the humero-ulnar joint. Passive flexion and extension are limited, but rotation is of full range and painless, showing that the radio-humeral and radio-ulnar joints are not involved. It is only in advanced arthritis that rotation is also limited. The *capsular pattern* at the elbow is rather variable, flexion is usually rather more restricted than extension, but sometimes the degrees of limitation are nearly equal. Ten degrees limitation of extension would correspond to about 30 degrees limitation of flexion; 30 degrees limitation of extension would correspond to perhaps 45 degrees even up to 80 degrees limitation of flexion; with this degree of arthritis some restriction of rotation would be beginning. Palpation of the joint may reveal warmth, effusion, synovial thickening, crepitus, or clicking.

Pain felt at the wrist on the extremes of passive rotation of the forearm incriminates the lower radio-ulnar joint.

The following types of articular disorder occur.

CAPSULAR PATTERN

1. Traumatic Arthritis

This shows itself in the humero-ulnar joint. After an injury of any severity to the elbow, flexion and extension are markedly limited and painful, but rotation is full range and painless. In other words, an arthritis exists at the humero-ulnar joint but not at the radio-humeral and radio-ulnar joints. Should rotation be painful in a patient with an acute traumatic arthritis at the elbow, the head of the radius is almost certainly chipped or cracked. The radiograph is then diagnostic.

The interesting question of the relationship between traumatic arthritis of the elbow joint and traumatic *myositis of the brachialis muscle* arises. On the one hand, resisted flexion of the forearm does not hurt in traumatic arthritis; hence, there is nothing to suggest a lesion of the brachialis muscle. Moreover, flexion is limited, not merely painful at its extreme— a point at which a tender part of the muscle might lie squeezed between humerus and ulna. These two findings suggest that the brachialis muscle is not involved in traumatic arthritis. On the other hand, two conflicting facts emerge, both of which suggest that there is some connection. These are: (1) traumatic arthritis may later develop myositis ossificans. If the late stage is an obvious affection of the brachialis muscle, what was the early stage? (2) in traumatic arthritis, resting the elbow in flexion in due course restores the range of extension at the joint. This position rests the brachialis muscle and, were an irritative lesion present, should let this subside. Analogy with other joints suggests that, in a purely articular disorder, fixation in flexion is not likely to lead to an increase in the range of extension. However intra-articular hydrocortisone quickly abates traumatic arthritis; such an injection could not influence a lesion of the brachialis muscle. This finding has considerable medico-legal import.

Treatment

Rest in Flexion

Whether the lesion is of the joint or of the brachialis muscle may not yet be agreed, but there is no difference of opinion on the treatment, which is *rest in flexion*. The elbow is immediately immobilized in flexion by a collar-and-cuff bandage. If full flexion is no longer attainable at the patient's first attendance, the elbow is held as flexed as possible, and flexed more daily until full flexion is achieved. This position is held for, say, a fortnight; then the elbow is rested in slightly less flexion. If, three days later, examination shows the range of flexion to remain full, the forearm is allowed to drop a little farther.

Enough range at the elbow is usually regained after six weeks to enable the patient to wear a sling instead of collar-and-cuff bandage. At the end of two or three months, a full range of painless movement has returned to the joint.

Efforts to speed recovery by massage, exercises or, worse, passive stretching of the joint defeat their own ends. They lead to irritation of the joint and increased limitation of movement. They are widely regarded as encouraging the development of myositis ossificans, and it would be scarcely possible to defend a medico-legal action were this 'treatment' given and a bony mass found later.

Hydrocortisone

Rest in flexion is still widely practised, but is in fact out of date. All that is required is two intra-articular injections of 2 cc. hydrocortisone suspension, the first on the day the patient is seen. The arm kept in a sling for a few days; and the second given 7 days later. In about a fortnight the joint has recovered. If there is any blood in the joint, it is aspirated first.

There are many approaches to the elbow joint. A simple technique is for the patient to lie prone on a couch, his arm by his side and the forearm supinated. During full extension of the elbow the groove between the humerus and the head of the radius is easily felt posteriorly, and a 2-cm. thin needle can be accurately introduced between them.

2. Myositis Ossificans

It is widely believed that myositis ossificans results from improper treatment of a damaged elbow, i.e. by neglect of rest in flexion. My view is that the development of the bony mass is determined by the nature of the original injury. If the brachialis tendon is torn, rest in flexion, even from the outset, will not necessarily prevent ossification. If it has not been torn, improper treatment postpones recovery and increases pain, but does not cause myositis; a number of such cases have been encountered, some of whom had received quite strong manipulation from bonesetters.

In established myositis ossifications of the brachialis muscle, only a little movement to either side of the right angle is possible. Rotation is also markedly limited. The bony tumour is sometimes palpable and is shown clearly by X-rays.

No treatment avails. Excision of the bony mass seldom helps.

3. Osteoarthritis

This may come on for no apparent reason in late middle-age and is often bilateral. Alternatively, it may follow fracture involving an articular surface. Quite often the only symptoms are aching after considerable exertion and inability fully to extend the joint. Examination shows 10 degree or 20 degree limitation of flexion and extension, the movement ending abruptly with the sensation of bone-to-bone. Coarse crepitus is often palpable. Forcing is uncomfortable rather than painful. This discomfort and the slight limitation of movement differentiate osteoarthritis from the gross painless limitation of neuropathic arthropathy. In the latter, the radiograph is diagnostic. By contrast, X-ray evidence of osteoarthritis at the elbow is compatible with full range and painless function at the joint.

Treatment. As a rule no treatment is required. If overuse has superimposed a traumatic arthritis, an intra-articular injection of hydrocortisone suspension is indicated.

4. Monarticular Rheumatoid Arthritis

When other joints are also affected, the rheumatoid or spondylitic origin is clear. In acute or subacute monarticular rheumatoid arthritis, the joint is warm and the capsule thickened; this is best detected by palpation over the head of the radius laterally. Marked limitation of flexion, some limitation of extension and, in due course, some limitation of rotation supervenes in the untreated case. The end-feel is hard and the wasted muscles spring into spasm when the extreme of the possible range is reached. After some years of arthritis a characteristic silken crepitus becomes palpable on movement, quite different from the coarse grating of osteoarthritis. Decalcification and, later, erosion of cartilage are visible on the radiograph. Distinction should be made between involvement of the joint in Reiter's disease, psoriasis, gout, spondylitis, or lupus erythematosus.

Intra-articular hydrocortisone is the only effective treatment and can be repeated as often as necessary. I have never encountered steroid arthropathy in a joint that does not bear weight. The injection stops the pain but does not usually increase the range of movement much.

NON CAPSULAR PATTERN

1. Loose Body in the Joint

A displaced loose body jams the joint, either preventing full extension, but leaving flexion full and painless; or preventing flexion and leaving extension full and painless. When extension is limited by the displaced fragment, the end-feel is characteristically soft; in all other disorders of the elbow joint it is hard.

In Adolescence

From the age of fourteen, osteochrondritis dessecans, less often a chip fracture into the joint, leads to exfoliation of a fragment of bone covered by articular cartilage. These loose bodies are often multiple and two to six fragments may be encountered at operation. They have three effects.

1. *Attacks of Internal Derangement*
The young patient describes sudden twinges at irregular intervals and attacks of sudden fixation of the joint that gradually subside in a few days. It is curious that, although the joint usually locks suddenly, it does not unlock equally suddenly with a click, as happens at the knee. The range of movement returns by itself gradually in a few days; in due course, this series of events is repeated.

2. *Growth of the Loose Body*
In a growing adolescent, the loose body may grow too. The fragment, whose osseous nucleus may have been 1 mm. across at radiography at fourteen years of age, may become a centimetre across five years later. It then jams the joint increasingly, and should be removed. The loose body is covered with cartilage and is thus always considerably larger than the shadow on the X-ray photograph.

3. *Osteoarthritis*
If the loose bodies are left inside the joint, even though they cause no trouble, slight limitation of movement soon sets in at the elbow joint, and by the time the patient is eighteen or twenty, osteophyte formation has

begun to show radiographically. There may well be 5 degrees limitation of extension and 10 degrees limitation of flexion at the elbow, permanently.

Diagnosis

If, in the absence of obvious trauma, an adolescent complains of trouble at the elbow, this diagnosis suggests itself; for it is the common cause at that age. If the joint is locked at the time the patient attends, the mere fact that this came on suddenly and is known to be transitory is significant; examination shows the non capsular pattern and a soft end-feel. For the first couple of years nothing may be discernible between attacks, but the history is clear and the radiographic appearances confirmatory. By the age of twenty, slight limitation of movement appears, due to osteo-arthritis, now with a hard end-feel between attacks, but a soft end-feel when extension is additionally blocked by the displaced fragment. Loose body formation is the only non-traumatic cause of osteoarthritis in a young person; this fact alone suggests the diagnosis.

Treatment

Manipulative reduction seldom presents difficulties and should be carried out (see Vol. II). But removal is advised, since recurrence is very probable and, in any case, osteoarthritis is a strong likelihood unless operation is done early. Admittedly, such osteoarthritis is not at all painful, but limited extension at the elbow may interfere with a man's games or a girl's piano playing.

In Adults

The patient complains of attacks of pain at the elbow. If a loose body becomes impacted, it may cause a constant ache or pain whenever the elbow is exerted; if so, the trouble is regularly ascribed to a tennis-elbow. If such an elbow is manipulated in Mill's manner, a severe traumatic arthritis may be provoked. The distinction is therefore important.

Site of the Fragment

There are two possibilities. If the loose body lies in the triangle between humerus, ulna and radial head, it limits extension, while flexion is full and painless. Extension has a soft end-feel, and the limitation does not exceed a few degrees. If it lies between the coronoid process and the anterior aspect of the humerus, it limits flexion, extension being free and painless. Flexion has a hard end-feel, but is not as painful as in arthritis; it just will not go, since the coronoid process is engaged against the loose body. Flexion may be anything from 45 degrees to 70 degrees limited, at a time when extension is unaffected: a very clear non capsular pattern.

When the attacks begin in middle-age, osteoarthritis does not supervene (at any rate within ten years) even if the bouts of internal derangement continue. At this age too, many loose bodies are purely cartilaginous (presumably chip-fractures) and do not show by X-rays. Hence, if they show, well and good; if not, the diagnosis need not be mistaken; the fragment merely does not contain a bony centre. But to many, pain at the elbow and a normal radiograph in middle-age suggest tennis-elbow: an ascription easily disproved by clinical examination.

Treatment

A loose body limiting extension can usually be reduced, i.e. shifted to a part of the joint where it no longer blocks movement and lies silently (see Vol. II). If the attacks are not too frequent, this is all that need be done. If the patient prefers, and X-ray examination shows its position (and how many are present), removal is a satisfactory operation. Elderly patients' elbows do not take kindly to being opened; hence, removal is best avoided for fear of marked post-operative stiffness. Manipulative reduction must be carried out each time derangement occurs.

A loose body limiting flexion cannot be shifted by manipulation; hence treatment is removal or nothing, depending on the patient's age and preference. If nothing is done, the loose body may, it seems, become slightly embedded; in one patient with 60 degrees limitation of flexion the day after the shift, there was only 30 degrees ten years later.

2. Osteoarthritis with a Loose Body

Osteoarthritis is often complicated by the presence of one or more loose bodies, displacement of which gives rise to attacks of pain seldom lasting more than about a week. These attacks are not abrupt, they come on in the course of hours and subside even more gradually. The history is indicative; an elderly patient complains of slight, long-standing aching in the elbow, punctuated by attacks during which the elbow loses most of its movement. Between bouts, examination reveals merely the osteoarthritis (see p. 295). During an attack, gross limitation of recent onset usually of the non-capsular pattern makes the diagnosis clear. The radiograph is confirmative; for the loose body has a bony nucleus. However, it should be remembered that not all elderly patients with loose bodies in the elbow suffer attacks of internal derangement.

Manipulative reduction should be carried out (see Vol. II).

3. Sprain of upper Radio-ulnar Joint

This is a rare cause of pain at the elbow. Examination shows that passive supination evokes the discomfort; the other passive movements do not and the resisted movements at elbow and wrist are painless. The patient is always regarded as suffering from tennis-elbow.

One, or at most two injections of hydrocortisone into the elbow joint are curative within a few weeks. Untreated, or aggravated by active measures, the disorder is apt to last several years.

It should be remembered that in bicipital tendinitis occurring at the radial tuberosity, full passive pronation squeezes the tender tendon against the shaft of the ulna. Passive pronation hurting alone must thus not be regarded as an articular sign unless—unexpectedly—bicipital tendinitis is absent.

Limitation of passive pronation alone is a rare and curious articular sign. It appears to continue indefinitely and intra-articular hydrocortisone has no effect. I am not at all sure what the lesion is in these cases and regard it as incurable.

4. Ligamentous Sprain

Sprains of either collateral ligament set up traumatic arthritis; they do not show as an isolated lesion. Calcification in either collateral ligament giving rise to slight limitation of movement is rare, and is not amenable to active treatment. The radiographic appearances are diagnostic.

5. Pulled Elbow

I have never met with a case myself. It occurs when children are pulled along by the hand too forcibly. The disorder is confined to children less than eight years old. The radius is displaced vertically downwards; this is best shown on a radiograph not of the elbow but of the wrist (which has been shown to me). The resulting articular disturbance at the elbow and the lower radio-ulnar joint naturally gives rise to limitation of movement and Magill and Aitken (1954) state that extension is 20 degrees limited and that forcing is met by rubbery resistance. Reduction is immediately secured by rotating the forearm rapidly to and fro, while pushing the radius upwards towards the humerus by pressing the elbow against a wall; the click of reduction is felt on full supination.

PAIN ON RESISTED MOVEMENT

If the passive movements show the joint to be normal, and the preliminary examination shows the region of the elbow to contain the lesion, the elbow is held at mid-range and the effect of resisted flexion, extension, supination and pronation is reported. The examiner must apply the resistance with his hand on the patient's lower forearm; for, should the movement be resisted by pressure against the hand, pain will also be elicited from the muscles controlling the wrist joint.

Pain may be felt or weakness discovered on resisted movement, always associated, except in rare double lesions, with full range at the joint.

1. Resisted Flexion

When this hurts a lesion of the biceps or brachialis muscle exists. If, as is to be expected, it is the former, there is pain also on resisted supination. When the biceps is affected, the lesion may lie at one of four sites.

Biceps Muscle

(a) *At the long head of biceps.* The tendon is nearly always affected at the upper part of its extent in the groove on the humerus, and the patient states that the pain is felt at the shoulder. The only way to find out which

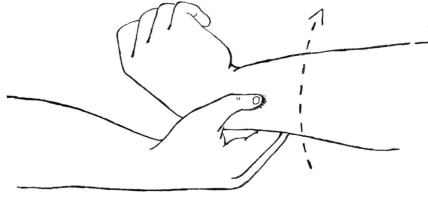

FIG. 45. Resisted supination at elbow joint. The examiner resists the supination movement by pressure exerted at the lower forearm

part of the tendon is involved is by palpation for tenderness along its course. Local anaesthesia affords no added precision. Finding the right point is vital; for cases of even ten or more years' standing, that have resisted every treatment, are permanently cured after three or four sessions of deep massage, given to the exact spot (see Vol. II).

Rupture of the long head of biceps causes no symptoms then or later. Clinical testing does not even reveal any weakness of the muscles flexing the elbow.

(b) *In the belly of the biceps.* Minor rupture of the anterior aspect of the belly causes no symptoms once the immediate discomfort and bruising have cleared. A symptomless swelling is then present at the lower arm, which contracts with the rest of the muscle forming what looks like a golf ball just above the elbow. When, however, a few muscle fibres tear at the posterior aspect of the belly, pain in the arm on certain movements results which may persist for months or years. Spontaneous cure usually takes two years in patients who avoid straining the muscle during this time; in those who continue at heavy work the symptoms may go on indefinitely.

The area of tenderness at the back of the belly must be sought by pinching the deep aspect of the muscle between finger and thumb; palpation from in front is no help. When the probable site of the lesion has been found, local anaesthesia should always be used as confirmation; for exact localization is otherwise difficult. The injection sometimes does lasting good in recent cases, and in any case shows the physiotherapist exactly where to give the deep massage. This is quickly effective (see Vol. II).

(c) *At the lower musculo-tendinous junction.* The pain is felt at the lower arm and palpation confirms its site. Local anaesthesia is usually required to confirm the diagnosis, but has no therapeutic value. Without deep friction, a lesion at this point in the muscle is apt to go on hurting indefinitely; for it has occurred at a point where the natural mobility of muscle is restricted by the presence of tendinous strands. The patient's active efforts merely strain the muscle afresh; there is no alternative to proper massage.

(d) *At the lower teno-periosteal junction.* At this level the position of the pain is distinctive and a localizing sign exists. The patient complains of pain felt to start at the centre of the front of the elbow, radiating down the front of the forearm as far as the wrist. Resisted flexion and supination elicit the pain; so does full passive pronation at the elbow joint, especially when this is held flexed. This sign indicates that tenderness is evoked by pressing the tuberosity of the radius against the ulna; in other words, that the lesion in the tendon lies at the tuberosity.

One infiltration with hydrocortisone is usually curative. The patient lies prone, his arm by his side, with the forearm in full pronation. In this position the radius is fully rotated, so that the tuberosity faces directly backwards. The lower edge of the head of the radius is now identified and a spot chosen along the shaft of the bone 2 cm. below this line. No particular tenderness is found. A needle 2·5 cm. long is inserted here and

2 ml. of hydrocortisone suspension is injected at slightly different places about the teno-periosteal junction, where the tip of the needle can be felt touching bone.

The alternative treatment is deep friction, but it is painful and takes several weeks (see Vol. II).

Weakness of the Biceps Muscle

This occurs in fifth and sixth cervical root-palsies; in the former, in conjunction with weakness of abduction and lateral rotation in the arm; in the latter, together with weakness of the extensors of the wrist.

The Brachialis Muscle

If resisted flexion hurts but resisted supination does not, the lesion must lie in the brachialis muscle. The tender spot is difficult to discover, and is usually at the lowest part of the muscle under the biceps tendon. Since hydrocortisone shows that traumatic arthritis of the elbow is not a lesion of the brachialis muscle, the stigma attaching to massage of this muscle has been lifted. Even so, it would be unwise for medico-legal reasons, to give massage to this muscle, unless a full passive range of movement is present at the joint, or it might be falsely alleged that the limitation of movement was the result of the massage—a notion that some present opinion would support. In fact, massage to the affected area in a lesion of the belly is quickly curative.

2. Resisted Extension

Triceps Muscle

This seldom sets up pain, since lesions of the triceps are uncommon. If this muscle is affected, the usual site of the lesion is the musculo-tendinous junction; deep massage is quickly curative. If the tendon itself or the teno-periosteal junction is affected, infiltration with 1 or 2 cc. of hydrocortisone suspension is indicated. If the olecranon is fractured, pain is severe and accompanied by gross weakness and marked articular signs at the elbow joint.

Pain felt near the shoulder on resisted extension at the elbow has the same significance as a painful arc. When the triceps contracts, the humerus is pulled upwards towards the scapula. If a tender structure lies between the humeral head and the acromion, this upward movement may pinch it and cause pain, especially in subdeltoid bursitis.

Weakness of the triceps muscle occurs in two disorders:

(a) *Radial palsy.* This is usually due to pressure from a crutch or sleeping with the inner side of the arm pressed against an edge ('Saturday-night paralysis'). If so, extension of the hand is even more obviously weak; wrist-drop may occur. By contrast with the obvious weakness, there is little or no pain.

(b) *Seventh-root palsy.* In sixth-cervical disc lesions, the triceps may be found weak in isolation, or in conjunction with the flexor muscles of the

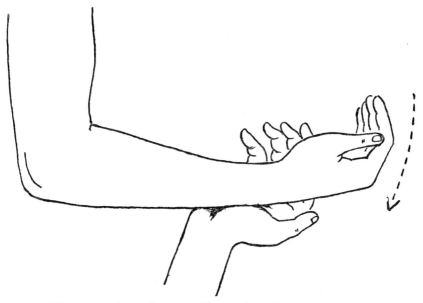

FIG. 46. Resisted extension at elbow joint. The examiner resists the movement by pressure directed upwards at the patient's lower forearm.

wrist. The pain is severe; the weakness by comparison is slight. The neck movements set up scapular pain.

3. Resisted Supination

If this movement hurts, resisted flexion must also be tested. If this hurts too, the biceps muscle is at fault (see above). If flexion against resistance is painless, the *supinator brevis* muscle is at fault. Local anaesthesia induced at the muscle posteriorly between the upper radius and ulna confirms the diagnosis and is occasionally followed by lasting relief. If, as more often happens, the pain returns, deep massage soon brings about full recovery (see Vol. II).

4. Resisted Pronation

The common cause of pain on resisted pronation is a golfer's elbow. The origin of the pronator teres muscle merges with the common flexor tendon. Hence strain here deceptively gives rise to pain on resisted pronation as well as on resisted flexion at the wrist. This should therefore be tested.

Very rarely, the lesion actually affects the belly of the pronator muscle. The tenderness is usually at its mid-point and a few sessions of adequate deep massage are curative.

Incapacity to perform alternate rotation movements of the forearm quickly is a most useful early sign in paralysis agitans. The first few rotations can be carried out fairly rapidly; after that, the affected forearm flags and finally stops.

BURSITIS AT THE ELBOW

Olecranon Bursa

Pain at the elbow may occur in the absence of any pain on passive or resisted movement. The pain may be provoked by leaning the elbow on a table, or on a flexion movement at the elbow only when a coat is worn. This is typical of olecranon bursitis, and tenderness should be looked for about the tip of the olecranon. A blow may induce haemorrhage into the bursa. Palpable thickening of the bursal wall may or may not be present, but it is very sensitive to pressure. Rheumatoid disease, gout and xanthomatosis affect this bursa.

Septic Olecranon Bursitis

As the result of a local abrasion of the skin, cellulitis at the back of the elbow may result. This involves the olecranon bursa which may fill first with clear fluid; eventually sepsis may set in and pus require evacuation. Miners refer to this condition as 'beat elbow'. In the earliest stage, when heat or redness of the skin are not yet obvious, confusion may arise, since resisted extension of the elbow is painful.

Epicondylar and Radio-humeral Bursae

Two other bursae may give rise to vague symptoms at the elbow— the superficial epicondylar and the radio-humeral. Epicondylar bursitis, in my experience, was always secondary to rheumatoid arthritis of the elbow joint. One bursa formed a large painless swelling which aspiration showed to contain 15 ml. fluid. In another, an area of calcification half-an-inch across was shown on the radiograph. In none of the cases was an appreciable degree of pain mentioned. Radio-humeral bursitis can be detected only if calcification has made it visible on the radiograph and even then the distinction between this condition and calcification in the radial collateral ligament is by no means clear. Bursal affections have been mistaken for tennis elbow, but as no pain results from resisted movements at the wrist joint, examination distinguishes tennis-elbow immediately.

Treatment

Aspiration followed by protection is called for. When the bursa contains blood, aspiration suffices. Septic bursitis requires wide incision and antibiotics.

When tenderness or swelling persists, a bursa may be excised. According to Carp (1932), the radio-humeral bursa can be burst by manual pressure against the head of the radius.

Large round swellings attached to the posterior aspect of the shaft of the ulna about $1\frac{1}{2}$ in. below the olecranon occur in (1) tophaceous gout, (2) rheumatoid arthritis, (3) xanthomatosis. If they cause annoyance, surgical removal is indicated. Multiple xanthomata gradually disappear on prolonged treatment with clofibrate, which reduces the plasma level of cholesterol and triglycerides.

NERVES AT THE ELBOW

The Ulnar Nerve

Friction against the sheath of the ulnar nerve at the medial humeral condyle gives rise to little or no aching at the elbow, but to paraesthesia at the fourth and fifth fingers. In recurrent dislocation of the ulnar nerve, the patient feels something go out and in at the elbow with a paraesthetic twinge. Structural abnormalities at the elbow, such as the cubitus valgus that may occur developmentally or as the result of a mal-union of a condylar fracture, may cause friction here on account of the altered stresses on the nerve. Some cases result from a fall on the elbow, bruising of the nerve-sheath setting up an irritability that elbow-flexion habits may now maintain. Many cases are postural, the patient sleeping with his elbow bent up under him, or he may hold a telephone receiver to his ear for hours on end, or enjoy lying with his hands at his occiput.

Examination in the first place reveals that the patient is not suffering from (a) a seventh cervical disc lesion; (b) first rib pressure on the lower trunk of the brachial plexus; (c) a ganglion in connection with the flexor carpi ulnaris tendon; (d) occupational pressure on the ulnar nerve at the proximal part of the palm.

An old injury to the elbow is soon apparent when the joint is examined. If the joint itself is normal, the elbow should be kept bent for some time; this may bring on the pins and needles. Unfortunately, no such test as stretching the nerve by a full radial deviation movement of the hand, while the elbow is kept fully flexed has proved helpful in diagnosis. Friction on the nerve-trunk is suggested by finding tenderness of the nerve-sheath; the two sides must always be compared. Thickening, especially in cases of recurrent dislocation, may be great enough to produce a spindle-shaped swelling of the nerve at the back of the elbow. Local anaesthesia provides the only satisfactory diagnostic criterion in early cases; in late cases, an ulnar-palsy makes the diagnosis obvious.

If ulnar neuritis occurs apparently causelessly, it should be remembered that such mononeuritis may result from diabetes.

Treatment

1. The Avoidance of Postural Strains or Pressure

Keeping the elbow bent for any length of time, or resting the inner side of the flexed elbow on the arm of a chair or on a desk while writing, must be avoided. A cushion under the forearm to raise the elbow off the desk may suffice. The substitution of a hard for a soft arm to the chair enables the olecranon to bear all the weight of the arm. It is important to study the patient's daily routine and to explain to him which of his activities is maintaining the pressure.

2. Hydrocortisone

An injection of hydrocortisone suspension about the nerve desensitizes its sheath and can afford lasting relief, as long as conduction has not yet become impaired and structural changes are absent at the elbow. After the injection the patient must avoid the postural strains or minor traumata that originally caused the disorder.

The injection must be made not into the nerve but about it, since it is the external surface that is primarily affected. The patient lies prone, his arm by his side, palm on couch. The condylar groove is identified and a site 2 cm. from it chosen. A needle 4 cm. long is inserted horizontally and guided towards the groove. It reaches the edge of the bone and is then manœuvred so as to lie deeply within the groove, between nerve and bone. Since the needle passes parallel to the nerve it will push it aside rather than enter it. One millilitre is injected here.

3. *Anterior Transposition of the Nerve*

When the frictional element is due to structural changes at the elbow, undue stress on the nerve cannot be avoided. Thus, in cubitus valgus deformity, transposition is called for without too much delay. Indeed, once ulnar weakness has begun, there is no point in waiting for it to become more severe before operating.

Medial Cutaneous Nerve of Forearm

This nerve becomes superficial at mid-arm and supplies the skin from the inner aspect of the elbow as far as the wrist. It crosses over the median basilic vein at the elbow and is subject to trauma there by extravenous injections of pentothal. Numbness lasting some months results, but pain and hypersensitivity of skin at the antero-medial extent of the forearm may continue for up to a year.

TENNIS-ELBOW

By tennis-elbow is meant a lesion, situated near the elbow, of the extensor muscles controlling the wrist. Hence, the movement that hurts the *elbow* is resisted extension of the wrist (Fig. 47).

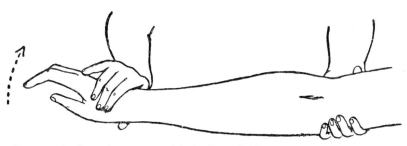

FIG. 47. Resisted extension at wrist. While the elbow is held in extension, the wrist movement is resisted by the examiner's hand pressing on the dorsum of the patient's hand

The condition is frequently misunderstood. Its notoriety with the public is due to the east with which the layman arrives at a correct diagnosis, its frequency and its refractoriness to treatment. A tennis-elbow may be provoked by any exercise involving repeated and forcible extension movements at the wrist—not neccessarily tennis—and bears this name only because it was first described as a tennis-player's disability. Rarely, a direct injury to the epicondyle sets up a traumatic periostitis that the repeated irritation of muscle-pull prevents from subsiding.

Historical Note

The tennis-elbow syndrome has been recognized for almost a century and received its name more than eighty years ago: Runge described the first case (1873). In an article on writer's cramp—from which he distinguished it—he cited a case of two years' inability to write associated with tenderness on the lateral condyle of the humerus. As rest for three months and electrical treatment had no effect, he cauterized the skin over the tender area and rested the elbow until the ulcer had healed; this took six weeks. The patient was now well, and remained so a year later. Runge ascribed the cramp to a traumatic inflammation of the periosteum in this position due originally to a forcible supination effort and kept chronic by the continual pull of the extensor muscles attached to the lateral condyle.

The condition was first named by Morris (1882), who called it 'lawn-tennis arm' and noted its similarity to rider's sprain. An annotation in the *Lancet* (1885) drew attention to the number of sufferers from 'tennis-elbow' whose plaintive letters had recently appeared in the lay press. Remak (1894) and Bernhardt (1896) agreed that it was a periosteal tear due to occupational overuse of the extensor muscles arising from the lateral condyle; the latter had collected thirty cases. Couderc (1896) called it a ruptured epicondylar tendon: Féré (1897) 'epicondylalgie'; Franke (1910) 'epicondylitis'. Osgood (1922) suggested radio-humeral bursitis, thereby incriminating the bursa described by Monro in 1788. Schmidt (1921), on the other hand, believed the fault to lie in the superficial epicondylar bursa, first described by Schreger in 1825. On the whole, English writers have called it 'tennis-elbow' while continental authors have preferred 'epicondylitis'. The former name is preferable, since in by no means every tennis-elbow does the lesion lie at the epicondyle.

Pain

Pain starts at the outer side of the elbow when, as in nine patients out of ten, the lesion lies at the common extensor tendon; and the patient has usually found for himself that the epicondyle is tender. The pain is referred along the back of the forearm often as far as the wrist and the dorsum of the hand. Occasionally, the long and ring fingers also ache. Rarely, there is no pain in the forearm, the pain spreading up from the elbow to the shoulder. The pain is brought on by grasping and lifting—indeed, by any exertion involving extension of the wrist; sometimes there is also a constant ache, worse at night, with stiffness of the elbow on waking.

At the moment when he gives himself a tennis-elbow, the patient feels nothing. Some days after the causative exertion, he notices an ache in the forearm on certain movements. This gets worse and after a fortnight he cannot take a backhand stroke at all. It is thus not the tear in the tendon that causes pain; the symptoms result from the painful scar that forms later. Tennis is by no means the only cause of tennis-elbow; a right-handed golfer gets a left-sided tennis-elbow in the same way as a tennis-player with a strong forehand drive can give himself a golfer's elbow. Using an axe, a hammer, a fishing-rod or even scouring pots and pans can strain the extensor muscles enough to lead to post-traumatic scarring. A curious feature of tennis-elbow is sudden twinges, so severe that the grip is rendered momentarily powerless involuntarily; the patient drops even a light object held in the hand, e.g. a teacup.

Examination

Since the common age for a tennis-elbow is forty to sixty, it is highly probable that any patient old enough to suffer from this disorder will have X-ray evidence of 'cervical spondylosis' as well. Hence the view has been expressed that tennis-elbow is a result of such 'spondylosis'. No one denies that pain in the elbow can arise from the neck, but it is impossible for pain in the elbow evoked by wrist movements to have such an origin. Hence clinical examination distinguishes the two sources.

Whatever the type of tennis-elbow, on examination, although the elbow hurts, there is nothing amiss at the joint or the muscles controlling it. The negative signs are: (a) passive movement of the elbow is of full range and painless. (b) the resisted movements of the elbow are of full power and painless. The positive sign is that the pain at the elbow is reproduced on resisted extension, but not resisted flexion, at the wrist. Care must be taken that the elbow is held in full extension while the resisted wrist movements are tested, otherwise a false negative result may be obtained. In the ordinary teno-periosteal variety, the pain is such that the patient often winces and lets his hand go when asked to extend it vigorously against resistance. Further examination shows that resisted radial, but not ulnar, deviation hurts. If the fingers are held flexed actively so that the extensor digitorum is thrown out of action, the extension movement at the wrist still hurts. In this way it can be proved that the only muscles at fault in tennis-elbow are the extensores carpi radialis. If, as is usual, the tenderness is at the epicondyle itself, the extensor carpi radialis brevis is at fault, since the longus is inserted higher up.

Two facts warn that one of the unusual sorts of tennis-elbow is present: (1) no wince, the patient can hold his wrist extended against strong resistance, feeling pain insufficient to make the muscles give way; (2) a history lasting longer than a year in a patient under sixty years of age.

Palpation

When it has been established by selective tension that a tennis-elbow is present, precision is lent by search along the radial extensor muscles for tenderness. The origin of the longus is palpated above the epicondyle along the supracondylar ridge; then the anterior aspect of the epicondyle; then the tendon level with the joint-line and over the head of the radius; finally, the uppermost extent of the muscle bellies. When tenderness is sought here, it must be remembered that the brachio-radialis muscle lies

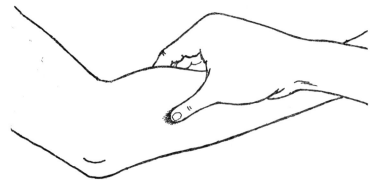

FIG. 48. Palpation of the bellies of extensor muscles in upper forearm. Since pressure of the muscle bellies against the radius is normally painful, palpation must be carried out in the manner shown.

superficially and is always tender in normal people. Since it is a muscle not involved in extension at the wrist, such tenderness must be ignored and palpation confined to the muscles lying deeply to it (Fig. 48).

Palpation usually identifies the lesion at (1) the anterior aspect of the lateral humeral epicondyle, at the origin of the common extensor tendon from the bone, i.e. the teno-periosteal junction—90 per cent; (2) the upper extent of the muscle belly, level with the neck of the radius—8 per cent; (3) the supracondylar origin of the extensor carpi radialis longus and the part of the extensor tendon lying level with the head of the radius— 1 per cent each.

Double lesions can occur in tennis-elbow; the findings on palpation are then very difficult to interpret and diagnostic local anaesthesia may become imperative. Alternatively, the more obvious of the two lesions can be treated and the forearm muscles then examined again.

It should be remembered that, in cases of the teno-periosteal variety, *associated tenderness* of the type well recognized in 'styloiditis radii' may be found at the *back* of the lateral humeral epicondyle. Since the patient's pain is elicited by a resisted extension movement at the wrist and no part of this extensor mechanism is attached to the posterior aspect of the epicondyle, tenderness here represents no relevant lesion.

In tennis-elbow, the radiograph is normal.

Pathology of Tennis-elbow

The muscular and tendinous types are examples of ordinary overstrain such as may occur anywhere. On the other hand, the far commoner teno-periosteal type is an injury to which no exact parallel exists elsewhere in the body. Much evidence has been brought forward (Cyriax, 1936; R. S. Garden, 1961) to show that the usual lesion is a tear between the common extensor tendon and the periosteum of the lateral humeral epicondyle. Examination of the resisted wrist movements shows clearly that the trouble lies in one of the radial extensor muscles of the wrist. Since the tenderness is at the epicondyle, the fault cannot lie at the origin of the long radial extensor muscle, which is attached to the supracondylar ridge. Hence the tear lies at the origin of the extensor carpi radialis brevis muscle. In the early stages, just as often as the tear begins to unite, so often does the patient, by using his hand, pull the healing surfaces apart again. The result, as might be expected, is that a painful scar forms at the teno-periosteal junction. This view, first expressed in 1936, was confirmed by McKee (1937), when operating on cases of tennis-elbow.

The onset of a tennis-elbow is always slow. This shows that the minor tear in the tendon is not itself a source of appreciable pain. It is only when endlessly repeated attempts at union have been broken down again and again during daily use of the hand that a chronically inflamed scar appears and causes the symptoms.

Spontaneous Cure

In patients with a teno-periosteal tennis-elbow, recovery seldom takes more than a year if the patient is under sixty; two years if he is older. The uncommon varieties, with the lesion above or below the epicondyle, show no such tendency and often go on indefinitely. At the teno-periosteal junction, a second attack is rare, and freedom from recurrence for as long as 25 years has been reported (Cyriax, 1936). Injection of hydrocortisone inhibits the mechanism of spontaneous cure. Hence it is not uncommon for patients to remain well after an injection for some months and then to need another, and so on for several years. Left untreated, the tennis-elbow would have got well by itself in twelve months.

Spontaneous cure appears to result, in the case of teno-periosteal tear, from a gradual widening of the gap between the two edges. Finally, the two surfaces cease to lie in apposition and tension on the scar ceases. The gap now fills with fibrous tissue and heals with *permanent lengthening*. In consequence much strain no longer falls on that part of the tendon connected to the extensor carpi radialis brevis muscle. Recurrence is prevented by this structural alteration. Moreover, several muscles are attached here; hence slight permanent lengthening of the section of tendon relevant to only *one* muscle does not weaken the power to control the wrist.

Treatment

The different types of tennis-elbow need different treatment. This fact is by no means widely accepted, all tennis-elbows being regarded as requiring treatment directed to the epicondyle, owing to the idea that there exists only one type of tennis-elbow—teno-periosteal. This is the common variety, it is true, but there are three other positions for the lesion, accounting for 10 per cent of all cases.

1. Teno-periosteal Variety

This is the common site for the painful scar. Two different approaches exist: (1) to remove the inflammation from the scar and leave a painless scar; (2) to separate the two surfaces between which the scar exists, thus avoiding tension on it; this imitates the process of natural cure. Triamcinolone has the first effect; manipulation the second.

Before treatment, the patient, if less than sixty years old, should be told that spontaneous cure is highly probable within a year. He may, if he knows this, prefer merely to wait, sparing his elbow as much as possible meanwhile.

(1) *Injection of Triamcinolone*
Since hydrocortisone was first suggested for tennis-elbow (Cyriax and Troisier, 1952), there have been many cases in which various steroids have been injected without success; yet an injection of triamcinolone suspension has proved curative. It is clear, therefore, that many different techniques exist, some of them unsatisfactory.

Hydrocortisone is not the steroid of choice. It is successful, but causes two days' severe after-pain, whereas triamcinolone is just as effective and sets up much less discomfort, for only 12–24 hours.

The injection procedure is as follows:

(a) Is a tennis-elbow present? The passive movements of the elbow are full and painless; the resisted movements do not hurt. Resisted extension at the wrist, but not resisted flexion, hurts at the elbow.

(b) Is the lesion at the teno-periosteal junction? If not, steroid injection will not help. Tenderness is found at the anterior aspect of the lateral humeral epicondyle, and tenderness is absent at the origin of the extensor carpi radialis longus, at the tendon and the upper bellies.

(c) The exact limits of the tender area are carefully defined, while the elbow is held flexed to a right angle with the forearm fully supinated. Pressure is exerted with the tip of the thumb, the fingers encircling the medial aspect of the elbow. The position of the hand is the same as that for giving friction to the epicondyle, illustrated in Vol. II.

(d) A tuberculin syringe is filled with 1 ml. triamcinolone suspension, and fitted with a very fine needle 2 cm. long. Neither a local anaesthetic agent nor a hyaluronidase is added.

(e) The tendon has thickness as well as position. Hence the needle is thrust through the skin 1 cm. in front of the epicondyle and advanced until the resistance of the common extensor tendon is felt. One droplet of the suspension is injected here. The needle is then pushed on till the tip touches bone and another drop injected there. It is then half withdrawn and reinserted a millimetre away until some ten infiltrations have been made at the teno-periosteal junction, and another ten or so at the same part of the tendon but nearer its surface.

(f) Throughout the infiltration the physician keeps his thumb on the tender spot. As each droplet is injected, he can feel exactly where the little bulge forms, and can thus be sure that the point of the needle is embedded in just that part of the tendon that he is aiming at. Since the steroid is insoluble, it works where it lies, but not elsewhere; hence it is vital to infiltrate the lesion throughout its entire extent and thickness during direct palpation, without wasting any of the suspension to either side.

After-treatment consists in avoiding all exertion for seven days, allowing the anti-inflammatory action of triamcinolone to proceed undisturbed. The patient then returns to his ordinary activities. He is seen again after a fortnight. If resisted extension at the wrist is entirely painless, no more need be done. If it is slightly uncomfortable, the degree of discomfort not causing any inconvenience, the injection must nevertheless be repeated, otherwise complete relapse occurs within a month.

Permanent cure with one or two injections is achieved in two-thirds of all cases.

(2) *Manipulation*

The intention is to pull apart the two edges of the tear and thus relieve the painful scar lying between them from tension, imitating the mechanism of spontaneous recovery. This allows the self-perpetuating post-traumatic inflammation to subside, and healing with permanent lengthening. Henceforth the intact part of the tendon takes all the strain, thus affording protection against the recurrences that are sometimes a problem when steroids are used.

The method is that described by Mills in 1928. His intention was to shift the annular ligament, which he regarded as out of place; in fact, it applies the greatest possible stretch to the extensor carpi radialis muscles, and, carried out with a sharp jerk, tends to open the tear in the tendon and abolish tension on the tender scar by converting a tear shaped like a V into separation of the torn surfaces, i.e. a U (see Vol. II). This manipulation is performed two or three times a week until the patient is well—some four to eight sessions may be required. Analgesia should be supplied by deep friction to the anterior aspect of the epicondyle first for ten or fifteen minutes. Apart from the reactive hyperaemia, this massage has the further advantage of softening the scar-tissue that the manipulation proposes to rupture. Local anaesthesia is not recommended; for when induced at the epicondyle, two days' severe pain follows, thus setting up more discomfort than it avoids.

General anaesthesia is contra-indicated. Indeed, under pentothal anaesthesia, full muscular relaxation prevents the traction falling on the tendon; instead, the elbow joint takes the brunt of the forcing. This is not only useless, but may well set up a traumatic arthritis. Nitrous oxide anaesthesia carried to the point of unconsciousness, but not of muscle relaxation is satisfactory. However, Mills's manipulation is over so swiftly that it is best carried out without analgesia; moreover, it has often to be repeated several times and few patients accept repeated anaesthesia.

Mills's manipulation must in no circumstances be performed unless extension at the elbow is of full range and painless. This must be ascertained at the patient's each attendance; for Mills's manipulation, imperfectly performed (i.e. with the patient's wrist not held fully flexed throughout), may lead to slight traumatic arthritis at the elbow. If the joint is rested for a week or two, it recovers, and treatment can safely begin again, whereas immediate repetition of the manipulation can set up serious trouble. If osteo-arthritis, a loose body in the joint or traumatic arthritis limit extension at the elbow, Mills's manipulation is out of the question and one of the alternative measures must be employed.

(3) Cock-up Splintage

Distraction by muscle pull of the two edges of the tear can be prevented by immobilization of the wrist (not the elbow) in full extension in a splint or in a plaster cast; the elbow must not be included. This treatment is worth a trial if the history is short, say a month or less. The plaster splint should be retained until attempted extension of the hand against the resistance of the cast is painless. If this is not being achieved by the end of two months, the immobilization is hardly worth continuing. The only theoretical objection is that, since healing occurs without any permanent lengthening, the patient may develop a tennis-elbow again later, but this also applies to steroid injections. It is a matter of some importance to professional tennis-players.

Cock-up splintage is sometimes called for in the treatment of tennis-elbow in patients so neurotic that they cannot stand active measures.

(4) Tenotomy

If a teno-periosteal tennis-elbow proves incurable and goes on for several years, the only treatment left is tenotomy (Hohmann, 1926). This appears to cure about half of all cases submitted to open division. Garden (1961) lengthens the extensor carpi radialis tendon just above wrist rather than at the epicondyle.

Subcutaneous tenotomy under local anaesthesia is very simple. The skin over the epicondyle is infiltrated with 1 ml. of 2 per cent procaine and another 1 ml. is used for the common extensor tendon. After a minute, resisted extension at the wrist is tested; if the correct spot has been infiltrated, this movement has become quite painless. The tenotome is then thrust through the skin and the tendon divided down to the bony epicondyle across its whole width. Mills's manipulation is then carried out to ensure complete separation of the two cut ends.

This little operation is not always successful although it is difficult to understand how division—open or closed—can fail. However, one happy result in these failures is that a lesion hitherto refractory to steroids becomes amenable, and cure results from one or two further injections of triamcinolone.

2. Muscular Variety

Local anaesthesia is the treatment of choice. Even though the patient may have had pain for five or ten years, two to four weekly injections into the right spot nearly always permanently cure. The great difficulty is to find the right spot and infiltrate it thoroughly.

Technique of Injection

The elbow is bent to a right-angle and the forearm supinated. The tender spot lying deep to the brachio-radialis muscle is identified, usually lying level with the neck of the radius. A 10-ml. syringe is filled with 0·5 per cent procaine solution and a needle 5 cm. long fitted. It is introduced vertically, until the point lies at the lesion in the extensor carpi radialis belly, which is held pinched between the fingers. As the fluid is forced in, the solution is felt to expand the belly, and shows that the point of the needle is correctly situated. The resisted movement is tested some minutes later; if it is painless, the right spot has been infiltrated. Caution should be exercised in giving this injection to, say, a concert pianist. If the needle by chance pierces the deep branch of the radial nerve, a month or two's weakness of the extensor muscles of the wrist may rarely occur.

3. Tendinous Variety

The lesion lies in the body of the tendon, level with the head of the radius. Adequate massage is effective in four to eight sessions, however long the symptoms have lasted.

4. Supracondylar Variety

When the origin of the extensor carpi radialis longus at the supracondylar ridge above the epcondyle is at fault, two to four treatments by deep massage always cure (see Vol. II). This is the easiest tennis-elbow to relieve; unfortunately, it is seldom encountered.

GOLFER'S ELBOW

This is a lesion of the common flexor tendon at the medial epicondyle. In the right-handed, golfer's elbow occurs at the right elbow in those who play golf; at the left elbow the lesion produced by golf is a tennis-elbow. Again, those who play tennis with a strong forehand drive can develop a golfer's elbow—and both disorders affect those who play neither game. The names are useful to indicate the condition, but they should not be given aetiological weight; they are justified only historically.

Golfer's elbow is less common than tennis-elbow, and much less disabling. The pain is felt clearly at the inner side of the elbow and does not radiate far, seldom beyond the ulnar side of the mid-forearm. Severe pain on using the flexor muscles and paralysing twinges—both common in tennis-elbow—are seldom experienced.

Examination

The signs are:

(1) A full range of painless movement at the elbow.

(2) All resisted movements at the elbow are painless except, occasionally, pronation, since this muscle takes origin from the common flexor tendon.

(3) Resisted flexion, but not extension, of the wrist sets up pain at the elbow. Rarely, flexion of the fingers rather than of the wrist elicits the symptoms best.

N.B. The movement should be tested while the elbow is held extended, or a false negative result may be obtained.

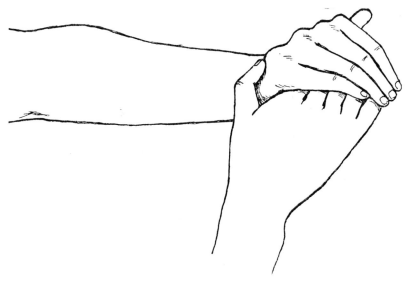

Fig. 49. Resisted flexion at wrist. The patient flexes his hand at the wrist against the resistance of the examiner's hand. The elbow is kept extended.

Treatment

The teno-periosteal tear is best treated analogously to tennis-elbow by a *local injection of steroid suspension*, thereby transforming a painful into a painless scar. The alternative is *deep localized massage* breaking up the scar-tissue; this is not followed by manipulative stretching as in tennis-elbow. Manipulation is without effect and in any case unnecessary; for the massage suffices. Indeed, tennis-elbow is the only teno-periosteal tear in the body insusceptible to massage alone, and the only one where manipulation has any effect. When the musculo-tendinous junction of the wrist-flexor group is at fault, the only successful treatment is adequate massage.

Technique of Injection

The patient fully extends his elbow, the arm held in full lateral rotation so as to bring the inner side of the elbow into an accessible position. Facing the patient, the exact spot is singled out by palpation with the index, in the same position as for massage (see Vol. II). A tuberculin syringe with 1 ml. triamcinolone suspension, is fitted with a fine 2-cm. needle. The needle is inserted from in front and thrust in until the re-sistance of the tendon is felt. Some twenty droplets are injected all over the affected area of tendon, within both the superficial and deep fibres, with the tip of the needle against bone. The patient must not use the hand strenuously for a week and, when seen after a fortnight, if any ache on resisted wrist-flexion persists, a second infiltration must be given, other-wise the trouble will recur.

ISCHAEMIC CONTRACTURE

Permanent contracture (Volkmann) of the flexor muscles of the forearm results from persistent spasm of the brachial artery, caught against the edge of the humeral shaft in supracondylar fracture of the humerus. The elasticity of the muscle bellies is largely lost and extension of the fingers remains possible only after the wrist has been flexed—the constant length phenomenon. Resisted flexion of the fingers does not hurt.

In a patient with such a fracture, the first sign of this complication is often pain in the forearm, increased on passive extension of the fingers. Then the radial pulse ceases. If this is lost after a fracture at the elbow, and does not return when the patient is warmed, the artery should be exposed and painted with papaverine (Kinmonth, 1952). For the established condition a muscle-sliding operation is required.

14

The Wrist and Hand

LOWER RADIO-ULNAR JOINT

Lesions of the radio-ulnar joint are rare, and cause pain felt at the wrist only. Hence it is easy to forget the existence of this joint and to look only at the wrist. It is part of the routine examination of the wrist to perform full passive supination and pronation at the lower radio-ulnar joint, before examining the passive and resisted movements at the wrist itself. The lower forearm must be grasped when testing these two movements, to prevent any strain falling on the carpal joints.

Rotation through 180 degrees is present at a normal radio-ulnar joint, the ulna remaining stationary as the radius revolves round it.

Capsular Pattern

If both passive extremes are painful, arthritis is present.

A mal-united fracture just above the wrist leads to osteoarthritis later. If there has been no injury, non-specific arthritis must be present. Its nature is not at all evident; the only clear facts are: (a) all endeavours to stretch the joint out aggravate the condition, whereas (b) one injection of hydrocortisone into the joint affords full, and nearly always permanent, relief.

In a patient who already has rheumatoid arthritis this joint may become affected too, often bilaterally. If so, hydrocortisone is again effective, but may have to be repeated at six- to twelve-monthly intervals.

Technique of Injection

The patient's forearm is fully pronated; the prominence of the lower end of the ulna is now clearly visible. The joint line is identified by palpation, the examiner pushing the radius and ulna backwards and forwards on each other and feeling for the plane at which this occurs. A point is chosen on this line not more than 5 mm. above the upper edge of the lunate bone, since the joint extends for only 1 cm. upwards from that edge. A syringe containing 1 ml. hydrocortisone suspension is fitted with a fine needle 2·5 cm. long. It is thrust in vertically and strikes bone; it must then be withdrawn a short distance and a number of tiny adjustments made until it is felt to pass between the radius and ulna. The injection is then given.

Noncapsular Pattern

Pronation is of full range and painless; supination is limited by painless bony block. This results from mal-union of a Colles's fracture and consequent shortening of the radius. The limitation of movement is of course permanent.

If this phenomenon is accompanied by pain at one or both extremes, osteoarthritis has supervened. The symptoms are not severe, and a bandage about the wrist may ease discomfort. Hydrocortisone intra-articularly is well worth a trial.

When teno-synovitis of the extensor carpi ulnaris muscle exists at the groove at the base of the ulna, full passive supination is apt to hurt for no very obvious reason.

Resisted Movements

When these hurt, the fault does not lie locally. The examiner must resist the movement by grasping the lower forearm, to avoid stress on the wrist. Resisted pronation causes pain felt at the upper forearm in golfer's elbow, very rarely as the result of an actual lesion of the pronator teres muscles. In my experience, the pronator quadratus is never affected. Resisted supination hurts at the elbow and upper forearm in lesions of the biceps and supinator muscles; again no local lesion is responsible.

THE WRIST JOINT

Lesions at the wrist result from injury, overuse or arthritis, usually rheumatoid. The history is seldom distinctive, and examination, clinical and radiological must be relied on for diagnosis. Since pain is not referred appreciably from tissues lying at the distal extent of a limb, patients with wrist trouble know quite well that their symptoms originate there.

Inspection

This may reveal swelling. If there is a history of trauma, fracture should be suspected; if not, rheumatoid arthritis, which is usually bilateral. A ganglion is visible and palpable, and can often be burst and can always be punctured, disappearance confirming the diagnosis. Multiple large ganglia occur in longstanding rheumatoid arthritis.

Routine Examination of Movement

Examination comprises:

1. The radio-ulnar joint—two passive rotations.
2. The wrist—four passive movements; flexion, extension, ulnar and radial deviation.
3. The wrist—the same four movements carried out against resistance.
4. The thumb—passive movement at the trapezio-first-metacarpal joint and the resisted thumb movements.
5. The fingers—resisted abduction and adduction. These movements must be included, since patients with a strained interosseous muscle at its proximal extent usually complain of pain at the wrist.

In teno-synovitis the evidence obtained when the passive movements of the wrist are tested is open to a misconstruction. A movement that might be regarded as merely relaxing a tendon often, in fact, pushes it painfully down its sheath; hence the discomfort elicited in this way may be misinterpreted.

Crepitus

One of the classical signs of teno-synovitis is crepitus. Fine creaking when the tendon moves inside its sheath indicates roughening of gliding surfaces such as follows overuse, and is common only at the abductor and extensor tendons where they curl round the lower radius. In hyper-acute cases, the crepitus on movement may be felt even at the bellies in the upper forearm—myosynovitis. A much coarser creaking is palpable in tuberculosis and advanced rheumatoid disease. Crepitus does not have to be sought; it obtrudes itself. However, in slight or chronic teno-synovitis or in teno-vaginitis, crepitus is often absent, and it must not be thought that the absence of crepitus shows the tendons to be normal or excludes a diagnosis of teno-synovitis.

Passive Movements at the Wrist

Flexion, extension and ulnar and radial devitation must be tested. Limitation of movement in each direction indicates arthritis; limitation in one direction only suggests a disorder localized to one joint or persistent carpal subluxation. In these conditions the resisted movements are painless. The following disorders occur:

Capsular Pattern

The capsular pattern is about the same amount of limitation of flexion as of extension at first. However, in long-standing severe arthritis, fixation in flexion supervenes unless this is prevented by immobilization in the mid-position.

Traumatic Arthritis

In my experience, this does not occur in the absence of a carpal fracture. I have never known a case of simple traumatic arthritis last more than a day or two.

The clinical diagnosis of carpal fracture is usually simple, whereas the radiograph taken soon after the injury may reveal no lesion. There is a history of trauma, not necessarily severe. The whole wrist is swollen. Passive flexion and extension movements are limited by muscular spasm, coming on with a vibrant twang. The patient should be asked on which side of the wrist he feels his pain. If a passive deviation movement towards the painful side hurts more than that away from this side, it is clear that squeezing the carpal bones together causes pain: further evidence of fracture. Palpation of the site of tenderness shows which of the bones has been damaged. The bone most often fractured is the scaphoid, since it spans the joint between the proximal and distal rows of carpal bones. The above signs are constantly present and are more reliable in pointing to the diagnosis than the radiograph taken immediately after the accident. One taken two weeks later reveals the damage to bone. Fractures of the scaphoid bone require treatment by immobilization at once; hence, when the above signs are elicited, a plaster cast should be applied immediately, holding the joint in mid-position but in radial deviation; this posture ensures that the fractured surfaces are pressed together. A second radiograph is taken a fortnight later. So long as the diagnosis remains uncertain, physiotherapy, active exercises, etc., are contra-indicated.

Rheumatoid Arthritis

This is common. In addition to the limitation of movement, the joint is visibly swollen, warm to the touch and the joint-capsule is the site of much soft thickening. The chronic stage may progress to virtual ankylosis in flexion; the swelling then diminishes but seldom disappears and the local warmth ceases. The disorder usually affects both wrists, often after the fingers have been affected. Except in the most chronic stage, the blood sedimentation rate is greatly raised. Gout, dermatomyositis, Reiter's and gonococcal arthritis must be excluded.

In the acute stage, if pain is severe, immobilization of the wrist for some weeks by an elastoplast bandage or a cock-up splint is indicated. In the subacute or chronic stage, hydrocortisone is usually very successful. No attempt is made at intra-articular injection, but the areas of capsular thickening and tenderness are identified and infiltrated each in turn until the whole affected region has been treated. The actual injection is very painful, but the result, especially in the chronic case, excellent.

Generalized osteoarthritis of the wrist may follow severe injury, or the use of vibrating tools; in the elderly no cause is usually apparent. Limitation of movement without appreciable capsular thickening is accompanied by crepitus when the wrist is moved within the possible range.

The radiograph shows osteophytes and one or more diminished joint spaces with sclerosis of the bony margins. Diffuse cystic change may be noted. By contrast, minor osteoarthritic change seen on the X-ray photograph is compatible with perfect function.

No treatment has appreciable effect; the symptoms seldom warrant arthrodesis.

Noncapsular Pattern

Persistent Subluxation of a Carpal Bone

The sign that draws immediate attention to internal derangement at the wrist joint is limitation of movement in one direction only. This is found when carpal subluxation occurs at the wrist, muscle spasm limiting extension of the wrist while the other movements remain of full range, though not necessarily painless. The site of the subluxation is easily found by looking at the wrist when held in flexion (see Plate 16); the projection can be seen and felt with ease, and the ligaments about the capitate bone are tender, especially at the lunate-capitate and capitate-third-metacarpal joint lines. Clinically, the capitate bone has subluxated. However, radiography reveals no displacement. It is easy to argue that postulated osseous subluxations which do not show radiologically are imaginary; but the edge of the capitate bone merges with the others and cannot be separately visualized on the radiograph, nor can its position be measured against the superimposed margins of the other bones. Moreover, (a) the clinical signs of an intra-articular displacement are clear; (b) the undue projection is visible on full flexion; (c) manipulative reduction is accompanied by a click and the immediate restoration of full range, and (d) there is a liability to recurrence. It has been argued that the manipulation ruptures an adhesion; but what adhesion placed at the dorsum of the joint can limit extension, and why should a ligamentous adhesion, once ruptured, lead to recurrence?

Manipulative reduction is easy to perform during traction and consists

M

in separating the proximal from the distal row of bones and then gliding them antero-posteriorly (see Vol. II). If the subluxation has been present for several months, some of the ligaments about the capitate bone remain strained and, though a full range of movement is restored at once, the extremes of movement remain painful. One or two sessions of adequate deep massage then afford full relief. A recurrence is treated by immediate reduction.

Disorder at an Isolated Joint

Three conditions give rise to solitary limitation of extension at the wrist, but all show clearly radiologically. They are Keinboch's disease (aseptic necrosis of the lunate bone), un-united fracture and isolated osteo-arthritis. In the first case, sclerosis and deformity of the lunate bone are obvious by X-rays; in the lunate-capitate joint, localized disappearance of articular cartilage (seldom with osteophytes) is seen. Localized osteo-arthritis comes on some years after an un-united fracture, especially of the scaphoid bone. The projecting osteophytes can be seen and felt; marked limitation, more particularly of extension, resulting. Sometimes there is little or no pain.

Ligamentous Sprain

There are several different sites.

Ulnar Collateral Ligament

This follows imperfect reduction of a Colles's fracture, or fracture of the styloid process of the ulna. Inspection reveals the radius united with deformity, and examination of the passive movements at the wrist shows that only radial deviation hurts. Spontaneous cure takes a year; but an injection of hydrocortisone is rapidly curative.

Radial Collateral Ligament

Sprain here is very rare and is characterized by pain felt only on the extreme of passive ulnar deviation. In fact, the condition usually present when a sprain here is suspected is teno-vaginitis of the thumb tendons at their carpal extent. Trial of the resisted movements prevents error. An injection of hydrocortisone affords lasting relief.

Lunate-capitate Ligament

This is common, and may occur without subluxation at the joint; alternatively, it may persist after a subluxation of some months' standing has been reduced. There is pain felt at the dorsum of the wrist at the extreme of flexion, all the other passive movements proving of full range and painless. Search for tenderness reveals the exact site of the sprain. Deep massage, is always curative in a few weeks, even if the condition has persisted (as it often has) for several years.

Differential diagnosis is difficult between a severe sprain of this ligament and a minor degree of bony subluxation at the lunate-capitate joint. In a doubtful case, no harm is done by an attempt at reduction, followed at once, if it is found that there is nothing to reduce, by deep massage.

Occasionally other ligaments are sprained; perhaps the radio-lunate, the capitate-third-metacarpal or the ulnartriquetral (cuneiform). The site of tenderness is always carefully sought, remembering that these sprains are often multiple, the search continues even after the most obvious spot has been found. Unless *all* the sprained ligaments are given adequate massage, the patient is condemned to a permanently troublesome wrist; for there is little or no tendency to spontaneous recovery and hydrocortisone is not effective at these ligaments.

Chronic ligamentous sprain at the wrist differs from that at all other joints (except the coronary ligaments at the knee and the deltoid ligament at the ankle) in that, forced movements, with or without anaesthesia, afford no benefit. Indeed, they further overstretch the painful ligament and tend towards aggravation. By contrast, the scar can easily be mobilized by deep massage with recovery; all other methods are of no avail, including manipulation, hydrocortisone injections, many months' immobilization in plaster, or operation. Indeed, permanent minor disability will be avoided only when deep massage is recognized as the only effective treatment for these ligamentous strains at the wrist.

Ligamentous Rupture

This follows a severe flexion injury and leads to permanent instability of the wrist. The ligament that usually ruptures is the capitate-third-metacarpal; a depression can be palpated at this point on full wrist flexion, and the bone can be seen not to flex with the rest of the wrist. After a month, the symptoms cease, but recur if the patient exerts the wrist much. Care and a wrist-strap are called for, but the joint remains unstable permanently; for the ligament does not unite and cannot be reconstituted by surgery.

One patient ruptured this ligament and kept subluxating her capitate bone. She was treated by three injections of the same sclerosing agent as used for the lumbar ligaments, with considerable increase in stability. Subluxation occurred every month or two, but by being somewhat careful, there has been no attack for a year since treatment. The injection itself was very painful and each time the wrist remained sore for ten days.

Volkmann's Contracture

Ischaemia of the forearm owing to traumatic occlusion of the brachial artery leads to diffuse fibrosis of the flexor muscles of the forearm. As a result, extension of the wrist is limited when the fingers are held in extension, but the restriction ceases when the fingers are flexed. This is a good example of the constant length phenomenon, the amount of movement of which one joint is capable depending on the position in which another joint is held.

Resisted Movements at Wrist

Extension, flexion, radial deviation and ulnar deviation at the wrist are all tested against resistance, with the elbow held in extension. If this condition is not observed, false negative responses may be elicited in cases of golfer's or tennis-elbow. The resisted thumb and finger movements follow since the thumb tendons also move the wrist, and the interosseous muscles, if damaged proximally, cause pain felt at the wrist.

Pain felt on movement resisted at the wrist may be felt in two places—at the elbow or at the wrist. This differential localization by the patient indicates correctly where the lesion lies. If the pain is felt in the upper forearm or lower arm, a golfer's or a tennis-elbow is present. If one (or two congruous) movements cause pain near the wrist, a tendinous lesion is present.

Pain on Resisted Extension

If the pain is felt at the wrist, the extensor tendons of the wrist, seldom of the fingers, are affected. Crepitus is occasionally felt when the carpal extent of the extensor indicis muscle is involved. If the fingers are kept flexed voluntarily, the extensor digitorum longus muscle is thrown out of action; now, should the resisted movements towards extension still hurt, the carpal extensors are involved. Whether resisted radial or ulnar deviation hurts indicates whether the extensores carpi radialis or the extensor carpi ulnaris is involved. In the former case, the lesion is sought with the wrist held in full flexion and will be found at the insertion of the tendons into the bases of the second and third metacarpal bones (sometimes one, sometimes both). This is a pure teno-periosteal strain, therefore incurable by any operation slitting up the tendon-sheath; there is no teno-vaginitis or teno-synovitis. If the extensor carpi ulnaris tendon is at fault, the lesion has by contrast three possible sites, identified by discovery of the site of tenderness while the wrist is held in full radial deviation: at the base of the fifth metacarpal bone (teno-periosteal); at the extent of tendon between the triquetral (cuneiform) bone and the ulna; at the groove in the lower extremity of the ulna. It is when the tendon is affected in this groove that the puzzling phenomenon occurs of pain elicited at the extreme of passive supination of the forearm.

If the disorder is due to strain or overuse, both deep massage and hydrocortisone injection are extremely successful. If the tendon is warm to the touch, swollen or nodular, the inflammation is probably rheumatoid; if so, massage is harmful but hydrocortisone succeeds. Tuberculous and gonorrhoeal teno-synovitis have virtually disappeared but an occasional gouty case is encountered.

Weakness on Resisted Extension

When testing resisted extension at the wrist reveals painless weakness, full neurological examination is required.

Bilateral Weakness

If this is confined to the extensor muscles at both wrists, lead poisoning is suggested. If this is not a factor, carcinoma of the bronchus should be suspected.

Unilateral Weakness

This occurs in: (a) Radial pressure palsy from, e.g., a crutch or the edge of a chair impinging on this nerve in the arm or fracture of the humerus at mid-shaft. (b) Sixth or (seldom) seventh cervical root-palsy. In the former, the flexors of the elbow also lose power; in the latter, the triceps and wrist flexor muscles are much weakened. (c) In eighth cervical root-palsy, the extensor and flexor carpi ulnaris become weak and, when the resisted extension movement at the wrist is tested, the hand deviates radialwards. If so, the extensors and adductor of the thumb are also weak.

Pain on Resisted Flexion

If the pain is felt in the lower forearm, the flexor tendons of the wrist or fingers are at fault. Resisted flexion of each finger and resisted radial and ulnar deviation are tested, and the affected tendon defined. When the flexor digitorum profundus is affected, the tender extent is usually about 4 cm. long at the lower forearm. When the flexor carpi radialis is affected, the whole distal extent of the tendon is usually tender, sometimes including the teno-periosteal junction at the base of the second metacarpal bone. When the flexor carpi ulnaris is affected, tenderness must be sought at two sites: proximal and distal to the pisiform bone. In the latter instance, deep palpation through the thickness of the hypothenar muscles is required.

Both hydrocortisone injection and adequate deep massage quickly afford full relief at all these sites.

Rheumatoid Teno-vaginitis

This disorder is apt to involve one flexor tendon near the carpus. During the first few weeks the distinguishing feature is diffuse swelling and local heat palpable at the front of the forearm, combined with tenderness over an extent of tendon greater than is expected in cases due to overuse. Usually within a month, the swelling resolves into a series of nodules on the tendon; local heat persists. Treatment is by one or two infiltrations with hydrocortisone, which gives lasting quiescence. Rheumatoid arthritis does not supervene, at any rate for the next fifteen years.

A swelling, similar to that causing trigger-finger, sometimes forms at a flexor digitorum tendon at the wrist. This sets up pressure on the median nerve where it passes under the transverse carpal ligament and is one of the causes of the carpal tunnel syndrome.

Tuberculous Teno-synovitis

This is a disease of the past in Britain. A swelling forms that can be made to fluctuate from palm to lower forearm—'compound palmar ganglion'.

Foreign Body Teno-synovitis

An uncommon cause of tendinous trouble at the wrist is movement of a foreign body embedded in the forearm. Even after many years—the longest period that I have so far encountered was thirty-two years—a small fragment of metal, e.g. lead shot or shrapnel, may suddenly work its way out of the fleshy mass of muscle in which it has lain and, in the course of some hours or a day, move down and lodge at the wrist. Crepitating teno-synovitis results. This condition should be suspected if the forearm is scarred and the patient believes that fragments of metal remain. The position of the foreign body should be identified by palpation. It is then pushed downwards by the fingers. When it has reached the middle of the palm, it disappears; it can no longer be felt and it ceases permanently to trouble the patient.

Weakness on Resisted Flexion

This finding indicates a seventh cervical root-lesion and is associated with marked loss of power in the triceps muscle. The triceps jerk is seldom sluggish.

An eighth cervical root-palsy leads to weakness of both the ulnar deviators of the wrist. In such a case during the resisted flexion movement, the hand is seen to deviate radialwards. Corroboration is found in associated weakness of the extensor and adductor muscles of the thumb.

THE THUMB

Since both arthritis and teno-vaginitis at the thumb give rise to pain felt at the wrist, no examination of the wrist is complete without a study of the passive and resisted movements at the first carpo-metacarpal joint.

A small thumb since birth may indicate a congenital deformity at the lower cervical spine of the Klippel-Feil variety. Widening and shortening of the distal phalanx of the thumb occurs in the distal absorption of bone that may complicate psoriasis.

In arthritis at the trapezio-first-metacarpal joint, the thumb is often visibly fixed in adduction; the osteophytes can be seen and felt.

Passive Movement

T rapezio-first-metacarpal Joint

Only one passive movement need be tested at the trapezio-first-metacarpal joint: backward movement during extension. Since the anterior aspect of the capsule of the joint is that most affected, this is the movement that always hurts in arthritis even when the others do not; limitation of movement is largely confined to abduction. Tenderness is most obvious at the front of the joint. In osteoarthritis, crepitus can usually be elicited by pressing the bones together and moving the first metacarpal bone to and fro over the trapezium. The radiograph shows the condition clearly. It is often bilateral, sometimes in association with osteoarthritis of the fingers. In traumatic arthritis, the X-ray photograph reveals no abnormality; pain may go on for months.

Deep massage to the capsule of the joint on alternate days relieves traumatic arthritis within about a fortnight; in osteoarthritis, hydrocortisone injected into the joint often eases the pain for many months. In severe osteoarthritis, arthrodesis provides a strong and painless thumb with some limitation of movement, whereas excision of the trapezium gives more mobility but a weaker though painless joint.

Technique of Injection

A small syringe with a very thin needle 2 cm. long is filled with 1 ml. hydrocortisone suspension. The physiotherapist opens the joint-space by grasping the patient's thumb and pulling hard, applying counteraction with her other hand at the elbow. The distraction enables the groove between the bones to be felt easily (except in gross rheumatoid swelling) and the needle is inserted at right-angles to the first-metacarpal shaft. The point of the needle becomes intra-articular at about 1 cm.

Resisted Movements

Arthritis at the carpo–first-metacarpal joint may be simulated by teno-vaginitis at the base of the thumb (de Quervain); for the passive movements slide the tendon up and down within its sheath, thus setting up painful friction. Hence there is often pain on some of the passive wrist and thumb movements; but, when the resisted movements are tested, extension and abduction are found to hurt, thus incriminating the tendons.

Pain on Resisted Extension

This is associated with pain on resisted abduction; resisted flexion and adduction are painless (Fig. 50). The pain may be felt only in the lower fore-arm; if so, the abductor longus and extensores pollicis tendons are affected where they cross the shaft of the radius just above the wrist.

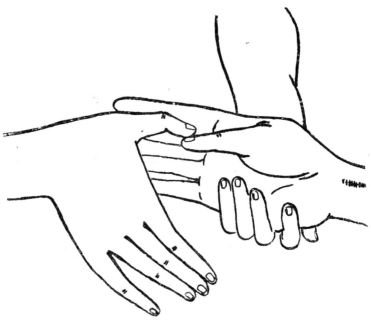

Fig. 50. Resisted extension of thumb. While the patient's hand is held steady, he presses his thumb upwards against the examiner's thumb.

Crepitus is present in recent cases; the tendons are tender over an extent of 4 cm. If the pain is felt diffusely, radiating down to the thumb and up the forearm, the tendons of the extensor brevis and abductor longus are probably affected at their carpal extent. If so, crepitus is absent, but a localized thickening can be seen at the radial side of the wrist and there is a small area of great tenderness at the radial styloid process. This is an example of the phenomenon I named 'associated tenderness'. The bone is more tender than the tendon itself, though this area of bone has no connection with the tendons. When the teno-vaginitis ceases, the bony tenderness ceases too; so they must be related.

Tenderness of the abductor longus and extensor brevis tendons in their common sheath occurs in three places: (1) at the level of the carpus; (2) at the insertion of the abductor longus into the base of the first metacarpal bone; (3) at the groove on the base of the radius. The tenderness of the styloid process of the radius must be ignored, since no lesion exists at this point. The condition is quite disabling since it hurts considerably whenever the patient grasps anything.

The extensor longus pollicis is very seldom affected at the wrist. Cure by massage takes about a fortnight.

'Styloiditis Radii'

Sometimes the pain at the styloid process is so noticeable that the patient says his wrist is painful and tender at that point, but does not mention pain on moving the thumb. This is very puzzling unless the relationship of an abductor and extensor teno-vaginitis of the thumb to tenderness of the styloid process is kept in mind. When associated with pain on resisted extension and abduction movements of the thumb, tenderness at the styloid process merely indicates that the carpal extent of the tendons is at fault; no lesion at the actual process is present. The condition has been described under the misnomer 'styloiditis radii'; this is putting the cart before the horse, because the teno-vaginitis is the primary lesion and the bony tenderness continues until the tendons recover.

Treatment

Hydrocortisone. Before steroid treatment existed, this condition caused much trouble. Now one, at most two, injections of hydrocortisone cure. The only difficulty is to place the injection correctly, along the gliding surfaces between tendon and tendon-sheath.

The patient sits with the radial side of his wrist uppermost, the hand held in ulnar deviation with the thumb well flexed. A small syringe with a very fine needle 2 cm. long is filled with 0·5 ml. hydrocortisone suspension. The tendons are now identified and the needle thrust in almost horizontally, parallel to them, just above the base of the first meta-carpal bone. The needle is guided to the free surface between sheath and tendon, and as the fluid is injected a little sausage forms along the tendons as far as the styloid process. The patient is seen ten days later and, if not fully recovered a second injection is given.

Operation. This is effective, but obsolete. The tendon-sheath is ex-posed at its carpal extent and slit open longitudinally over a 3-cm. length. Since the tendon now runs in a sheath that no longer fits, the patient is cured; but he has had an anaesthetic, two days in hospital and a scar 5 cm. long for a disorder easily put right by conservative means.

Massage. This is effective in three months, but also out of date, except at a hospital where hydrocortisone is not used and the cold orthopaedic surgical waiting-list is over two months long.

Immobilization. This is useless, even when persevered with for months.

Awaiting Spontaneous Cure. This is certainly not worthwhile since the disorder takes three to four years to resolve, with considerable disablement during all that time.

Rheumatoid Teno-vaginitis

This may occur at the carpal extent of the abductor longus and extensor brevis pollicis tendons. Marked soft swelling of the tendon-sheath provides the first sign. The gross thickening contrasts with the slightness of the symptoms, thus distinguishing the disorder from that described above, where the pain and disability are far greater than might be expected from the minor degree of swelling. Treatment by one or two injections of hydrocortisone is successful; recurrence is unlikely, and there is no par-ticular tendency to later rheumatoid arthritis.

Pain on Resisted Flexion

Pain felt when this movement is tested by resistance exerted at the distal phalanx shows the flexor pollicis longus tendon to be at fault. If it is affected at its metacarpal extent, an injection of hydrocortisone is effective, but deep massage useless. If it is affected at the wrist, crepitus is sometimes palpable and hydrocortisone or deep friction is equally successful.

Trigger-thumb

A swelling on the flexor pollicis longus tendon may become engaged in the tendon-sheath, during active flexion of the thumb. The patient then cannot voluntarily extend the thumb again, it being fixed in flexion at the interphalangeal joint. He straightens the thumb by using the other hand there is a snap and movement is restored. The swelling can be felt moving up and down as the patient flexes and extends the thumb; it lies just proximal to the head of the metacarpal bone.

An injection of hydrocortisone is often effective symptomatically although the node remains. If the symptoms recur, a small plastic operation slitting up the tendon-sheath longitudinally in the region of the swelling affords immediate and lasting relief.

Weakness of the Thumb Muscles

Weakness of abduction and extension of the thumb characterizes a disc-herniation at the seventh cervical level with consequent eighth root-palsy. It is associated with weakness of ulnar deviation at the wrist.

Weakness of abduction is scarcely perceptible even when the abductor pollicis brevis muscle is markedly wasted as the result of a cervical rib compressing the lower trunk of the brachial plexus. Wasting with some weakness of the thenar muscles denotes severe pressure within the carpal tunnel.

Weakness results, of course, when a tendon ruptures; this is usually obvious. Rupture of the extensor longus pollicis is an uncommon complication of fracture at the lower end of the radius. After a Colles's fracture, the tendon may become frayed by the bony irregularity at the fracture line, finally parting during, as a rule, the second month. The treatment is surgical. Tendons may also rupture in advanced rheumatoid arthritis.

Ischaemic contracture may affect the belly of the flexor longus pollicis muscle; if so, the metacarpophalangeal and the interphalangeal joint can each be extended singly, but not simultaneously—an example of the constant length phenomenon.

CARPAL TUNNEL SYNDROME

Irritation of the median nerve near the wrist was briefly discussed in a paper (Cyriax, 1942) in the *British Medical Journal* under the heading 'median perineuritis'. One case was recorded in which such severe twinges were felt in the thumb that two fruitless operations had been performed for a suspected foreign body in the pulp; cure (which lasted twelve years before I lost sight of the patient) followed two local anaesthetic injections about the median nerve at the wrist. However, the condition remained rather a nebulous entity until the appearance of Brian, Wright and Wilkinson's article (1947) in the *Lancet*.

The first symptom is pins and needles felt at the front of the outer three and a half digits of, usually, the right hand. The fact that the radial, but

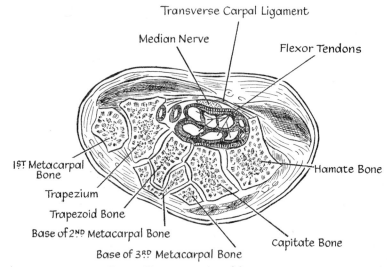

FIG. 51. Transverse section of the carpus.

not the ulnar border of the ring finger is paraesthetic, combined with the fact that only the palmar surface of the fingers is affected, strongly suggests pressure, exerted at the distal part of the limb, on the median nerve. In, for example, sixth cervical root-palsy due to a disc lesion or in cervical rib of median development, such accuracy is not attained. The patient notices that using the hand increases the symptoms and rest gives temporary relief. Advantage can be taken of this fact in diagnosis. If splinting the patient's wrist for a few days abolishes the paraesthesia, pressure on the median nerve at the wrist is confirmed. If the other hand becomes affected too, as happens in about a third of all cases, the complaint of pins and needles in both hands is very reminiscent of the thoracic outlet syndrome. After the condition has been present for many months, pain may come on in the palm and forearm, but the pins and needles remain in the hand only.

Diagnosis

The problem is to differentiate a cervical disc lesion, the thoracic outlet syndrome and pressure on the median nerve in the carpal tunnel. The history is the most informative and the radiograph the least, since this is a disorder of middle-age—when X-ray changes in the cervical spine are to be expected in normal individuals.

In the carpal tunnel syndrome, the pins and needles are increased by use of the hand and appear at the anterior aspect of three and a half digits. There is no paraesthesia above the wrist, though there may be aching.

In cervical disc lesion, the pins and needles come and go, day or night, in an erratic fashion, and do not actually last more than an hour at a time. Nothing in particular brings them on and they are felt within the hand and fingers, not at any aspect.

In the thoracic outlet syndrome, at least for the first few years, the pins and needles are strictly nocturnal, waking the patient after some hours' sleep. Usually all the digits are affected, not on any aspect.

When the carpal tunnel is at fault, examination of the neck for articular signs or of the thoracic outlet for the release phenomenon is negative. By contrast, when the wrist is held extended and the patient flexes and extends his fingers while the physician presses at the front of his wrist, the pins and needles may be evoked and recognized by the patient as his familiar sensation. The physician may feel a swelling on a digital flexor tendon (analagous to that causing the trigger phenomenon) which, as it moves under the transverse carpal ligament, sends a shower of pins and needles down the digits. So does keeping the wrist flexed for a minute and suddenly extending it.

Wasting and weakness of the thenar muscles are not expected in the early case; however, it is occasionally encountered. In Stevenson's (1966) series of 120 patients, two-thirds of whom had symptoms for six months to several years, wasting was noted in 29 per cent.

Any diagnosis based largely on negative findings is tentative. Hence, therapeutic confirmation is always required. Hydrocortisone is injected into the carpal tunnel and the patient seen ten days later. Relief may not be permanent but, in the short run, is diagnostic.

Technique of Injection

The patient sits, with wrist fully extended. A syringe containing 2 ml. hydrocortisone suspension, is fitted with a needle 4 cm. long. A spot on the palmar aspect, 3 cm. above the wrist, is chosen and the needle thrust in almost horizontally, so that it travels in the tunnel parallel to the tendons and nerve. It thus passes along them and does not penetrate the nerve. The needle is advanced to almost its full length and the injection given with its point under the ligament.

Six Varieties of Compression

1. Subluxation of the Lunate Bone

As the result of injury, not necessarily very severe, the patient's wrist becomes suddenly fixed. Extension is impossible; a few degrees of flexion can be obtained. Median paraesthesiae come on at once, leading to numbness within a few days and obvious muscular weakness within a week or two.

Radiography does not reveal the subluxation at all clearly, since the lesion is a fixed rotation of the lunate bone.

Surgery is required at once.

2. Rheumatoid Arthritis, Gout, Myxoedema, Sespsis, Acromegaly and Pregnancy

Thickening of the transverse carpal ligament and of all the tendons in the tunnel, may result from the general disease of fibrous tissue occurring in rheumatoid arthritis. Division of the transverse carpal ligament is required.

In an acute gouty attack affecting the flexor tendons, such swelling may result that the median nerve is severely compressed and, even if the attack is quickly controlled by indomethacin, butazolidine or colchicum, conduction may take six months to recover. In these cases, cutaneous analgesia is more marked than muscle weakness.

Murray and Simpson (1958) put forward evidence that the paraethesia in the hands that often accompanies hypothyroidism results from an accumulation of myxomatous deposits within the carpal tunnel; they found thyroid extract was usually effective. The same occurs in acromegaly, and (Oates, 1960) in pyogenic infection of the hand. It has also been described in pregnancy.

3. Swelling on a Digital Flexor Tendon

If the swelling is large, a characteristic symptom is mentioned. The patient complains that he cannot flex his fingers actively on waking in the morning but has to work them up and down with the other hand at first. This loss of active movement coming on after a period of immobility is accompanied by median numbness. Search for the swelling must not be confined strictly to the territory of the carpal tunnel; for it may lie several inches up the forearm. If the swelling lies close to the palm and in connection with the tendon running to the fourth or fifth finger, the thenar branch of the median nerve escapes pressure and the pins and needles occupy the index, long and ring fingers only.

Treatment consists in acupuncture. About half of all such cases are relieved, at any rate for some years, by careful location of the swelling and the passage of a needle right through it. Presumably, a small fluid core is liberated by the needle. If acupuncture fails, division of the transverse carpal ligament is indicated.

4. Colles's Fracture

When immobilization of the wrist ceases, say six weeks after the break occurred, and the patient begins to move his wrist again, the median nerve may catch against the callus.

5. No Palpable Abnormality

These are the cases favourable to treatment by hydrocortisone and account for about half the total. One injection, perhaps another a fortnight later, suffice to afford lasting relief. It is uncertain whether the sheath of the nerve is lastingly desensitized or inflammation of the tendons leading to local swelling is abated. If injections fail, the transverse carpal ligament should be divided.

Electromyography is helpful in prognosis; for Stevenson (1966) found that a motor latent period exceeding 7 milliseconds from wrist to thumb showed that the effect of conservative treatment would be temporary only.

6. Occupational Causes

Repeated use of the hand while it is held in extension at the wrist grinds the median nerve against the carpal bones. Hence scrubbing on hands-and-knees or using clippers is often the aetiological factor. After the harmful exertion, the nerve stays tender, being apt to produce pins and needles on very little provocation for some weeks afterwards.

Avoidance of the causative work, aided by local hydrocortisone, is indicated. Division of the transverse carpal ligament is without avail.

Three Partial Syndromes

1. Direct Trauma

A fall on the outstretched hand may bruise the branch of the median nerve to the thumb, at the point where it crosses the medial aspect of the trapezio-first-metacarpal joint. For many months afterwards the patient suffers pain and paraesthesia in the thumb alone. The symptoms are usually thought to be psychogenic.

Although it is not easy to find the exact spot with the point of a needle, one injection of 2 ml. 0·5 per cent procaine solution is lastingly curative. But it may take two or three attempts to infiltrate about the nerve correctly.

2. Stick Palsy

A patient, perhaps with chronic nervous disease or osteoarthritis in both hips, may habitually squeeze that part of the median nerve running to the index and long fingers by holding his walking-stick the wrong way. Instead of gripping the curved handle of his stick across his palm, he may grasp it longitudinally in line with his forearm. All the pressure is then borne at the exact point of emergence of the median nerve from under the distal edge of the transverse carpal ligament. Persistent paraesthesia in the index and long fingers results, which division of the ligament does not alter.

3. Palmar Flexor Tendon Swelling

Pins and needles in the long and ring fingers result from a largish swelling on a digital flexor tendon at its emergence just beyond the distal edge of the transverse carpal ligament. The trigger phenomenon is absent and the swelling easy to miss. It should be trimmed surgically; division of the ligament is of no avail.

PRESSURE ON THE RADIAL NERVE

This is rare. A minor subluxation of the scaphoid bone may lead to stiffness of the wrist and paraesthesia at the dorsum of the three and a half radial fingers owing to pressure on the nerve in the anatomical snuff-box. Examination of the wrist shows the pattern characteristic of internal derangement—limitation of extension only. Manipulative reduction restores movement at the wrist and abolishes the pins and needles simultaneously.

An osteoma projecting dorsally at the base of the third metacarpal bone (sometimes the result of an accessory centre of ossification there) may engage against the branch of the radial nerve to the index and long fingers. When the hand is then moved from side to side during wrist flexion, a sharp twinge is felt as the nerve engages against the projection and rides over it; the dorsum of these fingers then tingles for several minutes. The exostosis can be removed if the symptoms warrant.

If the sensory branch of the radial nerve catches against the lower edge of the radius, the patient describes a characteristic movement as bringing on the paraesthesia. This movement consists in bringing the arm backwards from the dependent position and then twisting it into full medial rotation; with the elbow straight he then flicks the forearm into full pronation and the wrist and fingers into flexion. This position stretches the radial nerve to the maximum and a sharp tingle results. An injection of hydrocortisone suspension is given where the nerve crosses the edge of the radius.

THE HAND

Pain in the hand usually results from local trauma or overuse. Much weight should be given to the history and the site of pain, which is usually felt exactly at the site of the lesion. Conversely, when pain in the hand is referred from above, the patient knows it. Inquiry is made for changes in colour such as suggest a circulatory disorder, e.g. Raynaud's disease or a cervical rib pressing on the subclavian artery or vein.

Paraesthesia

Numbness and pins and needles in the fingers are a common symptom which has been named 'acroparaesthesia'. They are felt in the hand irrespective of the level at which the causative pressure is exerted, hence the relevant nerve-trunk—identified by which fingers and which aspect are affected—must be examined from neck to hand. Pins and needles in all four limbs characterize disorders such as peripheral neuritis, diabetes, pernicious anaemia, and central cervical disc lesions.

Localized Paraesthesia. The main diagnostic points are—which fingers? Which aspect?

Thumb alone: numbness only—occupational pressure on the digital nerve at the outer side of the thumb; pins and needles—contusion of the thenar branch of the median nerve.

Thumb and index finger: fifth cervical disc lesion.

Thumb, index and long finger: fifth cervical disc lesion or thoracic outlet syndrome.

Thumb, index, long and adjacent side of ring finger; palmar surface—median nerve in carpal tunnel; dorsum—radial nerve.

Thumb and fifth finger: tumour of humerus.

All five digits of one or both hands: thoracic outlet syndrome.

All five digits of both hands: cervical central disc protrusion.

Index and long fingers: palmar surface—trigger-finger or stick-palsy; indeterminate—sixth cervical disc lesion; dorsal surface—carpal exostosis or subluxation.

Index, long and ring fingers: sixth cervical disc lesion or carpal tunnel syndrome, 3.

All four fingers: sixth cervical disc lesion.

Long finger alone: ditto

Long and ring fingers: ditto, stick-palsy.

Long, ring and little fingers: seventh cervical disc lesion.

Ring and fifth fingers: seventh cervical disc lesion or thoracic outlet syndrome.

Ulnar side of ring and whole fifth finger: pressure on ulnar nerve at elbow or palm.

As always, when a nerve twig, trunk or root is pressed on, even if the paraesthetic area appears to identify the one affected, the whole nerve must be examined from spine to digit; the above indications are probabilities, not certainties. When an area that does not correspond to any one cutaneous nerve is described, the lesion must lie above the differentiation of the brachial plexus.

Muscles of Hand

The muscles most often strained are the interosseous bellies. They may receive a direct injury and are in any case bound to be damaged when a metacarpal shaft is fractured. Musicians, especially violinists and pianists, sprain these muscles by an over-vigorous movement during fingering, and, unless treated, may be permanently unable to play perfectly again.

When, as is commoner, a dorsal interosseous muscle is strained, the pain in the hand is elicited by a resisted abduction movement of the extended fingers. The tender spot in the muscle must be found—the patient's sensations are a good guide—and deep massage given there. Even after months of disablement that has resisted every conceivable treatment, a musician can be confidently assured that he will be able to play again tomorrow night. Two or three sessions of massage are curative.

Tendinitis of an interosseous muscle at the base of one of the first phalanges may be difficult to distinguish from a strain of the joint itself. Though the tender spot is level with the joint and that side of the joint is slightly swollen, some of the passive movements at that joint hurt, others do not; i.e. the noncapsular pattern. It is then that pain elicited by a resisted movement clarifies the diagnosis.

Differentiation is important; for three to six sessions of adequate deep massage cure a tendinitis, however long-standing, but have no effect on traumatic arthritis.

Occasionally an abduction sprain of the thumb overstretches a thenar muscle, most often the origin of the oblique abductor muscle at the base of the second or third metacarpal bone.

Considerable ingenuity is required in testing the small muscles of the hand and in finding the tender spot in the structure thus identified. The physiotherapist too must take considerable trouble to find the position that allows her finger the best access to the tissue at fault, perhaps by pressing one metacarpal bone forwards and the adjacent one backwards.

All the intrinsic muscles and their short tendons respond immediately to adequate massage, but not to hydrocortisone. On the long flexor tendons in the palm, by contrast, massage has no effect, but hydrocortisone is successful.

Joints of the Hand

Arthritis occurs at any of the hand joints and gives rise to limitation of movement. The pattern for the joint is an equal degree of limitation of flexion and extension; except in severe arthritis rotation is painful at extremes rather than limited in range. The history, combined with the appearance of the joint provides the clearest pointer to the type of arthritis present. The relevant points are: whether the onset is apparently causeless, traumatic, or the result of immobilization because of neighbouring sepsis; whether the affection is multiple or single; whether the distal or the proximal joints were affected first; whether the capsule of the joint is swollen or not; whether the joint changes colour or not; whether there is a family history of gout or Heberden's nodes.

Rheumatoid Arthritis

This never begins at the distal interphalangeal joints, whereas osteoarthritis usually does. Rheumatoid arthritis often begins as stiffness of the fingers on waking in the morning; at this stage no clinical signs may be perceptible, but the sedimentation rate is markedly raised. Sooner or later one or more metacarpo-phalangeal or proximal interphalangeal joints of one or both hands develop the familiar spindle-shaped swelling. Later on, ulnar deviation of the fingers is characteristic. The mechanism is as follows: during gripping, as the fingers flex they also deviate ulnarwards in the normal individual, partly owing to the slight tilt on the metacarpal heads, partly because the tendons of the interosseous muscles lie at the medial side of the joint. By dint of much gripping, the ulnar deviators become stronger than the radial deviators. The deviation in rheumatoid arthritis is initiated by these two factors, and the effect is then enhanced by the extensor tendon gradually shifting towards the ulnar side of the joint and pulling the phalanx over each time the muscle contracts.

An identical picture is presented by multiple subacute arthritis complicating Reiter's disease, gonorrhoea, chronic gout, psoriasis, and the early stage of scleroderma. In psoriasis the nails are ridged.

Care should be taken not to assume too readily that the symptoms in a patient with rheumatoid arthritis are due to the rheumatoid disease. A trigger-finger is a common complication, since the tendons are also very apt to be affected. Sometimes the swelling becomes large enough to prevent active, but not passive, flexion of a finger. Since movement is easily restored by a small plastic operation on the tendon-sheath, correct diagnosis is important. A ganglion lying between the head of the second and third metacarpal bones must not be mistaken for rheumatoid arthritis.

Treatment

Intra-articular hydrocortisone is the treatment of choice and is very successful when only a few joints are affected and the patient not in an acute phase. Recently, surgery has been advocated in the early stage, in order to obviate the invasion of bone, cartilage and ligament by the inflamed synovial tissue, so as to avoid irreversible change. Once the rheumatoid synovium has been removed surgically, it seldom grows again; hence distension of the joint and stretching of the ligaments ceases. Invasion of subchondral bone with formation of cysts and destruction of articular cartilage is also prevented by this means. A good case can therefore be made out for early surgery, the difficulty being that some half of all cases do well without. It is thus a question of selecting the cases that will do badly.

Vaino (1967) considers that the indications for operation are: (1) patients under forty years old, specially women; (2) raised E.S.R. at the onset; (3) abnormality of the albumin/globulin ratio at the onset; (4) rapid development of bony erosion visible radiographically. Moberg (1967) states that two areas of synovial hypertrophy appear early in rheumatoid arthritis, the larger on the dorsum of the joint, the smaller lying anteriorly. Each develops close to the nutrient foramen causing obstruction, and cells appear to be released from these areas of hypertrophy which degenerate with the release of an enzyme that attacks cartilage. Early synovectomy prevents this damage.

Osteoarthritis

This may result from a severe injury; if so, only one joint is affected. In the apparently causeless cases of multiple involvement that occur in elderly patients, usually women, a strong familial trend is evident. The distal joints are affected first; after many years the disorder spreads to the proximal interphalangeal joints, very seldom to the metacarpophalangeal joints. The knobbly appearance of the joint is quite different from rheumatoid arthritis; for the base of the distal phalanx can be seen projecting abruptly as two small rounded bosses at the dorsum of the joint. A varus deformity, usually at the index, may develop at a distal joint. Both hands are usually affected more or less symmetrically. The radiograph shows the osteophytes and erosion of cartilage clearly. From time to time, a new node forms at an affected joint; while it is growing there is pain for a month or two and occasionally the finger-tip goes pink. This mottled pink is different from the shiny red of gout. After a month or two the discoloration passes off and the node stops hurting.

Heberden's nodes and osteoarthritis cause little in the way of symptoms. They are unsightly and cause aching and clumsiness. Since the distal finger-joints fix in 45 degrees flexion in the end, arthrodesis seldom brings much improvement unless an intractable painful traumatic arthritis supervenes after injury. Some patients are pleased to have the exostoses removed surgically for cosmetic reasons.

Traumatic Arthritis

This is common, and results from direct contusion, indirect sprain, chip-fracture or reduced dislocation. The history is characteristic; the joint itself is swollen in the spindle shape resembling rheumatoid arthritis. After severe trauma, the joint is often warm to the touch for about a month. Movement is limited; the active, passive and resisted movements must all be tested in case a tendinous lesion coexists.

All treatment is futile. The joint recovers, whether treated or not, in six to eighteen months, depending on the severity of the original trauma and the age of the patient. Whether the patient uses the joint enough to make it ache or not has no effect on the ultimate result. Hydrocortisone, so useful in traumatic arthritis at the toe joints, gives no benefit in traumatic arthritis at the fingers. Immobilization is, of course, strongly contra-indicated.

Unreduced Dislocation

At the interphalangeal joint of the thumb, dislocation is sometimes mistaken for traumatic arthritis; it is extraordinary how the local swelling obscures the deformity. Examination shows the joint to be fixed in full extension, quite different from arthritis in which flexion and extension are equally limited.

In late cases, reduction is impossible and arthrodesis in 45 degrees of flexion gives a good result.

Immobilizational Stiffness

Before the days of antibiotics this was the common result of splintage for sepsis. The fingers must not be splinted for a day longer than is absolutely necessary, and never in full extension.

Gout

Involvement of the hands is usually a late manifestation of the disease. The familial predisposition and the history of recurrent attacks, clearing up completely, beginning at the big toe and later spreading to other joints, is diagnostic. The shiny red appearance of the joint is characteristic.

When chronic gout comes on gradually in an old man, the onset and the clinical appearance of the joints may perfectly mimic rheumatoid arthritis. Tophi in the ears and a raised blood uric acid level finally appear, but are of little diagnostic aid in the early, doubtful case. Therapeutic testing with butazolidine is the quickest way to a clear answer.

Treatment

Indomethacin, 25 mg. four times a day; or phenylbutazone 200 mg. three times a day, have displaced colchicum. They cause subsidence of the acute attack within a day or two.

Tendons of the Hand

Teno-synovitis

The flexor tendons in the palm may develop much coarse grating in advanced rheumatoid arthritis. Such chronic teno-synovitis causes little or no symptoms. If the discomfort warrants, hydrocortisone injected into the affected tendon-sheath is effective.

Trigger-finger

A swelling on any of the digital flexor tendons may form just proximal to the metacarpophalangeal joint. When big enough, this gives rise to trigger-finger or trigger-thumb. When the digit has been fully flexed actively, the swelling engages within its sheath and becomes fixed in this position. The affected finger, usually the third or fourth, can then no longer be extended by muscular action; the patient has to free it by pulling at it with his other hand, whereupon it disengages with a snap. The swelling on the tendon is easy to feel in the palm or thenar eminence, just proximal to the head of the metacarpal bone. Some cases are apparently causeless; others due to multiple minor traumata (e.g. using a pair of clippers); yet others complicate rheumatoid arthritis. If necessary a small operation enlarging the relevant part of the tendon-sheath by slitting it up affords permanent cure, but many patients are hardly disabled enough to wish this done. In minor cases an injection of hydrocortisone usually abolishes symptoms for months or years.

Rarely, the swelling may become so large that active flexion of the finger stops at half-range. The fact that passive flexion is not limited draws immediate attention to the digital flexor tendon. Equally rarely, the swelling may form on the proximal part of the tendon in the palm and interfere with the branch of the median nerve running to the index and long fingers, causing pins and needles at the adjacent surfaces of these two digits.

A small tender swelling may form on the flexor tendon level with the proximal crease of the finger. It causes no symptoms unless the patient carries a suitcase; the local pressure then hurts.

Ruptured Tendon

Mallet-finger

Any injury that forcibly flexes the distal finger-joint while it is actively held in extension may cause rupture of the extensor insertion at the base of the distal phalanx. A cricket ball is often the culprit. The distal joint can be fully flexed voluntarily; the elastic rebound of the tissue takes it back to 45 degrees; the last 45 degrees cannot be actively performed, although the passive movement remains full. The dorsal aspect of the base of the phalanx is tender and swollen.

Treatment should be instituted at once. In young persons the affected finger should be fixed in full flexion on the palm of the hand by one piece of strapping running along from the dorsum of the finger to the front of the wrist covered by another piece of strapping encircling the hand (Fig. 52). This position ensures full relaxation of the distal part of the tendon (since the distal joint is held in full extension) while the tendon is held taut proximally by fully flexing the proximal interphalangeal joint. The strapping is kept on for four weeks; union between tendon and bone is then firm. In elderly patients, keeping the metacarpophalangeal joint fully flexed may lead to undesirable stiffness; hence it is best to fix the distal joint in full extension and the proximal joint in full flexion by a small plaster gutter, leaving the metacarpophalangeal joint free. This is kept on for a month, but union is less sure. Attempts to suture the tendon

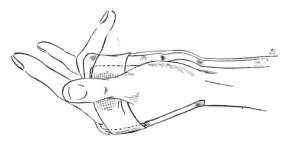

FIG. 52. Strapping for mallet-finger. One piece of strapping extends from the dorsum of the hand, along the finger to the front of the wrist. This fixes the affected finger in flexion at the metacarpophalangeal and proximal interphalangeal joints. A second piece of strapping encircles the hand, pressing the finger-tip into the palm. This ensures that the distal interphalangeal joint is kept in full extension.

to the bone operatively are so seldom successful that the late case is best left untreated.

Ruptured Flexor Tendon

Rupture of the flexor digitorum longus at its insertion into the base of the distal phalanx is a rarity. The whole tendon recoils into the palm where it lies bunched up, giving rise to a swelling superficially resembling Dupuytren's contracture. The distal finger-joint cannot be actively flexed, although the passive movement is retained. Arthrodesis is called for if the patient's work is interfered with.

Ganglion

A ganglion sometimes forms between the heads of the second and third metacarpal bones, and is nearly always mistaken for rheumatoid arthritis. It gives rise to vague local aching. Inspection of the hand shows the swelling to project between the bones; movement at the two adjacent metacarpophalangeal joints is of full range and painless; the radial side of the second and the ulnar side of the third metacarpophalangeal joint are clearly not swollen, and palpation reveals a fluctuant swelling. Acupuncture affords permanent relief; I have yet to meet a recurrence.

A ganglion may form on the front of the palm just distal to the hamate bone. It lies hidden under the hypothenar muscle bellies and causes no symptoms until it becomes large enough to compress the ulnar nerve. Ulnar paraesthesiae and weakness result, for which no cause can be found as the nerve is followed down from the base of the neck, until this swelling is detected in the proximal part of the palm. If the sensory branch to the ulnar fingers and to the hypothenar muscles has already been given off, weakness without cutaneous analgesia results, affecting the adductor pollicis, the interosseous and the two medial lumbrical muscles. Up to 5 ml. of mucus may be obtained on aspiration. If the ganglion fills up again quickly, as it is apt to do, it should be removed before the palsy becomes too severe. I have encountered only one instance of a swelling on the flexor digitorum tendon running to the fifth finger, prominent enough to compress the ulnar nerve. The condition was bilateral and the enlargement lay 4 cm. above the wrist joint.

An ulnar palsy of similar nature comes on in workmen who repeatedly hit a lever with the front rather than the side of the ulnar border of the hand. Thrombosis of the ulnar artery has also been recorded, after similar repeated local minor traumata.

Multiple Xanthomata

These occur in the extensor tendons of the fingers at the dorsum of each hand and along each proximal phalanx. The tendons present a number of closely spaced, discrete nodules, causing visible projections that can be seen to move up and down with the tendons. No symptoms result and no tendency to rupture. Coincident bilateral involvement of the tendo Achillis is almost a certainty. Finally, large nodes form on the extensor tendons at the dorsum of the foot and on the front of the upper tibiae and the back of the upper ulnac. The blood cholesterol level is usually greatly raised, to twice or three times the normal level (200 mg).

A corn-oil diet has been shown (Jepson, 1961) to diminish the cholesterol level in the blood, and, if the patient regards treatment as worthwhile, should be continued indefinitely. Mason and Perry (1965) treated four patients with large xanthomata on knees and elbows with clofibrate (2 gm. daily for two years) with disappearance of the swellings and the serum cholesterol fell from 1100, 500, 460 and 325 to under 250 in each case. Bengal Grain is now under trial.

If the projections on the long bones annoy, they can be excised.

Bones of the Hand

Clubbing of the distal phalanges occurs in pulmonary disease. Since clubbing occurs mainly in disease of the lungs and upper colon, especially ulcerative colitis—both tissues innervated by the vagus—the suggestion has been made that, in some obscure way, the disorder is mediated via the vagus nerve. This is given considerable confirmation by Flavell (1956) who reported that the clubbing disappeared after section of the nerve and was confirmed by Holling *et al.* (1961).

Swelling of the terminal phalanges with radiographic evidence of erosion at the tip of each bone occurs in psoriasis. The whole skeleton of the hand enlarges greatly in acromegaly. In sclerodactyly the bones of the fingers are narrow and tapering, with the skin stretched tightly over them; the joints are contrastingly prominent.

Fractures are common.

Post-traumatic Osteoporosis

This is a curious and rare sequel to injury, first described by Sudeck in 1900. It nearly always follows a fracture of the forearm near the wrist (e.g. Colles's) or of the leg near the ankle. Cases have been described, however, after an otherwise unexceptional sprained ankle, not even treated by splintage.

A week or two after the accident the wrist and fingers swell and there is considerable pain on movement. The distal part of the limb becomes cyanotic and cold; the lower leg becoming almost black when left dependent for a few minutes. The range of movement at carpus (or tarsus) and fingers (or toes) diminishes rapidly. Trophic change supervenes and the nails stop growing. The radiograph, which showed no such change just after the injury, reveals severe osteoporosis involving the distal part of the broken bone and the entire hand or foot, far more than can be accounted for by immobilization. Union of the fracture proceeds normally.

The cause is unknown. No treatment to the hand makes any difference; recovery (which may never be complete, some stiffness remaining permanently) takes one to two years. Active use of the injured hand or foot should be enjoined. The radiograph shows a degree of atrophy so extreme as to suggest that the bones of the foot might easily give way under the stress of weight-bearing; moreover, softening, such that the affected bones can easily be cut with a knife post-mortem, has been described. Nevertheless, no harm results from ordinary weight-bearing activities and I have seen no case of subsequent deformity.

Palmar Fascia

A painless contracture of the palmar fascia, named after Dupuytren

(1832), but first described by Astley Cooper in 1822, may develop slowly, usually towards middle-age, and lead to fixed flexion deformity of the fingers. It affects the ring finger most often, but sooner or later the third and fifth fingers also become involved. It is usually bilateral, but considerably more advanced on one side than the other. The palmar fascia thickens, becomes adherent to the skin and the cause of the deformity is obvious. The disorder is familiar; four-fifths of the patients are men. Rarely the plantar fascia is also affected.

In the early stage, the patient should himself be taught to stretch out his finger daily so as to elongate the palmar fascia as fast as it contracts. Later, a plastic operation using a Z-shaped incision is indicated, followed by splintage in extension of the fingers.

Digital Nerves

Occupational pressure on the radial side of the thumb leads to numbness rather than pins and needles at the outer border of the distal phalanx. The workman is found to steady his hand against the edge of his bench. Recovery usually takes six months. Rarely the ulnar side of the little finger suffers in the same way.

Swelling on a digital flexor tendon in the palm may squeeze a digital nerve and set up paraesthesia felt at the contiguous sides of two fingers.

Direct trauma may bruise the thenar branch of the median nerve where it crosses the trapezio-first-metacarpal joint leading to pins and needles in the thumb.

A ganglion adjacent to the hamate-fifth-metacarpal joint may lead to an ulnar palsy.

Many nervous diseases begin by setting up symptoms referable to the hand: e.g. cervical rib, cervical disc lesion, neuroma, syringomyelia, paralysis agitans and chorea.

WRITER'S CRAMP

This is an occupational neurosis, the patient finding himself able to do everything effortlessly with his hand, except write. It is thus evident that the mental concept of writing interferes with the act of writing. Inability to write is often the first symptom in paralysis agitans. If so, repeated quick rotation of the forearm to and fro cannot be performed on the affected side.

There are two types of complaint: (1) pain, and (2) involuntary movements.

1. *Pain*

If the pain comes on as soon as the pen is grasped, the source of the symptoms must lie in the cerebrum. In such cases, physiotherapy and psychotherapy have each proved valueless.

If the pain comes on after a time, it may be caused by ischaemia. Arrest of circulation in the forearm is possible if such great and continued force is used in grasping the pen that the muscles are kept in tetanic contraction. In such cases, the physiotherapist can help the patient by re-educating muscular relaxation. She holds his upper forearm while he sits writing, and stops him each time she feels the contraction become excessive.

The carpo-pedal spasm of tetany (often set up by hyper-ventilation) must be distinguished from painful writer's cramp.

2. *Involuntary Movements*

After some words have been laboriously written, the patient finds his hand straying away, lifting the pen from the paper. Alternatively, sharp jerks may occur. These cases must be differentiated from the slow writing of early Parkinsonism. In my experience, treatment is futile but McGuire and Vallance (1964) claim relief by aversion therapy using electric shocks. If this fails, the patient must learn to use a typewriter.

OEDEMA OF THE HAND AND FOREARM

Angioneurotic Oedema

When oedema of the dorsum of the hand occurs without apparent cause, it is termed 'angioneurotic'. It may be allergic, but in some cases the chief underlying factors are psychological. The oedema is usually most marked on waking, disappearing as the day goes on. Pitting is easily produced. No treatment appears to make any lasting difference, unless an allergic sensitivity is discovered. The antihistamine preparations may be tried.

Interference with Lymph or Venous Return

Thrombosis of the axillary vein, or interference with the drainage of lymph as the result of operation, or carcinomatosis of the axillary glands should be considered.

Post-traumatic Oedema

The cause of this uncommon sequel to injury to the hand is obscure.

The distinguishing feature is that the oedema stops abruptly at the wrist or elbow instead of gradually fading away. The ridge formed by the upper extremity of the oedema is clearly palpable. The patient may allege much pain and disablement, and may add that the grip is weak and the hand numb. The oedema is clearly real, but there is a full range of movement at every joint, and no weakness or wasting of the muscles is discernible. Radiography reveals at the most some disuse atrophy. The supposition that the condition is an hysterical manifestation has received support from the work of Scott and Mallinson (1944), who cured a number of patients by psychotherapy, some in a few weeks.

In some (possibly all) cases the oedema is an artefact, produced by the application of a tight band. It was much commoner during the war years of 1939–45 than it is now.

15

The Thorax and Abdomen

Symptoms referable to the thorax arise from a wide variety of disorders, not all of them visceral. Preoccupation with visceral disease leads to neglect of the somatic causes of thoracic pain. Thoracic disease may give rise to symptoms felt wholly outside the thorax, in the abdomen perhaps, or in a limb only. If the patient's symptoms depend on activity and posture rather than on visceral function, their provenance from the moving parts should be particularly considered.

Clinically, *the thoracic spine begins at the third vertebra*, the upper two thoracic joints and nerve-roots being best examined as part of the neck. Moreover, the upper two thoracic segments form the inner aspect of the upper limb, thus being most easily examined with the cervical segments that make up the rest of the limb.

SOURCES OF THORACIC PAIN

The common sources are:

1. The Neck

Displacement of part of the third or fourth cervical intervertebral disc sets up pain felt to radiate as far as the root of the neck; at the fifth and sixth levels, pain felt as far as the mid- or inter-scapular area is commonplace; at the seventh level the pain is often wholly mid-thoracic, sometimes at its most intense at the lower angle of one scapula. Great opportunities for mistaken diagnosis thus exist; for the extrasegmental reference of pain from the dura mater is a puzzling phenomenon.

Even more misleading reference occurs at times. Instead of a cervical disc lesion setting up scapular pain it may give rise to pectoral pain only. This is no greater a transgression of the rules of segmental reference than the pain being felt in the third or fourth thoracic dermatome posteriorly. Being a rare site of reference, however, the true diagnosis may not even be considered.

2. The Thoracic Joints and Dura Mater

Internal derangement at a thoracic joint gives rise to pain felt centrally or to one side of the posterior thorax. If the intercostal nerve-root is compressed, pain is usually felt posteriorly first, then spreading anteriorly. Deep breathing may hurt. In disc lesions of primary postero-lateral evolution, the pain may be unilateral and anterior only, in the thorax or, less often, the abdomen. Occasionally, a thoracic disc lesion sets up sternal pain only. In first and second thoracic disc lesions the ache is felt at the lower scapular area radiating to the ulnar side of the palm or the inner arm respectively.

Compression phenomena occur at the intervertebral joints, causing central posterior or bilateral pain, sometimes referred round to the side of the lower thorax.

Ligamentous pain occurs in ankylosing spondylitis and vertebral hyperostosis felt at the interscapular or sternal area. Rarely, sternal pain may arise from the manubriosternal joint.

3. The Ribs

Fracture is common and results in localized pain lasting six weeks at most. Disease is rare and is usually due to bacterial invasion or secondary malignant deposits. Tietze's painful swelling of a costochondral junction is uncommon.

4. The Muscles

The intercostal muscles are, of course, slightly torn when a rib breaks; they may also be bruised or strained by direct contusion. Bruising of the digitations of the serratus anterior occurs. In these cases, the pain is very localized.

A more diffuse thoracic pain, often referred to the arm as far as the elbow, results from strains involving the pectoralis major or latissimus dorsi muscles. Athletes may strain the posterior inferior serratus muscle.

5. The Bones

An angular kyphos is often very difficult to palpate at the thoracic spine. Wedge fracture of a vertebral body, if uncomplicated, causes symptoms for not longer than three months. For the first week there is often girdle pain. Kyphotic compression of the anterior aspects of the vertebral bodies gives rise to a postero-central bone-to-bone ache that can go on unchanged for decades. Senile osteoporosis causes no symptoms unless, as may happen, pathological wedge-fracture occurs.

Osteitis deformans, aortic aneurysm, tuberculous caries and secondary malignant deposits in the spine or sternum naturally set up pain arising from diseased bone.

6. The Nerves

Neuritis of the long thoracic or suprascapular nerve gives rise to a constant unilateral scapular pain lasting three weeks. In herpes zoster, the vesicles appear after three or four days. Early in the course of neuralgic amyotrophy, bilateral upper thoracic pain is felt, but it spreads to one or both arms within a few days.

In the early stages of a thoracic intra-spinal neuroma, the symptoms may be posterior thoracic only.

7. The Diaphragm, Pleura and Lung

Diaphragmatic pain (C 3, 4, 5) is often felt at the shoulder at each breath, i.e. at the fourth cervical dermatome, in correspondence with the main embryological derivation of the diaphragm. Pain arising from that part of the pleura not in contact with the diaphragm is also brought on by respiration but is felt in the chest. The lung is insensitive, but large tumours invade the chest wall, setting up local pain and causing spasm of the pectoralis major muscle, with consequent limitation of elevation of the arm. They may also cause limitation of thoracic side-flexion away from the affected side.

8. The Myocardium

The heart is developed from the first, second and third thoracic segments. Hence pain originating here may be felt spreading from the thorax to the root of the neck and to the upper limb as far as the ulnar border of the hand on the left or on both sides. Alternatively, there may be thoracic pain only; or, less often, pain confined to the left or both upper limbs.

9. The Aorta

Thrombosis of the lower aorta leads in due course to intermittent claudication in the legs and absence of the femoral pulses. An occasional case is encountered of posterior lower thoracic pain only, before blood-flow in the iliac arteries is much diminished. Such cases are very puzzling and the diagnosis remains in doubt until femoral pulsation becomes impaired later.

Haematoma formation after intra-aortic injection of contrast material sets up left-sided lower thoracic pain.

10. Venous Thrombosis (Mondor's Disease)

Unilateral pain at the front of the thorax may coincide with the appearance of a tender cord running from the pectoral area to the umbilicus, rendering full elevation of the arm painful. The cause is thrombosis of the thoraco-epigastric vein. Spontaneous recovery takes a month or two.

THORACIC DISC LESIONS

Since most cervical and lumbar symptoms are nowadays generally regarded as having an articular origin, the question naturally arises: are thoracic symptoms also caused by disc lesions? In my view, they are (Cyriax, 1950). The marked signs that eventually serve to clarify the diagnosis in cervico-lumbar protrusions seldom appear at the thorax, however long a patient is kept under observation; hence this theory is correspondingly difficult to prove. Moreover, operation, which has established the pathology of disc lesions in the lumbar and cervical regions so firmly, is very seldom necessary at the thoracic spinal joints.

At the cervical and lumbar joints an alternation exists that simplifies diagnosis. A minor degree of protrusion interferes with the joint, not yet with the nerve-root; hence local pain and articular signs are at their most obvious when neurological signs are lacking. By contrast, when the protrusion has passed postero-laterally and interferes little with joint movement, it exerts its maximum pressure on the nerve-root; hence root-pain and clear neurological signs supervene as the articular symptoms and signs fade.

Disc lesions occurring at the thoracic joints by no means show this characteristic sequence. There is an extraordinary variation in the mode of onset; moreover, the articular signs are seldom obvious, and neurologic signs are conspicuous only by their absence. Clinicians therefore properly hesitate to inculpate a thoracic joint as the source of what used to be called 'fibrositis', 'pleurodynia' or 'intercostal neuritis'. It should be noted that pain on deep breathing occurs just as readily when a disc lesion compresses the dura mater *via* the posterior ligament as in pleurisy; connection with respiration has then no differentiating significance, though doubtless this fact is responsible for the invention of 'pleurodynia'.

N

Diagnosis is always difficult, confusion with visceral disease being excusably very frequent. Indeed it is always safest to approach diagnosis from two aspects, the absence of signs of visceral disease balancing and confirming those of an articular plus nerve-root disorder.

Spontaneous Cure

Though scapular and lumbar pain can go on indefinitely when caused by a cervical or low lumbar disc lesion, unilateral root-pain has a set period and seldom lasts more than four and twelve months respectively. No such tendency exists at the third to twelfth thoracic levels and root-pain, usually at one costal margin, with or without a posterior component, can continue unchanged for many years. The length of time that root-pain has continued determines reducibility at cervical and lumbar levels; by contrast it presents no such criterion at the thorax; a disc lesion, even in a young person, may well prove reducible after constant root-pain for ten years.

Symptoms

These form five groups:

1. Thoracic Lumbago

The patient bends or twists and is suddenly fixed in flexion by severe posterior lower thoracic pain, central or unilateral. A deep breath usually hurts more than coughing; the reverse is true in lumbar lumbago, when a cough hurts but a deep breath is seldom uncomfortable. A few days in bed ensure recovery but recurrence is to be expected, brought on by bending or twisting the trunk, especially during compression of the joint, i.e. when carrying a weight.

The pain may be at one side of the posterior thorax on one occasion, on the other the next time; movement of the loose fragment across the midline is common. The same phenomenon may be noted during manipulative reduction; a click may be felt that makes the pain change sides. (This is one of the phenomena that made me realize twenty years ago that thoracic pain was caused by disc lesions.)

The pain often radiates along the relevant dermatome, as in cervical and lumbar disc lesions, i.e. round to the front of the chest, usually at about the level of the lower costal margin, but also to the side of the sternum or to the abdomen in high and low lesions respectively. Central disc protrusion may cause radiation round to both sides of the anterior thorax.

2. Sternal Pain

Occasionally, upper or mid-thoracic lumbago causes pain felt anteriorly only, at the sternum or epigastrium. Since the onset is sudden, during say lifting, the symptoms suggest coronary thrombosis and differential diagnosis may not prove easy at first, especially as this type of onset is apt to occur in middle age. A quick test is to ask the patient to take a deep breath, which aggravates the pain in disc protrusion but not when the myocardium is at fault.

3. Thoracic Backache

Slow protrusion causes posterior thoracic backache, often coming on after sitting for some while in flexion, and is commoner in patients who already have excessive thoracic kyphosis. The pain may be central or unilateral, most often at the lower part of the thorax, and the history discloses a clear relation to posture and exertion. The pain is often inter-mittent, according to what the patient does, and often absent for months on end.

The nuclear self-reducing lesion is common in those who sit for long periods each day, e.g. typists. The patient wakes comfortable and for the first few hours up feels nothing. Then sitting brings on the posterior thoracic ache which increases as the day wears on. Standing and lying abolish the ache in a few minutes. The cause is a posterior bulging of the joint contents, which recede as soon as excessive flexion is no longer maintained.

Symptoms of pleural, intercostal muscular, costal and dural provenance are all increased on coughing or deep inspiration; hence respiratory exacerbation serves to rule out cardiac pain only. Pressure on the dura mater at any thoracic level does not, as at the lower lumbar levels, give rise to limitation of straight-leg raising, but the pain caused by a lower thoracic protrusion may be increased, or the pain on neck-flexion aggra-vated, during *full* straight-leg raising.

4. Root-pain

Primary Postero-lateral Protrusion

This takes place at the thoracic joints no less than at the cervical and lumbar. In these cases, the posterior component is absent and the unilateral pain confined to the front of the chest or to the abdomen. There is no correlation with visceral function but clear correspondence with posture and activity. These cases give rise to much diagnostic difficulty and are responsible for the idea that manipulators can cure angina, gastritis, cholecystitis and the like, by doing something unspecified to the spinal joints that they declare alters autonomic tone.

If the eleventh or twelfth thoracic nerve-root is compressed, there is pain in the iliac fossa perhaps radiating to the testicle. Occasionally, the abdominal component is absent and pins and needles in groin or testicle may be the only symptom, leading to a diagnosis of 'testicular neuralgia'.

In upper thoracic disc protrusion the symptom may be merely a band of unpleasant tingling as the patient runs his hand down the front of his chest. Another unusual symptom is impingement against the nerve-root, only when the dura mater is drawn upwards. The patient states that he feels nothing unless he bends his head right forward, when he notices a sharp stab of pain at one side of the sternum, sometimes accompanied by pins and needles in the mid-pectoral area.

Secondary Postero-lateral Protrusion

This is the commoner type of onset, but now the history of posterior unilateral pain, later radiating to the costal margin, naturally draws atten-tion to the back of the trunk. Even so, the fact that a deep breath and, some-times, a cough aggravate the pain often misdirects attention to the pleura.

In general, the likelihood of anterior thoracic and abdominal symptoms stemming from pressure on an intercostal nerve-root is forgotten. Obviously, most thoraco-abdominal pain has a visceral source, but when symptoms at the front of the trunk are independent of visceral function, and alter with posture and exertion, the possibility of thoracic root-pain should be considered more often than is the present habit. Manipulative reduction can then be performed within the medical sphere.

5. Spinal Cord Symptoms

Pins and needles come on in both feet, gradually spreading to include the legs and thighs. Then weakness and some numbness of the legs sets in. There is no backache to speak of, but vague girdle pains are usually mentioned. Pressure from a central protrusion on the thoracic cord clearly accounts for some cases of what used to be called transverse myelitis.

Physical Signs

Inspection

The patient stands with light falling evenly on his back, its general shape being noted. The angular kyphos characteristic of a collapsed vertebral body is quickly seen and can later be palpated; a flat lower lumbar spine and excessive upper lumbar-lower thoracic kyphosis suggests a past adolescent osteochondritis. Absence of the lumbar lordosis with a marked thoracic kyphosis suggests ankylosing spondylitis. Scoliosis and kypholordosis dating since adolescence are immediately visible, of course, but neither has any significance; for disc lesions are not more common in patients with these postural deformities than in others. Scoliosis confined to the upper thorax and lower neck suggests unilateral cervical rib or congenital vertebral deformity of the Klippel-Feil type.

Active Movements

Upper Thoracic Pain

Since the common cause of upper thoracic pain, especially posterior, is a *cervical* disc lesion, examination must begin at the neck, and only if this is negative need a local origin be considered at all. Moreover, scapular pain can result from a scapular lesion or from disorders like long thoracic or suprascapular neuritis, the signs of all of which are revealed only on examination of the upper limb. Lesions at the apex of the lung may affect the first thoracic root, and are identified only when the strength of the small muscles of the hand is tested. Hence, not only the neck movements but the whole routine testing of the upper limb must be completed before the thorax is examined.

Neck-flexion has two results; movement at the cervical joints and stretching of the dura mater. The fact, therefore, that neck-flexion provokes a thoracic pain is no evidence that it has a cervical origin, whereas if any of the other movements of the neck hurt, a cervical lesion is highly probable.

Scapular movement also has two results. In a local lesion this may be uncomfortable, but scapular approximation pulls on the first and second thoracic nerves, and tends to stretch the dura mater upwards just as does neck-flexion. Hence in a thoracic disc lesion at any level, this movement is apt to hurt *via* this unexpected mechanism and must not be thought to incriminate a scapular muscle.

Lower Thoracic Pain

Pain arising from the neck or upper two thoracic joints does not reach below the sixth thoracic dermatome. Pain felt below this level, particularly if it lies fairly close to the spine, has a thoracic source, and the thoracic joints are examined. The movements tested are: (1) flexion, (2) extension, (3) both side-flexions, (4) both rotations. Range is tested; the normal range of active rotation of the thorax on the pelvis is 70 degrees in each direction. If pain is provoked, its site must be noted. Care is taken to inquire for pain occurring at half-range; for a painful arc, especially on rotation, is common and pathognomonic of a disc lesion.

Passive Movements

The patient sits, his hands on his abdomen. The examiner stands, grasping his shoulders, holding his knees between his own. His pelvis is thus fixed while the passive rotation is carried out. Rotation to 90 degrees in each direction exists at the thoracic joints in all but the elderly—more than can be performed actively. It follows that in thoracic articular lesions much more discomfort can be elicited by passive than by active movement.

Passive extension is tested with the patient prone. Each joint is pressed towards extension with a slight jerk in the hope that it will hurt at one more than another, or that greater resistance will be encountered, thus identifying the exact level of the lesion. Unfortunately, the same amount of discomfort or stiffness is apt to be elicited at several adjacent levels.

Stretching the Dura Mater and Nerve-roots

Neck flexion

This stretches the dura mater upwards, since the neck is 3 cm. longer in full flexion than in full extension. In consequence, this movement is apt to tauten the dura mater against an intraspinal projection or to lift up a nerve-root until it impinges. Hence, the symptoms of any intraspinal space-occupying lesion at a thoracic level may be exacerbated by neck-flexion. The sign is common to disc lesions, small benign tumours and disseminated sclerosis (in which connection it was described by Lhermitte in 1929).

Sometimes, although neck-flexion does not cause or increase symptoms, it aggravates the pain after it has already been elicited by passive rotation, when the thorax is held twisted to the extreme of range. It can then be deduced that an articular lesion exists, interfering with dural mobility. This can be only a posterior projection, i.e. a disc lesion.

Scapular Approximation

For a long time it has been obscure why scapular approximation is apt to increase the pain caused by a disc lesion at any thoracic level. In the past, this finding has been repeatedly misinterpreted, and has led to disc lesions being attributed to trouble in the trapezius or in a rhomboid muscle. That the fault lies in the muscle is easily disproved, for passive approximation of the scapulae (which relaxes these muscles) hurts just as much.

Scapular approximation pulls on the first and second thoracic nerve-roots and sets up scapular pain, of course, in first and second thoracic nerve-root pressure. But it thereby lifts also the whole thoracic extent of the dura mater upwards. This movement is apt to elicit pain when even a lower thoracic disc lesion is present. Indeed, as manipulative reduction proceeds, it may be the last sign to disappear.

The First Thoracic Stretch

Another sign exists, positive only when the mobility of the first thoracic root is impaired.

The patient is asked to bring his arm out horizontally in the coronal plane, and to bend his elbow until his forearm points vertically upwards. This should not alter the symptoms. He is then asked fully to flex his elbow, putting his hand behind his neck. This stretches the ulnar nerve, which pulls on the first thoracic nerve-root, setting up the pain in the scapular area or arm.

Parenchymatous Involvement

Conduction along an intercostal nerve is seldom appreciably affected in thoracic root-pressure caused by a protruded disc; hence, articular signs with root-pain without signs of impaired conduction is the usual combination. A small area of cutaneous hypersensitiveness or analgesia is occasionally demonstrable anteriorly; alternatively, a wide band is found with borders so ill-defined as to afford no real help towards indicating the level of the protrusion. Occasionally a small patch of analgesia in the groin characterizes pressure at the twelfth thoracic level. Paralysis of one intercostal muscle would, on the contrary, be highly significant, but I have yet to detect this phenomenon. Electromyography might help here.

Disc-protrusion at the first thoracic level should provide a welcome exception, since clear signs of a first thoracic root-palsy would obtrude as soon as the strength of the small muscles of the patient's hand is tested. However, I have not yet encountered a case of unilateral first thoracic root-pressure severe enough to weaken the muscles. Cases with neurological signs were all found to suffer from other conditions: e.g., secondary malignant deposits in this vertebra, pulmonary sulcus tumour, pressure by a cervical or first rib, or on the ulnar nerve at the elbow or wrist.

Spinal Cord Signs

Pressure on the spinal cord is rare, but in all cases of suspected thoracic disc protrusion the signs of an upper motor neurone lesion should be sought, whether articular and nerve-root signs are present or not. If the posterior displacement lies strictly centrally and has come on slowly, articular and nerve-root signs are absent, but in large postero-lateral protrusions, the signs of both disorders may be combined.

Pins and needles felt in both lower limbs on neck-flexion may prove the only symptom or sign, occurring equally with a central cervical, as with a central thoracic (but not lumbar) protrusion. In a recent minor case, not severe enough to warrant immediate laminectomy, much anxiety is naturally aroused. Some progress and require operation, but there are cases of slight spastic uni- or diplegia, caused by a thoracic disc lesion, with symptoms and signs that remained unaltered for up to twenty years. Even osteopathy has in some cases proved harmless, though it has also precipitated catastrophe requiring immediate laminectomy.

Resisted Movements

At the thorax, the resisted movements have particular importance. Unlike the cervical and lumbar regions where muscle lesions scarcely occur, the muscles of the thorax and abdomen can suffer strain leading to post-traumatic scarring and persistent symptoms. A pectoral or intercostal muscle may be affected in this way, as may the latissimus dorsi, the inferior posterior serratus, the rectus or the oblique abdominal muscles.

Resisted rotation is best tested sitting as for passive rotation, and the result compared with the response to active and passive rotation. Side-flexion is best tested with the patient standing, the examiner resisting the movement by applying his hip to the patient's, grasping his far shoulder, and asking him to bend away from the side where the examiner stands (Fig. 53).

Resisted flexion is best tested with the patient sitting, while the examiner holds his knees and presses against his upper sternum. The response to active, passive and resisted extension can be simply contrasted by asking the prone patient to: (a) lift his chest off the couch with his arms behind his back, (b) push himself up with his arms letting the back sag (press up), and (c) attempt extension against the examiner's pressure at the base of the neck and at the knees.

Psychogenic symptoms at the thorax are not uncommon. By the time the neck has been examined, then the arm down to the hand, then the active, passive and resisted thoracic movements, followed by the lumbar spine, sacro-iliac joints and lower limbs, the patient is hopelessly confused and has put forward a self-contradictory pattern. Pain provoked by resisted thoracic movement is a particularly likely allegation in such cases; for the patient is apt to equate effort with pain. Hence, a pattern indicating an inconceivable series of lesions emerges.

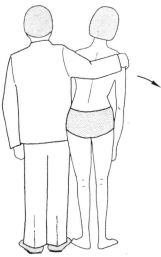

FIG. 53. Resisted side-flexion. The patient applies his hip to the examiner's and bends away from him as hard as possible. The examiner resists the movement by holding on to his far shoulder.

Radiology

This seldom affords any help in disc lesions. The physical signs show that a protrusion is causing symptoms, but I am unable to reach greater clinical accuracy than to estimate the level as upper, mid- or lower thoracic. Should an isolated joint within the requisite bounds chance to show a markedly diminished joint space or much larger osteophytes than the others, this may be taken tentatively to indicate the joint affected. Calcification of one or more discs has no significance.

Myelography is urgently indicated when signs of pressure on the spinal cord are present; it reveals the level of the obstruction. Postero-lateral protrusions are difficult to demonstrate unless Jirout's technique of dynamic pneumomyelography is employed (see page 466). In any case, myelography is called for only preparatory to laminectomy; an operation that the degree of these patients' disablement seldom warrants. Surgery is apt to prove dangerous, and should be advocated with reserve.

RESULTS OF EXAMINATION

The pattern that emerges when a thoracic disc lesion is present is, as elsewhere, the partial articular pattern characteristic of internal derangement.

Pain, therefore, is to be expected, and perhaps limitation, on some but not other of the thoracic active movements; more pain when these movements are carried out passively; no pain when the same movements are attempted against so great a resistance that the joint stays motionless.

As always in internal derangement, the partial capsular pattern emerges. One side-flexion or rotation movement is limited, the other not. As a rule two, three or four of the active movements of the thorax hurt; correspondingly four, three or two do not. Often the articular movements elicit the posterior ache only, not affecting the anterior component which is apt to be increased on neck-flexion alone. In difficult cases comparing the results of passive and resisted extension may prove helpful. A combination of articular with dural signs is common, but either may exist alone. Not only neck-flexion but approximation of the scapulae often brings on the pain, because this movement pulls on the dura mater via the upper two thoracic nerve-roots.

One rotation, often both, especially when carried out passively, nearly always hurts in a lower or mid-thoracic disc lesion. In a minor case, this may be the only painful movement. Even so, if passive rotation hurts and resisted rotation does not, a clear articular sign has emerged. If neck-flexion now increases the ache present on full rotation, the diagnosis is clear.

So little movement is possible at the upper two thoracic joints owing to rigidity of the first and second ribs and sternum that, in lesions at these two levels, the articular signs may be wholly absent, only the movements stretching the nerve-root increasing the pain.

Muscle lesions do not radiate pain from the posterior thorax to the anterior; this fact taken alone exculpates the muscles. If a resisted movement hurts and the passive movements—other than the one that fully stretches the muscle—do not, a muscle lesion is present. If no movement hurts, the pain is unconnected with the moving parts, and renewed search for a visceral origin must be undertaken.

Caution

There is one pattern of which the examiner must beware. Active side-flexion away from the painful side is *limited* and painful; both passive rotations are full and painless. Neoplasm of the lung or even in the upper abdomen may be present, alternatively, there is an intraspinal neuroma at a lower thoracic level. The last three cases I saw with this sign had respectively, carcinoma of the hepatic flexure of the colon, neoplasm of the lower lung, and a dumbell neuroma at the tenth level, lying partly inside and partly outside the spine.

Treatment

Postural Prophylaxis

In kyphosis, the posterior aspect of each of the joints between the vertebral bodies gapes and the anterior aspect is narrowed. This if, of course, the position of the joint most favourable to retropulsion of the intra-articular contents. The cervical and lumbar lordoses have the welcome effect of reversing this inclination of the joint-surfaces: they thus serve to prevent displacements at the upper and lower extent of the vertebral column. These lordoses happily placed at the more mobile spinal joints necessitate the existence of an intermediate compensatory kyphosis; otherwise the centre of gravity of the body would lie too far anteriorly. In consequence, kyphosis has developed at the thoracic part of the spine, where movement and, by corollary, the likelihood of displacement of a fragment of disc, is greatly restricted by the rigidity of the thoracic cage.

It should be realized that even in individuals so supple that they can bend backwards and put their head between their thighs, the thoracic spine, owing to the inextensibility of the sternum, has been shown by radiography never to extend beyond a straight line. Hence, it is quite hopeless to expect a patient to maintain a thoracic lordosis; no such achievement is possible. Any patient with a lower thoracic disc lesion should avoid flexing his back and, more important, should not rotate it during flexion, especially if lifting a weight; he must avoid prolonged compression of the joints, i.e. carrying, and should maintain as great a degree of extension as possible during weight-lifting.

Those who sit all day and develop the—usually upper—thoracic ache due to posterior nuclear bulging must have their work rearranged so that the maintenance of kyphosis is no longer necessary. To this end, papers should be placed higher on an inclined plane so that the office worker has to lean away from them, i.e. backwards. A music stand supporting paper above the typewriter forces a typist to look upwards. A drawing board may be held almost vertically.

Swimming is the only advantageous sport in thoracic (or lumbar) disc lesions. When the body floats, all compression strain on the joint ceases, and keeping the head out of water involves some degree of trunk extension: the beneficial posture. This does not apply to diving, since this involves trunk-flexion.

Manipulative Reduction

This is attempted in all cases, unless a contra-indication exists.

Contra-indications

Pressure on the spinal cord precludes any attempt at manipulation, i.e. a spastic gait, incoordination of the lower limbs, extensor plantar responses. Such patients should be left severely alone and laminectomy considered.

Paraesthetic feet show that the lesion has begun to touch the spinal cord. In such cases manipulation is contra-indicated but traction is well worth trying, and, in cases of not too long standing, may well succeed.

Indication for Manipulation

The articular signs are of the expected type, some hurting, some not, usually unilaterally, and one or both rotations prove painful. Limitation, if present, is usually of one rotation only. Dural signs are elicited but spinal cord symptoms and signs are absent. No signs of interference with an intercostal nerve-root are detected.

All the findings that, at cervical or lumbar levels, show that manipulation will fail, have no bearing on lesions lying between the third and twelfth thoracic vertebrae. Whether the root-pain came first or followed posterior aching, how long the root-pain has been present, whether the history suggests a nuclear or a cartilaginous protrusion—none of these considerations is material. Nuclear protrusions are most uncommon and come to light only when the attempt at manipulative reduction fails; if so, the protrusion is usually centrally placed in a patient with considerable thoracic kyphosis.

Technique

Manipulative reduction should be carried out: (a) without general anaesthesia; (b) during traction. The actual manipulations are described in Vol. II, and only general principles require mention here.

Traction is applied either by two assistants—one pulling on the patient's arms or head (depending on the level of the lesion), the other at his feet. If two physiotherapists trained in this work are employed, they can help the manipulator a great deal by altering their line of pull at the same moment as he forces the requisite movement.

After each manipulation, the patient stands up and states what difference (if any) he notices; the manipulator notes any objective alteration in the range of movement at the affected joint. This precaution prevents patients being made worse, as is sometimes unavoidable during general anaesthesia. As long as any particular manipulation does good, it is repeated. When it ceases to help, the manipulator passes on to the next one. This goes on until full reduction has been secured, or the patient has clearly had enough for one day, or it becomes evident that the protrusion is irreducible.

Once well, the patient should attend again quickly if he suffers a recurrence; indeed, it is an exceptional patient with a thoracic disc lesion who attends less often than once every year or two. It is only at the upper four thoracic levels, where disc lesions are uncommon, where so little joint movement is possible that reduction is normally permanent. However, many patients are kept continuously comfortable, by having their protrusion reduced by manipulation at once whenever it recurs.

Oscillatory Technique

The to-and-fro movements devised by Maitland are particularly useful in two sets of circumstances. (1) A thoracic disc lesion may cause considerable aching, but very minor articular signs; this is particularly apt to happen secondary to wedge-fracture. (2) The patient has such severe thoracic lumbago that the ordinary manipulations are difficult to tolerate. Oscillatory manœuvres continued for, say, fifteen minutes often reduce the displacement to the point where the ordinary manœuvres become possible.

Sustained Traction

Thoracic disc lesions seldom protrude centrally and remain fixed in that position. If they do, especially if the patient has a postural kyphosis or an old crush fracture, manipulation may be dangerous or unlikely to succeed, or both. Alternatively, a history of gradual onset may suggest a pulpy protrusion. Or, manipulative reduction, when tentatively begun, may aggravate the symptoms. When pins and needles are felt in the feet, manipulation is avoided and traction is indicated.

In such cases, reduction by sustained traction should be attempted at once (see Vol. II); it seldom fails. The traction lasts 30 to 45 minutes daily; a small woman may need 35 kg., a large man 70 kg.

Prevention of Recurrence

The same precautions must be taken as are set out under postural prophylaxis (p. 365).

Corsetry

Whereas a corset is a great protection against recurrence in lumbar disc lesions, there is no corresponding benefit from wearing a corset with steels extending from the lower buttock to the upper thorax. This is always prescribed, but is the reverse of what is required. If the thorax is to be immobilized, the more the lumbar spine is free to move, the better. Hence the cloth part of the corset can enclose the pelvis or not, as the patient and corset-fitter prefer, but the steels must start at the mid-lumbar region only (for a lower thoracic disc lesion) or at the lowest thoracic level (for a mid-thoracic lesion).

Ligamentous sclerosis

Since the thoracic spine is devoid of lordosis, the patient, though he must do his best, cannot always keep his intervertebral joint so tilted that it is open wider in front than behind. This is particularly so after wedge-fracture of a vertebral body, for consequent kyphosis at the joints either side of the fracture is considerable, and the supra- and inter-spinous ligaments on each side of the fracture are grossly overstretched.

In all cases in which a marked tendency to recurrence becomes manifest, sclerosing injections into the ligaments joining the spinous processes should be given. The result may not become apparent until a couple of months after the third infiltration, but there is a good chance of enhanced stability.

Recumbency

This is the traditional treatment for all pain of spinal origin felt at the posterior aspect of the trunk. If manipulation and traction both fail, prolonged rest in bed is the only alternative. Happily, this wearisome treatment is very seldom required but, when it is, the outlook is indeed poor; for each recurrence then has to be dealt with by renewed recumbency.

In elderly patients, the capsular contracture of osteoarthritis prevents the bones from coming apart when weight-bearing ceases. If so, recumbency is fruitless.

Operation

Laminectomy is feasible only when contrast myelography reveals the site of the protrusion. In early cases of spinal cord compression, laminectomy must be considered and, if the lesion is progressive, carried out. But the cases of recurrent thoracic pain with increasing pins and needles in the lower limbs that render the patient more and more unable to carry on are best treated by arthrodesis. The myelogram is usually negative, since the protrusion is not yet large enough to indent the dura mater sufficiently to interfere with the flow of contrast material, but clinical examination can determine the level within two or three joints. Arthrodesis carried out over four or five joints has been conspicuously successful in several cases of this kind.

Osteopathy and Chiropraxy

The difficulty in distinguishing between visceral disease and root-pressure set up by a thoracic disc lesion is responsible for many diagnostic errors. This has served to strengthen laymen's claims that visceral disease results from vertebral displacements and is curable by their reduction. The osteopath or chiropracter is himself misled when the patient, after his spine has been manipulated, declares that his, say, 'cholecystitis' or 'angina' has ceased. A doctor has diagnosed visceral disease. Finding that his spinal treatment has relieved it, the manipulator naturally imagines that he has really cured a visceral disorder; so does the patient. In consequence, all sorts of theories exist on the effect of vertebral manipulation on the autonomic system.

The many vocal and satisfied patients of lay-manipulators—most of them by no means the neurotics so often supposed—combine to show how often a thoracic disc lesion remains unsuspected.

COMPRESSION PHENOMENA

Since some degree of kyphosis is universal at the mid- and upper-thoracic joints, symptoms due to gradual retropulsion are common, especially in individuals with a marked thoracic kyphosis.

1. Posterior Bulging at the Thoracic Spinal Joints

Mid- or upper-thoracic central aching is apt to come on in those who sit bent forward for long periods on end. The discomfort is probably caused not so much by an actual disc lesion as by a gradual and slight movement backwards of the entire intra-articular contents at several adjacent joints. After some years, this pressure stretches the posterior longitudinal ligament, bulging it backwards against the dura mater. The greater the patient's thoracic kyphosis, the longer he sits bent, and the more he compresses the spinal joints, the greater the likelihood of this occurring.

Diagnosis

This is made largely on the characteristic symptoms. The patient wakes comfortable; as the day goes on, the posterior thorax begins to ache centrally. The ache gets slowly worse, spreading bilaterally until most of the back of the chest is painful. Carrying anything heavy or sitting for some time increases the symptoms; lying down for a few minutes, later for some hours, brings relief. While the pain is bad, a deep breath usually hurts. This pain goes on appearing by day and ceasing at night, coming on earlier in the morning as the years go by, and taking longer to abate with recumbency. Improvement follows change in the patient's circumstances, e.g. leaving a kyphotic occupation (such as sewing) or acquiring domestic help.

Examination shows minimal articular signs and an absence of all other signs. The patient who describes a complaint that gives rise to practically no signs, and then is found to have practically no signs, must be believed. He is not suffering from psychoneurosis; for hypersensitive patients have multiple symptoms and display exaggeration and incongruity in their signs, not a consistent negative.

For the first ten to thirty years, the radiograph reveals no abnormality. Finally, anterior erosion takes place, as described below.

Treatment

In the early stages this should be to change the patient's occupation to one more suitable, combined with explanation on how the pain is produced and, by corollary, avoided. Later, as the condition develops, lying down for an hour in the late morning and again in the afternoon may keep the pain within bounds. If this does not suffice, sustained traction is indicated and is best given daily for, say, a fortnight, then at weekly, finally monthly, intervals. Traction can finally be stopped, but relief seldom lasts more than six months, when it must be repeated. Alternatively, a 'lively' corset made in two halves, the upper and lower parts of which are held distracted by a strong spring (Coplans, 1956), can be worn, but only if the compression lies at a lower thoracic level. Manipulation is contra-indicated; for no reducible fragment is present.

2. Anterior Erosion

Finally, a thoracic kyphosis leads to such continued pressure on the anterior aspect of each disc that the front of the bodies of two adjacent vertebrae wear it through and meet. Where bone touches bone, a localized anterior osteophyte appears on each vertebral body, with bone sclerosis at the point of contact. Though this outcrop can be called an osteophyte, its existence does not mean that the whole joint is osteoarthritic in the sense that a patient may be said to be suffering from osteoarthritis of hip or ankle. It is a localized pressure phenomenon. Bone contains nerves and is a sentinent structure. Hence bone pressing against bone can well cause pain. The osteophyte is not the cause of pain, but the result of the disc-erosion that has enabled the bones finally to grind together painfully, and the pain would have appeared had no osteophytes formed.

Anterior erosion of the disc takes years to develop; hence, patients with this condition are nearly always middle-aged or elderly, possess a rounded thoracic kyphosis and give a past history of posterior articular bulging (see above). The intermittent thoracic ache finally becomes constant, and analgesic drugs become necessary. The radiograph shows the typical changes. Not all patients with this radiological appearance suffer much discomfort; the degree of pain caused is extremely variable and more attention should be paid to the patient's statements than to the X-ray appearances.

Clinical examination shows very little. The characteristic kyphosis is noted; the limitation of movement is obvious but the joints are often so stiff that the active movements prove painless and only the passive movements elicit the articular pain.

A conservative treatment sometimes effective is traction, repeated at such intervals (if it succeeds for the time being) as the symptoms warrant. Daily neck suspension provides an alternative.

3. Lateral Erosion

Exactly the same mechanism occurs in long standing severe scoliosis. At the concave side, the intra-articular disc becomes worn through and bone touches bone painfully with the same local sclerosis but less pronounced osteophytes. Unilateral pain felt in the erector muscles of, usually, the lower thorax is the first symptom. Since the bulge is lateral, not posterior, and thus cannot press on the dura mater or a nerve-root, no symptoms arise until bone touches bone. The ache is purely local and unilateral, without radiation to the front of the trunk. A deep breath is painless, and dural signs are absent. Finally, the pain becomes constant by day, and is aggravated by any exertion tending to press the joint surfaces together, e.g. carrying. For many years a night's rest brings relief, but ultimately the ache may persist all night.

The passive movements at the relevant spinal joints hurt; the stiffness is such that the active movements are grossly limited but more or less painless. The resisted movements do not hurt. Sustained traction is the only conservative treatment worth attempting, but often fails. If the symptoms warrant, extensive operative fusion is indicated.

PATHOLOGICAL WEDGING

The bodies of the thoracic vertebrae become wedged as the result of a number of different pathological processes.

1. Adolescent Osteochondritis

This occurs at the lower half of the thoracic spine (and in the upper lumbar region). Between the ages of fourteen and eighteen, an osteo-chondritis may appear at the end-plate of one or two adjacent vertebrae. Osteochondritis is merely a descriptive label; as at other epiphyses, both the cause and the nature of the disorder are unknown. The end-plate disappears anteriorly and nuclear material erodes the now unprotected bone; marked wedging results. The process is painless and in itself insignificant, but it leads to a permanent increase in the degree of kyphosis at the affected joints. This posture tends to eventual retropulsion of disc-substance, and posterior bulging due to compression occurring in patients who may still be quite young.

The lateral radiograph (Plate 35) shows the condition clearly, but since the disorder often causes no symptoms, X-ray evidence of vertebral osteochondritis, past or present, must not be regarded as significant, unless the symptoms and clinical signs point to an articular lesion at the affected level.

When adolescent osteochondritis occurs to a rather lesser degree but over many vertebrae, the disorder is named Schauermann's disease.

I have never seen a case of Calvé's osteochondritis of the vertebral body itself with consequent wedging.

2. Fracture

Flexion injuries may cause fracture of a vertebral body. The immediate pain usually encircles the trunk at the appropriate level; this girdle pain lasts a week or two. At the end of three months symptoms have ceased; no treatment is necessary unless the patient is seen during the first few days, when a week in bed may be required. If the bone alone has been damaged, no further trouble need be feared. If the disc has also suffered, endless trouble is to be expected. Permanent kyphosis exists at the joint on each side of the fracture, and manipulative reduction is apt to prove very temporary. Such patients, when involved in law-suits, are apt to be described as suffering from compensation neurasthenia; some are, it is true, but many others are not. They are suffering from a lesion that the radiograph cannot reveal, and force sufficient to break bone may well injure adjacent cartilage as well. The flexion deformity may give rise to considerable ligamentous aching in the overstretched supra- and inter-spinous ligaments and to a feeling of insecurity on bending forwards. In either case, sclerosing injections are indicated. If fixed flexion deformity eventually leads to a compression phenomenon, pain is apt to return, perhaps years later. Occasionally, post-traumatic ossification in the liga-ments leads to fixation of the joint and permanent cure.

The convulsion of E.C.T. may, by hyperflexing the spine, drive the nucleus pulposus into the body of a vertebra. No wedging results and slight and transitory pain in the bone from the minor fracture is the only symptom. The radiograph is diagnostic.

3. Senile Osteoporosis

This disorder affects the whole thoraco-lumbar spine and pelvis of elderly persons, more often women (see Plate 37); the neck and the bones of the limbs are not appreciably affected.

The bodies of the vertebrae soften; hence the first radiological sign is a marked biconcavity of the vertebral body, caused by disc-substance pushing its way evenly towards the spongiosum. At this stage, *there are no symptoms*, and it is a common mistake to suppose that, if a patient has a backache and the radiograph shows senile osteoporosis, the lesion accounts for the backache. The same appearance is seen in young patients who once suffered from severe rickets, and in tropical osteomalacia. Later on pathological wedging may occur. If this takes place suddenly, fracture with girdle pain results, leading after a week or two to localized bone pain. After three months, the fracture has united and symptoms have ceased unless the flexion deformity gives rise to retropulsion of the articular contents as a compression phenomenon. If the wedging takes place gradually, it may cause no symptoms, but in due course the compression phenomenon may ensue. Palpation for the kyphos should be followed by radiography.

Nordin (1959), working with the radio-isotope 47Ca, showed that the rate at which bone was laid down was not reduced and that osteoporosis was caused by enhanced resorption of bone, the result and not the cause of a negative calcium balance. Steroid therapy is well known to induce such a negative balance, with increased loss, mainly faecal, of both calcium and phosphorus. Rose (1965) states that fluoride and calcium therapy is with-out avail. In my experience, 1 gm. of calcium gluconate three times daily together with an anabolic steroid often prevents further deformity and should be continued indefinitely. Testosterone appears to have no such effect. Calcitonin may prove useful; for it lowers the plasma calcium level.

4. Pathological Fracture

The angular kyphos is palpable and radiography shows the cause. When this is due to isolated myeloma of the vertebral body, X-ray therapy may be permanently effective. Tuberculous caries has been regarded as calling for immobilization and arthrodesis but Konstam and Blesovsky (1962), working on unpromising clinical material in Ibadan, published a review of 207 cases of spinal tuberculosis treated with isoniazid and para-amino-salicylic acid without plaster, the patients remaining ambulant. Even the 56 with paraplegia were allowed to get about as much as they were able. Complete recovery was obtained in 178 cases of the 207, and in 51 of the 56 paraplegics.

Schmorl's Nodes

These appear for the first time at about the age of sixteen at the lower thoracic and upper lumbar levels and represent small invasions of the vertebral body by nuclear disc-material protruding vertically. They never cause any symptoms, at the time of their occurrence or later. By fixing the annulus in the centre of the joint and thus preventing a tendency to pressure directed posteriorly they may well protect the patient against posterior protrusion.

THORACIC SCOLIOSIS

Congenital Scoliosis

The mother notes that the baby lies always on one side, but the rotation deformity often remains unnoticed and is regarded, when it is perceived, as an infantile scoliosis.

Adolescent Scoliosis

This starts at about the age of ten, when the rate of bone-growth increases. It is commoner in girls, and the prominent convex side is more often the right. The deformity increases until vertebral bone growth ceases at sixteen to eighteen years of age. It then remains static till middle-age, when the discs begin to wear away on the concave side; the deformity then increases again. When they are completely eroded and bone touches bone, pain appears for the first time. It is remarkable how seldom the ordinary type of thoracic disc lesion with attacks of intermittent displacement of a loose fragment complicate thoracic scoliosis.

Orthopaedic surgeons disagree on whether treatment makes an appreciable difference to the outcome of scoliosis. Early stapling or arthrodesis obviously can stop an increasing deformity from getting worse, but it is very doubtful if exercises and corsetry do much for the child; their chief virtue appears to me to be giving the parents the feeling that 'something is being done'. After the age of sixteen, nothing further is required, since growth of the vertebrae ceases then.

Secondary Scoliosis

Hemivertebra, neuro-fibromatosis, thoracoplasty and anterior polio-myelitis affecting the trunk muscles asymmetrically are the likely causes.

It had always been thought that, in scoliosis complicating neurological disorders, the deformity resulted from unequal muscle pull, the stronger muscle naturally lying on the concave side of the curve. Kleinberg (1951) pointed out that this was not necessarily so. The contrary can happen; moreover, the degree of deformity is not necessarily proportional to the severity of the muscle weakness. Purdon Martin (1965) described fourteen patients with post-encephalitic Parkinsonism who had developed a scolio-sis. Some patients deviated towards, others away from, the more rigid side. In two cases, the curvature was corrected when operation on the glo-bus pallidus relieved the rigidity. He therefore suggests that the scoliosis is the result of positive neuro-muscular action.

THORACIC ANKYLOSING SPONDYLITIS

In ankylosing spondylitis, the distinctive feature is pain coming and going irrespective of what the patient does. During a good period, no degree of exertion has any effect; during a bad period, the back may ache without provocation. When the thoracic spine is affected, the pain is posterior and central, but when the anterior longitudinal ligament be-comes involved, it may be epigastric or sternal and worst on waking. A deep breath does not hurt, but there may be a feeling of tightness, owing to the onset of rigidity of the costo-vertebral joints.

Realisation that the symptoms stem from thoracic spondylitis depends on examination of the whole spine.

A flat lumbar spine associated with an upper thoracic kyphosis is suggestive, and marked limitation of side-flexion in each direction at all the lumbar and thoracic spinal joints is pathognomonic. Sacro-iliac and lumbar involvement sometimes proceed painlessly; even so, with rare exceptions, the lumbar spine becomes rigid before the thoracic joints stiffen. Since spondylitis in the sacro-iliac joints never begins after the age of forty and usually begins during the twenties, the restriction of lumbo-thoracic movement is detected long before the age when limitation from advanced osteophyte formation can have set in. When spondylitis has omitted the lumbar spine and has jumped from the sacro-iliac to the thoracic joints, diagnosis is very difficult; for thoracic aching due to the spondylitic process begins while a full range of movement remains at the lumbar spine; moreover, there has not been any gluteal or lumbar discomfort. The hint is given by the complaint of an ache worse on waking, coming and going for years without apparent cause or connection with exertion. Clinical examination shows that the range of passive thoracic rotation is limited to 45 degrees or 60 degrees (normal 90 degrees), and that at the extreme of the possible range the movement stops with a hard end-feel and a great deal more pain than would be provoked if merely a minor long-standing disc lesion were present. Repeated radiographs have revealed no abnormality at the thoracic joints, but these clinical findings naturally call for X-ray examination of the sacro-iliac joints, at which the tell-tale sclerosis is seen.

Treatment consists of relief from pain and stiffness by means of either butazolidine or indomethacin, and surprisingly small doses often suffice. If there is pain only in the mornings, 100 mgs. of butazolidine taken last thing at night may enable the patient to wake comfortable. Other patients prefer indomethacin and 25 mgs. three times a day are often prescribed, but except during an exacerbation, one or two tablets a day are often enough. During a remission, all drugs are avoided.

Surprisingly, fixation of the chest, with consequent reliance purely on the diaphragm for breathing, does not lead to increased incidence of pneumonia, etc. Zorab (1966) states that in a Ministry of Pensions analysis of the cause of death in seventy cases of advanced spondylitis only five were from an acute respiratory disorder.

LESIONS OF THE THORACIC CAGE

The intrinsic thoracic muscles, notably the intercostal muscles, are liable to direct bruising. The muscles connecting scapula and humerus to the thorax may be painfully strained, especially in athletes. Hence an essential part of the examination of the thorax is to test the resisted movements of the neck, scapula, arm, thorax and abdominal wall.

It should be remembered that diaphragmatic, intercostal or abdominal muscular symptoms and signs, when accompanied by fever, may result from epidemic myalgia, less often from infestation with Trichina spiralis.

Intercostal Muscles and Ribs

Damage to one or more intercostal muscles follows direct bruising, nearly always at the front of the chest. The ribs may or may not remain intact. Fracture of a rib must involve some muscle fibres tearing close to the break. When there is no displacement of the fractured ends, the surfaces fit and movement here is not a cause of appreciable symptoms. Nevertheless, breathing and other active movements set up pain, clearly of muscular origin. The patient points to the spot in a characteristic way; he places one finger on the exact place. In other painful affections at the thorax the pain is diffuse and he indicates the site of symptoms with the palm of his hand.

Referred pain does not arise from an intercostal muscle, for it is developed at the distal end of one short segment; moreover, it lies superficially.

The main diagnostic difficulty is the primary postero-lateral disc protrusion causing anterior pain only; in the other types the pain is posterior as well as anterior and no confusion can arise. Full active trunk extension stretches the affected intercostal muscle and resisted flexion and rotation of the trunk also usually hurt. Luckily these are the very movements that do not hurt a patient with a thoracic disc lesion. Springing the chest wall by pressure on the rib at a distance from the injured point hurts in fracture but not in a disc lesion. Palpation has no diagnostic value, since a referred tender area can always be found at the front of the chest wall in any case of disc lesion with anterior pain. If, however, a fractured rib or a strained intercostal muscle is found, local tenderness defines its exact site.

Medico-legal considerations apart, when the intercostal muscles are damaged by direct bruising, it makes no difference whether an uncomplicated fracture of one or more ribs is present or not. The cause of pain and the treatment are the same.

Clicking of a costal cartilage is painless. Momentary discomfort, however, is felt when the point of one of the lower ribs hits the iliac crest, as may happen on side-flexion of the trunk in patients with exceptionally long floating ribs or with marked scoliosis. Quite severe pain lasting as long as a minute occurs when the point of a rib becomes loose anteriorly and is forced into the substance of the abdominal muscles on trunk flexion. The attacks are recurrent and the patient often supplies the diagnosis himself. Painful swelling of a costo-chondral junction (Tieze, 1921) is visible and palpable.

Treatment

Muscles

The intercostal muscles respond very quickly to massage. Especially if he is elderly, the patient cannot mobilize the muscle himself however deeply he breathes; hence pain persists indefinitely, but the scarring is broken down by transverse massage in a very few sessions (see Vol. II).

Fractured Rib

As already pointed out, it is tearing of the intercostal muscle, not the broken ribs themselves, that sets up pain in uncomplicated fracture. In recent cases the best immediate treatment is local anaesthesia induced at the affected muscle. The pain on breathing may be such as to cause shock, which the anaesthesia immediately abates. The severe pain very seldom returns. Further relief from pain can be achieved by strapping the affected side of the chest. The criterion for its application is the degree of pain, not the fact of fracture; hence, strapping is equally indicated in recent inter-costal lesions, whether or not associated with fracture.

Non-elastic strapping is applied horizontally; it must cross the mid-line at the sternum and at the spine, and must be applied very tightly at the extreme of a full expiratory movement (Fig. 54). Fractured ribs unite enough to become painless in four to six weeks and union is invariable; thus, pain persisting after this period has elapsed must arise in the inter-costal muscles. Should pain persist longer than a month, deep massage is indicated.

Loose Rib

If a loose rib or long floating rib causes sufficient symptoms, its anterior extent can be removed.

Muscle Lesions

Minor Trauma to the Diaphragm

These cases are uncommon. They result from blows on the chest with transmitted stress. The pain is on respiration only; no pain is elicited when trunk movements are performed while the patient holds his breath. It is my impression that the central fibres of the diaphragm give rise to pain felt at the point of the shoulder whereas the fibres near the ribs give rise to local pain only.

I have encountered one case only of a painful scar occurring at the attachment of the diaphragm to the back of the xiphisternum. The spot was just within finger's reach. The symptoms had been taken for indigestion for ten years and treated by drugs and finally cholecystectomy. Deep massage at this point gave lasting relief.

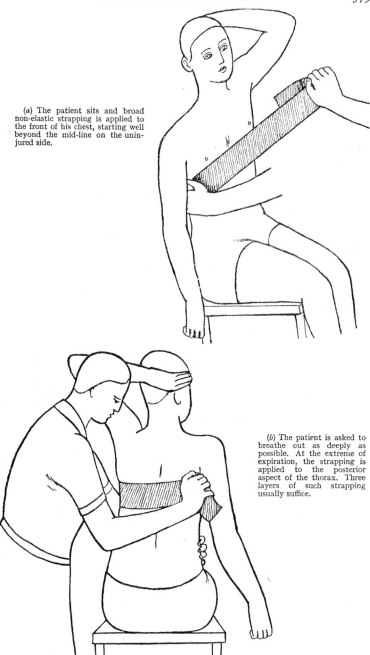

(a) The patient sits and broad non-elastic strapping is applied to the front of his chest, starting well beyond the mid-line on the uninjured side.

(b) The patient is asked to breathe out as deeply as possible. At the extreme of expiration, the strapping is applied to the posterior aspect of the thorax. Three layers of such strapping usually suffice.

FIG. 54. Strapping for fractured ribs.

Stitch

This is supposed to arise from the diaphragm and may be an ischaemic phenomenon akin to claudication. The alternative theory is tugging on the diaphragmatic origin of the peritoneal ligaments suspending stomach and liver. Running soon after a meal predisposes to stitch, which may be a recurrent phenomenon, coming on at the same moment in race after race.

Examination of the patient between attacks reveals no abnormality; after a race deep breathing hurts for a few minutes—nothing else. Lying down stops the pain.

It is alleged that keeping the arms into the sides during exertion postpones or avoids pain. As a rule, nothing avails.

Lesions of the Pectoralis Major and Latissimus Dorsi Muscles

These are dealt with in Chapter 11 since they are muscles controlling the arm. In the former case, the pain comes on gradually and is felt in the pectoral area, usually spreading down the inner side of the arm to the elbow. Full passive elevation of the arm stretches the muscle and hurts; it hurts also when a rib is fractured close to the pectoral origin and in Monder's phlebitis. Resisted adduction of the arm also hurts but resisted medial rotation usually does not. The best way to elicit pain in lesions of the pectoralis major muscle is to ask the patient to bring both arms horizontally forward and then press his two hands together as hard as he can (Fig. 39). The two areas most often affected are the inner fibres just below the clavicle or the lowest part of the outer edge close to the ribs. When the differentiation between an intercostal and a pectoral pain is required, and pain on a resisted adduction movement of the arm is not clearly elicited, the following test is useful. The patient places his hand on his hip and tenderness is compared while the pectoralis major muscle is in contraction and in relaxation. In the case of a pectoral lesion, the tenderness is greater on contraction. The pectoralis minor muscle appears never to suffer comparable strain, though it may be involved in contracture of the costo-coracoid fascia.

Treatment consists of local anaesthesia or deep massage (see Vol. II).

When the thoracic extent of the latissimus dorsi muscle is affected, the pain is localized. Resisted adduction and full passive elevation of the arm both hurt; the thoracic movements are painless. Local anaesthesia often has some lasting effect, and deep massage is quickly curative (see Vol. II).

COSTO-VERTEBRAL JOINTS

Movement at these joints lessens as age advances; in consequence, the respiratory excursion of the chest wall diminishes. A thoracic kyphosis, emphysema or a liability to asthma increases the tendency to early stiffness. In such cases, the joints should be kept as mobile as possible by passive forcing, whereupon the patient practises deep breathing exercises that maintain the added range. To this end the physiotherapist places her hands on the lower ribs and increases the respiratory movement of the chest wall by manual pressure (Fig. 55).

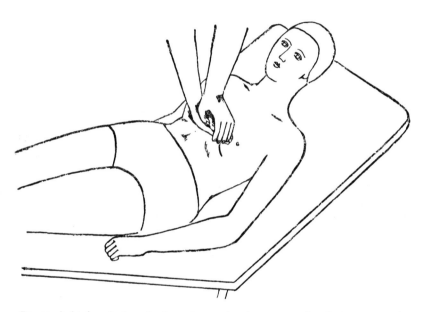

FIG. 55. Assisted expiration. As the patient reaches the extreme of expiration, pressure is exerted strongly at his lower sternum. This mobilizes the costo-vertebral joints.

In ankylosing spondylitis, the costo-vertebral joints eventually become fixed as part of the ligamentous ossifying process. During the involvement, which may take years, pain may be felt at one or both sides of the sternum or of the thoracic region posteriorly. It is apt to be most troublesome after some hours' sleep or on waking in the morning, i.e. after relative immobility. Breathing is uncomfortable and the patient feels the respiratory excursion of his chest to be restricted—as indeed it is. The trunk-movements do not alter the pain, but make the diagnosis clear; for side-flexion of the lumbar spine is largely or fully lost by the time the costo-vertebral joints are affected. Pressure on the sternum while the patient lies supine reproduces the pain. If one costo-vertebral joint only is affected, an endeavour should be made to inject hydrocortisone into it. Certainly, when the injection is correctly placed, relief is secured within twenty-four hours and usually lasts many months. If many are affected, indomethacin 25 mg. twice daily or butazolidine 100 mg. twice daily is indicated.

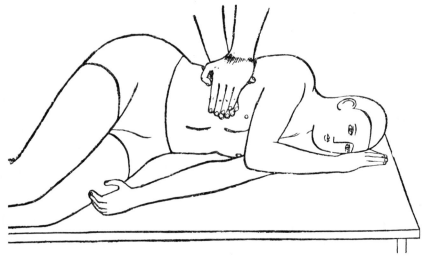

FIG. 56. Assisted inspiration. As the extreme of inspiration is reached, pressure is exerted on the lower ribs. This mobilizes the costo-vertebral joints in the opposite direction to that shown in Fig. 55.

Post-operative posture and respiration provide an important field for the physiotherapist. The patient's position in bed is most important, e.g., after thoracoplasty. After operations of any severity on the chest and abdomen, the vital capacity is much diminished. Breathing exercises, postural drainage and manual shaking greatly diminish the incidence of post operative pulmonary complications.

THE STERNUM

Most sternal pain has a visceral origin, but there are other sources.

Lesion of Bone

The sternum may be fractured; if so, an upper thoracic vertebra is often wedged as well. It may also be painfully invaded by metastases. In either case, the bone itself is tender and the radiograph diagnostic.

Manubrio Sternal joint

The cause of trouble at this joint is seldom an injury; monarticular rheumatoid arthritis or ankylosing spondylitis is more commonly responsible. The patient knows exactly where the pain is and the manubrio-sternal ligaments are swollen and tender. Hydrocortisone injected at the joint is most successful.

Tietze's Syndrome

The costo-chondral junction may become strained, especially in patients with a persistent cough, e.g. chronic bronchitics. The pain is brought on by a deep breath and cough and is felt to one side of the sternum, about 4 cm. from its edge. A small swelling is palpable at the affected junction, and the tenderness is on the bone. If the intercostal muscle or membrane is strained, the tenderness lies between the two bones and if the pain has lasted longer than a month, fracture of a rib cannot be responsible.

Pressure on the sternum or at the lateral aspect of the thorax usually reproduces the unilateral pain, and the site of tenderness is diagnostic. One infiltration with hydrocortisone is curative.

Pain Referred to the Sternum

An upper thoracic disc lesion protruding centrally may give rise to sternal pain only. If so, diagnosis is often difficult, since the upper thoracic joints possess little mobility, confined as they are by ribs and sternum. Hence the active thoracic articular movements may be misleadingly painless, only passive forcing reproducing the sternal ache. But the dural signs are usually clear, neck-flexion and scapular approximation reproducing the symptom well.

When the anterior longitudinal ligament is affected in ankylosing spondylitis, the pain may be purely sternal.

LESIONS OF THE ABDOMINAL WALL

An accurate, detailed history is essential in differentiating visceral disorder and thoracic disc lesions from anterior muscular pain. Except in athletes or after an operation for inguinal hernia, anterior abdominal pain seldom results from a muscular lesion; hence this ascription should be made unwillingly.

Examination of Abdominal Movements

When the abdominal muscles are affected, little information is supplied by the trunk movements of the standing patient; for only extension hurts in lesions of the abdominal musculature. The resisted abdominal movements are tested as follows.

The patient lies supine; then, resting his hands on his lap he sits up. The examiner places one hand on his feet and the other against his sternum, and a strong trunk-flexion movement is resisted (Fig. 57). Pain on such

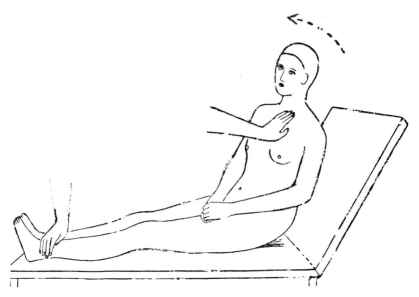

FIG. 57. Resisted flexion of trunk. The examiner supports the patient's legs with one hand while resisting the patient's attempt to sit up by pressure on his chest. Test for the rectus abdominis muscle.

resisted movement may be felt in the abdomen, in which case it arises from the rectus abdominis; or in one groin, in which case it arises from the flexor muscles of the hip. The sitting patient is next asked to twist his trunk against the examiner's resistance applied at both shoulders (Fig. 58). Pain on such a movement away from the painful side suggests a lesion of the external oblique muscle; towards the painful side, of the internal oblique muscle.

The structure defined by which movement proved painful should be examined for tenderness near the area where the pain is felt.

If the rectus abdominis muscle is at fault the lesion is most frequently above the umbilicus. Then, full active elevation of the ipsilateral arm, when the patient stands or lies flat, often stretches the muscle and causes

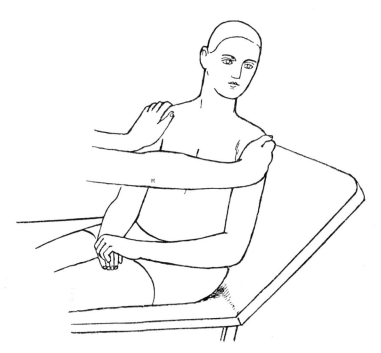

FIG. 58. Resisted rotation of trunk. The patient tries to twist his trunk against resistance applied at his shoulders. Test for the oblique abdominal and serratus posterior inferior muscles.

the abdominal pain. A small haematoma can often be felt. Tenderness at the pubic insertion suggests fracture or puerperal subluxation of the symphysis pubis rather than a muscular lesion.

When the origin of either oblique muscle from the ribs is affected, tenderness is best elicited by bringing the finger under the costal edge and pressing upwards and forwards. As some tenderness here is normal, the two sides must be carefully compared. The belly of an oblique muscle is involved as a rule at one or other iliac fossa. Chronic appendicitis may then be closely simulated. The following test serves to determine whether the source of pain is in the muscle or viscera.

The semi-recumbent patient is asked to raise his head and shoulders from the couch, i.e. to contract his abdominal muscles—and pressure is applied at the spot which has already been found to be tender. The patient is then asked to lie back and relax, and pressure of the same degree is applied again. If the pain is accentuated in the former event—namely, when the pressure is exerted against taut muscles which protect the underlying viscera—its source must be in the muscles or fasciae of the abdominal wall. If, on the other hand, it is greater when the patient relaxes, the source must lie inside the abdomen.

Gross weakness of the abdominal muscles results from advanced myopathy or anterior poliomyelitis.

The treatment of muscle lesions of the anterior abdominal wall is deep massage (see Vol. II).

SYMPHYSIS PUBIS

Puerperal subluxation results in pain and tenderness felt exactly at the symphysis as soon as the patient gets up after the confinement. Resisted trunk-flexion sets up local pain (Fig. 57). Radiography while the patient stands first on one leg, then the other, demonstrates the laxity, which allows up to half an inch of movement between the bone ends.

A tight binder is worn until the patient is usually symptom-free in six weeks. Obstetricians report that, after division of the symphysis pubis in difficult labour, fibrous union is complete in two months. In men, pain arising from this joint is a rarity; it is usually relieved by an injection of hydrocortisone.

The symphysis may be seen radiologically widened in the pubic osteitis that may come on one to two months after prostatectomy. A line of calcification at the centre of the symphysis due to deposition of calcium pyrophosphate occurs in pseudo-gout.

THE FEMALE BREAST

Retraction of the Nipple

Weller pointed out that stimulation of the back of the new-born baby's palate by the tip of the nipple initiates the wish to suck and swallow. The nipple must, therefore, pass the 2 cm. gap formed by the gums and reach 2·5 to 3 cm. beyond, by the length of the nipple itself and the amount of stretch in the areola. This is the minimum elastic yield that must be imparted for the establishment of the baby's eagerness to suck. Primipara's nipples should be examined and treatment should be undertaken during the seventh month of pregnancy. The nipple should be everted until it is more prominent than the areola and the expanded tip grasped between the thumb and two fingers. The physiotherapist shows the mother how to apply continued traction.

ANTENATAL AND POSTNATAL EXERCISES

Such antenatal exercises as are alleged to mobilize the sacro-iliac joints are at best valueless. Luckily they do not have this effect, otherwise the patient would suffer pain in the buttocks. They do however mobilize the lumbar spine towards flexion; this is a real disadvantage particularly when it is remembered how many backaches follow childbirth. The length of

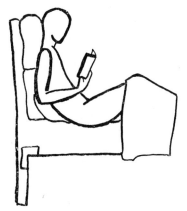

Fig. 59. The 'nursing mother's position'. Note the lack of support at the lumbar region which remains in kyphosis all day long. Disc protrusion is thus encouraged.

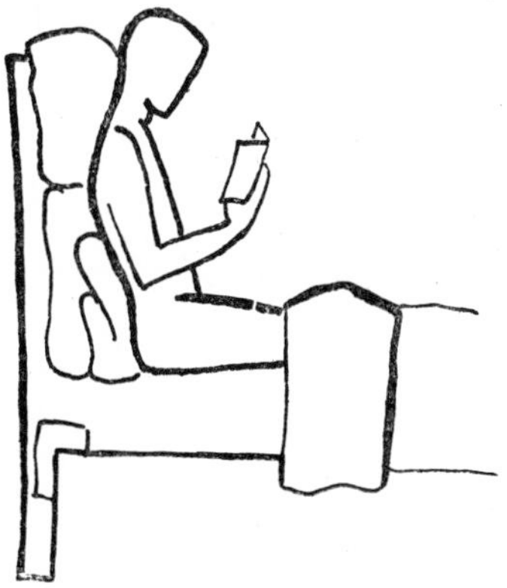

Fig. 60. The correct way to sit up in bed. A special pillow maintains the lumbar lordosis, and the posterior longitudinal ligament is spared.

labour, the call for analgesic drugs, the incidence of perineal laceration and the forceps rate is the same whether exercises have been carried out or not. This was proved by statistics from various hospitals, including St. Thomas's, and was confirmed by Rodaway (1957) and by Davidson (1962). On admission to the labour ward the demeanour of the patient prepared by prenatal classes is, however, noticeably happier and more confident, and it is clear that the explanation of the processes of birth and instruction in general relaxation that are given at these classes are as valuable as the exercises themselves are futile.

Since so many women state that they first developed backache soon

o

after the birth of a baby, it is obvious that great care should be taken of the lumbar spinal joints during the puerperium. Disc protrusion often begins from prolonged, severe stretching of the posterior longitudinal ligament at its lumbar extent by 'the nursing mother's position' (Fig. 59). Lying for days with a lumbar kyphosis tends to retropulsion of the disc and to stretching of the only ligament that holds a damaged disc in place. Such kyphosis is easily and comfortably avoided by a pillow placed in the lumbar region (Fig. 60). It is a further advantage if the patient turns to lie prone for several periods a day. Such simple attention to posture in bed is even more important in patients who have already suffered backache or lumbago.

Postnatal exercises contrast with the uselessness of antenatal exercises and should never be omitted; they should begin the day after the birth unless some obstetric contra-indication exists. In particular, the levator ani muscle should have its strength quickly restored; for it suffers overstretching during labour, and, unless its tone is restored by the time the patient gets up, the beginnings of retroversion, cystocele, stress incontinence and rectocele are laid down.

Exercises for the equally overstretched and flabby abdominal muscles follow. These should be performed statically or against resistance during lordosis rather than by active trunk-rotation movements during flexion, so as to avoid damaging the lumbar spine. Finally, exercises to the quadriceps and foot muscles are given to maintain their strength until the patient gets up, and to the calf muscles for the prophylaxis of venous thrombosis.

16

The Lumbar Region

Lumbar disc lesions are responsible for well over ninety per cent of all organic symptoms attributable to the lower back. This is a very different belief from twenty years ago. It was then taught, and believed, that affections of the muscles and fasciae of the lumbar area were the usual source of pain. This idea arose from Sir William Gower's lecture in 1904 when he postulated the existence of a disease called 'fibrositis', which, attacking the fibrous tissues of the lower back, caused lumbago. This notion was adopted and unchallenged for forty-one years until a fresh approach to lumbago was proposed (Cyriax, 1945). The new view is now widely accepted and it is largely agreed that a disc lesion causing internal derangement is the cause of lumbago. Indeed, Mixter and Barr stated in 1946 that disc lesions could cause backache only. Schiotz (1958) points out, however, that my father, Edgar Cyriax, wrote in *The Practitioner* in 1919 that 'the pathology of the vertebral cartilages has received but little attention. . . . As regards the intra-articular cartilages, I can find no mention of any investigations on their morbid anatomy. Presumably the laws that govern the general pathology of fibro-cartilage are applicable to the vertebral cartilages as well . . . In the vertebral column, symptoms are sometimes found that so exactly resemble those induced by cartilaginous displacement elsewhere that it can with safety be assumed that these occur in the spine'. He regards him as the first to consider the possibility that disc lesions cause painful internal derangement.

'Fibrositis' proved a much more stubborn belief at the upper trunk, thought it was discredited twenty years ago (Cyriax, 1948). The concepts set out in these two papers have now been enthusiastically adopted. But, the pendulum has swung too far and the diagnosis of a disc lesion is now made too readily at the lower part of the vertebral column. There are a number of causes of pain in the back and lower limb other than disc lesions. They are all uncommon and form a small group dealt with in Chapter 18.

'Osteoarthritis' of the lumbar spine has been challenged for the last fifteen years in successive editions of this book; yet even now remains a common ascription. It was still considered the commonest cause of backache at the symposium held at the Mayo Clinic in 1951, although Beneke (1897) and Kahlmeter (1918) had already pointed out that vertebral osteophytosis was secondary to disc degeneration.

Nomenclature

In this book, the undermentioned terms are used as follows:

Backache. Discomfort in the lower back.

Lumbago. A sudden access of pain in the lower back causing some degree of fixation and twinges on attempted movement. During recovery from lumbago, a moment is reached when the patient has merely backache. There is no exact point at which this change takes place; hence the differentiation is clear enough at extremes but merges indefinitely at the centre.

Sciatica. Pain felt radiating from the buttock to the posterior thigh and calf. There is no name for pain felt only in the buttock, nor for pain of third lumbar provenance felt along the anterior aspect of the limb. Many cases of such radiation are labelled 'sciatica', but I regard such an extension as unhelpful.

THE ERECT POSTURE

Why disc lesions are so common? Dillane, Fry and Kalton (1966) found in their practice that every year 2·4 per cent of their patients suffered from a lumbago severe enough to request medical help. Indeed it is rare to reach middle-age without attacks of internal derangement at one or more spinal joints. Why does ordinary use of the joints of the spine cause pain so readily, when the other joints of the body can so often withstand lifelong exertion without causing trouble?

The answer is man's acquisition of the erect posture. The cerebellum has caught the vertebral column unprepared, the capacity to maintain equilibrium on two legs outstripping the evolution of the spine. As soon as man learned to stand, the function of the spine altered; hence the whole column should have been redesigned.

In the long evolutionary period from fish to quadruped, the spine had served to maintain the distance apart of the front and hinder parts of the living creature. It never had to bear any compression strain. Moreover, a quadruped has no occasion to bend forwards since his forefeet are already on the ground; in consequence, little reason existed for the development of a structure able to withstand flexion strains. But sagging of the spine as it hung between its anterior and posterior supports was undesirable, hence the column became a mechanism strong against extension stress. As soon as the erect posture was assumed the strains of compression and of flexion were imposed on a structure not designed to withstand either. Worse still, the spinal nerves emerged opposite the weakest part of the column— namely, the joints—instead of the exit for each pair lying (as might just as easily have happened) opposite the vertebral body. Worst of all, each spinal joint (except the two uppermost) contained a disc; a ring of fibro-cartilage with a pulpy centre. This arrangement stopped the cervical spine from being driven up into the brain when an individual fell on to his head or, seated, on to his buttocks; for the downward momentum of the skull and the upward impetus of the body were cushioned by twenty-two elastic washers. The likelihood of a vertebral fracture at any level was also much diminished. This buffer was quite satisfactory so long as the spine was kept horizontal and suffered only extension strains, since movement in this direction tended to push the articular contents ventralwards, away from the nerve-roots, but as soon as the maintenance of the erect posture forced the joints to bear weight and to accept flexion strain, the system broke down.

Though the discs protect the central nervous system from vertical impact, they are clearly not required by the joints as such. Indeed, the two joints that bear the greatest weight are the ankle and the talo-calcanean. As the patient walks, these joints support alternately more than twice the compression applied to any lumbar joint; yet they hold up perfectly for a lifetime, in spite of the absence of any buffer. Again, no symptoms necessarily result from such complete erosion of disc-substance that the lumbar vertebrae lie in virtual apposition, bone to bone. Hence it is most arguable that the existence of the intervertebral discs often causes more trouble than it prevents.

THE LUMBAR LORDOSIS

It is puzzling that the spinal column, though a weight-bearing structure, has been designed in a series of curves rather than as a vertical pillar. There are individuals who possess a perfectly straight spinal column from sacrum to neck; they have a graceful carriage and move well. A straight vertebral column is therefore not impossible to construct; indeed, general mechanical principles would suggest that at the spine as at the limbs, a vertical line is ideal for weight-bearing. Aesthetic considerations strengthen this view; for a straight back leads to an agreeable posture, where an exaggerated lordosis leads to prominence of the belly and buttocks.

For years the view has therefore been held, on apparently logical grounds, that the lumbar lordosis should be as slight in degree as possible.

It is my belief that the lumbar and cervical lordoses were developed to protect—albeit not with great success—the posterior longitudinal ligament from excessive strain and to exert an anteriorly directed pressure on the contents of the intervertebral joint. Biologically speaking, the development of the lordosis must be recent and subsequent to the emergence of

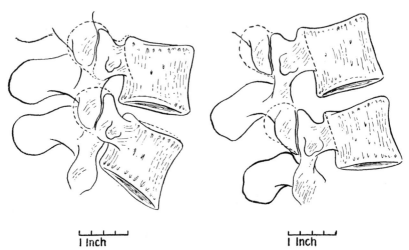

FIG. 61. Lumbar extension. Tracing of a radiograph taken in trunk-extension. Note that the front of the intervertebral joint gapes widely ($\frac{1}{2}$ inch) whereas the posterior aspect is narrowed ($\frac{3}{16}$ inch). When the articular surfaces are thus tilted, the pressure of the body weight forces the contents of the joint forwards.

FIG. 62. Lumbar flexion. Tracing of a radiograph of the same individual taken during trunk-flexion. Note that the inclination of the joint surfaces is now reversed. The anterior aspect of the joint-space ($\frac{1}{4}$ inch) has now become less than the posterior ($\frac{5}{16}$ inch). The intra-articular contents now tend to be forced backwards. This is the dangerous tilt.

the capacity to maintain the erect posture; for the spinal curves are absent at birth and during the first year of extra-uterine life. The spinal joints most subject to internal derangement are the fifth and sixth cervical and the fourth and fifth lumbar—the areas of the spine where the normal lordosis is most marked. The primary thoracic kyphosis present at birth is thus retained as a compensatory mechanism whereby the erect position can be maintained in spite of lordosis above and below. The existence of the cervical and lumbar lordoses means that the joint-space is wider in front than behind. In this way a slight pressure, directed forward, is constantly exerted on the intervertebral disc during weight-bearing. Figures 61 and 62 show the difference in the tilt on the joint, when a normal subject holds his lumbar spine, first extended, then flexed. In patients with a flat spinal column, the intervertebral disc has no such protection, and it is noticeable that patients with a lumbar spine devoid of anterior convexity are more apt to suffer from backache than those with a normal degree of lordosis. Clearly, if the joint-surfaces lie parallel when the patient stands erect, a slight degree of trunk-flexion begins at

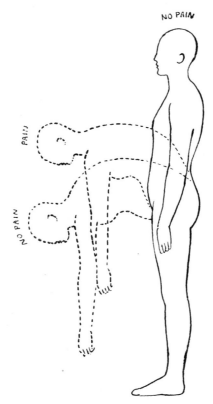

FIG. 63. Painful arc on trunk-flexion

once to squeeze the disc backwards; whereas the existence of a lordosis ensures that the trunk has to be well flexed before the angle is reversed and the back of the joint becomes wider than the front.

The phenomenon of a painful arc (Fig. 63) on trunk-flexion throws light on intra-articular mechanics. Discography (Lindholm, 1951) with contrast material injected into a lumbar intervertebral joint shows how the nucleus tends to move backwards during trunk-flexion, both in normal and in abnormal joints. When patients with a normal lumbar curve stand erect, the disc is pushed anteriorly. As trunk flexion proceeds the moment comes at the half-flexed position when the surfaces have moved enough to reverse the tilt. At this point a mobile fragment of disc moves sharply backwards, jarring the dura by pressure transmitted through the posterior longitudinal ligament. Further trunk-flexion may not alter the position of the disc again; the remainder of flexion is then painless. Alternatively, the pain may reappear at the extreme of trunk-flexion, if the loose part is squeezed yet farther backwards. Hence a painful arc is pathognomonic of hypermobility of a fragment of the intra-articular disc in a spinal joint.

Practical Bearing

In the past, the prescription and technique of postural exercises have been too much guided by aesthetic considerations. In fact, the prevention of future backache has the prior claim; it is such a universal symptom that prophylaxis is worth while from a child's early days. It is to the gymnasts who teach at schools that we must look first for a reversal of policy. No endeavour must be made to persuade children to bend down and touch the floor. Those who can, well and good; those who cannot must not force their trunks, nor have them forced, towards flexion. Lessons on how to sit and lift maintaining the lordosis should become part of gymnastic school training everywhere. Once such postures become second nature, they can be carried on into working life indefinitely.

The control, therefore, that aesthetic considerations used to exercise over the child's posture should be tempered by knowledge of the frequency and mechanism of disc-protrusion. Once growth has ceased, postural exercises are powerless to alter the shape of the bones. However, they may well be harmful if they include movements towards flexion, for they are still capable of stretching ligaments and moving a loose fragment of disc to an unfavourable position. There is a sort of fetish that no one is healthy unless he bends to touch his toes a number of times every morning. Many disc lesions are the result of acting on this extraordinary idea. Hospitals still exist in England where flexion exercises are ordered for back trouble under the physiotherapist's supervision. Even when the sufferer from backache finds that flexion exercises increase his discomfort, alas he congratulates himself on affecting the right spot. The potential harm inherent in postural exercises based only on 'health and beauty' concepts should be explained to all.

'Postural Pain'

Posture is a concept, a shape, not a disease. Hence the phrase 'postural pain' adds nothing to what is already said when a patient complains of backache. In all lesions of the moving parts, the posture adopted by the part at fault influences symptoms. When standing with the knee fully extended hurts a patient with arthritis in his knee, he is not regarded as suffering from postural knee-ache; if this posture hurts, it is agreed by all that a lesion exists at the knee. Backache arising from the moving parts varies according to posture; in other words, the pain alters as the stress on some lumbar structure is altered. A change in symptoms corresponding to the stresses acting on the lesion is common to all disorders of the moving parts. If the pain is then called 'postural', the most that this adjective has said is that the pain due to the unnamed lesion alters with the position of the affected part. Nevertheless, the idea is widespread that, if an individual with backache has a 'bad' posture, the two are connected. This popular notion is an obvious misconception; for not only do many people with 'good' posture suffer from backache but an equal number with a 'bad' posture do not. There is only one posture that enhances the likelihood of backache—namely, a flat back—and this is the one long regarded as 'good'. This view has been confirmed by Hult (1954). He studied 1,200 workers and found that the incidence of back trouble and of radiographic signs of disc-degeneration was the same in those with scoliosis or kypho-lordosis as in other individuals.

Backache arises, whatever the posture, as the result of some lesion. The diagnosis must state the nature of this lesion, and name the tissue responsible for the pain. 'Postural' does neither. Indeed, the many different ideas about backache are mostly dependent on uncertainties about the mechanics of the lumbar region. The application of simple anatomical fact to the problem of backache is set out below.

THE INTERVERTEBRAL DISC

History

When a syndrome has become widely recognized, it is always found to have been described before in papers that attracted no attention at the time.

Vesalium was the first to describe the appearance of the intervertebral disc in 1555. Cotugno wrote a book on sciatica in 1764 (*De Ischide Nervosa Commentarius*), and Lassègue had already noted wasting of the muscles in the affected limb by 1864. In 1838, Key reported two cases of paraplegia caused by protrusion of an upper lumbar disc. Virchow (1857) reported a herniated disc post mortem; he regarded it as caused by trauma.

In 1888, Charcot described the characteristic spinal deformity in sciatica and Ribbert (1895) produced protrusion in rabbits by puncturing the intervertebral disc. Kocher (1896) described a case of rupture of the second lumbar disc after a fall on the heels. In 1916 Elsberg drew attention to 'spinal chondromata', and in 1919 Goldthwait described one case, and Middleton and Teacher two cases, of flaccid paraplegia with paralysed sphincters resulting from 'exaggerated prominence of the fifth lumbar disc' of traumatic origin. The latter put a segment of spine into a vice and reproduced the expulsion of the disc experimentally. Dandy (1929) described two cases of paraplegia caused by extrusion of disc substance. Glorieux of Bruges gave the first full account of disc lesions in *La Hernie postérieure du Ménisque intervertébral*—a book published in 1937. His myelographic plates are particularly clear. Though this was the first complete account of lumbar disc lesions, it attracted no attention and is omitted from nearly all bibliographies.

Cartilage and Pulp

Between the bodies of each two lumbar vertebrae lies the disc. The structures here are:

1. *The End-plate*
This consists of hyaline cartilage covering the articular surfaces of each vertebral body.

2. *The Annulus Fibrosus*
This consists of fibro-cartilage and is attached to the end-plate, the vertebral bodies and the anterior and posterior longitudinal ligaments; it surrounds the nucleus. The lamellae have been compared to the layers of an onion, but run in different directions, crossing each other; this arrangement gives the annulus great strength. Round the circumference, the fibro-cartilage sinks into the vertebral body forming a strong band. The spongy structure of cartilage provides hydrostatic lubrication (Mc-Cutchen, 1964). Were the liquid contained within cartilage not retained by viscous resistance, it would be squeezed out as soon as the disc bore weight. The disc would then be reduced to an inelastic solid, half its original thickness. Cartilage contains neither blood vessels nor nerves; hence all damage is permanent, union and regeneration being impossible. Being devoid of nerves, the lesion of itself cannot cause pain; fracture or degeneration of the disc cannot cause symptoms unless some other tissue is secondarily affected.

3. *The Nucleus Pulposus*
At birth the nucleus occupies the centre of the intervertebral joint. But during growth the anterior aspect of the vertebral body grows faster than

the posterior. Hence in adult life the nucleus has come to lie slightly behind the centre. It consists of softish, gelatinous material and forms the cushion between the vertebrae, during compression exerting hydrostatic pressure, uniformly distributed. It bulges when cut. In the young it is quite distinct from the annulus, less so in adults, and by late middle-age has disappeared completely. The disc has then become uniform throughout its substance and consists of the familiar 'crab-meat' removed at laminectomy. For this reason, nuclear disc protrusion is rare in the elderly.

The function of the nucleus is partly to act as shock-absorber, and partly to change shape when the vertebrae tilt on each other, thus maintaining a uniform distribution of stress throughout the joint.

Bearing on Treatment

Cartilage is hard and its displacement, in whatever joint of the body it occurs, is often susceptible to manipulative reduction. This should be done at once in all suitable cases, so as to minimize ligamentous overstretching at the back of the joint.

Nuclear material is soft and usually cannot be successfully manipulated back into place. If a manipulation is attempted, the technique is different; sustained pressure replaces the sharp jerk, since it is now the intention to squeeze rather than to click the displacement back into position; but the endeavour is apt to fail. Most pulpy protrusions are reducible only by traction or by rest in bed.

THE AGING OF CARTILAGE

Cartilage is an avascular structure; hence it cannot unite or regenerate after it has been damaged. This applies to the intervetebral disc no less than to the meniscus at the knee, where it is admitted on all sides that a tear never heals. Even in articular (as opposed to intra-articular) cartilage, Davies, Barnett and Palfry (1962) showed by electron microscopy in young adult rabbits that no evidence of cell division is discernible. Tonna and Cronkite's radio-isotopic studies show cartilage to be a static tissue. They found that in rats no detectable multiplication of cells took place after the first month of life. Nine months after injection of tritated thymidine, cartilage cells were still loaded with it, whereas it disappeared in a month from rapidly dividing tissues. Professor Burnett's (1965) research with the electron microscope in Tasmania has led him to state: 'Articular cartilage turns out to be a remarkably static tissue.' In Portugal, Miniero (1965) devoted a book to a detailed description of the vertebral arterial and venous supply. His photographs of injected specimens from foetal life to eighty years old show consistently that the disc itself is entirely devoid of blood-vessels. Yet one of the arguments put forward for the treatment of lumbago by rest in bed is 'to allow the disc to heal'. This impossibility is important medico-legally, since there is (1) no certain relation in time between damage to a disc and the first attack of internal derangement; (2) a permanent liability to recurrence. Once a loose fragment of fibro-cartilage has moved, the crack cannot unite so as to prevent another displacement.

The nutrition of articular cartilage appears to begin from the surface and penetrate towards the bone, not the reverse. The permeability of cartilage lessens with age, and Stockwell showed that in a three-month-old rabbit silver proteinate passes quite readily into articular cartilage from its free surface, but penetrates much less at two years old. Lowered cell nutrition and reduced elasticity lead to damage to the gliding surfaces which are then no longer adequately covered by the film of synovial fluid on which virtually friction-free movement depends. This is how Stockwell considers that osteoarthritis is caused.

Many patients are distressed at being told that they are suffering from one or more 'degenerate discs'. This suggests an irreversible and crippling phenomenon. The term should be discarded; for disc-degeneration is universal as age advances and causes no symptoms. Disc protrusion is painful whether degeneration has set in or not. Degeneration without displacement compresses nothing and so cannot cause symptoms. The phrase is therefore pathologically inaccurate and psychologically undesirable.

THE PRESSURE WITHIN THE DISC

Many calculations had been made, some leading to impossibly large theoretical loads on the joint. Nachemson carried out valuable research by *in vivo* discometry. Between 1960 and 1965, he published a book and four further papers setting out the results. He measured the intradiscal pressure by means of a needle thrust into the nucleus, thus directly assessing the pressure when the individual adopted different postures. Initially, he found that in an excised lumbar spine the ligaments about the joint exerted a pressure of 0·7 kg. During sitting, 10 to 15 kg. pressure per square cm. was exerted. This was reduced to two-thirds of this figure when the individual stood, and halved when he lay down. Leaning forward 20 degrees increased the load by 30 per cent. These findings correspond with the clinical facts that a patient with severe lumbago can lie and stand without too much discomfort, but can neither sit nor bend forward without increased pain. In moderate degeneration of the disc, as evidenced by an irregular outline on the nucleogram, the increase in pressure on sitting was the same as in those with a normal nucleus. By contrast, on bending forwards, the pressure on the posterior aspect of the disc was twice as great in individuals with moderate degeneration as in those with a normal nucleus.

The intradiscal pressure is dependent on the load. Movement of part of a disc depends on the state of the disc, the inclination of the joint surfaces and the centrifugal force acting on the disc. Strong muscles tend further to squeeze the joint and to enable heavier loads, i.e. more centrifugal force, to act on the disc. This situation—i.e. that however strong they are, the lumbar muscles contribute nothing to the prevention of lumbar disc lesions—is not yet appreciated, and the generalization that the stronger the muscles the more stable the joint is erroneously accepted. In probably every hospital in the country exercises are blithely ordered for both prophylaxis and treatment.

Damage to the Disc

If it is entire, the disc cannot protrude unless the posterior ligament ruptures. When time and the multiple minor traumata of ordinary active life have initiated damage, the cartilage becomes slightly, then more, cracked, but being devoid of nerves there is no warning discomfort. In the end, a fragment forms that is either completely detached within the joint or lies hinged. The stage is now set for the first attack of internal derangement, i.e. of lumbago if the loose piece lies centrally, or of root-pain if the fragment lies postero-laterally within the joint.

Since the two end-plates lie nearly parallel, a displaced fragment of disc can occupy an indefinite number of positions. The situation is not the same as at the knee where the semi-detached fragment of meniscus can lie only at one or other side of the dome of the femoral condyle, i.e. either 'in' or 'out'. At the knee, therefore, displacement and reduction are both sudden phenomena, heralded by a click. At a lumbar joint, by contrast, although the onset of lumbago is often instantaneous, spontaneous reduction during rest in bed is usually a slow process. The displacement recedes a little day by day, the symptoms and signs waning correspondingly. Manipulative reduction is often as sudden as the onset, and the click may be heard and felt.

The nucleus sometimes pushes past the annulus; if so, pure herniation of pulp with an intact annulus results (Fig. 65). If the annulus is cracked and part of it moves, the centrifugal force always acting on the nucleus may push pulpy material into the breach. As a result, any cartilaginous dis-

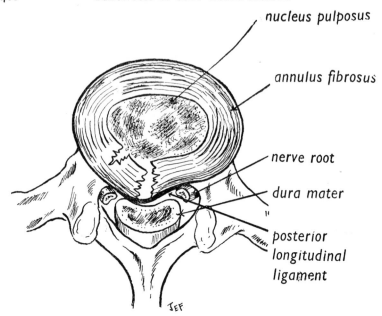

FIG. 64. Cartilaginous disc lesion. An annular crack has led to posterior displacement by hingeing. The posterior longitudinal ligament is bulged out backwards and pressure exerted on the dura mater; lumbago results. No nuclear material has extruded; hence reduction by manipulation is simple.

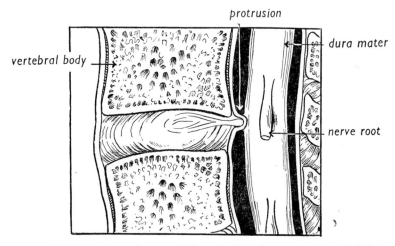

FIG. 65. Pulpy disc lesion. Nuclear material has pushed past the intact annulus and is bulging the posterior longitudinal ligament backwards until the dura mater is pressed upon (after R. H. Young). Backache or lumbago results. Reduction by manipulation is often impossible; the treatment of choice is sustained traction.

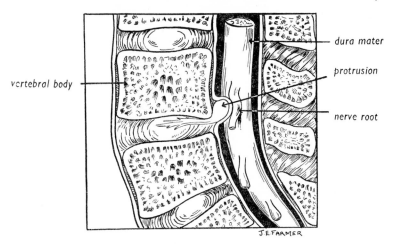

FIG. 66. Sciatica caused by herniation of nuclear material at the fourth lumbar level. The protrusion has passed postero-laterally and now impinges on the nerve-root (after R. H. Young). In to longer presses on the dura mater; hence the backache ceases when the pain in the limb comes on.

placement of sufficient size and standing becomes aggravated by secondary herniation of pulp into the gap. This may take the shape of a collar-stud, the narrow track at the annulus forming the stem of the stud. If so, manipulative reduction becomes impossible.

HYDROPS OF THE DISC

There is a theory that lumbago is caused by sudden swelling of the disc as the result of rapidly absorbing fluid. This ignores several obvious facts.

1. If the disc were to swell, it would force the vertebral bodies apart. Since two-thirds of the intervertebral joint lies anterior to the axis about which flexion and extension take place, the spine would be fixed in extension, whereas in lumbago the spine is fixed in flexion.

2. Radiography in recumbency, i.e. without compression strain on the joint, does not show an increased width of the joint space during lumbago. Moreover, some patients deviate *towards* the painful side.

3. Intra-articular cartilage is avascular; hence it cannot suddenly change its nature and become absorbent. The meniscus at the knee is not found swollen when removed during an effusion into the joint. In any case, where would this fluid suddenly appear from? A more reasonable hypothesis would be haemarthrosis, which can, after all, come on in a few

moments. But evidence of past haemorrhage is a rare finding in laminectomy.

4. Fluid suddenly permeating the disc would not come on with a click
during trunk-flexion. Still less would it disappear with another click
during manipulative reduction.

The evidence therefore strongly opposes this hypothesis.

RADIOLOGY

X-rays are today frequently studied to decide whether or not a disc
lesion exists. Nothing could be more fallacious. What the radiograph
shows is whether the disc is thick or thin and whether osteophytes are
present or not. But a disc can atrophy without displacement; alternatively,
protrusion can occur at a joint where the space is of full width. Osteophyte
formation is itself symptomless; it merely indicates some degeneration, as
is almost universal in elderly people, some of whom have never had backache in their lives. What matters is whether or not a displacement is
present—and this the straight radiograph cannot show. Another error is
to state that a normal radiograph excludes a disc lesion. No-one would,
after inspecting the X-ray photograph of a young man's knee, say whether
his meniscus was torn or not, nor would radiographic evidence of displacement be expected. Similarly, the X-ray appearances of the bones of the
back cannot be expected to exclude damage to the cartilage.

Osteophytosis with or without a diminished joint space is secondary to
disc-degeneration and results from ligamentous traction lifting up periosteum. Bone then grows out to meet its limiting membrane. Most osteophytosis is directed laterally or anteriorly and does not matter. Rarely an
osteophyte projects posteriorly, compressing the dura mater or a nerve-
root. This finding is often significant and connected with symptoms.

The real use of a lumbar radiograph is negative—to show that no other
disorder is present. Degeneration of a disc, once it becomes considerable,
appears as a diminished joint space with osteophytosis on the radiograph.
When a disc is ground to pieces entirely, the joint space disappears and
bone all but touches bone, only the end-plates intervening (Plate 24); in
many such cases the mushroom phenomenon supervenes. If the disc is
reduced to rubble and passes anteriorly, its remnants can often be seen
lying enclosed by two bony breaks (Plate 25). The nucleus can herniate
into the body of a vertebra; this phenomenon causes adolescent osteochondritis and Schmorl's nodes (Plate 35). Complete absence of the joint
space is compatible with painless function, but not with a full range of
movement. The fact that the joint space is of normal or diminished width

does not indicate where the posterior—the important—part of the disc happens to be lying. Hence the appearance of the disc-space on the radiograph adds nothing for or against a clinical diagnosis of displacement of a disc-fragment. This view has since been confirmed by Soderburg and Andren (1956). They began with the idea that a diminished disc-space with osteophytosis reduces the risk of protrusion, but finally found no correlation between the clinical and radiological findings.

When a firm diagnosis of disc lesion has been made, the fact that this or that joint space is diminished does not even prove that the lesion lies at the narrowed level. For example, at laminectomy for sciatica, it sometimes happens that a patient's symptoms are the result of protrusion at, say, the fourth level (where the joint space is of normal width) and the contents of the fifth joint (where the space is much diminished) are not responsible for any symptoms, degeneration with thinning having gone on silently for years. Moreover, some twenty per cent of patients subjected to laminectomy are found to have two protrusions (R. H. Young), not necessarily at the levels the X-rays appeared to indicate.

Markedly diminished joint spaces at the upper lumbar levels are often seen in elderly patients, but disc lesions causing symptoms at the first or second lumbar level are a great rarity. Semmes (1964), at laminectomy on 1,500 cases, found one first and two second lumbar protrusions; Collis's discograms detected one at the second lumbar level and none at the first in 1,014 cases. It is clear, therefore, that mere thinning of the disc affords no evidence of protrusion past or present.

Multiple erosion of disc-substance leads to considerable loss of height as age advances. Each lumbar disc may well be 1 cm. thick originally. If all five are reduced to a thin wafer the patient becomes 5 cm. shorter.

Calcification of a ligament shows that it has probably suffered damage some years before (Plate 29); bleeding into an intervertebral joint may be followed by intra-articular calcification. Calcification of the disc itself occurs in chondro-calcinosis (pseudo-gout).

SPONTANEOUS RECOVERY

Pain in the neck, posterior thorax or lumbo-gluteal area caused by a disc protrusion in the midline can continue indefinitely. This does not apply to accute torticollis or to sudden thoracic pain or to lumbago; in these disorders the tendency to spontaneous recovery in a week or two is considerable. But neckache, scapular aching, posterior thoracic aching and lower backache can go on for many years. The same applies to cases of bilateral root-pain. However, the moment the protrusion moves to one side, compressing a nerve-root, with easing of the pressure exerted via the posterior ligament against dura mater, a mechanism leading to spontaneous recovery is set in motion. This takes six to twelve months at the three lower lumbar levels; three to four months at cervical levels; an indeterminate time at the first and second thoracic levels. Spontaneous recovery from root-pain may not occur at all at the third to twelfth thoracic levels.

In sciatica, the more marked the neurological weakness, the sooner the patient loses his pain in the limb. Time must be counted from the first appearance of strong unilateral root-pain coupled with cessation of central pain in the trunk; mere lumbar aching radiating slightly to one limb does not suffice, and the time that has elapsed since the pain in the trunk or gluteal area began is wholly immaterial. It is important to realize that the central backache must cease before one can begin counting. If it is not lost, or the symptoms are projected to *both* limbs, there is no limit to how long root-pain can last.

There are four ways in which spontaneous recovery is secured; the anatomical result in each case is different.

1. Reduction

The displaced part of the disc may return to its bed spontaneously, either during rest in bed or merely because the patient maintains his lordosis, since he finds that trunk-flexion is painful. Reduction can also be secured by manipulation, traction or recumbency. Once back in place, the loose fragment is not more or less firmly in place because it took place slowly during rest in bed or quickly during manipulation, and recurrence is not avoided more by one method than the other. Reduction implies that the damaged tissue no longer protrudes, but what has displaced itself once can do so again. Recurrences are thus to be expected.

Some believe that the click which often signals reduction at a lumbar joint indicates that the loose fragment has been shifted away from the dura mater or the nerve-root by becoming even further displaced. Were this so, recurrence would be obviated; for what is not restored to its original position cannot displace itself again and, when a patient who had had twenty attacks of lumbago in his life came to laminectomy, twenty small fragments of disc would be found lying free in the intervertebral canal. This is not so.

2. Erosion

A large postero-lateral protrusion (Fig. 66) pressing against a nerve-root lies in close contact with the dura mater. This pulsates, and jolts the protrusion against the back of the vertebral body at each heart beat. The bone is therefore eroded (as occurs on a larger scale in an aortic aneurysm) painlessly and the protrusion is finally accommodated (Fig. 67). I am indebted to my colleague R. H. Young for explanation of this important phenomenon. The protrusion now ceases to compress the nerve-root and the patient recovers fully. What is more, the protrusion now lies in a

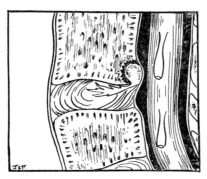

FIG. 67. Spontaneous recovery. The postero-inferior aspect of the vertebral body is eroded and the protrusion accommodated (after R. H. Young). When this process becomes complete, dura mater and nerve-root are no longer subjected to pressure. Symptomatic recovery is now established.

position from which it cannot become dislodged, and I regard patients in whom recovery has been awaited as the result of this mechanism as no more subject to further attacks than a normal individual. Hence they can resume heavy work and need not wear a corset.

3. Root-atrophy

Root-pressure from a protruded disc goes on hurting so long as the sheath of the root remains sensitive. Extreme pressure so deprives the compressed extent of root-sheath of its blood supply that it loses sensitivity.

As ischaemic root-atrophy becomes complete, the pain abates, the appropriate cutaneous area goes numb, stretching the root returns to full range and the root-palsy, sensory and motor, reaches a maximum. In other words, the patient has become subjectively better by getting anatomically worse.

Good recovery from the palsy is to be expected when only one root is paretic, but when two adjacent roots atrophy, some lasting loss of power of the weakest muscle may persist. There is very little tendency to recurrence.

4. Disc-shrinkage

Surgeons report that at laminectomy on patients who had severe sciatica years ago, inspection of the disc shows a normal hard cartilaginous surface, level with the bones. The protrusion has receded. It would seem that its extra-articular position deprives the fragment of its nutrient synovial fluid; hence the protrusion slowly shrivels. This must be the mechanism operating in those cases of postero-lateral protrusion which recover spontaneously in a year without the supervention of any neurological deficit. This mechanism is not brought into play when the displacement lies centrally, causing pain felt chiefly in the back, presumably because the protrusion still lies intra-articularly, confined by the posterior longitudinal ligament.

THE MUSCLES

It is an accepted orthopaedic principle that the stronger the muscles about a joint, the more stable it is. This is a sound generalization, but there are exceptions.

This principle does not apply to internal derangement. Who puts the cartilage out in his knee? The professional footballer, whose exceptionally strong muscles and vigorous movements strain the joint in a way unlikely in a weaker man. Strong muscles protect the bones they join against displacement; they do not protect against intra-articular subluxation. Indeed, it can be argued that a man whose muscles enable him to put a 100 kg. compression strain on his lumbar joint, is more apt to damage his disc than a weaker individual who can lift only 50 kg. Strong muscles do not prevent internal derangement at a lumbar joint, rather the contrary. Stability here is determined only by the interlocking of the lateral facets and the strength of the many ligaments. The sacrospinalis muscles lie along the postero-lateral aspects of the vertebrae; hence the first effect of their contraction is to squeeze these bones together, thus compressing the intervertebral joints. Only when all the play in these joints has been taken up is the spine moved towards extension. Thus the stronger the sacrospinalis muscles, the more the joint is compressed. It is then the strong man who puts the greater compression stress on his lumbar joint during lifting. Retropulsion of disc-material may ensue, rendered more probable by his muscular prowess. As a corollary, patients whose lumbar muscles have been weakened by poliomyelitis seldom develop lumbar disc-lesions.

An extension movement from the standing position is initiated by the sacrospinalis muscles. As soon as the thorax passes behind the vertical line, the movement continues by the force of gravity. The abdominal muscles pay out to allow the movement to be carried to its extreme. Pain elicited at the extreme of range is not derived from the muscle by active contraction. For this reason, standing trunk-extension, being a passive movement, must be regarded as a test of articular function. If pain of muscular origin is suspected, the spinal movements must be tested against resistance. In fact, myofascial lesions are very uncommon at lumbar levels and result from direct trauma only. In young men, early disc lesions are often called 'sprained muscle', but not by those who test muscles by resisted contraction.

When an individual bends forward to pick up a heavy object, the sacrospinalis muscles pay out and at the extreme of range are fully stretched. When he strains upwards to lift, three forces act on the lumbar joint while it is held in flexion. First, as soon as the lumbar spine on its journey upwards passes the horizontal line, the weight of the trunk begins to compress the joint; secondly, the weight of the object lifted compresses the joint further; thirdly, both sacrospinalis muscles contract and compress the joint further still. Hence the stronger these muscles are, the greater the compression stress on the joint—in other words, the greater the liability to a disc lesion. Although flexion exercises have fallen out of favour, there is hardly a hospital department in the country where back exercises of some sort are not carried out in the 'treatment' of disc lesions, in the mistaken belief either that extension exercises encourage reduction, or that strong muscles beneficially support the joint. Though patients do recover in spite of such exercises, convalescence is delayed, and renewed protrusion during their performance—even if they are merely prone-lying trunk-extension exercises—is by no means unknown.

The ilio-psoas and the abdominal muscles are the flexors of the lumbar spine; the former flexes the spine when the femur is fixed; the latter flex it when the pelvis is fixed. In the standing patient, once the movement has been initiated by these muscles, flexion proceeds from the force of gravity, the hamstring and sacrospinalis muscles paying out smoothly to let the trunk down.

In acute lumbago, the flexed position of the lumbar spine is maintained by simultaneous contraction of the psoas and sacrospinalis muscles fixing the joint from both aspects in the neutral position. As a result of this flexed posture, the sacrospinalis muscles have to work hard against gravity to prevent the trunk toppling further forwards; since the patient is no longer poised vertically in line with his centre of gravity. This fact accounts for the mistaken idea that lumbago results from spasm or 'fibrositis' of the sacrospinalis muscles. One has only to remember that the muscles extend the joint to realize that spasm of the sacrospinalis muscles is neither the cause nor the result of lumbago. Were these muscles really in spasm, the joints would be held in extension, as happens in the opisthotonos of tetanus.

When 'fibrositis' was discredited (Cyriax, 1948), more plausible lesions of the non-articular structures were proposed. Fatty lobules are present in the sacrospinalis muscles and their herniation through the lumbar fasciae with strangulation was postulated as a cause of symptoms. Their existence in most normal persons is not denied. Alternatively, the word 'fibrositis' has been changed to 'fasciitis', 'myogelosis' or 'non-articular rheumatism'. That the muscles, fascia and fatty lobules are not affected in lumbago is proved again by the patient's posture; were any of these soft-tissue disorders really present, he would instantly relieve his pain by bending backwards and relaxing tension. Indeed, the mere fact that a pain in the back or buttock is increased on bending backwards shows that it arises from a joint and not from the now-relaxed extensor muscles of the lumbar spine and hip joint.

Strange (1966) has put forward quite a different reason for avoiding the word 'disc' and going back to the muscular theory of lumbago. He states that this diagnosis, 'imperfectly made, has been responsible for making tens of thousands of perfectly fit men and women into life-long invalids'. In his address he went on to decry 'thousands of unnecessary operations', 'hundreds of thousands of physiotherapists' hours wasted', 'millions of pounds won in totally improper compensation', 'millions of man-hours of work lost'. Every word of this arraignment earns approval except the plea for a return to a false pathology. If a rational attitude to disc lesions ('displacement of a piece of cartilage', frightens nobody) were promoted, if logical treatment were carried out at once as a matter of course, the word would soon lose the dire significance that it possesses for patients today.

THE BONES

The antero-posterior stability of the lumbar spine depends largely on engagement at the two lateral joints of the articular facets of one vertebra against the corresponding pair above and below (Fig. 68). If the pedicle is lengthened (Plate 32) or a fibrous defect replaces bone at each isthmus between the superior and inferior articular processes, this stability is endangered. Plate 33 shows the considerable displacement that can occur after excessive removal of bone at laminectomy. Bony defect at the pars intermedia of the articular process may not lead to untoward stretching; if so, the condition is known as spondylolysis (Plate 30). However, the fibrous tissue at the defect in the bone may lengthen; spondylolisthesis results (Plate 31). Since the stretching takes place antero-superiorly to the lateral articulations of the affected vertebra, the spinous process of the spondylolisthetic vertebra is held in its normal relationship to that of the vertebra below. The body of the vertebra above, however, follows the

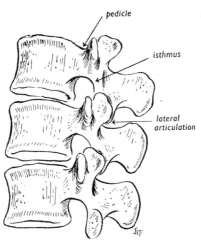

FIG. 68. Antero-posterior stability of the lumbar spine. This depends on the integrity of pedicle, isthmus and the engagement of facets at each lateral articulation.

body of the affected vertebra, and its spinous process therefore lies displaced anteriorly. For this reason, the irregularity of the spinous processes visible and palpable in spondylolisthesis appears at the vertebra above that shown on the radiograph to be at fault.

Congenital Abnormalities

Those who regard any congenital abnormality visible on the radiograph as sufficient explanation for backache are diminishing. Different observers have noted between fifteen and sixty per cent. incidence of congenital abnormality in the lumbo-sacral region of patients not subject to backache. Sacralization of the fifth lumbar vertebra has no local significance, but it shows this joint to be fixed and suggests that excessive strain has fallen on the fourth lumbar joint which has had to do the work of two. It occurs in some 10 per cent. of ordinary individuals. In sacralization, the likelihood of a disc lesion is enhanced at the joint above; recurrence is also more difficult to avoid. A lumbarised first sacral segment has no significance. Spina bifida occulta is a defect of the neural arch and thus unconnected with any joint; it has no significance. Sutow and Pryde (1956) found it

present in 28·5 per cent of normal adults, whereas Southworth and
Bersack's (1950) figure is 18·6, and Crow and Brogdon's 35·7 per cent.
These authors examined 936 young men and found only 40·2 per cent
devoid of all radiological abnormality. 'Osteoarthritis' of an abnormal
joint between the upper surface of the sacrum and the fifth lumbar transverse process is also symptomless.

In contrast, spondylolysis and spondylolisthesis (Plates 30 and 31) are
significant, since they may result in painful stretching of ligament or
nerve-root, but much more often in a disc lesion at the unstable joint.
Spondylolisthesis can exist for a lifetime without causing any symptoms.

Hemivertebra itself causes no symptoms. Spontaneous correction
above and below the angulation often leads to minimal postural deformity,
although the radiographic appearances are most asymmetrical. Hemivertebra may lead to a secondary disc lesion at the oblique joint. Alternatively, it can eventually result in the same painful bony contact of the
vertebral bodies as complicates long-standing scoliosis from any other
cause.

THE JOINTS

The axis about which antero-posterior movement takes place lies at
the junction of the anterior two-thirds and the posterior third of each
lumbar vertebral body.

The primary movements at the lumbar joints are flexion, extension and
side-flexion. Flexion is brought to a stop by the supra- and inter-spinous
ligaments, the ligamentum flavum and the capsule of the lateral articulations, which prevent the facets sliding any farther apart. Bouillet (personal
communication, 1961) noted at laminectomy, that at the level of the disc
lesion, the interspinous ligament is often torn, sometimes to shreds. He
had found a reliable guide to the level of the protrusion. Clinically, palpation may reveal a gap between two spinous processes if the supraspinous
ligament has parted. In wedge-fracture, the two supraspinous ligaments
are always overstretched. The posterior longitudinal ligament scarcely
limits flexion; for it lies so close behind the pivotal point of the movement.
Extension is limited by the abdominal muscles, the anterior longitudinal
ligament, bone meeting bone at the lateral joints, and the engagement
posteriorly (cushioned by the interspinous ligaments) of the spinous
processes. Side-flexion is limited by the deep lumbar fascia, the lateral
spinal ligaments, the ligaments of one lateral facet preventing further
movement apart, and the point of one lateral process meeting the lamina
on the concave side.

Very little rotation takes place at the upper four lumbar joints. Engagement of the inferior and superior articular processes largely prevents rotation. At the lumbo-sacral joint the angle of the facet surfaces is tilted usually to about 45 degrees, but the variation (0 degrees to 80 degrees) is considerable. Hence a little rotation is possible, limited by the ilio-lumbar ligaments. A little ligamentous play and a slight shearing play also exist at the facet joints; it is thus an exaggeration to say that rotation is wholly absent at the lumbar spine. Nevertheless, the range is very small and in Sollmann's cineradiographic film of a young woman dancing the twist, the lumbar spinous processes can be seen to remain vertically above each other, rotating with the pelvis but not on each other.

At the spinal joints, increasing limitation of movement is to be expected as age advances, unlike the joints of the limbs, where range alters little from childhood to senescence. Osteophyte formation and ligamentous contracture come to limit the range of movement at the spinal joints so much, that what would be gross limitation in a man of twenty-five is full range at seventy. This absence of an absolute criterion causes much difficulty in diagnosis.

A patient with a small but painless range of lumbar movement is unaware of any rigidity, whereas a patient with ample range but discomfort at extremes states that his back feels stiff. Stiffness at the lumbar spine is thus a subjective phenomenon, unrelated to the amplitude of movement present. This is fortunate; for the spinal joints are the only ones in the body at which a diminished range of movement is advantageous and unperceived by the patient. At all joints other than the spinal, the endeavour is to abolish symptoms by the restoration of as full movement as is possible; the reverse applies to those spinal joints that contain damaged discs.

'The Facet Syndrome'

These pairs of joints maintain stability; they do not bear weight. They withstand rotational and shearing stresses on the lumbar spine while allowing flexion, extension and side-flexion movements. They contain small irregular triangles of intra-articular cartilage that Töndury (1949) likens to menisci. Hence, in theory, any patient with unilateral pain and articular signs might just as well have a lesion of one lateral articulation as a postero-lateral disc protrusion.

The facet joints have come into prominence lately, not because of any scientific evidence that lesions here are a common cause of backache, but by becoming involved in a matter of prestige. The advocates of the 'facet syndrome' are the osteopaths and those medical men who embrace their ideas. Radiography had shown the 'displaced vertebra' of Still, pressing on an artery, later on a nerve, to be an untenable hypothesis. Emphasis then shifted to the sacro-iliac joint, minor subluxations here being preferred, since they could believably prove invisible on the X-ray photograph. After that, disc lesions had to be accepted, but they were a medical discovery and thus basically unwelcome. Hence the more forward-looking osteopaths are now shifting their ground again and concentrating on the facet joints. This ascription of common disorders to joints that (apart from fixation in spondylitis) doctors correctly regard as not setting up symptoms at all, restores osteopathic mystique and the esoteric nomenclature by which this is enhanced.

There are strong reasons for *not* ascribing lumbar symptoms to lesions of a lateral articulation. Severe lesions of these joints do not cause symptoms; hence it is reasonable to infer that minor trouble is equally painless. For example, patients with marked erosion of a disc have lost up to 1 cm. in distance apart of the vertebrae; gross incongruity of the facet joints must result, but there is no pain. In spondylolisthesis, marked osteoarthritis of both facet joints is not uncommon; again, there are no symptoms.

A lesion of a unilateral structure cannot cause central pain. The facet is so placed that it cannot compress the dura mater; hence, patients with central dural pain, extrasegmental reference of pain, or a cough or neck-flexion hurting, are ruled out; also those with limitation of straight-leg raising. If the facet lesion pinched a nerve-root—a doubtful anatomical possibility—both flexion and side-flexion of the trunk away from the painful side would stop the pain at once; this excludes a further large number of patients. Nor could the lumbar pain shift from the centre of the back to one side. Nor could the backache cease when the root-pain came on; the facet is not a movable structure, as is a fragment of cartilage lying detached in a centrally-placed joint. Nor would local anaesthesia of the external aspect of the dura mater stop the pain for the time being. Nor would removal of the disc protrusion, which is practised so successfully by surgeons all over the world, help if the pressure on the nerve-root arose at the facet joint. Hence, even in cases of unilateral pain confined to the back, although the mere discovery of articular signs at the lumbar spine cannot be held to incriminate one joint rather than another, many considerations combine to show that the lateral articulations are very seldom or never the source of pain. They are sensitive neither to gross incongruence nor to osteoarthritis. Moreover, the symptoms and signs present, when critically evaluated, rule out the lateral articulation in almost every case.

THE LUMBAR LIGAMENTS

The Posterior Longitudinal Ligament

This ligament plays an important part in disc protrusion. It occupies the mid-line but is deficient on each side; hence a protrusion initially present-ing centrally meets the barrier of a tough ligament. The resistance of the ligament to stretch tends to push the protrusion back again anteriorly, and accounts for the regular occurrence of spontaneous reduction in lumbago. After repeated attacks, the protrusion is apt to shift towards a zone of lesser resistance, i.e. to one or other side of the ligament. As a protrusion enlarges, therefore, it usually becomes unilateral. As a result, central pain in the back is replaced by root-pain in the lower limb.

Should the posterior longitudinal ligament rupture, it is then possible for the entire contents of the intervertebral joint to extrude backwards. If so, the cauda equina is subjected to strong pressure and severe bilateral sciatica results. In addition, the third and fourth sacral roots may be com-pressed and paralysis of the bladder ensue. This may become permanent unless early laminectomy relieves the pressure quickly.

Cases have been described of lumbar puncture being followed by a lumbar disc lesion. It is very doubtful whether the introduction of the needle bears any relevance to the disorder; for, were it a question of extrusion of nuclear material *via* the puncture in the posterior longitu-dinal ligament, manipulative reduction would prove impossible. In fact, manipulative reduction usually succeeds, and it is clearly the flexed position in which the patient has been maintained, not the needle itself, that has caused the displacement.

Ilio-lumbar Ligaments

These have an important bearing on patient's symptoms and signs. These ligaments anchor the transverse processes of the fifth lumbar vertebra to each iliac crest and to the sacrum. They therefore restrict side-flexion, which has a much smaller range at the lumbo-sacral joint than at the other lumbar joints. The fourth lumbar joint is capable of great side-flexion; hence, in a patient with a protrusion at this level, the joint can gape so much that the displacement is accommodated. In other words, he presents marked deformity and thus avoids most of the pain. The same degree of accommodation is not possible at the lumbo-sacral joint; in consequence, the deformity is slight but the pain correspondingly severe.

'Kissing Spinous Processes'

The space between the spinous processes is subject to great individual variation. Some authorities consider that trunk-extension can pinch the interspinous ligaments and cause pain—this notion is easily disproved by local anaesthesia of the allegedly affected ligaments, since the pain when they are pinched remains and clearly has another source. Congenital approximation occurs when the processes are unusually large, and causes some limitation of extension without discomfort.

LUMBAR 'OSTEOARTHRITIS'

'Osteoarthritis' of the lumbar spine is an imaginary disease. Not only does osteophyte formation at the intervertebral joint cause no symptoms, but it is beneficial, and is the mechanism whereby pain in later life is prevented.

Articular Insensitivity

For the proper comprehension of backache, the most vital point to grasp is that the lumbar joints are insensitive to osteophytosis and internal derangement. The analogy with the knee does not hold. Internal derangement of the knee hurts the sensitive knee-joint, which becomes the site of a painful traumatic arthritis. At the lumbar joints internal derangement is of itself painless, the ligaments of the joint being insensitive to the pressure exerted by the displacement. *Pain in lumbar protrusions is wholly dependent on whether or not the displacement presses on neighbouring sensitive structures.* The most obvious proof of this surprising state of affairs is the typical history given by patients suffering from primary postero-lateral protrusion of disc-material. Though they have suffered internal derangement at a low lumbar level from the first, they have not had, and will not have during the whole evolution of their disorder, one moment's backache, since the protrusion has, from the onset missed the dura mater and compressed the nerve-root only. Hence symptoms are felt only in the lower limb throughout the whole course of the disease. Another proof is afforded by the induction of epidural local anaesthesia. None of the solution gets inside any joint; only the dura mater and its investment of the nerve-roots is rendered anaesthetic, yet the pain disappears, although the protrusion is still present as an articular phenomenon. It has been argued that the pain in lumbago is caused by pressure on the posterior longitudinal ligament. This is not so; for, quite apart from the prominent signs of interference with dural mobility, epidural local anaesthesia destroys the pain for the time being and, though it might be thought to render the posterior surface of the ligament anaesthetic, it cannot reach the anterior surface against which the disc protrusion is pressing. It is the anaesthesia of the dural tube that secures relief. Moreover, when the posterior ligament ruptures and massive extrusion of the disc results, the backache does not cease.

It follows that the lumbar joints are insensitive. Hence, osteophyte formation cannot be expected to set up symptoms. If it did, nearly all elderly people would suffer intractable backache.

Osteophyte formation

Weight-bearing exerts a centrifugal force on the contents of each lumbar joint. When in middle-age degeneration of the disc begins, the bulging in each direction during weight-bearing pulls on the ligaments, especially laterally and anteriorly. Ligamentous traction now lifts the periosteum off the edge of the bone. Periosteum is the limiting membrane of bone and just as traction on the plantar fascia at its calcanean origin lifts up periosteum, whereupon new bone grows in to fill the gap, so does this familiar process affect the edge of the vertebral body. New bone gradually forms in the space between vertebra and periosteum, and in due course an osteophyte appears. The lumbar joint being insensitive, this is a painless process. Osteophyte formation brings two benefits. First, it replaces soft ligament with hard bone and the disc becomes cupped in bone—a strong hindrance to further protrusion. Secondly, the osteophytes limit mobility, thus preventing the very movements that might otherwise have resulted in an attack of internal derangement.

Anyone who still imagines that lumbar osteophyte formation causes a painful condition known as 'osteoarthritis' should visit a clinic where middle-aged heavy workers, e.g. dockers, are seen on account of a disorder unconnected with backache—say, renal calculus. He will see, on radiograph after radiograph of the urinary tract, gross osteophyte formation at all the lumbar vertebrae. Questioned, the patient insists that his back has never troubled him. The fact is that, sooner or later, heavy work results in lumbar trouble unless osteophyte formation comes into play as a protective mechanism. Those who carry heavy weights for a living and whose vertebrae adapt themselves by throwing out osteophytes are able to go on with such work until late middle-age, whereas those who do not develop 'osteoarthritis' develop disc lesions in the end and turn to other jobs. Admittedly, these osteophytes are not a perfect protection, and cases of discogenic pain are encountered notwithstanding marked osteophyte formation, largely because osteophytes have formed anteriorly and laterally but not posteriorly. When, as rarely happens, a posterior osteophyte enlarges enough to compress the dura matter or a nerve root, symptoms do of course result (Plate 18). The lumbo-thoracic spinal joints are not the only ones where osteophyte formation is symptomless, e.g. the cuneo-first-metatarsal joint.

Schmorl's Nodes

Another protective mechanism is the development of Schmorl's nodes. Unfortunately they are rarely seen where they are most needed, i.e. at the fourth and fifth lumbar levels, being common only at the lower thoracic

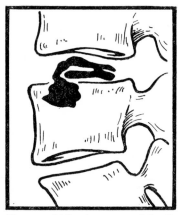

Fig. 69. Schmorl's node. The normal bilocular pattern of the disc is shown. The contrast material outlines the node, demonstrating the connexion.
(By courtesy of J. S. Collis and C. C. Thomas, Springfield, Illinois)

and upper three lumbar joints. This radiographic appearance indicates that the nucleus polposus has protruded vertically into the body of the vertebra. Erosion (Fig. 69) proceeds slowly and painlessly, greatly diminishing the centrifugal force exerted by the nucleus on the annulus and preventing it from tending to shift backwards. Hence it tends to fix the nucleus, but unhappily not at the joints where such protection is most desirable.

THE DURA MATER

This tough membranous tube runs from the foramen magnum of the skull to the caudal edge of the first sacral vertebra. The lower level varies a good deal and once in a hundred cases the theca ends at the second or even the third sacral level, being then pierced by the needle when epidural local anaesthesia is attempted via the sacral hiatus. It keeps the spinal cord, as far as the first lumbar level, then the cauda equina, buffered in a fluid medium. This liquid is continuous from ventricles to sacrum. A vascular jolt, e.g. coughing, momentarily enlarges the intradural veins and starts an impulse transmitted throughout cerebrospinal fluid.

Dural Mobility

The dura mater moves slightly in relation to the vertebrae it traverses. This has been unwittingly noted in two classical signs of meningeal irritation—neck retraction and Kernig's sign. Extension at the neck relaxes the dura mater as much as possible, and has its minor counterpart in local pain brought on by neck-flexion in a thoracic or a lumbar disc lesion. Occasionally a large mid-thoracic protrusion actually limits the range of neck-flexion. Kernig's sign is merely another way of demonstrating limitation of straight-leg raising, and has its counterpart in the patient with sciatica who cannot sit up in the bath without bending the knee of the affected leg. Whether the dura mater is immobilized by inflammation within or compression from without, the movement is limited because it stretches the dura mater from below, via the sciatic nerve. These signs have been accepted for decades, but their mechanism has not been elucidated, because hitherto the dura mater has not been regarded as possessing a mobility of its own, independent of movement at the joints it spans.

Dural stretching from above and below is painful in some patients but not in others with apparently identical lesions. The cause for this discrepancy was elucidated by Reid's (1958) anatomical studies in New Zealand. In the course of thirty-eight autopsies, he found that, in patients over twenty-five, no less than thirty-one had developed localized shortening of the dura mater. As a result, the dura mater had been drawn downwards so far that the thoracic roots could be seen running upwards to their respective foramina. Clearly, the presence or not of dural signs in any one case of lumbago will depend not only on the size of the protrusion but on whether or not the theca has undergone contracture.

Dural Sensitivity

The dura mater is often regarded as insensitive, chiefly because pricking the membrane during lumbar puncture is not felt by the patient. This is not an effective stimulus, any more than is acupuncture of the bowel. When laparotomy is performed under local anaesthesia of the abdominal wall, the intestine can even be divided without any pain. Yet no one denies the tension-pain of colic. The dura mater behaves in the same partly-sensitive way; it does not feel a prick but, when its mobility is impaired, resents stretching.

Edgar and Nundy (1966) made an important contribution to the study of pain arising from the dura mater. They investigated its nerve-supply and found that it was innervated from the sinu-vertebral nerve by three separate routes. However, these fibres all ran to the ventral aspect of the dura mater, no nerves being traced to, or discovered at, the dorsal surface of the membrane. This partial innervation confined to the anterior aspect of the dura mater explains why no pain is felt at lumbar puncture when the needle pierces the membrane. By contrast, a central disc protrusion bulges out of the posterior ligament enough to compress the sensitive anterior aspect of the theca.

The Main Dural Symptom

This is felt in the posterior aspect of the trunk on coughing; curiously enough, in the thoracic region, a deep breath evokes the pain better than a cough. It would not be surprising if the severe backache that sometimes heralds anterior poliomyelitis arises from the dura mater.

The Dural Signs

These are: (1) pain in the back brought on by neck-flexion; (2) pain in the back set up by straight-leg raising. This pain may then be further increased by neck-flexion. O'Connell (1956) made radiographic measurements in full flexion and full extension of the neck and his findings confirmed these views. He showed that in full flexion the length of the front and back of the cervical spinal canal increased by 1·5 cm. and 5 cm. respectively, compared with full extension. Neck-flexion thus stretches the dural tube upwards an average of 3 cm., and draws the thoracic extent of the dura mater with it. This is confirmed by Reid's (1958) postmortem studies.

Comment

In lumbar-disc lesions, the most remarkable feature is that the symptoms, although caused by displacement within a joint, arise from pressure transmitted indirectly to the dura mater and not from any pressure exerted on the articular structures themselves. For years, if the lumbar movements hurt, the common cause of backache was sought in the bones, joints, ligaments, muscles, fasciae—in other words, in the moving parts of the back. Unexpectedly, the intra-articular disc, invisible on the radiograph, provides the prime cause of backache, and the dura mater, formerly thought to lie inert and insensitive within the spinal canal, is the sensitive structure whereby derangements of the spinal joints made themselves felt. The experimental findings of Smith and Wright (1958) substantiate these views. By passing nylon loops around different structures in the back at laminectomy and pulling gently on these threads later, they found: (a) the nerve-root very sensitive, mere touch sufficing to provoke pain and limitation of straight-leg raising; (b) the dura mater only slightly sensitive, an ache appearing in three cases out of five; (c) the interspinous ligaments and the ligamentum flavum insensitive; (d) the posterior longitudinal ligament (tested in one case) sensitive. Unless this dual mechanism is understood, it is not possible to make sense of the signs presented by patients with, e.g., lumbago. The articular protrusion is the primary cause of pressure; it bulges out the back of the intervertebral joint. The ligaments are insensitive and nothing is felt until the bulge is large enough to compress the dura mater.

Since the mechanism is dual, the physical signs would be expected to be dual too. They are: dural and articular. It is possible painfully to stretch the dura mater by traction exerted from a distance—dural signs—and painfully to force the protrusion against the dura mater by movement at the affected joint—articular signs. For this reason, the sub-title of my paper in 1945 was 'the mechanism of dural pain'. Though the suggestion made then that lumbago is caused by internal derangement of a low lumbar joint is now widely accepted, the concept of dural pain has not filtered through appreciably.

Dural Reference

The mechanism of the production of pain in disc lesions is not merely academic; for readers of Chapter III will remember that the manner of reference of pain from the dura mater defies the rules of segmentation that all other tissues observe. False localizing symptoms are, therefore, commonplace, and deceptive. Indeed, there is no pain felt between the waist and the feet that could not originate from a lumbar disc lesion. The pain in acute central lumbago at a low lumbar level may spread to any of the following sites: the whole abdomen below the umbilicus; one or both groins; up the trunk posteriorly to the lower thorax; down the front, outer side or back of both thighs; to the coccyx. This clinical finding was experimentally confirmed by Fernström (1956) who found abdominal pain could be provoked at lumbar discography. Later in 1960, he reported pain in head, shoulders or chest in 1·3 per cent of patients undergoing discography. None of these symptoms has the slightest localizing value, and it must be remembered that, in lesions affecting the dura mater, ordinary anatomical tenets are regularly transgressed. Difficulty arises when pain in one buttock (first lumbar dermatome), one groin (twelfth thoracic dermatome) or the iliac fossa (lowest three thoracic dermatomes) is set up by a low lumbar disc lesion causing little or no concomitant backache. Renal pain, appendicitis or a lower thoracic disc lesion is then closely simulated and differential diagnosis becomes extremely difficult at times. The removal of the appendix for lumbago is no rarity, and by no means an easily avoidable error. Luckily, in those hospitals where it is carried out, epidural local anaesthesia provides a simple answer in all cases of doubt.

By contrast, the area occupied by the root-pain in the lower limb is highly significant; for the affected dermatome is clearly outlined.

LUMBAR INNERVATION

The authoritative research on the nerve supply of the vertebral column was carried out on monkeys by Stilwell in 1956. By means of intravital staining he was able to demonstrate even very delicate nerves in carefully prepared sections. He found the anterior and posterior longitudinal ligaments to be well supplied with nerves entering both from above and below and overlapping. In contrast to Edgar and Nundy, he found the dorsal aspect of the dura mater to be supplied with nerves exclusively from the autonomic plexus, whereas the ventral half was supplied by a recurrent branch from the sinu-vertebral ramus containing both autonomic and somatic fibres. This nerve travels back through the intervertebral foramen, composed of fibres derived from two roots.

The annulus fibrosus has nerves confined to a thin layer of connective tissue on its surface, continuous with the vertebral periosteum. No nerves penetrate the annulus. The interspinous and flaval ligaments possess nerves along their surfaces only, no fibres are detectable entering their substance. These fibres have two sources: the nerves to the overlying muscles, and the same nerves as innervate the dorsal aspect of the dura mater. The facet joints are supplied from the primary dorsal rami, which run to two adjacent joints; each therefore derives nerves from two segments.

THE LUMBAR NERVE-ROOTS

Obliquity

The lumbar roots emerge in pairs from the dura mater and reach the foramen of exit by passing downwards and outwards across the body of the vertebra and the postero-lateral aspect of the intervertebral joint. It is here that a protruded disc can impinge against them.

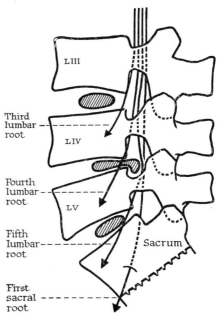

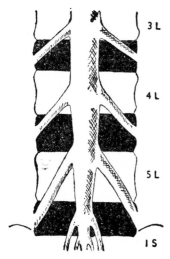

FIG. 70. Relation of the lumbar nerve-roots to the intervertebral discs (black)

(*From a photograph of a dissection: Burns and Young, 'Lancet', 1945.*)

FIG. 71. Compression of the fifth lumbar root by a protrusion at the fourth level. This diagram shows clearly that a herniation appearing just to one side of the posterior ligament misses its own nerve-root, since this had already passed too far laterally. It is apt to impinge against the root emerging one level below.

(*After G. Laurence in 'Revue du Practicien', 1955.*)

The downward slope of the lower nerve-roots has an important practical application. It is possible for a protrusion lying almost centrally at the fourth level to pinch the fifth root, whereas by presenting a little more to one side, it can compress only the fourth root (Fig. 71). A larger protrusion can, of course, squeeze both roots. Similarly, a protrusion at the fifth level may affect the first sacral or the fifth lumbar or both roots. A fourth lumbar palsy indicates that the lesion lies at the fourth level; a first sacaral palsy, at the fifth lumbar level; but a fifth lumbar palsy leaves the issue indeterminate. Hence, it is always best to confine the diagnosis to a statement on which root is affected.

The motor and sensory components of the nerve-root emerge separately; hence a purely motor (impingement from below), or a purely sensory (compression from above the root) paresis is common. A large protrusion affects both components of the root. Moreover, a protrusion emerging between, say, the fifth lumbar and first sacral root can compress the motor aspect of the lumbar root and the sensory aspect of the sacral root, causing a fifth lumbar motor, and a first sacral sensory, palsy. It is very rare for a third lumbar disc lesion to affect the third and fourth roots; at this level, the third root is affected alone. At the fourth and fifth levels, the third and fourth sacral roots may be compressed alone or in combination with the lower lumbar or upper sacral roots.

Dural Investment of Nerve-roots

The nerve-root draws out with it an investment of dura mater that extends, judging by clinical data, for at least 2 cm. The existence of this short sleeve derived from the dura mater was deduced on clinical grounds (Cyriax, 1949). The anatomical studies of Frykholm (1951) confirmed its presence and post-mortem specimens were illustrated (Brain, 1954) delineating the extent of the dural pouch. Hence reference of dural type is to be expected when a nerve-root is exposed to compression. Many observers must have been puzzled to note that the fourth and fifth lumbar dermatomes start in the lower thigh; yet the pain of sciatica usually includes the upper thigh and buttock. The pain occupies not only the whole extent of the relevant dermatome, but also a proximal area where the dermatome is absent. For example, a patient with a fourth or fifth lumbar root compression usually has pain in the buttock and upper thigh where no fourth or fifth segment of skin exists at all; he also has, of course, pain correctly felt in the distal extremity of the limb at the correct segmental area. This is an example of extrasegmental dural reference, analagous to the extrasegmental radiation of pain when the dura mater itself is compressed. The sciatic nerve-trunk beyond the dural sleeve is insensitive locally, and compression here merely gives rise to distal paraesthesia. It is a curious fact that only when the dural investment of the nerve-root is irritated does root-pain result and that, when it does, it is accurately dermatomal only in its distal extent. Pressure on any part of the whole of the rest of the nerve does not result in pain at all, merely numbness and pins and needles in the known cutaneous area of that nerve.

Sheath and Parenchyma

The nerve-roots consist of two parts, sheath and parenchyma, each with a different function.

Mobility of the Sheath

Each root has an external aspect—the dural sheath—which moves in relation to neighbouring structures. Experiments during laminectomy have shown that the lower two lumbar roots undergo an excursion of about half a centimetre during straight-leg raising. Restriction of mobility at these two roots limits the range of straight-leg raising, since the sciatic nerve lies behind the hip and knee joints. Restriction of mobility at the third lumbar root limits the range of prone-lying knee-flexion, since the femoral nerve lies in front of the hip-joint. Moreover, the occurrence of a painful arc on straight-leg raising (Fig. 72) shows that the nerve-root moves in relation to the posterior aspect of the joint. A bulge here may form a projection against which the nerve catches; if it is small, the root slips over it, causing momentary pain, after which the rest of the move-ment further stretching the nerve is painless.

Pain, whether in the back or lower limb, caused by straight-leg raising is often increased by neck-flexion. Now, if a pain brought on by straight-leg raising is aggravated by neck-flexion, the tissue whose mobility is impaired must run in a continuous line from the neck to below the knee, passing behind the hip and knee joints. There is only one such structure—the dura mater and its continuation, the sciatic nerve.

In sciatica, the lumbar spine may deviate in a manner calculated to minimise pressure on the sensitive sheath of the nerve-root. If a protrusion lies at the axilla of the root, the patient deviates towards the painful side, more so on trunk flexion, thereby avoiding dragging the root against the projection. This deviation is involuntary; the patient is unaware of the way he moves on bending forwards and cannot prevent himself doing so. If the protrusion lies lateral to the nerve root, he preserves the root by deviating away from the painful side.

Conduction

Each root has an internal aspect—the parenchyma—which serves conduction only; it is not concerned with mobility. Hence, interference with the parenchyma leads to a lower motor neurone lesion. Pressure on the sheath of the root, though painful, may not be great enough to affect conduction as well as mobility; if so, the tests for mobility show interference; for conduction, no interference. Greater pressure impairs both mobility and conduction. Pressure greater still may cause ischaemic root atrophy, whereupon the sheath loses its sensitivity and the protective reflex limiting straight-leg raising ceases. Then the hamstrings no longer contract to protect the nerve-root; in consequence, the range of the movement of stretching the nerve becomes of full range at the same time as the palsy becomes complete.

I have never met a case of an isolated sciatic neuritis (apart from neural-

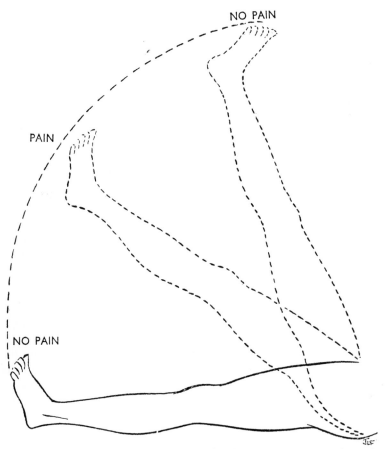

Fig. 72. Painful arc on straight-leg raising. This is found when the nerve-root catches against a small projection, and slips over it.

gic amyotrophy) at the lower limb, and doubt its existence. Were such a disorder to occur, only the parenchyma would be affected; hence mobility could not be restricted, only conduction.

The fourth sacral root lies centrally in the lumbar region, protected by the posterior longitudinal ligament. It is very seldom compressed by a protruding disc; for this tends to be turned off to one or other side by the strong central resistance. Interference with this root leads to perineal and lower sacral pain, weakness of the bladder, anal analgesia and numbness in the saddle area. This root is not stretched during straight-leg raising, and in isolated compression dural and nerve-sheath signs are both absent. More often, massive extrusion of disc-material compresses the entire cauda equina and severe bilateral sciatica accompanies the fourth sacral root palsy.

PRACTICAL BEARING

It follows from the matter set out in this chapter that a patient suspected of a lumbar disc lesion must be logically examined on the principles of applied anatomy. Fortunately this is quick and simple. The routine is:

The Bones
Inspection. Palpation. Radiography.

The Joints
Visible deformity standing still.
Lateral deviation on movement.
Range of movement.
Pain elicited at one or more extremes of movement; where is this felt?
Painful arc.

Dura Mater
Neck-flexion alone.
Straight-leg raising.
Neck-flexion during stretching of nerve-root.

The Nerve-roots
Sheath: estimating mobility.
Parenchyma: testing conduction.

This examination suffices for the identification of a disc lesion. It does not take account of differential diagnosis, which is dealt with in Chapter 18.

17

The Lumbar Region

PART II: EXAMINATION

The examination of a patient complaining of backache follows a logical sequence as given below.

The Patient Walks In

1. Inspection of gait and general appearance as he enters.

The Patient Sits

2. History.

The Patient Stands

3. Inspection of the posterior aspect of the trunk and lower limbs. Spinal deformity, pelvic tilt. The position of thigh and wasting are noted.
4. Asking the patient to point to the level and extent of his pain.
5. Noting the range achieved on each active movement at the lumbar joints.
6. Noting change in range or pain when the examiner aids the lumbar movement.
7. Noting if any movement alters a lumbar deformity.
8. Noting if any movement causes pain and if so where.
9. Noting the presence or absence of a painful arc.
10. Testing the muscles while the joints are held motionless, i.e. the resisted lumbar movements.
11. If any question of a weak calf-muscle has arisen, asking the patient to rise on tiptoe first on the good, then on the bad, leg only.

The Patient Lies Supine

12. Testing the mobility of the dura mater by neck-flexion, straight-leg raising, and neck-flexion during straight-leg raising.

13. Testing and mobility of the dural investment of the fourth lumbar to second sacral nerve-roots.

14. Testing conduction along the second to fifth lumbar nerve-roots.

The Patient Lies Prone

15. Testing conduction along the first and second sacral nerve-roots.

16. Testing the mobility of the dural sleeve of the third lumbar nerve-root.

17. Palpation for lumbar deformity.

18. Carrying out a series of small extension thrusts at each lumbar joint in turn, in order to determine at which level the symptoms are best reproduced. In addition, muscle guarding may be felt at the level of the lesion. Palpation for tenderness yields no useful information except when a fractured transverse process is suspected.

Further Measures

19. Radiography.

20. Sometimes, electromyography.

21. Sometimes, lumbar puncture.

22. Sometimes, myelography or epiduropraphy.

23. Sometimes, exploratory laminectomy.

When the function of every low lumbar structure has been fully tested, the hip joints with the muscles that control them, and the sacro–iliac joints, are examined. Occasionally, too, arterial examination is relevant.

Since backache is a common psychogenic symptom, the question of neurosis arises. Interspersed between the relevant observations, therefore, some tests are included to which ordinary patients' responses are uniformly negative. In this way, the examination singles out those who put forward the self-contradictory patterns characterizing pain partly or wholly of emotional origin. It also prevents the reverse error—namely, a mistaken diagnosis of psychogenic pain in an obviously neurotic patient who, nevertheless, happens to have a genuine lesion.

Preliminary Inspection

Before the history is taken, a glance is given at the overall picture presented by the patient. Does he walk in aided or unaided? How did he travel from his home to hospital? These findings may or may not tally with his account later of the degree of disablement. What is his posture and his gait? As he seats himself, does he do so easily, or with the caution that denotes the need to avoid severe twinges? If his seated posture is unexceptional, he must possess 90 degree range of flexion at hip and knee. A glance at his face gives an idea of how he has been sleeping and how badly the pain is affecting him; how does this compare with his account, perhaps, of severe pain and sleepless nights?

Patients brought in on a stretcher may well be suffering from severe lumbago or sciatica due to a disc lesion, but patients who arrive in a wheel-chair are usually suffering from spinal neoplasm or chronic osteomyelitis; for sitting is nearly always the most painful position in fourth and fifth lumbar disc lesions (but not at the third level, when the articular signs are often reversed).

HISTORY

Lumbar Symptoms

There is a tendency to become impatient with diseases that pass on neither to death nor to recovery. Many are uninterested in disorders that seldom lead to appreciable crippledom and yet run a variable chronic course over which it is difficult to achieve control. Most physicians and nearly all surgeons become bored by the backaches that are daily described to them. In fact, backache is a symptom hard to evaluate, and *all* cases of backache are in essence 'difficult'. Hence, every possible assistance is needed, and a detailed history in chronological sequence is the first stand-by. No effort should be spared to find out what the symptoms have been, and are now; when they started, and what vicissitudes the back has suffered during the years. Where was the pain originally; has it ever spread elsewhere; how did it begin; was it constant or intermittent; has it altered lately; what brings it on; is it affected by posture or rest or exertion? All this must be ascertained. How severe is the pain and what is the degree of disablement?

When the symptom is backache, the following questions are kept in mind:

(1) Is this a disc lesion or one of the uncommon causes of backache?

(2) If it sounds like a disc lesion, is the protrusion hard or soft, large or small, central or unilateral, stable or unstable? The behaviour of symptoms, as from their first appearance, is highly indicative. Is there any pointer to the level? If a postero-lateral protrusion is suggested, is it primary or secondary?

It must be realized that it is only the history that can suggest the mush-room phenomenon or a nuclear self-reducing herniation.

(3) What sort of a person is the patient? Does his account of his pain follow one of the well-known sequences? Do the activities that make the pain better or worse tally with the rest of the story? Do the described

degree of pain and his daily activities fit in with his appearance and with the disablement that he describes?

However simple the case seems, the patient should always be induced to talk about his reaction to his symptoms.

Time

This has both diagnostic and medico-legal bearing.

If a patient has had backache for years, progressive, serious disease is ruled out. Only a few disorders give rise to episodic pain, and only intermittent internal derangement repeatedly fixes a joint within its range of movement. Constant displacement of a part of the disc may get neither greater nor smaller for years; there is no limit to how long such a backache may last without recovery or aggravation. By contrast, a month or two of increasing backache, often in an elderly patient, may well signal lumbar metastases. In spondylitis, the pain spreads up the trunk.

A disc is damaged by prolonged wear and tear; it may also suffer in an accident. Should an annular crack be caused by an injury, it may not become complete for a year or two. Once it is complete, many months may elapse before the patient makes the movement that brings about displacement; now, for the first time he becomes aware of his lesion. Hence a gap of weeks, months or years may separate the accident from its eventual, nevertheless direct, result. This long interval between cause and effect causes great medico-legal difficulties and distresses Counsel and Judge who, naturally, expect guidance on the relevance of injury to a symptom beginning later. In fact, no theoretical limit exists to the interval between an accident and the onset of pain. Moreover, it is always arguable that the trouble is due to an antecedent injury or that the patient would in any case have developed symptoms as he grew older. There can be no certainty.

Similarity

When patients relate symptoms caused by a low lumbar disc lesion, the outstanding feature is the similarity of the accounts. Each is describing the effects on himself of events taking place in a closed cavity lying in the mid-line of the lumbar area. Since pain arises only from pressure exerted alternatively on the dura mater or on a nerve-root, there is a limit to the number of different events which can take place. 'All discs are alike, and all other disorders are different' is a sound working rule.

In general, the ache due to disc-trouble is increased by exertion, especially lifting, i.e. flexion during increased compression. The patient, even when free from all symptoms, can, if he chooses, bring his pain on by, e.g., digging for some time. Merely keeping the lumbar spine in kyphosis by sitting, driving a car or in an armchair, brings on backache relieved by standing up. Turning in bed often occasions a twinge. Avoidance of activity, recumbency and maintaining the lordosis lessen the backache.

By contrast, the way pain is referred from the back when a lumbar disc lesion is present is very variable, since the dura mater does not obey the rules of segmental reference, and pain spreading up to the scapulae, forward to the lower abdomen and down to the coccyx is as common as the proper segmental reference to the lower limbs.

Characteristic Histories

By lumbago is meant severe backache coming on suddenly and temporarily fixing the patient.

Annular Lumbago

The story is typical of internal derangement. The patient states that he bent down; as he came up again he felt a click and was seized with severe lumbar pain, locking him in flexion, less often in side-flexion. The pain is more often bilateral than unilateral. After some seconds or minutes, he could straighten up but agonizing twinges prevented any but the most cautious movement, and coughing and sneezing were very painful. A rare symptom is a momentary, painless giving-way of both legs, as if all postural sense had ceased in both lower limbs (neurologists describe this phenomenon in other disorders as the 'drop attack'). He retired to bed and the pain gradually eased, until, after some days or weeks, he was symptom-free. He remained so until a year or two later when a similar movement brought on the same train of events. The patient's account is the exact counterpart of internal derangement at the knee; a strain is followed by severe local pain and locking in flexion. A displacement lying at the back of his lumbar joint forces the patient to bend forwards, holding the joint in kyphosis so as to accommodate the protrusion; for, while erect, he squeezes the protrusion still further backwards, increasing the already painful pressure on the dura mater. Gradual reduction during rest in bed, i.e. during relief from the compression inherent in the erect position, follows the attack, but recurrence is very probable. Cartilage, having no blood supply, cannot unite once fractured, and a fragment that has moved once can always move again.

Nuclear Lumbago

The history in cases of nuclear herniation is equally characteristic. The patient did some heavy work involving much stooping and lifting, e.g.

laying a concrete path. After some hours he felt a slight backache but thought little of it. That evening after sitting for an hour or two in his armchair, the back felt stiff and ached. He slept comfortably, but woke next morning unable to get out of bed because of severe lumbar pain. He stayed in bed for a week or two and recovered. A pain that appears to be brought on by rest in bed and yet abated on further recumbency is puzzling. Sooner or later, he had another attack. This account describes to be the onset of a displacement slowly increasing in size and first giving rise to symptoms many hours after the maintenance of the causative posture, i.e. a nuclear protrusion. Pulp oozes; cartilage subluxates in an instant. The distinction has an important bearing both on treatment and on the maintenance of reduction. A hard fragment can be manipulated; a soft protrusion recedes most quickly with traction. A patient with a pulpy lesion can safely play tennis again; for, though he bends down, he comes up again instantly and the prolonged flexion that sets up nuclear movement does not come into operation. On the other hand, a patient with a cracked annulus has to be constantly on his guard.

Backache

A patient who declares that his lumbar pain was central or bilateral at first but is now unilateral, must have a disc lesion. His statement indicates that the lesion has moved from the centre of the back to one side. In order to move in this way, the lesion must occupy a central cavity; and there is only one such, the intervertebral joint, and the only tissue it contains is the disc itself. The converse does not hold; for a patient with either a disc lesion or ankylosing spondylitis may describe unilateral pain in the buttock later becoming central and lumbar.

Backache which changes sides is more often caused by a fourth than a fifth lumbar disc lesion; an ache in the buttock that alternates suggests sacro-iliac arthritis. Rather a similar story is recounted by patients with two low lumbar disc lesions, i.e., at both the fourth and fifth levels.

In very early disc lesions, or in those that remain minor, the characteristic feature is aching dependent on how much the patient exerts his back. This is the cause of the ordinary backache to which almost everyone is subject. Any work involving stooping is followed by pain or occasions sudden twinges; if he takes things quietly, he feels little or nothing. He may experience difficulty in straightening up after bending or in getting up out of an armchair or car (i.e., after the maintenance of kyphosis has allowed some posterior displacement of part of the disc). Turning in bed is often mentioned as occasioning a twinge awakening him.

A curious alternation sometimes takes place in long-standing backache caused by a disc lesion. For some or many years the patient wakes comfortable and then gets backache varying in intensity according to what he does: the expected pattern. Eventually, the situation reverses itself and he gets pain waking him in the early hours and easing when he gets up; an occasional patient is encountered who has had to leave his bed for half-an-hour before dawn for years. He may be able to do quite heavy work by day without discomfort. The second half of this history does ont suggest a disc lesion at all, but the first half of the history is characteristic, and the fact remains that the only effective treatment is epidural local anaesthesia. Rarely, a small chronic disc lesion sets up matutinal pain only, but the common cause of backache worst on waking is spondylitis ankylopoetica.

Compression Phenomena

A different account designates a self-reducing disc lesion. The patient, often in his twenties or thirties, wakes comfortable. After he has been up for some hours, the back begins to ache. This continues, often getting slowly worse as the day wears on. When he lies in bed the pain ceases after an hour or so. Again he wakes comfortable, and it is an essential part of the diagnosis that for the first hour or two up, the patient can bend in every direction and feel nothing, whereas the same movements performed in the afternoon are painful. The mere fact that a backache ceases when the patient is in bed is not evidence of a nuclear self-reducing type of lesion; he must be able to move his back fully and painlessly in every direction for the first hour each morning.

The mushroom phenomenon is also the result of compression. The patient is an elderly man, who after standing for ten or fifteen minutes gets backache. Further standing makes it severe, and if circumstances force him to stay upright for longer, bilateral sciation may be added to the backache. The moment he sits or lies down the pain ceases, never in longer than a minute. This sequence is also described in spondylolisthesis, both with and without a secondary disc lesion, but the patient is then usually much younger.

Pain on Coughing and Sneezing

This suggests interference with the dura mater, but is not pathognomic of a disc lesion. A neuroma is very apt to result in pain worse on coughing or sneezing, usually felt in the lower limb rather than the back. In active sacro-iliac arthritis, a cough raises the intra-abdominal pressure, thus momentarily distracting the sacro-iliac joints; hence, a cough hurts in one buttock.

Consistency

The following helps differentiate a nuclear from a cartilaginous displacement. Backache brought on *after* (some hours later, or even next day) rather than *during* exertion, suggests slow nuclear oozing. Pain in the back, buttock or lower limb increasingly evoked by sitting and relieved by restoration of the lordosis has the same significance. By contrast, backache coming on as soon as exertion starts suggests an annular lesion. If a click initiates or abolishes symptoms, the fragment is clearly cartilaginous.

Position

The patient is asked to indicate at what level he felt his pain at the onset, and to state whether it began centrally or to one side of the midline. He must describe any subsequent change in position of his pain and say whether it radiated elsewhere or shifted. Upper lumbar pain—'the forbidden area'—is very seldom the result of a disc lesion, whereas this is the common cause of purely low lumbar symptoms.

If a central pain becomes unilateral, a central lesion has shifted to one side: a possibility only if a loose body occupies a central cavity in which it is free to move to one side. This is just what happens in disc trouble.

Central pain cannot arise from a muscle or a facet joint, in which pain would be unilateral from the first.

Pain at one or other side of the sacrum, later leading to central backache, coming and going irrespective of what the patient does, characterizes spondylitis ankylopoetica. The same significance attaches to diffuse lumbar pain, often worst on waking, that spreads up to thoracic levels in the course of some years.

Stability

If a heavy worker gets an attack of pain in the back less than once a year, it is clear that the loose fragment of disc is pretty stable. In contrast, pain occurring each few months without any particular exertion implies great instability. Easy, successful manipulative reduction also suggests instability and the probability of early recurrence.

Central backache coming and going independent of exertion is most unlikely to be caused by disc trouble, but more probably indicates flare and subsidence in spondylitis ankylopoetica. Recent central backache slowly getting worse suggests spinal neoplasm or tuberculous caries.

Reducibility

If several weeks' rest in bed is needed before the patient can return to work, he suffers real economic hardship. If a couple of days suffice, his attacks hardly matter. If one manipulation puts him right each time, all he needs is a capable manipulator. However, a displacement insusceptible to manipulation that, untreated, lasts for months or is relieved only after some weeks' traction must be taken seriously and every endeavour made to prevent recurrence.

Size

Marked articular signs suggest a large protrusion. Fixation of the joint in deformity noticeable to the patient implies a considerable blocking of the joint. If he is fixed flexed by central pain, he is clearly describing a posterior displacement. If he states that one hip projects, he is describing deviation of the lumbar spine away from the prominent side. Tilt to one side suggests trouble at the fourth, rather than the fifth lumbar level; a fourth lumbar disc lesion is almost a certainty if the deviation varies in direction from one attack to another, or if it alternates from moment to moment. A lateral list implies that the dura mater has to be held to one side or another of a central projection.

Statement that the foot feels numb, or that it flops when the patient walks or that he finds that he cannot rise on tiptoe, naturally suggests a root palsy; this too is evidence of a large protrusion.

Neurosis

The patient with emotional trouble which he centres on his back does not really know what he ought to feel; he therefore describes not his symptoms but his degree of suffering. When asked to describe his trouble, he talks of 'it' or of feeling 'so bad', and can give no clear account of where his pain was at first, and is now, how long ago it began, and how it has altered since. Such a patient, if not interrupted, can talk for twenty minutes without mentioning his symptoms at all. He dilates at length on the circumstantial evidence for its reality: his disablement, and the reaction of his family to it, the number of different doctors consulted, diagnoses made and treatments undergone. When asked what took him to all those doctors in the first place, he rarely answers simply 'my backache' but explains that it was his inability to do things, or because his friends, perceiving his suffering, insisted on it.

When the question arises of how his pain has varied during the years, if it has spread and if so where to, what activities or postures make the pain better or worse, he becomes restive and makes it clear that he finds the physician's questions tiresome, irrelevant and displaying inexperience. This contrasts strongly with the patient with organic backache, who is only too pleased at last to have found a physician displaying an interest in his backache; he is only too delighted to give full details.

A genuine minor lesion in a neurotic patient presents a more difficult problem. He knows what to say; but the discrepancy between his symptoms and the degree of disablement, and then with the physical signs, is too great to pass unnoticed. He may be unable to go out or to work; yet he can travel up to hospital alone, walking into the clinic room with an easy gait. It must be remembered, however, that severe neurosis is no bar to the development of acute lumbago. In such a case, of course, the severe pain is balanced by equally marked physical signs.

Lumbago without Disc Lesion

There are six rare conditions in which a history of lumbago is described and yet internal derangement is not the cause—fracture, spondylitis ankylopoetica, afebrile osteomyelitis, tuberculosis, and tabes.

1. *Pathological Fracture*

A patient with malignant disease of the lumbar vertebra, senile osteoporosis or, yet more rarely, no predisposing lumbar disorder, may describe sudden lumbar pain on lifting an object, followed by difficulty in straightening up again. Though the history is similar, inspection of the lumbar spine shows the angular kyphos; the radiograph is diagnostic.

2. *Ankylosing Spondylitis*

When this disease attacks the lumbar spine, the patient can suddenly and painfully sprain the stiffening lumbar joints by lifting something heavy. The attacks simulate lumbago, but the pain may be *upper* lumbar and in any case, by the time these events are described, the range of both side-flexion movements at the lumbar spine is visibly impaired.

3. *Spondylitic Invasion of the Disc*

In the early stage of lumbar involvement by ankylosing spondylitis, postmortem studies have demonstrated (Bywaters, 1968) granulomatous invasion of the disc. This is weakened and becomes slowly replaced by vascular connective tissue. Such softening of the disc can clearly lead to fissures, fragmentation and, in due course, to sudden attacks of internal derangement at a time when no clinical limitation of movement is detectable. These bouts result from a disc lesion, the damage to which is secondary to the spondylitic process, not to ordinary wear and tear.

This disorder must be distinguished from a liability to lumbago in a patient who later on happened to develop spondylitis.

4. *Tuberculosis of the Disc*

This possibility is most deceptive, since it is caused by sudden central protrusion of a disc weakened, not as is usual by trauma or overuse, but by tuberculous disease. This disorder perfectly mimics the history and physical signs of a first attack of lumbago, caused by an uninfected disc, since, after all, it still is at that moment purely a disc lesion. The infection not yet having eroded bone, the radiograph reveals no abnormality and the sedimentation rate may well be normal. Naturally, such a case is bound to be treated at first for lumbago on standard lines, and it is only the lack of response to treatment that leads to radiography repeated later on. One such patient, treated by manipulation for a third lumbar disc lesion, remained pain-free for a year afterwards; the first radiograph to show erosion of bone was taken eighteen months after the onset.

Naturally, manipulation of a lesion that later proves tuberculous suggests negligence to the patient, and could lead to medico-legal difficulties. But it is doubtful if any real harm accrues to the patient with very early caries, even if manipulation accelerates the invasion of bone.

Until this becomes visible radiographically, no patient would accept nor doctor initiate the tedious treatment that tuberculosis necessitates. Hence, nothing effective can be done until the disease has reached the same stage either way.

5. *Chronic Afebrile Osteomyelitis*

The patient is sent up by ambulance as a case of acute lumbago. The story is of some weeks' increasing pain at the centre of the back coming on for no obvious reason. Severe pain stops the patient standing and nothing arouses suspicion at first except that coughing does not hurt; surprising in such an acute case. Examination, however, shows a complete absence of dural signs and epidural local anaesthesia does not abate the pain.

6. *Tabes*

Lumbago is occasionally mimicked by tabes. Cases occur of lumbar crises instead of gastric crises. The patient suffers periodic attacks of severe lumbar pain without vomiting, for which, on examination, there is no lumbar lesion to account. Absence of tendon reflexes at the lower limbs naturally leads to examination of the reaction of the eyes to light and to the serological tests for syphilis.

Root-pain

Pain caused by a lumbar disc lesion may be felt in the lower back only. Root-pain may supersede, or be added to it. Unilateral root-pain often occupies one clear dermatome, and is then an aid in diagnosis. Whether the lumbar pain disappears or not when the root-pain comes on is important in prognosis and treatment.

Extra-segmental Reference

In lumbago, the pain may spread up the back of the trunk to the scapulae, anteriorly to the abdomen and groins, down any aspect of the lower limbs, or to the coccyx. This radiation has no bearing on the level of the articular lesion, and is not as severe as the lumbar pain itself. When, as happens occasionally, referred pain only is present, diagnosis becomes difficult; for pain felt down both lower limbs or in one or both groins does not sound much like lumbago. Indeed, when the right groin only is affected, a diagnosis of 'chronic appendicitis' is often made.

There are two difficulties here. First, pain from a low lumbar disc lesion is often felt at the side of the sacrum or in the upper buttock. Yet the upper buttock is covered by skin of first, second and third lumbar derivation, and the lower buttock by skin formed from the first and second sacral segments. Hence, in theory, compression of the fourth and fifth lumbar nerve-roots cannot give rise to pain in the upper buttock— exactly where such pain usually begins. It is hard to find an explanation for this phenomenon, unless it is that the uppermost component of the root-pain is due to irritation of the edge of the dura mater and forms part of the extra-segmental reference from that tissue. The compression of the adjacent dural sleeve of the nerve-root can then be regarded as responsible for correct segmental reference to the distal part of the lower limit. Secondly, pain in the groin can arise in two separate ways. It may provide merely an example of extra-segmental reference, and thus possess no localizing significance. But it may also represent the proximal part of third sacral root-pain. If the pain spreads to the groin and along the inner aspect of the thigh to the knee, the third sacral dermatome is fully outlined, but if the pain is in the groin only, the significance is ambiguous.

Dermatomic Reference

Unilateral root-pain is a considerable help in diagnosis, giving a good pointer to which nerve-root is at fault. Pins and needles or numbness afford an even better clue, provided the patient can give a clear account of where they are felt.

Pain in the groin suggests third sacral root compression, not first lumbar root-pain. The latter is very rare and more apt to make the groin paraesthetic. Third sacral pain may travel along the groin and down the inner side of the thigh to the medial aspect of the knee. Pain at the front of the thigh characterizes a second or third lumbar root lesion; if the front of the leg is included the third lumbar root is singled out. Pain at the outer thigh and leg, crossing to the dorsum and inner aspect of the foot occurs with fourth and fifth lumbar root lesions. If the big toe is affected alone, either root may be responsible, but if the second and third toes are also involved, it is the fifth root. Pain reaching the outer two toes along the lateral border of the foot indicates that the first sacral root is affected, but pain from buttock to heel is common to the first and second sacral roots. Pressure on the fourth sacral root may give rise to perineal pain and weakness of bladder and rectum.

As a rule, when the root-pain comes on, the backache ceases; this is to be expected since a protrusion that moves from the centre to one side naturally stops compressing the dura mater at the same moment as it reaches the nerve-root. The determination of this moment is important in assessing the past and future duration of a root-pain, since calculation can begin only from the cessation of the lumbar pain and its transference to the lower limb. Backache continuing when the root-pain appears can go on indefinitely, especially when the back aches more severely than the limb. In elderly patients the backache seldom disappears when the sciatica comes on, and after the age of sixty no term can be put to a sciatic pain accompanied by some backache.

Primary postero-lateral protrusions usually come on slowly in patients aged twenty to thirty-five. They never impinge on the dura mater at all; hence premonitory backache is absent. The patient describes pain brought on gradually by sitting, felt at the calf, at the back of the knee, or at the posterior aspect of the thigh. After some weeks or months, the whole posterior aspect of one lower limb aches the whole time; the pain may extend to the buttock in the end. A cough hurts the limb. This history of such an onset is important, for such protrusions are always irreducible by manipulation.

Numbness is often described; if so, the distal extent enables the dermatome affected to be identified. Some days' or weeks' severe sciatica suddenly abating within a few hours, with the onset of a numb foot, characterizes root-atrophy. Some patients complain that the foot and leg feel cold. This is not a misinterpretation of numbness; for Stary (1956) showed by thermometry that the limb is often actually colder than its fellow, presumably as the result of loss of the circulatory pump in those with a weak calf muscle.

Bilateral sciatica, especially if it alternates, suggests the sacro-iliac arthritis of ankylosing spondylitis, less often it designates disc lesions at both the fourth and fifth lumbar levels. Rarely a disc may develop two protrusions, one at each side of the posterior longitudinal ligament, bilateral root-pain resulting. Massive extrusion of the whole disc after rupture of the posterior ligament compresses the whole cauda equina;

weakness of the bladder and perineal-anal-rectal-sacral numbness then accompany the bilateral root-pain. Bilateral sciatica without alternation characterizes spondylolisthesis, the mushroom phenomenon and malignant disease. Pain of similar distribution is described in bilateral osteoarthritis of the hip, intermittent claudication, spinal claudication and tabes.

Paraesthesia in the Lower Limb

Paraesthesia without root-pain can result from diseases like disseminated sclerosis, diabetes or pernicious anaemia. More often (in cases referred to the orthopaedic physician) the cause is pressure on the spinal cord from space-occupying lesions at any cervical or thoracic level, usually central disc protrusions. It is important to remember that such central protrusions may give rise neither to local pain (then or previously) nor to any interference with the mobility at the relevant joint. For example, a doctor with a spastic paresis of both legs for seventeen years never had any neckache. He had a full and painless range of movement at his neck, and yet myelography revealed a very large disc protrusion at the sixth cervical level, which was removed. Sometimes a clear sign emerges; one patient complained of pins and needles in his big toe only on bending his head forwards; this was abolished by manipulative reduction carried out at his neck. In other cases of pressure on the spinal cord, suspicion is aroused by the fact that the paraesthesiae are bilateral and neither spondylolisthesis nor the mushroom phenomenon is present. Alternatively, they may occupy an area not corresponding to any root or peripheral nerve area. For example, an elderly man whose cervical disc displacement was reduced (with some difficulty) had had neckache for ten years and one year's paraesthesia extending from both patellae to all the toes of each foot—an impossible anatomical distribution for any one pair of nerve-roots or nerve-trunks. Another patient whose mid-thoracic disc protrusion responded to traction had had eighteen months' pins and needles at the inner three toes of one foot, spreading to the same toes of the other foot for the previous three months.

Hence, pins and needles felt in one or both lower limbs without root-pain focuses attention on the spinal cord at cervical and thoracic levels rather than any low lumbar lesion (with the exception of spondylolisthesis).

Pressure Paraesthesia in One Lower Limb

Pins and needles, often with numbness over a lesser area, are apt to accompany root-pain when the protrusion compresses the sensory part of the root, by impingement from above. Accurate dermatomic distribution results. The possibilities are:

Front of thigh: second or third lumbar nerve-root; pressure on the middle cutaneous or obturator nerve.

Outer side of thigh: pressure on lateral cutaneous nerve, i.e., meralgia paraesthetica.

Front of leg: third lumbar nerve-root.

Outer leg: fourth or fifth lumbar nerve-root.

Big toe: fourth or fifth lumbar nerve-root; saphenous nerve at foramen below knee.

Big and second toes: fifth lumbar root, tight tibial fascial compartment, pressure on second digital nerve.

Big and two adjacent toes: fifth lumbar root.

All toes: compression of peroneal nerve at fibula; combined pressure on fifth lumbar and first sacral root.

Second toe and sole: loose body in knee.

Second, third and fourth toes: fifth lumbar root.

Fourth and fifth toes: first sacral root; Morton's metatarsalgia.

Heel, calf and posterior thigh: first and second sacral roots.

Saddle area, anus and scrotum: fourth sacral root.

Pressure Paraesthesia in Both Lower Limbs

Spondylolisthesis.
Spinal claudication.
The mushroom phenomenon.
Cervico-thoracic disc lesions protruding centrally.
Spinal neoplasms, benign or malignant.

EXAMINATION

Nothing is easier than to decide that the patient has a disc lesion. But it is by no means enough to say 'another disc'. This bare statement lacks all the detail essential to the formulation of an accurate prognosis and the prescription of proper treatment. Many relevant questions must first be answered. Is it large or small? Is it in place or out of place? Is it cartilaginous or nuclear or both? In which direction has it moved? At which level does it lie? Is it movable or fixed? Is it likely to get larger or to recede? Is it dangerously placed? Is it causing severe pain in the trunk or limb? Is there marked lumbar deformity which may become permanent? Is it interfering with a nerve-root enough to cause a palsy? If so, is one root compressed or two? In either case, does the palsy matter, and will it eventually recover by vertebral erosion, cartilaginous shrinkage, pressure atrophy or reduction, and, if so, how much longer will that take? Have adhesions formed about the root? Moreover, how stoical or hyper-sensitive is the patient?

Although the shift from postero-central to postero-lateral is slight anatomically, patients' signs vary in emphasis according to this change in position of the protrusion. In the former case, articular and dural signs predominate. When pain felt in the limb supervenes, the articular signs diminish and may disappear at the same time as the root signs become obvious. This happy alternation makes for ease in diagnosis.

If a patient is examined for a suspected disc lesion at a time when no displacement is present, nothing is found. He must be seen at a time when the symptoms are present, and the diagnosis must be a disorder from which full recovery is possible—not, e.g. osteophytosis.

Inspection

The patient's gait should be noted as he enters the room, together with the way he moves to sit down and the position which he prefers when seated. These important diagnostic aids are lost if the patient is first seen lying in bed at home or in hospital. The patient's face should be scrutinized to assess how badly the pain is affecting him constitutionally. The peaky facies and sunken eyes of ankylosing spondylitis may be seen. However, occasionally spondylitic patients are fat and cheerful, so too much reliance cannot be placed on appearances in this disease.

The patient stands with the whole posterior aspect of the body bared from head to foot. The light should fall from a source behind him, so that unilateral shadows do not give a false idea of the shape of his trunk. The following are noted:

1. The Position of the Pelvis

Is it horizontal or oblique? If it is oblique, the legs are not the same length. Seven per cent of normal people have a difference of 1·2 cm. or more in the length of the legs. Alternatively, fixed flexion deformity exists at the hip; if so, the knee on that side is held forwards, compared to its fellow; in more obvious cases, the heel is off the ground.

Boards are placed under the foot of the shorter limb until the pelvis becomes horizontal. If the lumbar tilt ceases when the iliac crests are rendered level, it is the result of the short leg. If it remains, the deviation is intrinsically lumbar. If the list to one side is accompanied by a lower thoracic or lumbar rotation deformity, it is unrelated to recent symptoms, representing merely a scoliosis present since adolescence. If there is no rotation, the deviation signifies a lumbar articular lesion.

If the patient has discomfort while standing, or on lumbar flexion or extension, his short leg is raised by a platform under his foot. If this eases or abolishes his pain, he should wear a raised heel indefinitely. The same applies to patients with shortening greater than 1 cm., to those with recurrent lumbago (when the frequency of attacks may be lessened by abolition of the shearing strain on the affected joint), and in those whose shoulders are markedly out of level.

2. The Shape of the Lumbo-thoracic Spine

Is there an angular kyphos? If so, a vertebral body has become wedge-shaped, as the result of tuberculous caries, neoplasm, fracture, localized osteitis deformans, or senile osteoporosis; alternatively, gross thinning of two adjacent discs gives rise to this appearance. Does the patient stand upright, or is he bent forwards at lumbar spine and hips? This flexed posture is typical of acute lumbago, but is also seen in bilateral arthritis at the hips.

Does he stand evenly on both legs? In sciatic root-pain due to a disc lesion or neoplasm of the ilium, the patient may be unable to put the foot on the painful side flat on the floor, and stands with all his weight on the painless limb, resting the other foot on tip-toe.

Is the back unduly flat? If so, is the thoracic kyphosis greater or less than usual? If it is less (i.e. the lumbo-thoracic column forms a vertical line), the cause is a failure in development, the infantile flatness of the lumbar spine persisting into adult life. This posture leads to a graceful carriage but an enhanced likelihood of disc protrusion. If the thoracic kyphosis is exaggerated, spondylitis ankylopoetica or adolescent osteochondritis should be suspected in the young; osteitis deformans or senile osteoporosis in the elderly.

Is there an excessive lordosis? If this is compensated by an equally excessive thoracic kyphosis, the postural deformity dates from adolescence. If there is no such compensation, the whole spine lying at a level anterior to the sacrum as the result of an acute localized lordosis, spondylolisthesis is present.

Is the lumbar spine regular? A mid-lumbar shelf in the spinous processes characterizes spondylolisthesis at the fourth lumbar level. The upper spinous processes lie at one level; then a step is seen, the lower two processes projecting level with it. Concealed spondylolisthesis occurs, visible and palpable when the patient stands, but disappearing when the joint is relieved of weight-bearing. Hence, radiography while the patient lies down does not reveal the displacement (Plate 34).

Is there any lateral deviation of the spine? If so, is it towards or away from the painful side? If the protrusion lies lateral to the nerve-root, this is drawn away from the projection and the trunk deviates away from the painful side; if the displacement lies medially, i.e. at the axilla of the root, the patient deviates towards the painful side. When the nerve-root is gripped by a protrusion embracing both sides like a nutcracker, the root cannot move either way and gross limitation of trunk-flexion without appreciable deviation results. Gross deviation results from fourth (plate 22) but very seldom from fifth lumbar disc lesions, on account of the stabilizing effect of the ilio-lumbar ligaments. Alternating deviation is diagnostic of protrusion at the fourth lumbar level. It indicates that the dura mater slips from one side to the other of a small mid-line projection; as he is unable to keep it perched on the apex of the protrusion, the patient cannot maintain a vertical posture. Long-standing lateral deviation without rotation occurs in hemivertebra (Plate 36). The angulation is sudden and often seen to have its apex at an upper lumbar or lower thoracic level. Though itself not a cause of pain, hemivertebra may lead to a disc lesion at the oblique joint, or to such complete erosion of cartilage that bone grinds against bone (as in scoliosis). In either case, symptoms then begin. Tuberculous caries may affect only one side of a vertebral body; if so, an angular lateral deformity arises without rotation.

Is there any rotation? Adolescent or congenital scoliosis is always accompanied by rotation. Hence, lateral deviation accompanied by rotation prominent on the concave side is long-standing and unconnected with a recent disorder; lateral deviation without rotation is recent and relevant. These antalgic postures were first described by Young, and later in the 1954 edition of this book. They were set out afresh by de Sèze in 1955, who pointed out that deviation away from the painful side commonly indicated a fourth rather than a fifth lumbar displacement. He confirmed the description of these three types of deviation: (1) towards the painful side; (2) away from the painful side; (3) alternating. There exist, however, three further undescribed postural effects of a protruded disc: (1) no deviation when the patient stands erect, but marked deviation, usually towards the painful side, on attempted trunk-flexion; (2) the reverse: deviation standing which disappears towards the extreme of trunk-flexion; (3) a momentary deviation at the arc, i.e. when the trunk is flexed halfway (Plate 21). This clinical finding was confirmed by Newman (1967).

Lastly, does the patient's posture conform to the alleged site of pain? Hysterical patients may allege lumbar pain and hold themselves bent sideways; yet the lumbar spine is held vertically, the tilt occurring at the thoracic and cervical spine. This is the reverse of a genuine deformity; if the lumbar spine deviates, correction is maintained by side-flexion in the opposite direction at the thoracic joints so that the shoulders are level and the head erect.

3. The Level of Pain

The patient is asked to point with one finger to the centre of pain. Care must be exercised against ascribing pain felt at the second or third lumbar levels to a disc lesion. When a disc lesion results in local pain, this is felt on a level with, or just below, the joint affected. Lower thoracic disc lesions are not uncommon and at the twelfth joint often set up pain felt at the first lumbar level. First and second lumbar disc lesions are extremely rare; third lumbar lesions contribute five per cent of the total. There thus exists an upper lumbar region about five inches wide—'the forbidden area'—where pain is very seldom the result of a disc lesion. Pain in the forbidden area suggests ankylosing spondylitis, neoplasm, caries, aortic thrombosis or reference from a viscus.

4. Muscle Wasting

Apart from myopathy and anterior poliomyelitis, wasting of the muscles of the trunk is a rarity. Visible wasting of the muscles of the buttock and posterior thigh occurs in arthritis at the hip and in first and second sacral root-palsies. In arthritis of any severity at the hip, the quadriceps muscles waste too. If the buttock on the painful side is the larger, neoplasm deep to the gluteal muscles is probably present.

5. Other Signs

If the foot turns a dusky red on standing but blanches on elevation, advanced arteriosclerosis is present, suggesting intermittent claudication as a possible cause of the patient's painful limb.

The patient's trunk may look compressed from above downwards, as if it had sunk into itself. This appearance suggests osteitis deformans, senile osteoporosis or advanced degeneration of the discs leading to diminished joint spaces at all the lumbar joints.

The recent development of genu varum in an elderly patient suggests osteitis deformans.

Spinal Movements

It is well to realize that the lumbar movements carried out voluntarily from the erect position are largely passive, not active, in their diagnostic import. Though the patient initiates the movement by muscular force, gravity then comes into play and does the rest. Only if, having bent as far as is comfortable, he is asked to bend a little farther, do the muscles contract again. If differentiation between a muscular and an articular lesion arises, the examiner should test the joint by gently forcing the required movement before performing the same movement against resistance.

The two questions that testing the lumbar movements helps to answer are: (a) Do the lumbar movements evoke or alter the symptoms? (b) What is the state of the lumbar joints?

The patient stands and four movements are investigated: extension, two side-flexions and flexion. Range is watched; painfulness ascertained. If pain is evoked, the patient is asked when and where it is felt. Since flexion is the movement that most often hurts, it is performed last, lest a persisting ache after this movement obscure the responses to the other movements.

Since lumbago and sciatica are variants of the same disorder, the signs are interchangeable. Occasionally, patients with sciatica are found who adopt the flexed posture of lumbago (Plate 19); in most of these cases, the pain in the limb is intensified by trunk-extension; whereas trunk-flexion and, later, straight-leg raising prove painless. By contrast, patients with only lumbar pain may show the lumbar deviation, limitation of trunk flexion and of straight-leg raising on one side that are more typical of sciatica. Painless clicking occurring at the lumbar spine on movement shows that a loose fragment of cartilage alters position but not enough to compress a sensitive structure.

Caution

Whether spinal movement is limited or not is most difficult to assess, because there is no absolute criterion. Whereas at most normal joints the range of movement is the same in childhood as in old age, this is not so at the lumbar joints. Thus, a young person may bend his trunk sideways until his upper shoulder lies vertically above his lower; the same individual, forty years later, may well possess only a few degrees of lumbo-thoracic movement. Yet he may feel no stiffness or discomfort, or indeed have anything the matter with his back at all. Hence, a range that would have been considered grossly pathological during adolescence may be normal in an elderly man. Any estimate of what is, or is not, likely to be pathological limitation of lumbar movements has to take into account the patient's age and habitus. This difficulty in separating the important from the harmless causes of limited lumbar movement is the reason why some request a radiograph in every case. This is justified, up to a point, but factors may appear in the history (e.g. pain of many years' standing) or the examination which clearly indicate that the lesion is not, in fact, osseous.

Extension

This may be limited or of full range, painful or painless. In acute lumbago, extension is lost altogether on account of the block at the back of the joint. Were it limited by muscle spasm, as many authorities maintain, it would be the abdominal and psoas muscles that were contracting, not the sacrospinalis. In fact, no such spasm can be felt to occur at the abdominal wall and flexing the hip joints does not increase the lumbar extension range.

In minor degrees of backache, extension is often painful at full range. Quite a common pattern in unilateral backache is: extension hurts centrally but full flexion hurts at one side of the back. Painful limitation of extension occurs in serious disease of the spine, including spondylitis ankylopoetica. Painless limitation of extension characterizes osteophyte formation. If a disc lesion and osteophyte formation co-exist, the extreme of such movement towards extension as is possible often proves painful.

If trunk extension sets up pain felt in the buttock or the lower limb, its origin must be articular, for in this position the lumbar joints are stretched, the sacro-iliac joint subjected to a rotation strain and the hip joint is extended, whereas the lumbar and buttock muscles are relaxed. Trunk extension hurting at the front of the thigh occurs in third lumbar disc lesions and arthritis at the hip. When trunk extension is severely limited by pain shooting down the back of the limb, the outlook for the success of conservative treatment is poor; many such cases require laminectomy. Rarely, when lumbar extension is attempted, it may cease abruptly long before full range is reached, the trunk bouncing forwards with a sharp twinge to the flexed position again. This is the same springy block as occurs when the meniscus is displaced at the knee and designates a buckled end-plate.

Side-flexion

All serious diseases of the lumbar spine result in limitation of the range of both side-flexion movements. A practised eye is required, since the range of this movement diminishes with the patient's age. Hence, knowledge of what range an individual of that age and shape ought to possess must be correlated with that actually found present.

Tuberculosis, malignant and benign neoplasm, chronic osteomyelitis, old fractures, and spondylitis ankylopoetica all give rise to marked painful limitation of these two movements. Painless limitation of side-flexion in an elderly patient denotes osteophyte formation, osteitis deformans or advanced osteoporosis. Limitation of side-flexion in one direction only is usually associated with visible lateral deviation the opposite way when the patient stands; it signifies a block lying at one side only of one joint—in other words, a lumbar disc lesion, usually at the fourth level.

One or both side-flexion movements may hurt. If each hurts on the side towards which the patient bends, he is clearly squeezing something painfully. This can result only from a lesion placed intra-articularly; for all the other structures on that side of the lumbar region are relaxed in this position. If it hurts on the side away from which he bends, he is stretching both joint and muscle; then, as elsewhere, it is the discovery later that the resisted movement in the opposite direction is painless that incriminates the joint. Alternatively, if extension and side-flexion away from the painful side both hurt, the symptoms must arise from the joint since full extension relaxes the sacrospinalis muscle. If side-flexion hurts on the side towards which the patient bends, an attempt at manipulative reduction is much less likely to succeed than when side-flexion away from the painful side hurts. If any lumbar movement other than flexion hurts in the lower limb instead of at the lumbar region or upper buttock, manipulation nearly always fails, especially if the patient is less than sixty years old.

A *painful arc* may be felt on side-flexion. It takes two forms. The early part of the movement hurts, but at full range the pain has ceased. Alternatively, the patient may complain of pain as his trunk passes the vertical on swinging from side to side. A painful arc is pathognomonic of a disc lesion; for it shows that the dura mater rides over an articular projection, usually at the fourth level.

Flexion

Patients with any serious disease of the lumbar spine flex from the hips, the lumbar spine being fixed in lordosis by spasm of the sacrospinalis muscles. This sign accompanies limitation of side-flexion (p. 446). In patients with considerable kypho-lordosis, the lumbar spine may stay extended when the patient flexes in what looks like the limitation of severe disease, but if side-flexion is of adequate range, this appearance can be disregarded. An occasional patient with lumbago flexes with a rigid back, but this must not be attributed to a disc lesion until radiography has demonstrated that no other disorder is present. A limited capacity to bend forwards without the intense spasm of vertebral disease, means that the patient is prevented from stretching the dura mater or a sciatic nerve-root.

Thus in central lumbago, pain limits standing trunk-flexion and, as a corollary, straight-leg raising often is later found bilaterally limited. This is by no means invariable, since in subacute lumbago trunk-flexion standing is often found limited, whereas straight-leg raising is of full range. The difference lies in the degree of protrusion present when the joint is, and is not, compressed by the body weight. This fact has an important medico-legal bearing; for it is *not* an inconsistency when a patient with lumbago cannot bend forwards but is found to possess a full range of straight-leg raising. What he cannot do is to sit up on the couch with his legs extended in front of him; for the body weight is then once more borne by his affected lumbar joint. Only this discrepancy is evidence of ill-faith. When manipulative reduction is carried out in lumbago, full straight-leg raising is often afforded by the first few manoeuvres, whereas it takes considerably more treatment to restore full trunk flexion from the erect position.

In lumbago, neck-flexion often hurts in the lumbar region, as this movement stretches the dura mater from above, just as straight-leg raising stretches it from below. Sometimes a pain created by flexing the trunk is, therefore, increased by neck-flexion. It might be argued that neck-flexion stretches the sacrospinalis muscles as much as it does the dura mater. This is true, but if resisted extension at the neck is tested, it proves painless, thus exculpating the muscle. If, in a patient with lumbar articular signs, neck-flexion increases the pain, the articular lesion must be such as to impair the mobility of the dura mater; in other words, a posterior projection exists at the joint.

In unilateral pain, whether in the lower back or the limb, the patient, though he stands upright symmetrically, may be found on flexion to deviate towards or away from the painful side, according to which side of the nerve-root the protrusion has passed. By contrast, other patients, who have a lateral tilt at the lumbar spine while standing upright, lose it at the extreme of flexion. This finding implies that accommodation for the block at the posterior aspect of the joint is no longer necessary owing to the increased distance apart of the articular surfaces. An alternating scoliosis may also be seen, the patient deviating one way as he bends down, but coming up deviating the other way. This means that the dura mater has to lie to one or other side of the projection.

Limitation of trunk-flexion because of pain felt in the limb posteriorly shows that the patient cannot stretch his sciatic nerve-root beyond a certain point. Usually this is associated with pain felt in the lower lumbar region or upper buttock on one or two of the other movements of the lumbar spine. However, usually in primary postero-lateral protrusion, limitation of trunk-flexion may prove the only sign, the other three lumbar movements being of full range and painless. In such a case the alternation between articular signs and root signs is seen at its clearest.

Pain appearing when full flexion is reached merely implies that some structure is painfully stretched or moved. In a disc lesion, the mechanism is two-fold. First, the dura mater lies stretched against the back of the intervertebral joint at full trunk-flexion; it may be applied more forcibly to any projection present by this movement. Secondly, when the intervertebral joint is held in kyphosis, its contents tend to be squeezed backwards; hence the projection may increase in size. For this double reason, full flexion nearly always hurts in lumbar disc lesions. If trunk-flexion causes central backache, the trouble must lie at the joint or its posterior ligaments. If trunk-flexion sets up unilateral pain felt in the buttock, although reference from the lumbar region is the common source, a torsion strain is applied to the sacro-iliac joint and the gluteal structures are stretched. Hence these tissues must be examined subsequently; if they prove normal, the pain has a lumbar origin.

Painful Arc

The patient feels the transient pain at mid-range, and may be seen momentarily to falter at this point. An arc shows itself in two ways. The patient may state that, as he reaches the half-way-down position, a momentary lumbar pain is felt. If this is not felt on the way down, it should be looked for on the way up from trunk-flexion; for this is the best means of eliciting the sign. Alternatively, the patient may be seen suddenly to deviate laterally at half-flexion, returning to a symmetrical posture as soon as this point is passed, up or down (Plate 21). He is quite unaware of this deviation. Usually pain is felt at the arc; occasionally it is visibly present but devoid of discomfort. A painful arc is usually associated with pain at the extreme of one or other of the lumbar movements, but it can be an isolated finding. Patients can induce the arc by tilting the pelvis to and fro on the lumbar spine rather than by flexing the spine on the pelvis; it is merely another way of doing the same thing.

A painful arc means that a fragment of disc lies loose in the joint and alters its position at the moment when the tilt of the articular surfaces reverses itself as the lumbar spine passes from lordosis to kyphosis. The pain, but not the visible deviation as the patient bends, is abolished by epidural local anaesthesia; hence, the mechanism must be a jarring of the dura mater *via* the posterior ligament as the fragment shifts. A painless momentary deviation at half range implies that the articular surfaces open to ride over a projection within the joint, but that the loose piece does not project enough to interfere with the dura mater.

A painful arc, whether on flexion or less often on side-flexion, is extremely helpful in diagnosis. It is pathognomonic of a disc lesion. It is a particularly valuable sign (a) in young patients with early disc lesions in whom the other lumbar signs are either not distinctive, or capable of more than one interpretation; (b) in medico-legal cases when it may be alleged that symptoms are caused by ligamentous strain (but at half-range no ligament is on the stretch); (c) when neurosis is suspected, since this is a physical sign which, in my experience, occurs only in organic lesions.

Interpretation

The distinctive finding in low lumbar disc lesions is the partial articular pattern that identifies internal derangement. Part of the joint is blocked, part is free; hence some movements prove painful at their extreme, some not. If there is limitation of range, its degree is unequal in different directions and the capsular pattern does not emerge. The severity of the signs depends on the size of the displacement, but the pattern has the same quality. The situation is the same as in the neck where acute torticollis (the analogue of lumbago) is characterized by gross partial articular signs, whereas in chronic disc lesions causing pain in one scapular area, they are minor, but still possess the same distinctive asymmetry.

The expected pattern is that of a partial joint lesion, and this usually emerges on examination. The pain may be shown to have a lumbar articular provenance, and yet be felt unilaterally. Of the four lumbar movements, only one, two or three may hurt. If they all hurt, as is common in severe lumbago, the pain on one movement may be much greater than on the others. Limitation of movement may be confined to flexion; or one side-flexion movement, not the other. In short, in minor degrees of displacement some movements are slightly blocked and, therefore, painful, but not limited; others are of full range and painless. In major obstruction, although all four movements may hurt, they hurt unequally and some are grossly limited, others not. Such articular signs may accompany central or unilateral pain, depending on the position of the displacement. Moreover, a painful arc is often present, especially in minor cases. This occurs at a moment when no ligament is on the stretch and is pathognomonic of an interarticular loose body shifting its position when the tilt on the joint surfaces is reversed.

THE PATIENT LIES SUPINE

How the patient moves to get on to the couch should conform with the degree of disablement reported in the history and indicated by the lumbar

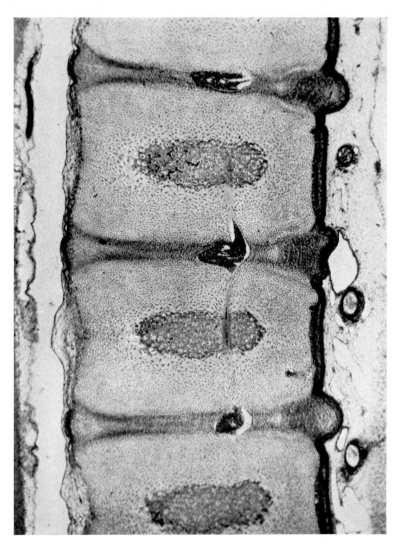

PLATE 17

Development of the discs. Microphotograph of spine of a 64-mm human embryo.
(By courtesy of Professor E. Blechschmidt (1961), *The Stages of Human Development before Birth*, Karger: Basel.)

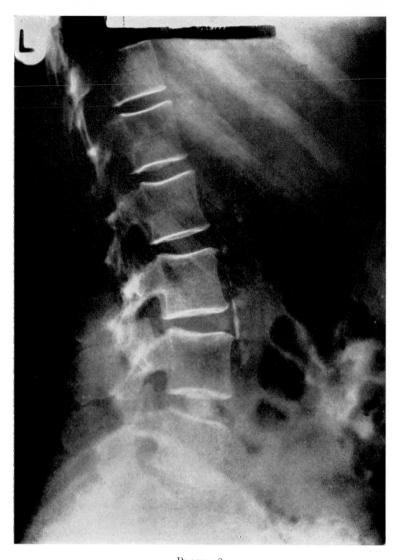

PLATE 18

Calcified nucleus. The size of the pulpy nucleus is clearly shown at the fourth lumbar level.

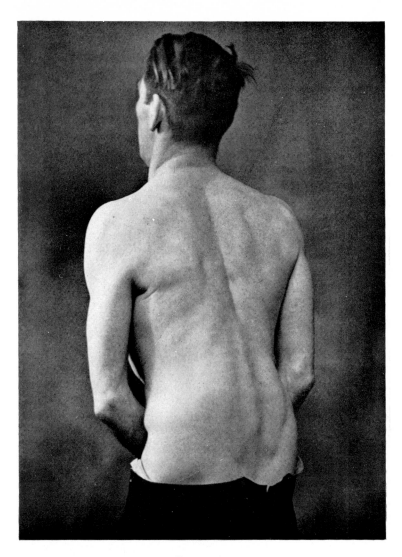

PLATE 19

Marked lumbar kyphos caused by posterior protrusion of part of a low lumbar intervertebral disc with left-sided sciatica. The patient is bending backwards as far as he can.

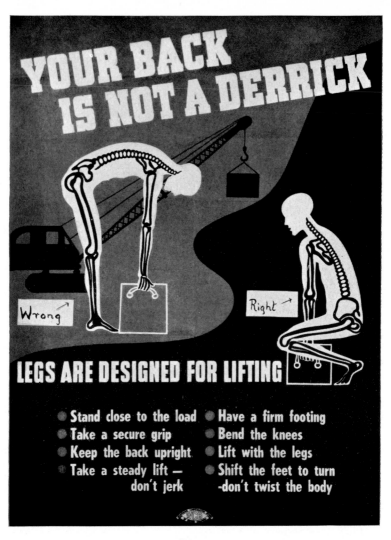

PLATE 20

A Canadian poster issued by the Workmen's Compensation Board in an endeavour to protect heavy workers from lumbar disc protrusion.

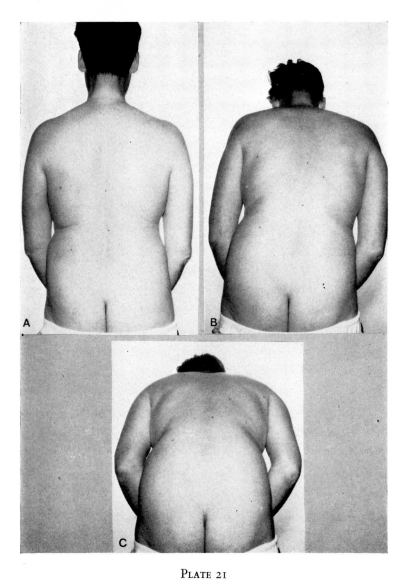

PLATE 21

Momentary deviation at the arc. A. Erect: no deviation. B. Deviation to right at half-range. C. Full flexion: once more symmetrical.

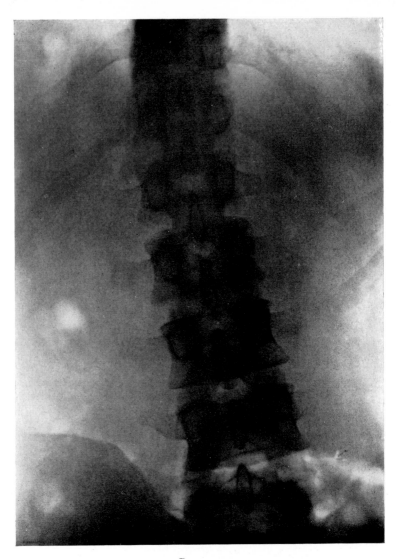

PLATE 22

Attempted side-flexion towards the patient's left does not even result in the spine reaching the vertical position. The block clearly lies at the left side of the fourth lumbar intervertebral joint, and a large cartilaginous fragment lying here was removed at operation.

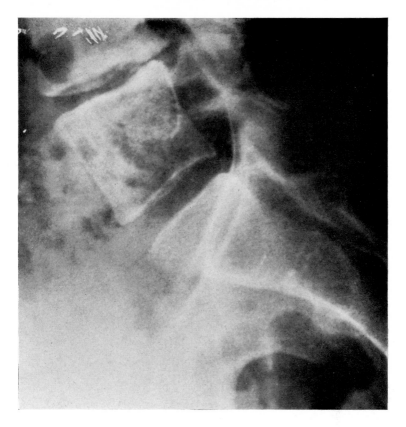

PLATE 23

Posterior osteophytosis. The osteophyte is clearly visible at the postero-inferior angle of the fourth lumbar body. A man of 36 had had recurrent lumbago for fifteen years and two years' constant backache.

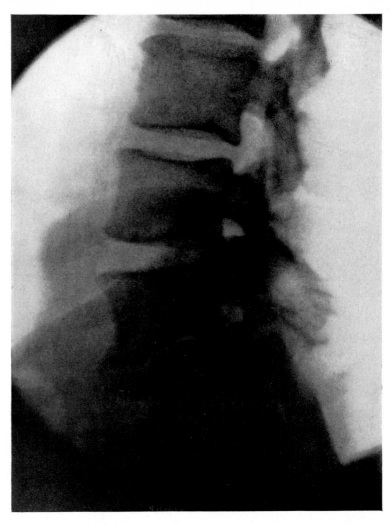

PLATE 24

Complete erosion of the disc at the fifth lumbar level.

movements. In suspected malingering, the patient is asked to sit on the edge of the examination couch, then to swing himself round, still sitting up, until his legs lie outstretched before him on the couch. If he sits in this position comfortably, a full range of straight-leg raising exists *while the lumbar joint is supporting the body weight*. It is fair to contrast this finding with the range of trunk-flexion already ascertained, and of straight-leg raising as determined later.

The sacro-iliac joints are now tested by pressure downwards and outwards on each anterior superior spine of the ilium. The range and painfulness or not of flexion, rotation and, if necessary, abduction and adduction at the hip-joints is determined next; the resisted hip movements may require testing for pain or weakness.

Testing the sacro-iliac joints, the hip joint and the muscles about it involves eight manoeuvres, none of which normally hurts a patient with minor lumbar trouble, although in acute lumbago almost any movement of the legs hurts the back; if so, the severe lumbar signs present overshadow these minor findings. It is true that full hip-flexion both flexes the lumbar spine and pulls slightly on the sciatic nerve-roots; it may therefore hurt a little. Medial rotation at the hip may set up discomfort in the buttock in an occasional case of sciatica, again by pulling on the nerve-root. However, the resisted hip movements cannot hurt the back in any circumstances. These eight tests therefore possess a dual purpose, partly to ascertain the integrity or not of the tissues under examination, partly to assess the patient's sincerity. If he alleges that all these movements set up or increase his backache, this is gross exaggeration.

Straight-leg Raising

History

Lassègue wrote his book on sciatica in 1864 without mentioning limitation of straight-leg raising, and it was his pupil Forst who drew attention to this sign in 1881 (Romagnoli and Dalmonte, 1965). In 1884, de Beurmann showed on a cadaver that straight-leg raising stretched the sciatic nerve-trunk. In 1901, Fajersztajn demonstrated on the cadaver that straight-leg raising on the painless side drew the dural tube downwards, thus exerting tension indirectly on the nerve-roots on the affected side. He suggested this was the reason why lifting the painless leg hurt the affected limb. In 1910, Zizina concluded that when crossed straight-leg raising hurt, the lesion must lie in the spinal canal. Yet for years, limited straight-leg raising was misunderstood and was considered the result of spasm of the pyriformis muscle squeezing the sciatic nerve-trunk. The fallacy should have been evident because: (a) when the muscle does contract fully,

Q

straight-leg raising does not become limited; (b) in sciatica, the thigh does not fix in abduction and lateral rotation as it would in pyriformis muscle spasm. These theories were finally confirmed by Smith and Wright (1958), who, by later pulling on threads placed round the nerve-roots at laminectomy, were able to reproduce root-pain and limitation of straight-leg raising on the conscious patient.

Technique

When straight leg-raising is tested, the patient's pelvis must not be allowed to rise off the couch, nor may the pelvis be allowed to rotate forwards, so that what now looks like straight-leg raising is really abduction at the hip joint. The leg is lifted as far as it will go, until muscle-tension prevents further movement. Whether the end-feel is abrupt or gradual is noted; in the latter case, an attempt is made to push the limb a little farther. The patient states if pain is produced and, if so, where it is felt.

The range of straight-leg raising is first estimated on the painless side. In disc lesions, at the extreme of range, pain is sometimes felt in the other thigh or buttock on account of tension transmitted *via* the dura mater, especially if the protrusion lies between dura mater and nerve-root at the fourth level. The range on the painful side is noted next. This is nearly always limited in pressure on those roots whose trunk passes behind the hip joint (i.e. the fourth and fifth lumbar and the first and second sacral). The examiner must not mind gently forcing straight-leg raising, as long as this causes only slight pain and the hamstring muscles do not terminate the movement abruptly. Otherwise he will miss a painful arc or those uncommon cases where pain begins at, say, 45 degrees and then goes on up to 90 degrees without increasing.

When the straight limb has been raised to the point where pain just begins, the patient is asked to flex his neck, keeping his trunk still. This often increases the pain by pulling on the other end of the nerve-root via the dura mater. It is a useful test, proving that the tissues whose mobility is painfully impaired runs from above the neck to below the back of the knee, and there is only one such structure: the dura mater continuous with the sciatic nerve trunk. Had this diagnostic manoeuvre been carried out regularly, the disputed question of sacro-iliac subluxation causing sciatica would have been resolved years ago; for by no stretch of the imagination can neck-flexion be regarded as altering tension on the sacro-iliac ligaments.

Some clinicians, when the straight leg has been raised as far as it will go, passively dorsiflex the foot. Whether additional pain is produced or not, this does not appear to yield any further information.

Significance.

Straight-leg raising tests the mobility of the sheath of the fourth and fifth lumbar and first and second sacral nerve-roots.

Hence, limitation of straight-leg raising indicates that the dural sleeve of the nerve-root cannot move properly; if any part of the nerve-trunk is affected beyond this sleeve, no limitation occurs.

In normal individuals, the range varies from 60 degrees to 120 degrees and, at the extreme, an uncomfortable stretching is always felt at the back of the knee. Straight leg exemplifies the constant length phenomenon which characterizes extra-articular limitation of movement; for the range of flexion at one hip differs from its fellow only when the knee is held in full extension. This proves that the tissue at fault spans at least two joints and runs behind both the hip and knee joints. If neck-flexion now increases the pain in the limb, the structure at fault must run up to the neck, spanning another twenty-four joints. The cause of limitation of straight-leg raising is spasm of the hamstrings; it is an involuntary protective mechanism preserving the lower intraspinal roots from painful traction analogous to the muscular spasm set up by appendicitis or arthritis. One has only to realize this useful purpose to shudder at the days (not so far in the past) when straight-leg raising was forced under anaesthesia.

Straight-leg raising is limited in meningeal irritation from any cause, and is known as Kernig's sign. This merely elicits limitation of straight-leg raising in a different way, by showing that the knee has to flex when the trunk is flexed on the thigh; the order in which the diagnostic movements are performed has merely become reversed. Again, in meningitis, neck-flexion soon does more than just hurt; it becomes impossible and in severe cases the neck is fixed extended to spare all tension on the dura mater.

Straight-leg raising is limited usually on both sides, though sometimes more on one side than the other, when the mobility of the dura mater is impaired by a large central disc-protrusion, i.e. in severe lumbago. The upward movement of either leg provokes lumbar pain and involuntary spasm of the hamstrings. Unilateral lumbago often causes unilateral limitation of straight-leg raising, or this is more restricted on the affected side. It is also limited, usually unilaterally, when the dural sleeve of a nerve-root from the fourth lumbar to the second sacral is unable to move freely. Sometimes, particularly in disc lesions at the fourth level, bilateral restriction is noted; alternatively, raising the limb on the painless side hurts down the good leg at full range. This finding designates an axillary protrusion, the nerve-root being drawn towards the projection lying at the medial side. This is more common at the fourth than the fifth lumbar level; and the same applies when straight-leg raising is only, or more, limited on the good side.

Straight-leg raising is not limited in minor backache; such cases show articular without dural signs. There is one exception to this rule: a rare form of chronic central backache in young people that persists for many years and is characterized by limitation of trunk-flexion and of straight-leg raising on each side, without any other signs. Straight-leg raising may provoke, in addition to the root-pain, pins and needles in the feet. Sometimes, neck-flexion during straight-leg raising also has this effect.

Straight-leg raising does not pull directly on the third lumbar nerve-root; indeed hip-flexion relaxes it. Nevertheless, at full range, pain may be provoked in the buttock or the front of the thigh by the pull from the roots below on the dura mater, but there is never limitation. The fourth sacral root does not reach the lower limb; hence, straight-leg raising does not stretch it and, when this root is involved alone, straight-leg raising is neither limited nor painful. More commonly, posterior sequestration of the disc when the ligament ruptures also catches the nerve-roots on each side, when bilateral sciatica with bilateral limitation of straight-leg raising is to be expected. Only rarely does the dural pull of full straight-leg raising exacerbate the pain of a severe lowest-thoracic disc protrusion; at this level the main dural sign is neck-flexion. Straight-leg raising cannot be limited in 'sciatic neuritis', since this is a purely parenchymatous lesion in which the exterior of the nerve-root takes no part. Straight-leg raising is less limited in degree than hip-flexion when the sciatic nerve trunk is invaded by a malignant tumour in the buttock.

Up to a point, the range of straight-leg raising varies inversely with the size of the protrusion, and when pressure is released it alters instantly. Though dura mater or nerve-root may have suffered compression for perhaps months and thus be regarded as likely to remain bruised for some days or at least hours after release, this is not so; straight-leg raising becomes full as soon as the pressure ceases. Hence it provides a most useful and delicate criterion during an attempt at manipulative reduction, showing from moment to moment how the protrusion is shifting. A full range of straight-leg raising is achieved before reduction is complete; once a displacement has largely receded, it may still cause pain on lumbar movements, tested standing, since the joint is subjected to pressure. The range of straight-leg raising is an equally sensitive criterion when reduction by traction is undertaken, but is not a reliable guide when tested immediately after a session ceases; it must be estimated each day *before* treatment starts. When reduction by recumbency is in progress, a full range of straight-leg raising suggests that the patient should begin to get up. Increase in the degree of protrusion beyond a certain point does not diminish the range of straight-leg raising, presumably because there is a certain amount of slack in the sciatic nerve trunk which has to be taken up before the root begins to move. Hence a patient with 30 degrees or 45 degrees of straight-leg raising with as yet no neurological signs may later develop a palsy, i.e. an increased degree of pressure on the root, without any corresponding further reduction in the range of straight-leg raising.

Epidural local anaesthesia abolishes the dural symptom—pain on coughing—and the two dural signs—pain on neck-flexion and on straight-leg raising—of lumbago for the duration of the anaesthetic agent. The protrusion is left unaltered, but it now impinges on a membrane rendered insensitive. After the injection, such articular signs as were visible do not change, and a lateral deviation or a momentary deviation at the arc can still be seen. However, these phenomena are now unaccompanied by any pain. In sciatica, a full range of straight-leg raising is usually restored for 90 minutes after the epidural injection, and the constant ache in the limb ceases for the same period.

A *painful arc* may appear on straight-leg raising, usually as the leg passes 45 degrees, movement above and below that point remaining painless (see Fig. 72). This sign implies that the nerve-root catches against a small protrusion and slips over it. It is quite a common phenomenon when a patient is nearly well in the course of reduction by sustained traction of nuclear postero-lateral herniation.

Rarely, straight-leg raising is severely limited on both sides in ankylosing spondylitis by pain felt in the back. A cough does not hurt and epidural local anaesthesia does not increase the range. Presumably the dura mater, possibly also the dural sleeve of the nerve-roots, is involved in the spondylitic inflammation. If this is not confined merely to the outer aspect of the dural tube and nerve-roots but affects its whole thickness, anaesthesia of the surface alone would have no effect.

The absence of dural signs in an apparent case of acute lumbago should make the examiner pause. If the pain in the back is so severe that the patient cannot move out of bed, yet there is no pain on coughing and a full range of straight-leg raising, afebrile osteomyelitis should be suspected. In cases of doubt, epidural local anaesthesia is diagnostic, since anaesthesia of the theca does not alter the pain of a bony lesion.

Straight-leg raising is not necessarily restricted in even severe sciatica, and it must not be thought that unless straight-leg raising is limited the patient cannot have a disc lesion. Indeed, there is one type of disc-protrusion in which trunk-extension is markedly restricted in range, attempted backward bending provoking severe sciatic pain; if so, trunk-flexion and straight-leg raising may even ease the constant ache.

In elderly patients with minor disc lesions causing as a rule backache *and* sciatica, a full range of straight-leg raising is usually present, sometimes not even painful at the extreme.

If the range of straight-leg raising is limited, the range of trunk-flexion, standing and of sitting with the legs outstretched must be restricted in equal degree. Inconsistency in this direction is a common finding in psychoneurosis and malingering. The converse does not hold; for many perfectly genuine disc lesions restrict trunk-flexion but not straight-leg raising, since in the former case the protrusion is greater owing to the compression strain on the joint. Unless this difference is appreciated, injustice may be done to patients with medico-legal claims. Similar considerations apply to gross lumbar lateral deviation visible when the patient stands but straightening out when he lies prone, or to limitation of trunk-extension standing but not lying. As soon as the joint is relieved of the compression of body weight, the pressure of the protrusion against dura mater or nerve-root eases, and the signs correspondingly diminish. These phenomena are thus organically determined and must not be thought inconsistencies and evidence of neurosis. By contrast, when the signs are greater when the body-weight is *off* the joint, this suggestion indeed arises.

The causes of limitation of straight-leg raising in other than disc lesions are: any other intraspinal lesion, e.g. tumour at or below the fourth level, malignant disease or osteomyelitis of the ilium or upper femur, fractured sacrum, ischio-rectal abscess, haematoma in the hamstring muscles. In all the above conditions affecting the buttock, hip-flexion is limited too; hence 'the sign for the buttock'—limitation both of straight-leg raising *and* of hip-flexion—emerges, and the physician is thereby warned (see Chapter 23).

Three Stages of Straight-leg Raising

1. *Limited Straight-leg Raising: No Neurological Signs*
This indicates a not very large protrusion. A minor degree of pressure exists close to the intervertebral foramen, interfering with mobility but not conduction.

2. *Limited Straight-leg Raising: Neurological Signs*
The range of straight-leg raising is largely independent of the degree of parenchymatous involvement; for it measures only the mobility of the dural sleeve of the nerve-root. This double finding indicates a great degree of pressure near the intervertebral foramen, enough to have compressed the parenchyma as well as the root sleeve, i.e. to impair conduction as well as mobility.

3. *Full Straight-leg Raising: Root-Palsy*

It may happen that a patient after some hours' or days' severe sciatica reports that his pain suddenly eased and, at the same time, his foot went numb. This indicates root-atrophy. The postero-lateral disc protrusion becomes maximal and compresses the root so hard that it becomes insensitive from ischaemia. When stretched, no protective reflex is evoked, since the root-sleeve is no longer sentient. Hence straight-leg raising reaches full painless range within a few days, at the same time as conduction along the root ceases; in consequence, the full syndrome of muscle-weakness, absent reflex and cutaneous analgesia appears. The patient has become symptomatically better by becoming anatomically worse.

Tests for Conduction

Conduction must be carefully tested both for diagnosis and to arrive at a proper choice of treatment. The magnitude of parenchymatous involvement must be assessed. The greater the degree of interference with conduction, the greater is the force compressing the nerve-root; in other words, the larger the protrusion. It is a safe rule that signs of interference with conduction, apart from minor paraesthesia, mean that an attempt at reduction by manipulation or traction will fail. By contrast, recent limitation of straight-leg raising without neurological deficit is an encouraging sign.

Often a root-palsy is incomplete. If the protrusion compresses the upper aspect of the root, a sensory palsy results; if the pressure comes from below, the palsy is motor. Large protrusions compress the whole root and cause both motor and sensory impairment; a full palsy is always present in root ischaemia.

A disc lesion, in general, affects only one nerve-root. A protrusion just to one side of the mid-line tends to compress the root below itself (Fig. 71, p. 421), whereas a more lateral protrusion catches the root at the same level as itself. Owing to the obliquity of the fourth lumbar to second sacral roots, it is possible for two roots to be compressed by one large protrusion. This happens at both the fourth and fifth lumbar levels; hence fourth-fifth lumbar, or a combined fifth-lumbar and first-sacral palsy can occur. Triple palsies are extremely rare, and so are combined third-fourth palsies; in either case, neoplasm should be suspected. When it compresses the nerve-root, the disc protrusion has moved to one side or the other of the posterior ligament; therefore, bilateral weakness of muscle is scarcely ever caused by a disc lesion, although both ankle-jerks occasionally disappear in unilateral sciatica.

Physiotherapist's Duty

It is the duty of the physiotherapist who treats a lumbar (or, for that matter, cervical) disc lesion by an attempt at reduction, to examine root-conduction before beginning manipulation or traction, and at intervals during treatment, especially if the patient is not doing well. A patient may be seen on one day and reduction advised; yet by the time treatment begins a few days later, a palsy may have supervened. The physician has no means of discovering this; it is the physiotherapist who must note and report this event, since the change makes attempted reduction futile. It is not uncommon to see patients in whom a lengthy course of treatment has been continued in the presence of the clearest signs that the endeavour is vain.

Resisted Movements

Resisted flexion of the hip is weak in second or third root-palsy. If contraction of the psoas muscle is both weak *and* painful, the physician must remember that he is testing part of the posterior abdominal wall and that neoplasm here, or at the upper lumbar spine itself, is the usual cause of this sign. Painless weakness of the psoas muscle is hardly ever caused by a disc lesion, except as the lesser part of a third root-palsy. If, then, this muscle is weak *alone*, serious disease at the second lumbar level must be suspected, e.g. neuroma; if the paresis is bilateral, secondary neoplasm. Secondary deposits at the upper femur also give rise to pain and weakness on resisted flexion at the one hip, but in that case the passive hip movements are restricted and painful.

The muscles controlling the foot are examined next. The tibialis anterior is tested by asking the patient to dorsiflex his foot strongly. Unless the examiner puts all his power into resisting this movement, minor weakness is not detected, since the normal individual's strength far surpasses the examiner's. The tibialis anterior muscle is derived largely from the fourth lumbar segment and is not appreciably weakened in a third or fifth lumbar palsy. The extensor hallucis is tested next; the examiner is stronger than the patient in this instance. It forms part of the fourth and fifth lumbar myotomes. Thus, although weakness of this muscle shows that the protrusion is big enough to have resulted in muscle weakness, it does not help to indicate whether it is the fourth or the fifth root. Eversion of the foot tests the peroneal muscles; normally, these are stronger than any examiner's resistance. They are supplied by the fifth lumbar and first sacral roots; hence weakness here is common to a lesion of either root. If the extensor hallucis muscle is also weak, the fifth lumbar root is at fault; if the calf muscles are weak, the first sacral root is inculpated.

During this examination, other diseases occasionally come to light, e.g. peroneal atrophy. Since the disorder is painless, minor degrees are scarcely noticed by the patient, and the discovery of long-standing bilateral weakness of the tibialis anterior and peroneal muscles may be thought recent and arouse a justified but mistaken suspicion of spinal metastases.

Sensory Signs

Search is made for cutaneous analgesia. If the third lumbar root is involved, this begins at the patella and continues along the front and inner side of the leg to just above the ankle. In fourth lumbar root-palsy, the big toe is often analgesic; in a fifth root-palsy, the big and two adjacent toes. When the first sacral root is affected, skin sensitivity may be impaired at that outer border of the foot as far as the two smallest toes. A second sacral root-palsy may give rise to a numb heel. Disc lesions very seldom give rise to bilateral neurological signs; hence if the paraesthesia is symmetrical, spondylolisthesis or neoplasm should be considered.

The *knee-jerk* is sluggish or absent in third lumbar root-lesions.

The *plantar reflex* should be tested in any patient who complains of upper lumbar backache, or that the limb drags or feels weak or heavy, or when muscular weakness of an unusual distribution is encountered, particularly bilaterally.

Arterial Examination

Pulsation should be felt for at the femoral, dorsalis pedis and posterior tibial arteries if intermittent claudication is suspected. In patients with claudication, pulsation is necessarily absent in the arteries at the ankle, but the converse does not hold, pulsation being absent for years without claudication appearing. Pitting oedema of one foot suggests venous thrombosis or angioneurotic oedema unless it is accompanied by gross neurological signs, when it usually indicates pelvic malignant disease. Inflamed varices at the ankle, empty and invisible when the patient lies, may cause local heat; if this is found, the ankle should be examined again while the patient stands and the veins show up. In thrombosis of the external iliac artery, the affected leg and foot are cold for many hours after exertion; after a day or two resting in bed, this difference on the two sides disappears. The tibia may be warm in osteitis deformans. Secondary deposits at the second lumbar level may affect the sympathetic supply, giving rise to a warm foot and markedly increased arterial pulsation at the ankle.

THE PATIENT LIES PRONE

The calves are inspected anew. Wasting may be visible in a first or second sacral root-palsy. Weakness of the calf muscles due to a disc lesion is never extreme enough to be detectable on plantiflexion against resistance, but can be demonstrated by asking the patient to stand tip-toe first on the painless leg then on the painful one.

The ankle-jerk is then tested. It becomes unilaterally sluggish or absent in fifth lumbar and first or second sacral root-palsy. Once having disappeared, in about half the cases it never returns even years after complete recovery. Hence in recurrent sciatica, its absence implies that the patient

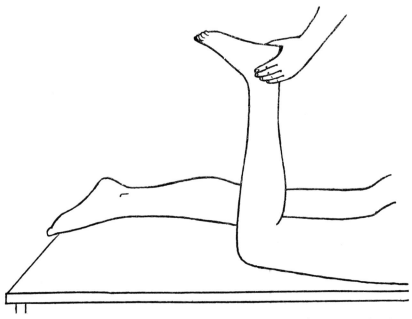

FIG. 73. Resisted flexion of knee. The examiner resists the movement by pressing against the patient's heel.

has had a root-palsy, but not necessarily that any large protrusion exists now. Bilateral absence of the ankle-jerk occurs in an occasional case of unilateral sciatica, and rarely the ankle-jerk disappears only on the painless side. Both ankle-jerks may disappear in spondylolisthesis, tabes, malignant disease and after some years of the mushroom phenomenon. Slow return of the foot after the tendon has been struck and the muscles have contracted suggests hypothyroidism. Not all individuals possess tendon-reflexes; bilateral absence of knee and ankle-jerks may or may not indicate some generalized disorder but has no significance in, e.g. a probable disc lesion.

Weakness of the quadriceps muscles is best tested with the patient prone; the two sides are compared. The patient should be stronger than the examiner. In a third lumbar root-palsy, the quadriceps is weakened, in severe cases in conjunction with the psoas muscle. Bilateral weakness occurs in myositis, localized myopathy and spinal neoplasm. Weakness accompanied by increased pain indicates a partial rupture of the quadriceps or a fractured patella.

The state of the hamstring muscles is best demonstrated by asking the patient to flex his knee against resistance (Fig. 73); this time the examiner is stronger than the patient. Weakness of the hamstrings shows that, if a disc protrusion is responsible, the first or second sacral root is compressed, i.e. that the lesion lies at the fifth lumbar level.

Weakness of the buttock muscles is seldom demonstrable by testing resisted extension at the hip, but wasting, sometimes gross, is often visible. It is best noted by asking the patient to contract his buttock muscles; the muscles on the normal side stand out prominently; those on the affected side remain flat and can be felt to remain very podgy on palpation. Increase in the size of the affected buttock is found in sarcoma of the ilium or a cold abscess originating from the sacro-iliac joint.

Prone-lying Knee-flexion

This is the test for the sheath of the third lumbar nerve-root (Fig. 74).

When a patient lies supine, flexion at the knee involves flexing the hip too; hence the quadriceps muscle and femoral nerve are relaxed above in proportion as they are stretched from below. However, when a patient lies prone, the hip remains extended as the knee flexes and the constant-length phenomenon comes into play. Limitation of prone-lying knee-flexion thus indicates a lesion connected with the muscles or nerves at the anterior aspect of the thigh. If the quadriceps is neither abnormally adherent to the shaft of the femur (e.g. after fracture of the femoral shaft) nor painful on resisted contraction, the muscle is exculpated and the limiting factor must be the nerve. In fact, prone-lying knee-flexion is to the third root what straight-leg raising is to the four roots below. Unfortunately, it is a far less constant sign than straight-leg raising. In most third-root lesions, it is painful at full range rather than limited. Since the extreme of this movement is uncomfortable in any individual, the question is the degree of pain: a very much less satisfactory criterion than visible limitation of movement.

If it is limited, the amount of movement obtainable varies according to the size of the protrusion (except in root-atrophy) in the same way as does straight-leg raising, and provides the same useful criterion during attempted reduction.

Palpation

The lumbar spine is palpated for any irregularity of the spinous processes. The physician should run his hand quickly down the central furrow of the spine feeling for any projection that arrests the progress of his fingers. Occasionally, congenital shortening or lengthening of one spinous process leads to unfounded suspicions.

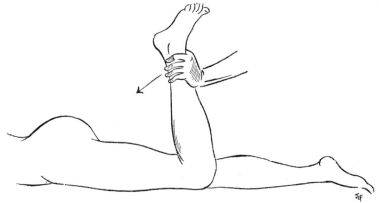

FIG. 74. Test for the third lumbar nerve-root. The patient lies prone, so that the hip remains extended. As the knee is flexed the third lumbar nerve-root is stretched via the femoral nerve. In disc protrusion at the third lumbar level flexion at the knee is unilaterally painful at its extreme, occasionally limited in range. Exceptionally, when a protrusion lies at the axilla of the root, full flexion of the knee on the painless side hurts the thigh on the affected side.

An angular kyphos indicates wedging of a vertebral body or complete loss of two adjacent disc spaces; a shelf indicates spondylolisthesis. In concealed spondylolisthesis the irregularity is visible and palpable as the patient stands, but can no longer be felt when the patient lies down (Plate 34). If an irregularity can be felt giving rise to acute lateral angulation of the spine, hemivertebra or asymmetrical erosion of bone in the course of tuberculous caries or secondary neoplasm should be suspected. As in all disorders affecting bone, radiography is then essential.

Rupture of a supraspinous ligament causes a palpable gap between the spinous processes, which feel farther apart than their fellows. At operation Bouillet has found this a good criterion for the level of a disc lesion.

The Resisted Lumbar Movements

These should be tested if three possibilities have arisen. (1) Was there direct unilateral trauma to the lumbar spine? If so, the last rib or one or more transverse processes may have been injured. These minor fractures show themselves clinically as muscle lesions, giving rise to pain on resisted contraction of the sacrospinalis muscle. (2) Is the patient suspected of psychogenic symptoms? If so, a comparison of the effect of active, passive and resisted movements may well prove informative. (3) Does the examiner believe in sprain of a lumbar muscle? Then the muscles must be tested separately from the joints.

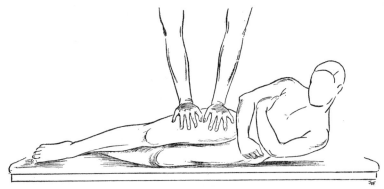

FIG. 75. Test for the sacrospinalis muscle. The patient lies on his painless side, his thigh supported by the examiner. He crosses his arms in front of him and lifts his thorax off the couch without using his elbow. This puts a strong strain on one sacrospinalis muscle. This movement is found painful in fracture of a transverse process.

The tests for the sacrospinalis muscles are three: resisted side-flexion standing, prone-lying trunk extension and side-lying trunk side-flexion. First, the patient lies prone and the examiner resists extension by placing one hand at the backs of the knees, the other at the upper thorax posteriorly. The response to this movement may be profitably compared with that to passive extension. To this end, the patient lifts his thorax off the couch by extending his elbows, letting his body sag. Secondly, the patient turns to lie on one side, crosses his arms in front of his chest and, without using his elbow, lifts his thorax off the couch. The physician steadies his thighs during the movement (Fig. 75).

If the resisted movements show that one or more transverse processes have probably been fractured, palpation helps to identify the level. Radiography is clearer still.

One difficulty in interpretation may arise. As was set out in the previous chapter, the first effect of contraction of the sacrospinalis muscles is to compress the lumbar joints. Hence, resisted extension may hurt even in a disc lesion. However, passive extension relaxes the muscles while straining the joint; hence, it is only the combination of painful resisted extension with painless passive extension that directs attention to the muscle. The same applies to side-flexion.

Forcing Extension

If examination of the trunk or lower limbs fails to show at what level a disc lesion lies, the attempt should be made by oscillatory forcing of extension. As the patient lies prone, a series of pressures towards extension is given, starting at the sacrum and repeated at each lumbar joint. The patient is asked to state at which level the thrusts provoke the greatest discomfort, and the examiner notes at which level muscle guarding is evoked.

Tenderness of the supraspinous ligament is no help, since whatever the level of the disc lesion, the fifth ligament is always the most sensitive. Looking for tenderness of muscle is, of course, quite pointless in an articular lesion.

DIAGNOSTIC LOCAL ANAESTHESIA

Sometimes the pattern obtained on examination shows merely that the symptoms arise from the moving parts of the back, but whether from a disc lesion or not is uncertain. Alternatively, testing the sacro-iliac joint and performing the lumbar movements both hurt, and it is not clear whether the lesion is lumbar or sacro-iliac.

In these cases, the induction of epidural local anaesthesia diagnostically should be carried out at once. The solution is confined within the neural canal by bone and ligament; it can escape only by the intervertebral foramina (Plates 47 and 48). Hence it anaesthetizes the dura mater and its investment of each nerve-root; it cannot reach the muscles or pass intra-articularly. If the symptoms arise from indirect pressure on the dura mater or a nerve-root because of minor displacement of a fragment of disc, the bulge presses on a surface now rendered insensitive; hence pain ceases for the duration of local anaesthesia. If this simple means of confirming or disproving a diagnosis of an early disc lesion were applied more universally the controversy around the disc *v.* the 'facet syndrome', sacro-iliac strain, lumbar muscle or ligament strain, 'fibrositis' and fatty nodules would be resolved; for this diagnostic infiltration, in a high proportion of cases, causes the pain to disappear for the time being. This implies that the lesion affects the dura mater or nerve-root. The facet joints, the muscles and fasciae, together with their fatty denizens, cannot in any circumstances touch the dural tube. If the injection does not alter the pain, diagnosis is difficult, sometimes impossible, and the alternative causes of lumbar pain must be considered.

THE RADIOGRAPH

The X-ray photograph has no positive value in disc lesions, since it cannot show the position of cartilage—a radio-translucent tissue. Its proper use is in differential diagnosis. Since bone disease is rare and nearly all backache arising in the moving parts has an articular origin, it suffices to demonstrate the absence of any bony disorder to draw attention to the joint, in other words, to disc-trouble. A diminished joint space shows the disc to be thinned but many discs atrophy as age advances without becoming displaced, and a normal disc space by no means excludes gross displacement of disc material. Even when a disc lesion is clearly present and the radiograph shows a narrow space, laminectomy may reveal that no protrusion exists at the level of the degenerate disc but that the lesion is recent and at an interspace of normal width radiologically. Middle-aged or elderly patients with psychogenic trouble often possess a symptomless diminished joint space, and excessive reliance on radiography then gives unwarranted credence to their allegations. By discography, Collis (1963) showed that 56 per cent of herniations arose at intervertebral spaces of normal thickness, 34 per cent at a narrow space, and 2·7 per cent at a space where posterior spondylolisthesis was visible.

Osteophytes also show, and indicate that the bulging disc has exerted enough ligamentous pull to lift up periosteum. The disc is now cupped in bone. The loose fragment of fibro-cartilage is therefore less likely to shift than before, but, as the osteophytes form chiefly laterally and anteriorly, they are not very usefully placed.

Posterior osteophytosis is of course important, if the bony projection becomes large enough to impinge on the dura mater. In fact, such a prominence is rare, and causes intractable backache, though seldom bad enough for the patient to accept laminectomy. Spondylolisthesis is a relevant X-ray finding in bilateral sciatica or paraesthesia in both feet; for the nerve-roots may catch against the shelf below. Much more often a disc lesion forms early in the unstable joint, and backache or unilateral sciatica in an adolescent often has this cause. Sacralization of the fifth lumbar vertebra is also significant; for immobility of the fifth lumbar joint leaves the fourth with double work to do; hence, a disc lesion there is apt to begin in adolescence.

Calcification of the disc has been described in pseudo-gout and can follow haemorrhage into the joint.

Myelography

A myelogram is seldom required, and need be considered at all only if laminectomy is contemplated. In a straight-forward disc lesion causing sciatica, it is unnecessary, since the surgeon will investigate both the fourth and the fifth lumbar levels in any case. Moreover, if the protrusion has passed well laterally, the dural tube is not indented and the protrusion does not show. Hence a negative finding does not exclude herniation. When a neuroma is suspected, contrast myelography is obviously indicated, and the investigation is also useful in patients with atypical signs in whom the alternative diagnosis is hysteria.

Jirout's Dynamic Pneumoradiography

Succeeding editions of this book have emphasised that compression of the intervertebral joint increases the signs of interference with the joint and with dural mobility. This is most obvious in sub-acute lumbago when the standing patient is found unable to bend forwards appreciably, but straight-leg raising (though often causing lumbar pain) is of full range. Again, a cough may hurt with the patient standing not lying. A marked lumbar deviation to one side may cease when the patient lies down. Such findings imply that the displacement—and with it the severity of the signs—protrudes farther during weight-bearing, and somewhat recedes when the joint is relieved of compression strain. My view since 1945 that the symptoms and signs of lumbago result from impingement upon the dura mater have met resistance, because a myelogram taken during lumbago usually shows no indentation of the dural shadow. Others have maintained that a protruded disc cannot reduce itself.

My deductions from clinical data have been confirmed by Jirout's work in Prague.

1. *Spinal Compression*

He noted that, at laminectomy, muscle-relaxation and relief from weight-bearing sometimes combined to allow a disc protrusion, already demonstrated by myelography, to disappear. He therefore applied a 40 Kg. longitudinal compression to the patient's spine by means of straps about shoulders and buttocks. After some ten minutes of such compression he was able to see the bulge re-appear.

2. *Pneumo-myelography*

Jirout's second method is a highly original piece of research and depends on the fact that, first demonstrated by him, the dura mater has an antero-posterior mobility. He appositely calls the method 'dynamic pneumo-radiography.'

With the patient in horizontal position lumbar puncture is performed and 40 cc of spinal fluid withdrawn. The table is then tilted to 30 degrees Trendelenburg position and only 20 cc of air are injected. While the tube is flaccid under such reduced pressure the anterior contour of the air column, i.e. the anterior wall of the dural sac at the level of L4 to S1 vertebrae shifts slightly backwards, so that the width of the anterior epidural space increases. A further injection of 60 ccs. of air is now given, strongly distending the theca and, in normal individuals, the second radiograph shows that the anterior contour of the air column has shifted anteriorly, the width of the anterior epidural space decreasing by an average of 3 mm. The dural membrane is now strongly applied to the posterior aspect of each vertebral body, outlining each bony concavity and the posterior margin of each disc. In disc protrusion, especially when it projects centrally, this dural movement is present above and below, but absent at the site of the obstacle. Such localized restriction of dural mobility is diagnostic of a space-occupying lesion, nearly always a pro-truded disc. Furthermore, on the second radiograph the projection has pushed the dura mater backwards and this can be seen to have lost its normal curve for several segments above and below. The air shadow shows the tube to run in two straight lines to the apex of the protrusion, where a dural angular kyphos is seen. Since the theca is already under such strong tension, it is not surprising that further stretching is resented—in other words, that in lumbago neck-flexion and straight-leg raising cause added pain. Pneumoradiography has thus enabled many disc displace-ments to be visualized which ordinary contrast myelography failed to reveal. Moreover, he has been able to show the protrusion to be mobile; for longitudinal compression of the lumbar spine increased the bulge; this was demonstrable in half of his 240 cases. Matthews' (1968) research at St. Thomas's Hospital has confirmed this mobility by an alternative method. Using epidural contrast radiography, he has shown the changes before, during and after traction most clearly (Plate 43).

In Jirout's book, entitled *Pneumoradiography*, radiographs clearly illustrate the increased protrusion caused by compression and the recession when this strain ceases. They also show the dura mater tightly stretched over postero-central displacements. Since so many regard protruded discs as irreducible, and many others do not consider the dura mater implicated in lumbago, the importance of this objective confirmation of deduction from clinical findings is manifest.

18

The Lumbar Region

PART III: DIFFERENTIAL DIAGNOSIS

An account follows first of the varieties and levels of disc lesion; then of the other conditions that predispose to disc lesions; finally, of disorders causing backache or pain to the lower limb unconnected with the intervertebral discs.

DISC LESIONS

A damaged disc can move in eight different ways at each joint, and in each case the displaced material may consist of nucleus, of fibro-cartilage or of both. Protrusion takes place at each of the five levels (though it is rare at the upper two). This amounts to more than a hundred possibilities in lumbar disc lesions alone.

The symptoms and signs that result are summarized below.

The Eight Ways

1. Gradual Small Posterior Displacement

The symptom is backache, brought on by stooping or lifting, relieved by staying erect or resting, such as almost everyone suffers from occasionally. If the protrusion compresses the dura mater centrally, the pain is central or bilateral. If it lies a little to one side of the mid-line, the symptoms are felt at one side of the lower back or in the upper buttock.

The signs are a full range of movement at the lumbar spine, some extremes hurting, some not; often, a painful arc. Straight-leg raising is of full range and painless. Examination of the lower limbs reveals no abnormality.

2. Swift Large Posterior Displacement

This results in lumbago. The patient is seized with severe pain in the lower back, coming on instantaneously during bending in the case of a cartilaginous displacement, often with a click; alternatively, coming on gradually hours after a period of stooping, and increasing for perhaps a day, when part of the nucleus pulposus protrudes.

There is a constant ache, punctuated by severe twinges on any unguarded movement. The pain may radiate to any part of the lower half of the body, including the abdomen (dural reference). The patient is immobilized in flexion or lateral deviation; he hobbles to bed. A cough and sneeze are agonizing: the dural symptom. The signs are (1) articular, (2) dural. The articular signs are fixed deformity at the joint and painful limitation of movement in the partial manner indicating an intra-articular block. The dural signs are bilateral limitation of straight-leg raising and lumbar pain on full neck-flexion.

3. Massive Posterior Protrusion

If the posterior longitudinal ligament ruptures, the whole disc may be extruded posteriorly, compressing the entire cauda equina against the anterior aspect of the two laminae. The sciatic nerve-roots are then squeezed on each side; in addition, the central component exerts such pressure on the third and fourth sacral roots in the preganglionic position that the bladder may become permanently paralysed. The symptoms are bilateral sciatica and severe lower sacral and perineal pain together with urinary incontinence. The signs are: bilateral limitation of straight-leg raising, often with a root-palsy on each side; analgesia at the saddle area, perineum and anus; weakness of the bladder.

4. Postero-lateral Protrusion

This may be secondary or primary; the former is the commoner.

Secondary

The patient suffers a number of attacks of backache or lumbago. This time, just as the pain in the back is passing off, it transfers itself to one aspect of the lower limb, front, outer side, or back, according to the level of the protrusion. In addition to the root-pain, pins and needles, numbness and aggravation on coughing may be mentioned.

The signs at the fourth and fifth levels are: limitation of trunk-flexion because of pain in the lower limb; one or two of the other lumbar movements may hurt in the lumbo-gluteal region; nearly always limitation of straight-leg raising; sometimes a root-palsy. In the elderly, the signs are less obvious. There is then often unilateral backache together with sciatica; the pain does not necessarily leave the back when it appears in the limb, as occurs in the young or middle-aged. Trunk-flexion may hurt in the lower limb, but is often of full range; the other lumbar movements hurt in the lumbar region; straight-leg raising is seldom limited, merely painful at full range; evidence of impaired conduction is uncommon.

In third lumbar disc lesions the movements are often reversed, since it is now bending backwards that stretches the nerve-root; hence trunk-flexion may even relieve the root-pain.

Primary

A young adult (18 to 35) develops an ache in the calf or posterior thigh on sitting. This gets slowly worse over a period of weeks or months, eventually spreading to the buttock and foot. There is no backache, and the root-pain is seldom really severe. Examination shows limitation of trunk-flexion, often with lateral deviation; the other three lumbar movements do not hurt; marked unilateral limitation of straight-leg raising; seldom appreciable signs of impaired conduction at the affected root.

5. Anterior Protrusion in the Elderly

Mushroom Phenomenon

The patient is elderly; my youngest to date is fifty-two. He complains that, after standing for ten to twenty minutes, increasing backache develops. In due course he notices that if he stands for longer, in addition to his backache, bilateral sciatica makes its appearance and after some years, prolonged standing may make both feet go numb. Occasionally, these symptoms are unilateral, sciatic pain and paraesthesia coming on in one limb only after standing for some time. Examination consists in making the patient stand until the pain starts; he is then asked to bend forwards. This abolishes the pain.

Anterior protrusion proceeds silently for years. Since there is no sensitive structure lying at the front of the joint, the displacement increases in size without compressing any sentient tissue. As the disc is slowly ground to pieces, the gravel passes forward and bulges out the anterior longitudinal ligament during weight-bearing. Periosteum is raised up by the ligament and two huge osteophytes form. On the radiograph, these two beaks can be seen enclosing a round ball of anteriorly displaced disc-substance (Plate 25); the disc becomes so narrowed that the vertebral bodies lie in apposition.

The mechanism of eventual pain is as follows: When the patient stands, the remnants of disc left at the intervertebral joint exert centrifugal force on the articular ligaments all the way round. The loss of thickness of the disc means that the ligament becomes lax and can bulge abnormally far out. In front and at the sides, this does not matter since there is nothing sensitive to compress; but the posterior component impinges against the dura mater *via* the ligament and finally also the nerve-roots. Bending forward opens the back of the joint and tautens the ligament, whereupon contact between ligament and dura mater or nerve-roots ceases at once. After years of this type of intermittent pressure, both ankle-jerks usually disappear.

This disorder has been named the 'mushroom phenomenon' (Cyriax, 1950) since it depends on bulging of the posterior longitudinal ligament at the back of the joint. It is often mistaken for intermittent claudication or for spinal claudication, since the patient gets the pain when standing, i.e. when walking, which is relieved when he sits down. Moreover, he is already at the age when poor pulsation in the arteries at the ankles may happen to be present. However, the mere cessation of walking does not alter this pain; he must sit; moreover, standing *without* walking induces the symptoms. This phenomenon may go on scarcely getting any worse for years. But, once it has begun, it goes on indefinitely.

The mushroom phenomenon must not be mistaken for younger patients' nuclear self-reducing herniation. However bad the pain in the former, lying abolishes it in less than a minute, whereas a self-reducing protrusion may take an hour or longer to return to its bed. Moreover, in the morning, whatever a patient does for the first hour or two, he remains pain-free, whereas a night's rest does not alter the timing of a compression pain.

If a young patient gives a history of backache followed by bilateral sciatica brought on by standing, spondylolisthesis is the probable cause.

6. Anterior Protrusion in Adolescents

Osteochondritis

Between the ages of fourteen and eighteen, the nucleus pulposus may burrow forwards between the cartilaginous end-plate and the bone of the vertebral body, which suffers pressure erosion. If the protrusion reaches the anterior longitudinal ligament, a small triangle of bone may be separated at the anterior corner of the vertebral body, which enlarges antero-posteriorly. After osteochondritis at a lower cervical level, the body may occasionally be seen on the lateral radiograph to be almost double the normal length. The phenomenon is common at lower cervical, mid and lower thoracic, and upper lumbar levels (Plate 35). Since excessive weight-bearing might well be supposed to help drive the nucleus pulposus into the bone, Wassman (1951) investigated the incidence of this type of anterior protrusion in the thoracic spine of young recruits.

He found it eight times more common in those from the country than from a town.

The disorder causes no symptoms and requires no treatment unless, as a result of the kyphotic posture of the joint consequent upon the vertebral wedging, posterior protrusion of disc-substance has begun. Manipulative reduction, which has to be repeated often at first, is then required.

7. Vertical Protrusion

This beneficent protrusion occurs, unfortunately, at the very lumbar levels where it is least wanted. It is not uncommon at the upper lumbar and lower thoracic levels; it is rare at the lower two lumbar joints at which it would be welcome.

There are two varieties:

(a) *Schmorl's node*. This is the only situation in the body where articular cartilage rests on trabeculae of cancellous bone rather than thick sub-chondral bone. During weight-bearing, the nucleus impinges against the articular cartilage of the vertebral body; this finally gives way and nuclear material invades the cancellous bone. This fixes the nucleus and diminishes the intra-articular centrifugal force, thus rendering posterior herniation less probable. No pain whatever is felt during this slow erosion of bone, but the radiograph shows clearly the irregularity of the joint-line. The node is first seen at the age of seventeen. The X-ray appearances do not alter appreciably later. Nachemson (1960) states that, after experimental fractures of the vertebrae, part of the nucleus pulposus may be forced through the end-plate. This diminishes the compressive stress within the disc, i.e. increased vertical and diminished tangential strain on the annulus. Again, this makes protrusion less likely.

(b) *Biconvex disc*. This phenomenon indicates softening of bone, and indicates past rickets, osteomalacia or senile osteoporosis. Normal pressure by the disc on soft bone results in a smooth curve at many adjacent bodies. The radiograph reveals that the causative force has been exerted diffusely so as to produce regular concavity at each surface of the affected vertebral bodies.

8. Circular Protrusion

During compression, a damaged disc may widen and bulge all the way round the joint. Outward pressure on the ligaments pulls on the perios-teum and lifts it off the bone. Bone grows till it meets its limiting mem-brane once more; hence osteophytes form. These bony outcrops are often large anteriorly and laterally, but slight or absent posteriorly; they cup the front and sides of the damaged disc and diminish the likelihood of displacement, but would clearly do so more efficiently if the posterior component were more marked. Moreover, they limit spinal mobility, and thus hinder the very movements that would otherwise have led the fragment of disc to move out of position again.

Osteophyte formation is a beneficent phenomenon, and is the chief reason why nearly all elderly patients do not suffer lumbar pain.

Disc Lesions at Each Level

First and Second Lumbar Roots

Frequency

Though radiological evidence of a narrowed joint space and/or osteophytosis is common in elderly patients at the first and second lumbar levels, disc lesions here causing symptoms are very rare. This view has recently been confirmed. Semmes (1964) found only one first lumbar protrusion and only two at the second lumbar level in 1,500 consecutive laminectomies. Collis's discography (1963), Armstrong's (1950) and Aronson and Dunsmore's (1963) findings on upwards of a thousand cases each are set out below:

Collis	Armstrong	Aronson and Dunsmore
L 1 : 0		L 1 0·29 per cent
L 2 : 1	L, 1, 2, 3	L 2 1·46 per cent
L 3 : 44	2·1 per cent	L 3 3·72 per cent

Disc lesions at the upper two joints behave quite differently from those at the other three levels. They are nearly always of the nuclear type, the symptoms gradually appearing when a certain posture has been maintained, and ceasing when the patient alters his position. Except when they are secondary to a lower lumbar arthrodesis, they seldom respond to manipulation, but often do well on traction.

First Lumbar Root

The patient complains of pain in the back radiating to the region above the trochanter and to the groin. Since this is a commonplace in low lumbar disc lesions, not only as a result of extra-segmental dural reference but also in pressure on the third sacral root, at first no suspicion of the unusual level is aroused. However, the patient may complain that if he maintains the posture that causes the pain in the groin, he develops numbness there, but I have yet to meet paraesthesia in the outer buttock, where the greater part of the first lumbar dermatome lies.

Examination shows that the patient points to the upper lumbar 'forbidden area' as the site of pain. The lumbar movements set up lumbar pain in the ordinary way, but it is felt in the upper lumbar region. Examination of the nervous system reveals no muscle weakness or alteration in reflexes, but cutaneous analgesia may be detectable at and just below the inner half of the inguinal ligament.

I have made this diagnosis only a few times (Plate 26 shows the radiological appearances in one such case). Since the diagnosis was made before the X-ray picture was available, and the two correspond well, it seems to have been correct.

Second Lumbar Root

The symptoms come and go in the same way. Standing for some time causes pain in the back radiating to the front of the thigh as far as the knee; sitting down abolishes it, or vice versa. This often goes on for years without change.

The lumbar pain is at an upper level; the lumbar movement hurts locally in the expected way; the painful limb is normal in every way except that a few patients show cutaneous analgesia along the front of the thigh. I have seen one case of a patient fixed in flexion by severe pain felt only at the front of one thigh. Any effort to straighten up or to walk was impossible, and she had been confined to her room for six months; during this time her condition had not altered. Manipulative reduction failed; sustained traction succeeded, and this elderly lady has now remained well for several years. Surprisingly, traction was also most successful in a case in which the psoas muscle was weak.

Only one of my cases of second lumbar disc lesion came to laminectomy. The patient was 46 years old and complained of anterior pain in the right thigh on lifting for four years. Two years later he noticed pins and needles in the right knee at night. His symptoms had been regarded as psychogenic. Examination showed a gross deviation of the lumbar spine to the left and trunk-extension hurt in the thigh. Provisional diagnosis was a neuroma at the second lumbar level and myelography suggested the same. At operation (McKissock), however, a second lumbar disc protrusion was disclosed. In a very similar case, a neuroma was found.

The common cause of upper lumbar disc lesions is arthrodesis at a low lumbar level. Some years after the operation, the joint above the fusion, which has been over-used owing to the immobility below, develops disc-trouble. Less common causes for upper lumbar disc lesions are fracture of a vertebral body or osteochondritis, each with coincident damage to the discs, either occurring at the time of the accident or resulting from the kyphotic posture of the joint secondary to the wedged body. Secondary malignant deposits favour the upper rather than the lower lumbar spine; here, they cause a gross limitation of lumbar spinal movements, together with such weakness of the psoas muscle that the patient may be seen to lift his thigh with his hands when he wants to shift his leg in bed. Lymphadenomatous invasion is a rarity. Meralgia paraesthetica must be considered, but posture, coughing and the lumbar movements do not affect the pain if the lateral cutaneous nerve of the thigh is at fault.

Third Lumbar Root

Four to eight per cent of all lumbar disc lesions affect this joint; the figures vary considerably. At 1,500 laminectomies, Semmes (1964) found a protrusion at the third lumbar level in only 2 per cent, but this may merely imply that third lumbar disc protrusions very seldom require laminectomy (which is, in fact, my experience). In 88 cases of root-pain in the lower limb, seven had signs of a third lumbar root-palsy (Cyriax 1965) and Troisier (1960) found seven out of 182 cases of root weakness to be third lumbar. Collis (1963) found that 44 out of 1,014 patients submitted to discography had a lesion at the third level.

The early symptoms are usually in the mid-lumbar region. The root-pain occupies the upper buttock, the whole front thigh and knee, spreading down the front of the inner side of the knee (Figs. 16, and 18) to just above the ankle. Numbness may be mentioned at the inner knee or anterior leg. The lumbar movements hurt the back in the expected way, but since the third root is stretched on trunk-extension and relaxed on flexion, the usual effect of these movements is reversed. Trunk-extension usually hurts in the anterior thigh. Flexion is of full range; though sometimes painful, it may be stated to relieve the pain; such patients sleep with their knees bent up towards the thorax. The full root-syndrome is: weakness of the psoas, weakness of the quadriceps, sluggishness or absence of the knee-jerk; pain at the front of the thigh on full straight-leg raising; limitation of prone-lying knee-flexion; cutaneous analgesia extending from the patella along the front or inner aspect of the leg to just above the ankle. As is usual in root-interference by disc lesions, all these signs are seldom present together.

Fourth Lumbar Root

About three-sevenths of all disc lesions occur at the fourth lumbar joint. Collis (1963) states that they comprised 42 per cent and fifth lumbar 37 per cent of his patients undergoing discography. The patient points to the mid-lumbar area or the iliac crest as the level of his lumbar pain.

When root-pain supervenes, it occupies the inner quadrant of the buttock, the outer aspect of the thigh and leg, and, crossing over the dorsum of the foot, it reaches the big toe, which often tingles.

Marked lateral deviation, consistent or alternating, characterizes fourth lumbar disc lesions, and, in such cases, gross limitation of one side-flexion movement is to be expected. In less severe cases, a painful arc on side-flexion is often experienced. The full root-syndrome is: limitation of straight-leg raising, often bilateral, the pain in the limb being further increased by neck-flexion; weakness of the tibialis anterior and extensor hallucis muscles; cutaneous analgesia at the outer part of the lower leg and the big toe. Neither the knee nor the ankle-jerk is affected. In 88 cases seen by me with various root weaknesses, the tibialis anterior was weak in twelve. All these signs are seldom present together.

Fifth Lumbar Root

About three-sevenths of all lumbar disc lesions occur at the fifth joint, but disc protrusions at either the fourth or the fifth level may equally compress the fifth root. A protrusion just off centre at the fourth level catches the fifth root, whereas one lying more laterally impinges on the fourth. Hence the discovery of a fourth root-palsy indicates a fourth lumbar protrusion, and of a first sacral palsy a fifth lumbar protrusion. However, the discovery of a fifth lumbar palsy has an equivocal significance and it is by noting the presence or absence of lumbar deviation and pain on crossed-leg raising that the probable level is selected. As the patient stands, the lumbar spine may be seen to deviate towards or away from the painful side. An attempt at trunk-flexion may increase the deviation, leave it unaltered or abolish it. Alternatively, the patient may stand with his lumbar spine vertical, but deviate when he bends forwards.

The lumbar movements hurt in the expected way. The full root-syndrome is: unilateral limitation of straight-leg raising, with increase in root-pain on neck-flexion, weakness of the extensor hallucis, peroneal and gluteus medius muscles, cutaneous analgesia at the outer leg and inner three toes; sluggish or absent ankle-jerk. Occasionally, a protrusion may compress the inferior aspect of the fifth lumbar root and the superior aspect of the first sacral root. In this event, weakness of the extensor hallucis and peroneal muscles is accompanied by paraesthesia at the outer border of the foot and fourth and fifth toes.

First, Second, and Third Sacral Roots

These three sacral roots can be compressed by a fifth lumbar disc-protrusion. Straight-leg raising is limited. The calf and hamstring muscles are weak; sometimes the peronei are also weak. Though weakness of hip-extension cannot be demonstrated, the gluteal mass is markedly wasted, and the patient cannot contract it. The outer two toes, the outer foot and the outer leg as far as the lateral aspect of the knee are analgesic.

In second sacral root-palsy, the signs are the same except that the peroneal muscles escape and the cutaneous analgesia ends at the heel.

In third sacral root pain, no palsy is detectable. The patient has pain in the groin running down the inner aspect of the thigh to the knee. Straight-leg raising is not limited and no muscular weakness occurs. Although the bladder is innervated also from the second and third sacral roots—the main supply is from the fourth—it is not my experience that the bladder or rectum is affected in second or third sacral root-syndromes.

Fourth Sacral Root

The twinges that are felt in the back in lumbago may be experienced deeply in the lower sacral area, and the patient may attribute his pain to rectal spasm. When this happens, the pain of proctalgia fugax is simu-lated, but I regard this event as an example of extra-segmental dural reference. The same misleading reference may well lead to pain felt at the lower sacrum or coccyx, but again this is not evidence of pressure on the fourth sacral root, which sets up pain felt to reach the penis, vagina, perineum, or testicles (one or both), often with paraesthesia. Hence pain in the perineum or genitals, weakness of the bladder or rectum, pins and needles felt in the saddle area, scrotum, vagina, testicle(s), analgesia of the anus, or impotence—all indicate that the fourth sacral root is menaced. This is serious. It is important in this connection to establish whether a patient's frequency of micturition is caused by such weakness of the bladder that he cannot hold his water, or by a strong urge. If the latter, the fourth sacral root is not at fault. In all cases of lumbago, the state of vesical function or presence of paraesthesia must be ascertained.

Since it is central protrusion that endangers the fourth sacral root, the pain is felt all over the sacrum and in an isolated palsy does not radiate to the lower limbs. Nothing, therefore, arouses suspicion until the patient mentions that during his attacks of lumbago he has difficulty in passing, or retaining, urine, or he gets pins and needles in his scrotum, or his saddle area feels numb or his rectum lacks expulsive power. These symptoms suggest a considerable bulging of the posterior longitudinal ligament; indeed, it may be on the point of rupture. By contrast, the signs may be very slight and the discrepancy between the severe pain and the minor signs may suggest that the patient is exaggerating. Examination reveals rather minor articular signs indistinguishable from those of ordinary cases of unimportant lumbago. In lumbago straight-leg raising may be limited as a coincident dural phenomenon, but the fourth sacral root is not stretched by this test; hence it is often of full range and painless. It is therefore a full history rather than the examination which inspires caution.

Bilateral sciatica suggests that the fourth sacral root is menaced, particularly if the second or third sacral roots are affected on each side. This event shows that the posterior ligament is being subjected to pressure from both sides, and may well have become overstretched, then torn at each side; finally, the central strands rupture. When this occurs, massive sequestration of disc substance—sometimes the entire disc—forces the cauda equina backwards against the laminae. Bilateral sciatica then appears at the same time as the fourth sacral palsy becomes manifest. Now straight-leg raising becomes bilaterally limited, neurological signs appear and the situation becomes obvious. In Jennett's twenty-five cases of discogenic paralysis of the bladder, fourteen began with bilateral sciatica.

Pressure on the fourth sacral root is exerted at a level proximal to the posterior ganglion and permanent paralysis of bladder function can ensue. So far, I have encountered twelve cases, in all of which a laminectomy was performed within twenty-four hours; all recovered bladder function. Jennett (1956), reviewing a thousand cases of laminectomy, of which twenty-five were for paralysis of the bladder, noted that operation some months later cured only four. Matheson (1960) mentions four cases, two coming on immediately after manipulation under anaesthesia; and one of my patients developed severe bilateral sciatica and vesical paralysis with retention some hours after manipulation by an osteopath. She was seen the day before when she requested, but was refused, manipulation because the fourth sacral root was in danger. Due care in selection of cases and in manipulative technique can single out these dangerous protrusions and avoid potential disasters.

Any suggestion that the fourth sacral root is menaced by a disc protrusion provides an absolute bar to manipulation by any method, and even traction is not wholly safe. Bilateral sciatica especially with third sacral root-pain, should make one cautious about manipulation except in patients over sixty. Once a fourth sacral paresis has begun, however slightly, laminectomy is indicated. Even if bladder function is returning as the sacral numbness is wearing off, this remains the correct treatment, for there is no guarantee that lasting incontinence may not follow the next attack of lumbago.

Those anxious to deprecate manipulation as a treatment emphasize the danger of permanent urinary incontinence, as the result of pressure on the fourth sacral root. It is a rarity but remains a remote possibility; however, when manipulation is carried out without anaesthesia and with the safeguards recommended here such a·catastrophe has never yet occurred. If it were ever provoked it can still be retrieved by immediate laminectomy.

Three interesting, perhaps unique, cases, are recorded:

The patient began lumbago at the age of 32. Aged 40, while standing, she felt a sudden click in her perineum. Instantly her left labium went numb, together with a small area to the left of the anus. This analgesia had persisted unchanged when she was seen thirteen years later. From the moment of the click she lost her libido, which never returned. There was neither dyspareunia nor bladder weakness.

A medical man, aged 23, fell heavily on to his buttocks and hurt his back severely. It ached for a week and intermittently after that. A year later, numbness appeared on the left at the medial aspect of the lower buttock and the uppermost three inches of the inner thigh. The left side of his penis and scrotum became analgesic; when erect, his penis deviated to the left. Libido was little affected and the bladder did not become weak. His anus became anaesthetic on the left and defaecation was felt as a unilateral phenomenon only. These symptoms largely disappeared after two years, but when he was seen for his recurrent lumbago at the age of 33, slight cutaneous analgesia at these areas was still detectable.

The third case was similar. Another medical man developed analgesia of the left side of the penis and anus at the age of twenty-six. He too noted leftward deviation during erection. The condition lasted two months. He began frequent attacks of severe lumbago, and at the age of 42 he was suffering from right-sided sciatica with a severe fourth and fifth motor-root palsy. Laminectomy was performed.

ADHERENT ROOT

Ordinarily, sciatica without appreciable neurological deficit gets well spontaneously in about a year. The herniation, deprived of its nutrient synovial fluid, shrivels and laminectomy years after an attack of sciatica reveals a normal appearance at the posterior aspect of the joint originally affected. When, with the passage of time the projection recedes, straight-leg raising reaches its full height again. However, the disorder occasionally continues past the allotted period for no clear reason; cases of sciatic pain and very limited straight-leg raising may continue indefinitely. However long-standing epidural local anaesthesia often restores the full range of straight-leg raising within a few minutes, thus indicating that the root is not adherent. By contrast, rare cases occur of adherence of the nerve-root to the posterior margin of the joint. The patient's sciatica gets slowly less and after about two years his pain may be gone, but he complains that he cannot bend forwards and examination shows about 45 degrees range of straight-leg raising on the affected side. Attempted trunk-flexion causes no pain; he just cannot bend, and heavy work produces no symptoms in the back or limb. The condition can last a lifetime.

Root adherence is suggested when a sciatica, particularly in a young man, goes on and on, the symptoms abating but the signs continuing; hence nothing special suggests this event during the first year or so of a root-pain. Continuation after that arouses suspicion; if so epidural local anaesthesia is diagnostic. Although the patient feels the root-pain down the limb during the injection, the anaesthetic solution cannot force its way between two adherent surfaces, but only between two surfaces in free contact. Hence, the injection does not alter such root-pain as is present nor restore for the duration of local anaesthesia the range of straight-leg raising. There is no other way of making this diagnosis—apart from inspection during laminectomy.

SPONDYLOLISTHESIS

Spondylolisthesis is not present at birth, although the lack of fusion at the pars intermedia which will bring it about is a congenital deformity. It first appears clinically and radiologically at about the age of fourteen. The appearance of the lumbar spine in a girl of twelve suggested spondylolisthesis, but the radiograph revealed no shift of the vertebra. Three years later the same shelf was noted and the spondylolisthesis was radiologically visible.

This developmental abnormality sets up pain in two separate ways: (1) commonly; by causing a disc lesion at the unstable joint; (2) rarely: by stretching the ligaments and the nerve-roots. It should not be forgotten that spondylolisthesis may cause no symptoms during the whole of a patient's lifetime. Crow and Brogden showed that 4·5 per cent of normal young adults who have never had backache have radiological evidence of spondylolisthesis, and a further 7·6 per cent have spondylolysis. My own figure for the incidence of spondylolisthesis in patients with symptoms attributable to the lumbar spine is 3·9 per cent.

Spondylolisthesis with Secondary Disc Lesion

Nothing in the history arouses suspicion unless the patient states that he has had trouble since childhood. He suffers backache or attacks of lumbago, unilateral or bilateral, indistinguishable from those occurring without spondylolisthesis, merely beginning at an early age. If he later develops sciatica, this is unilateral. Epidural local anaesthesia abolishes the backache for the time being. Laminectomy occasionally shows that the disc lesion lies at a non-spondylolisthetic joint.

It is only when inspection and/or palpation discloses the irregularity of the spinous processes that the presence of spondylolisthesis is suspected and confirmed by X-ray photography. The lumbar movements hurt in the manner characterizing a disc lesion; indeed, the signs and treatment are those of the disc lesion causing the symptoms. The only difference is the much enhanced liability to recurrence for slight reasons.

Spondylolisthesis of Itself Causing Symptoms

The induction of backache by spondylolisthesis shows that the ligaments about the lumbar intervertebral joints are not wholly insensitive. After years of stretching, they begin to set up discomfort. The ache is always central and largely unconnected with exertion; some days the back aches, other days it does not, for no clear reason. Prolonged standing is apt to cause either backache or discomfort at the outer aspect of both thighs; sitting or lying abates the pain. The patient may suffer vague crural numbness at night, but awakes comfortable. Thus the history may suggest a pulpy self-reducing disc lesion, but the aggravation by standing rather than by stooping or lifting should be a warning.

Inspection may reveal the irregularity. When the patient's lumbar movements are tested, unlike the effect when a displaced fragment of disc impairs articular mobility, usually none hurts, even though the back is aching at the time of examination. This finding should lead to renewed scrutiny and palpation of the lumbar spinous processes as the patient stands. When he lies prone, this palpation is repeated, in order to discover if the irregularity continues or disappears when weight-bearing ceases; the latter is a rarity. Epidural local anaesthesia cannot reach the ligaments about the intervertebral joint and does not affect the pain.

Spondylolisthesis also causes bilateral sciatica, with or without premonitory backache. After standing for, say, half an hour the patient develops increasing sciatic pain and paraesthetic feet, sufficient to compel him to sit or lie down. This may continue unchanged for years; the symptoms are the same as in the mushroom phenomenon, but the patient is much younger. The forward movement of the listhetic vertebra drags on the nerve-roots, which engage painfully against the shelf formed by the stable vertebra below. Alternatively, Gill et al. (1955) showed that a fibro-cartilaginous mass is apt to form at the defect in the pars interarticularis, leading to adhesions about and compression of the nerve-root. Good results followed removal.

Concealed Spondylolisthesis

The patient describes the typical history of backache, perhaps followed by bilateral sciatica, brought on by standing for some time, abolished by sitting or lying. Inspection of the back shows the irregularity; its presence is confirmed by palpation. When the spinous processes are palpated later with the patient prone, no irregularity is detectable. Relief from weight-bearing has allowed the bone to slide back into place again. Since most lumbar radiography is carried out in recumbency, the patient brings with him radiographs that disclose no abnormality (Plate 34). Unless he is X-rayed standing up, the displacement is not revealed.

Posterior Spondylolisthesis

This is usually symptomless and is more often seen at the upper lumbar and lower thoracic levels than at the fourth or fifth lumbar joints. It results from congenital laxity or gradual stretching of the ligaments at the lateral articulations.

During spinal extension the lateral facets of the upper vertebra tend to move backwards, partly owing to the force of gravity and partly because the surface of the lamina slopes downwards and backwards and thus, when the end of the articular surface is reached by the point of the facet, this is carried backwards as far as ligamentous laxity allows. By bending his trunk forwards, the patient approximates the surfaces of the facet joints once more. This instability is well shown in Morgan and King's paper (1957). Such instability at these lateral joints, although itself symptomless, leads to attrition of the disc. At the upper lumbar levels, this is usually a benign phenomenon but, particularly at the fourth level, may give rise to disc symptoms—backache, lumbago and sciatica.

In the case illustrated in Plate 33, which followed interference with the lateral articulations at laminectomy, considerable bilateral root-pain had been present for years, disappearing only when the patient lay down.

SPONDYLOLYSIS

This also causes no symptoms unless a secondary disc lesion with protrusion results. It is detectable only radiologically, when the defect in the pars intermedia on each side is shown in the oblique views. In the case illustrated (Plate 30) there was considerable intractable backache for some years; arthrodesis was advised but refused.

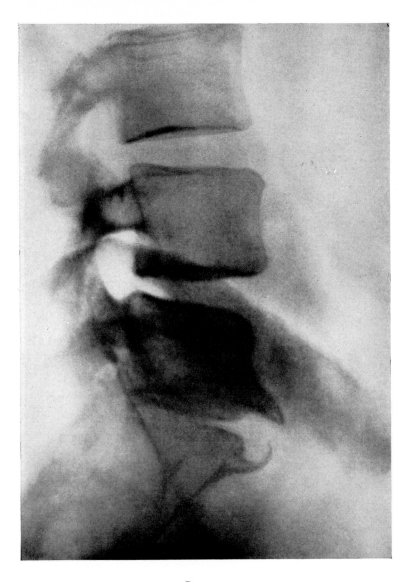

PLATE 25

Anterior disc protrusion. The fifth lumbar disc has been reduced to rubble and the intervertebral bodies lie in contact. Remaining disc-substance has become displaced forwards, where it lies enclosed by the two huge osteophytes that have formed in consequence of the traction exerted by the anterior logitudinal ligament. Since the protrusion does not impinge on a sensitive structure, for many years nothing is felt; finally compression causes the 'mushroom phenomenon' (see text).

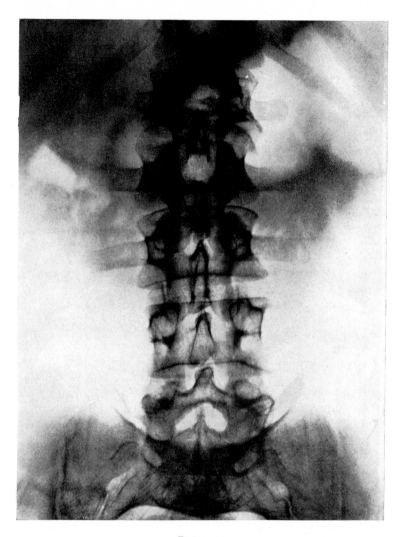

PLATE 26

First lumbar disc lesion. Radiograph of a man aged 31, whose upper lumbar pain and cutaneous analgesia in the left groin were ascribed on clinical examination to this rare lesion.

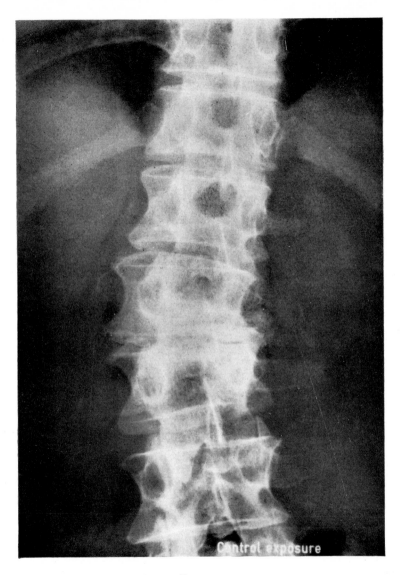

Control exposure

Plate 27

Osteo-arthritic compression of the second lumbar nerve-root. A woman of 57 had for two years suffered pain and pins and needles at the front of the right thigh down to the knee, after standing some time. Symptoms ceased as soon as she sat or lay down.

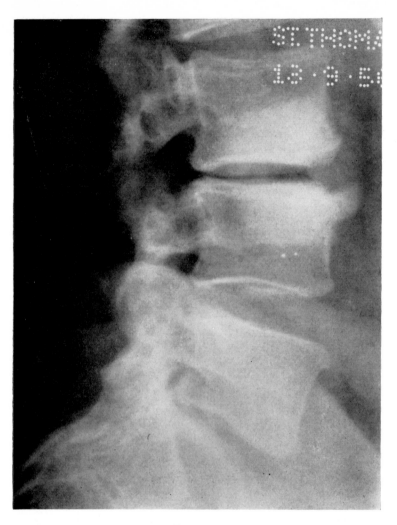

PLATE 28

Third lumbar root compression. A man of 48 had for six months noticed pins and needles at the inner aspect of the lower thigh on standing, relieved at once by sitting or lying.

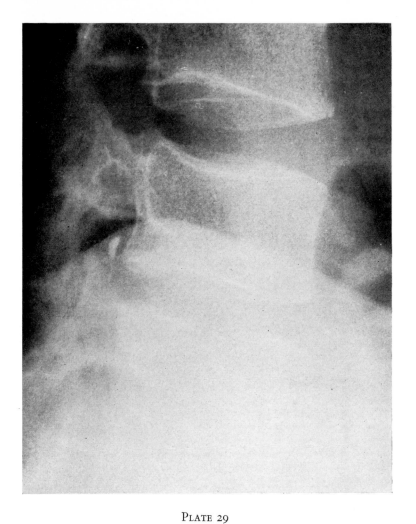

PLATE 29

Calcified posterior longitudinal ligament. It has been raised from the vertebral body by a large disc protrusion causing sciatica.

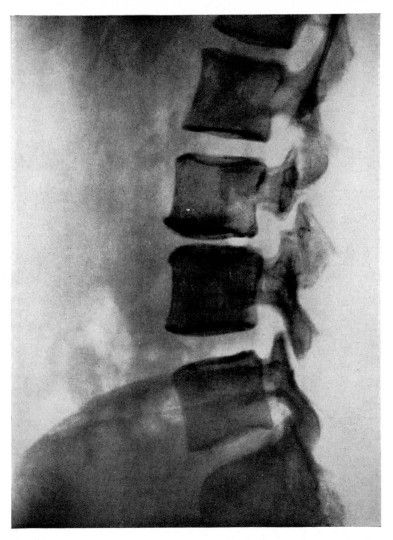

PLATE 30

Spondylolysis. Fibrous defect at the isthmus of the third lumbar vertebra without the deformity of spondylolisthesis. The patient was a woman aged 40 who had suffered from three years' backache. Though the radiograph suggests that the symptoms are due to a secondary disc lesion, examination showed capsular stretch to be responsible.

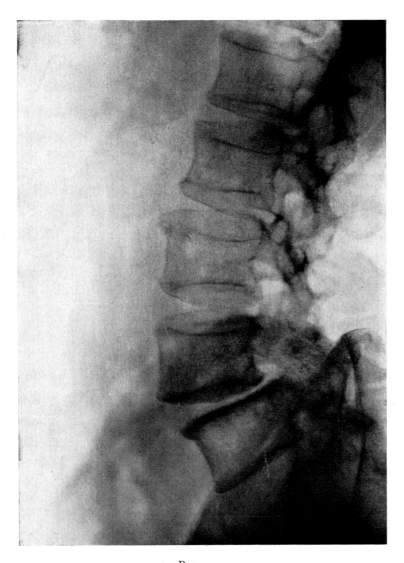

PLATE 31

Spondylolisthesis at the fourth lumbar level. This patient was a waiter whose deformity remained symptomless until it gave rise to bilateral sciatica at the age of 64 years.

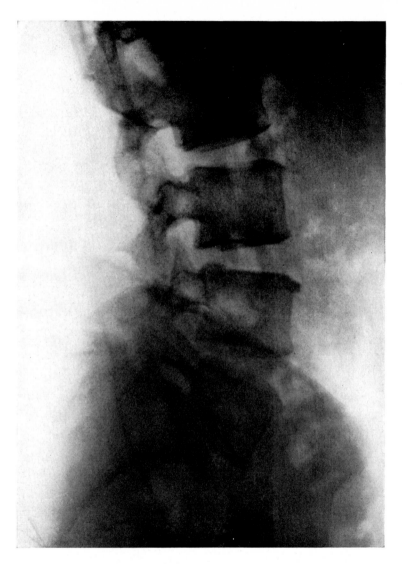

PLATE 32

Spondylolisthesis at the lumbo-sacral joint. The patient had suffered for twenty-five years from pain and paraesthesiae in his right lower limb after standing for some time. As soon as he sat down the symptoms disappeared. Note the forward displacement of the fifth lumbar vertebral body on the sacrum and the long pedicle. There was no complaint of backache. The sciatica was ascribed to stretching of the fifth lumbar nerve-root against the shelf formed by the upper edge of the sacrum.

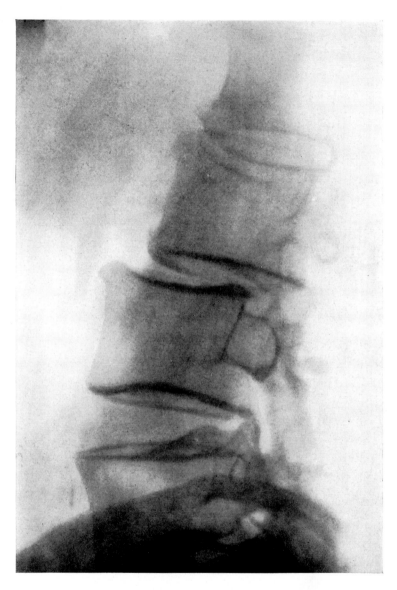

PLATE 33

Posterior spondylolisthesis at the third lumbar level. This followed a laminectomy at which the lateral articulations had been encroached upon. This patient had suffered several years' bilateral root-pain at the front of the thighs.

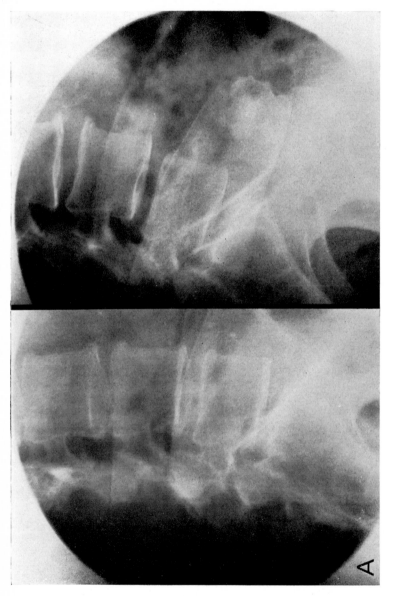

PLATE 34

Concealed spondylolisthesis. A man of 61 had had two years' backache and pins and needles in the toes of both feet. A lumbar shelf was visible and palpable as he stood, disappearing when he lay down. The forward shift of the fourth lumbar vertebra is well shown when standing (B) as compared to lying (A).

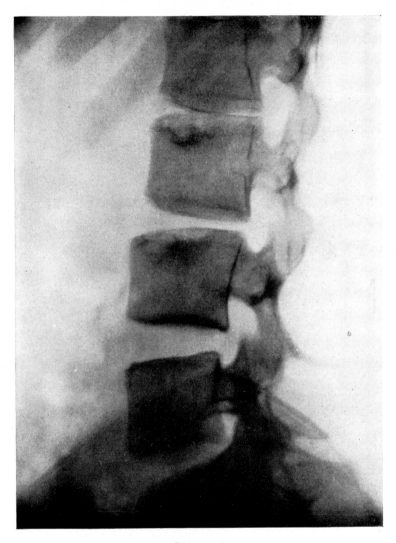

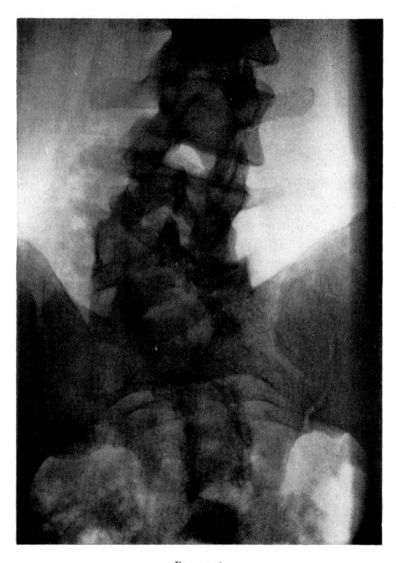

PLATE 36

Lumbar hemivertebra. This patient had had six months' aching at the back of both thighs.

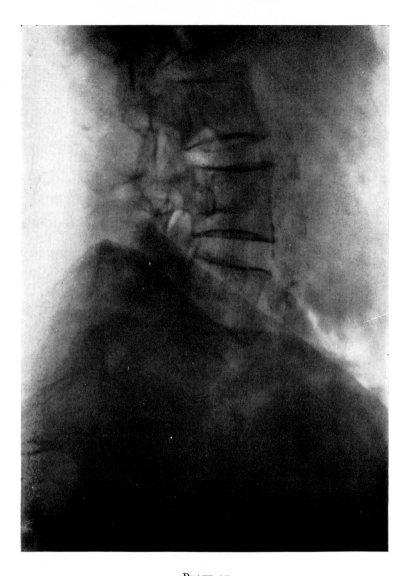

PLATE 37

Senile osteoporosis. Note the extreme degree of rarefaction of the lumbar vertebrae, contrasting with the calcified areas in the aorta. There were no symptoms.

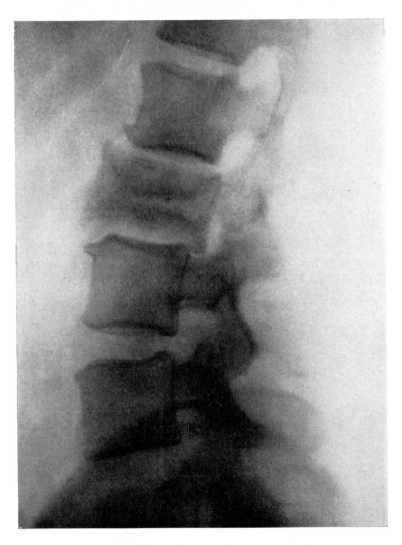

PLATE 38

Localized osteitis deformans at the second lumbar level. This man, aged 46, had had six months' backache. An upper lumbar angular kyphos was visible and palpable. Note that collapse continues until cortex touches cortex at the vertebral body. The pelvis showed the typical appearances of osteitis deformans.

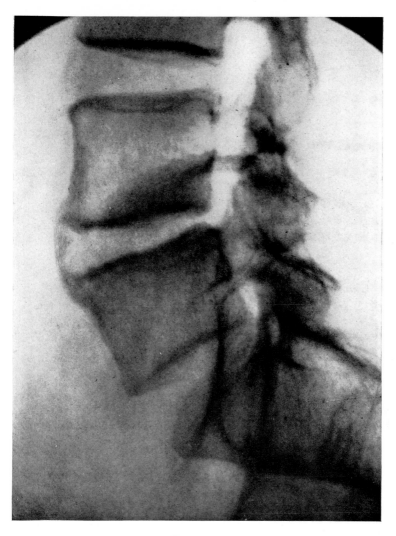

PLATE 39

Septic arthritis at the fourth lumbar joint. This man, aged 42, was first seen by me after six months' increasingly severe backache. The radiograph then revealed no abnormality, but the lumbar movements were markedly limited. At the end of a year the ankylosis by bone became clearly visible (see text).

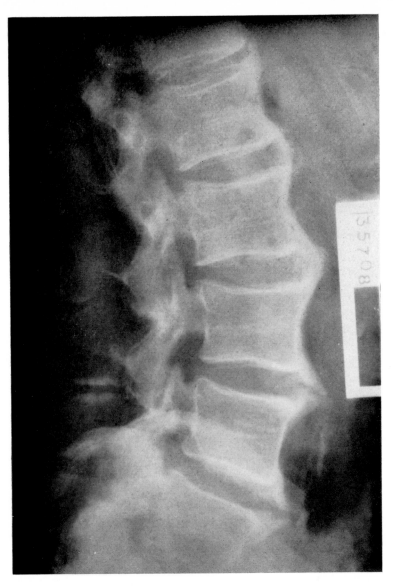

PLATE 40

Vertebral hyperostosis. A man of 58 had had five years' lumbo-thoracic backache. The anterior longitudinal ligament has ossified, and the disorder has involved the adjacent margins of the spinous processes.

WEDGING OF A VERTEBRAL BODY

This results from fracture, osteoporosis, adolescent osteochondritis, neoplasm, osteitis deformans and tuberculous caries.

Fracture Causing Wedging

This occurs at the upper rather than the lower lumbar vertebrae. Until the fracture has united, there is bone pain; it is severe for only a week or two and has certainly ceased in three months. Any pain after that is due to a coincident disc lesion. Naturally, force sufficient to break bone often also damages the discs above and below the fracture. Hence recurrent attacks of pain follow the injury. Moreover, there is now a permanent kyphosis at the joints above and below the wedged bone. This explains why some patients with a fractured body later have severe trouble, while others are symptom-free. It is not what happens to the vertebral body but the state of the discs, not visible radiologically, that determines whether symptoms persist after the fracture has united.

Inspection reveals a small angular kyphos; slight limitation of movement may be detected. The kyphos is palpable and, as the supraspinous and interspinous ligaments have sometimes ruptured, a depression can be felt between two spinous processes. Radiography identifies the wedged vertebra.

Many patients who know a vertebral body has been fractured allege pain; in some it is organic, but in many it is assumed or psychogenic. Examination to detect neurasthenia is then required. Such cases provide thorny medico-legal problems on which no light is thrown by mere inspection of the radiograph, which only shows the vertebral body united with minor angulation. The radiograph cannot show whether a disc is damaged or not; only detailed, possibly repeated, clinical examination enables an objective opinion to be formulated.

Senile Osteoporosis

Elderly patients, usually women, with marked generalized rarefaction of the spine may sustain a pathological fracture of one or more vertebral bodies. This is more frequent in the thoracic than the lumbar region. The wedging may come on slowly; it is then often symptomless unless a secondary disc lesion develops on account of the upper lumbar kyphosis at the joints to either side of the collapse. If wedging comes on suddenly, bone pain results; it may be severe for a week or two and ceases in two or

R

three months. The kyphosis is visible and palpable; radiography discloses the reason. Osteoporosis itself does not appear to me to cause aching unless disc protrusion or fracture supervenes.

Adolescent Osteochondritis (Schauermann)

In Crow and Brogden's (1959) series of 935 normal men who had never had backache, evidence of past Schauermann's disease in the lumbar region was present radiographically in 20·7 per cent. It comes on between the ages of fourteen (Plate 35) and eighteen, as the result of anterior disc protrusion. The end-plate is perforated, often at more than one upper lumbar level. Bone is eroded by the nuclear protrusion and wedging results. Since osteochondritis at other sites causes discomfort and at the spine involves bone, I used to suppose that this was a painful condition. However, twenty years ago, when examining a girl of fifteen with osteo-chondritis of six months' duration, a painful arc was found present. This was inconsistent with the concept of bone pain, and it seemed possible that the cause of symptoms was disc-pressure at one of the affected and, therefore, kyphotic joints. This proved so; for manipulative reduction was heralded by a click with instant disappearance of pain. This concept has since been confirmed on further cases.

Calvé's osteochondritis of the epiphysis of the body itself also gives rise to wedging with results similar, I imagine, to fracture. The disorder, of which I have no experience, is most uncommon.

Neoplasm

Rapidly increasing backache, in usually an elderly patient or one who is known to have had an operation for cancer, arouses suspicion. Limited movement due to muscle spasm and neurological signs in the lower limbs without root-pain make the suspicion a virtual certainty. A palpable kyphos confirmed by radiography completes the picture.

Osteitis Deformans

One vertebra may collapse leading to a palpable kyphos. Radiography to determine the cause reveals Paget's disease in the isolated vertebra and in the pelvis.

Tuberculous Caries

The symptoms are often slight at first, but inspection shows the be-ginnings of an angular kyphos or, if one side of the body is eroded alone, acute lateral deviation of the same type as occurs with hemivertebra. The lumbar spine is kept extended when the patient is asked to bend forward and the range of both side-flexions is markedly limited. These findings naturally call for immediate radiography, which usually reveals the lesion clearly. Four times in my experience, however, the disc was affected alone at first and the original radiograph revealed nothing.

LESIONS UNCONNECTED WITH DISCS

A large number of non-disc lesions give rise to pain in the back, groin and lower limb; they are much less common than a disc lesion, and are considered below.

Lumbar Pain

1. Fractured Transverse Process

This occurs only after direct injury to the back. The pain is unilateral, localized, and in the mid or upper lumbar region, since the fifth process is scarcely ever broken. The history and the discovery of pain elicited by resisted movements when the patient lies prone gives the clue, and the radiograph is diagnostic. If pain persists for more than a fortnight, it must be remembered that force sufficient to break a transverse process may also have injured a disc; alternatively, the idea of a 'fractured spine' may be so attractive to a patient that psychogenic symptoms supervene. A rare cause of fracture is manipulation of the back. The snap is felt quite clearly, and a week's discomfort is to be expected.

2. Ankylosing Spondylitis

If, as occurs in seven-eighths of all cases, the preceding sacro-iliac arthritis has caused no symptoms, the first complaint may be backache. It comes and goes according to its own vagaries, and is often worst on waking; exertion, however severe, does not bring on an attack although it may aggravate pain already present. As a rule, all the lumbar spinal joints become involved at much the same time. Hence the patient, instead of indicating one spot, points to the whole lumbar region centrally. Examination shows a flat lumbar spine with, perhaps, the beginning of an upper thoracic kyphosis, combined with limitation of side-flexion at the lumbar joints. By now active inflammation in the sacro-iliac joints has ceased and clinically they are painless, but X-rays of these joints—*not* of the lumbar spine—reveals the tell-tale sclerosis.

3. Osteitis Deformans

In advanced cases the pain is all over the elderly patient's back. On inspection, the trunk has a shortened appearance as if the thorax had come too far down towards the pelvis. Genu varum may be visible. Movement of the lumbo-thoracic spine is grossly restricted. Palpation of femur or tibia may show expansion. The radiograph of the pelvis is diagnostic.

Sometimes one vertebra is affected alone. If so, the body softens, broadens and collapses just as occurs on invasion by neoplasm, but does not proceed beyond cortex touching cortex. Localized backache results and inspection shows the angular kyphos. Plate 38 shows the typical appearances. The differential diagnosis is made largely by seeking evidence of osteitis deformans elsewhere.

4. Neoplasm

Neoplasms are nearly always secondary, although myeloma is encountered. In myeloma the sedimentation rate is seldom less than 100 mm. in the first hour. There may be a history of previous operation for malignant disease, but undue weight must not be given to this fact; for such patients, like other individuals, often suffer from ordinary disc lesions. Much distress is caused, and effective treatment not given, when a disc lesion is mistaken for secondary malignant deposits; hence it is an error hardly less grave than the converse.

In disc lesions, the neurological signs are minor and the root-pain severe; in neoplasm the reverse obtains.

The first suggestion of malignant disease lies in the history, which is not of pain varying with exertion but of steady aggravation irrespective of activity. A short period of increasing central backache in an elderly patient is always suspect. Then the pain spreads down both lower limbs in a distribution not corresponding to any one root. Moreover, the backache becomes worse when the sciatica, soon bilateral, appears. In a disc lesion, the backache eases when unilateral root-pain comes on. If examination does not yet reveal a kyphos, muscular spasm markedly limiting movement is seen at the lumbar spine, most obvious on attempted side-flexion. Neurological examination reveals signs that more than one nerve-root is involved, e.g. the knee-jerk is affected as well as the ankle-jerk; the psoas muscle is weak together with muscles of lower lumbar derivation; the muscle weakness and the site of cutaneous analgesia belong to separate segments; the signs are bilateral and asymmetrical.

In a disc lesion causing muscle weakness, the patient must have had considerable root-pain in the lower limb. Severe weakness without root-pain is very suggestive of spinal metastases. So is gross weakness with a full range of straight-leg raising, without a history of recent acute sciatica. At the upper two lumbar levels, neoplasm may interfere with the sympathetic nerves; if so, the foot on the affected side is warmer than its fellow. These signs often appear before the radiograph shows erosion or collapse of one or more vertebral bodies. Indeed, there may be no X-ray changes only a few weeks before vertebral bodies can be crushed by the fingers at post-mortem. Hence, *in the short run*, X-ray photography is not reliable. In a doubtful case, epidural local anaesthesia abolishes temporarily the pain due to a disc lesion, but not that due to metastatic invasion. The patient must be observed and X-rayed at monthly intervals until the diagnosis becomes clear, while a search for the primary growth is initiated.

5. Sacral Neoplasm

This is more difficult to detect than lower lumbar metastasis, because the spinal joints retain a full and painless range of movement. The patient complains of sacral pain, sometimes of coccygodynia only. However, invasion of the nerve-roots at the front of the sacrum, although (as the dural sleeve is not affected) it does not provoke root-pain or limitation of straight-leg raising, gives rise to gross weakness of the muscles of one or both feet. Such paresis in the absence of root-pain naturally suggests a tumour, and the radiograph usually discloses a sacral defect. The symptoms are slight at first and the patient is apt to present himself late in the evolution of the disease.

6. Afebrile Osteomyelitis

Acute

Afebrile osteomyelitis may come on quickly—in the course of, say, a week. The history is then identical with nuclear lumbago: rapidly increasing lumbar pain. After some days, when asked to stand for a moment to have his back examined, he cannot do so owing to severe pain. This is perfectly consistent with severe lumbago. But in central disc protrusion as marked as this, the dural signs are as conspicuous as the articular. Examination, however, reveals a full range of straight-leg raising; moreover, no pain is felt on coughing. This combination is typical of a severe spinal lesion, not affecting the mobility of the dura mater. Infection is suspected, and epidural local anaesthesia is induced at once, for confirmation. This has no effect on pain caused by osteomyelitis, thus confirming the diagnosis. The only objective sign is usually a raised sedimentation rate (40–60 mm.). The last such patient I saw lay in bed for two months before the abscess in the body of his fourth lumbar vertebra was revealed radiologically and was drained (Urquhart).

Chronic

The patient, always in my experience male, complains that a slight, constant, central backache came on some months previously and gradually became more severe. Examination at this stage reveals no diagnostic signs, but a disc lesion is excluded when epidural local anaesthesia fails temporarily to abolish the pain. Fever is absent. Radiography reveals no abnormality, but the ESR is raised. Under observation, the pain gradually worsens while restriction of side-flexion at the lumbar spine appears. The pain on movement and the increasing limitation of range may suggest ankylosing spondylitis but the onset is too swift, and the X-ray shows the sacro-iliac joints to be clear. The history is too long for a radio-invisible neoplasm. Once these points are established, the patient should be regarded as suffering from chronic osteomyelitis.

Plate 39 shows the appearance at the end of a year in a patient first seen six months after the onset of symptoms. Although the clinical signs were clear, the radiograph was still normal. In due course X-ray evidence of septic infection of the joint appeared.

Typhoid fever and brucellosis can give rise to spinal osteitis.

7. Posterior Osteophytosis

The early history is that of a disc lesion, since it is damage here that is responsible for the bulging of the posterior longitudinal ligament that in due course draws out the osteophyte. When this becomes large enough, a constant backache sets in (as often happens also in disc lesions without osteophyte formation). Clinical examination is not distinctive, the pattern of articular and dural signs suggesting a minor disc-protrusion. The diagnosis remains obscure until inspection of the lateral radiograph shows a large osteophyte jutting out backwards from the margin of the vertebral body and forming a bony projection (plate 23).

During the early stage of its formation the osteophyte causes no symptoms, but when it is large enough to irritate the dura mater, the constant backache can be relieved only by removing it at laminectomy.

8. Ligamentous Overstretching

This is most uncommon except in spondylolisthesis. In myopathy or anterior poliomyelitis affecting the muscles of the lower trunk, the patient has to balance himself bent slightly backwards. This puts a severe strain on the anterior longitudinal ligament; after some time a backache results that is immediately abolished by sitting down or bending forwards. Occasionally after laminectomy a flexion injury may painfully overstretch the fibrous tissue replacing the interspinous ligaments.

Rupture of a supraspinous or interspinous ligament increases the range of flexion at an intervertebral joint, thus predisposing to, or aggravating, damage to a disc. These ligaments are grossly overstretched on either side of a vertebral fracture with wedging. This tension may set up a central ache abolished for the time being by local anaesthesia.

9. Gastric Ulcer Adherent to Lumbar Spine

The symptoms are often remarkable, being connected with both eating and with posture. The pain may be lumbar or felt in one or other iliac fossa; it is not in my experience epigastric. One patient had to eat standing by the mantelpiece; another could not stand up straight after a meal. One patient with only upper lumbar pain obtained ease by frequently drinking hot water. He had twice had his stomach investigated by a barium meal, and it was only when this was repeated in the Trendelenburg position that the ulcer on the lesser curvature was revealed.

Trunk-extension stretches the scar tissue at the front of the spine and may cause central discomfort—a most misleading finding. However, the lumbar symptoms are felt in the forbidden area; they are not brought on by exertion although they are influenced by posture, and they are clearly connected with abdominal visceral function. This combination brings the diagnosis to mind.

10. Aortic Occlusion

D. L. Filzer (1958) pointed out that occlusion of the lower aorta or of the common iliac arteries may cause backache. Usually the claudication in one or both limbs overshadows the minor backache, which is felt in the upper lumbar region—the 'forbidden area'. The patient is regarded as suffering from sciatica, but the history is characteristic—limb pain occurs *only* on walking. The femoral pulse is absent and the diagnosis obvious. One patient with aortic thrombosis merely complained of numbness without pain at the front of both thighs after walking 50 yards.

Difficult cases are those with central upper lumbar or lower thoracic backache, unaltered by any movement of the spine. I examined such a patient once a week for a month before the femoral pulses ceased, clarifying the diagnosis. Another disorder difficult to identify is pressure, usually on the left third lumbar root, exerted by a slowly dissecting aneurysm. Severe left-sided pain in the back and limb without articular or root signs in an elderly patient should lead to suspicion. No relief is afforded by epidural local anaesthesia and myelography is, of course, also negative.

11. Spinal Claudication

Activity in a limb is accompanied by arterial dilation at the corresponding segments of the spinal cord. Hence pressure hindering such increased bloodflow can set up cord symptoms, as was recognized by Déjerine in 1906. In such cases, the patient's lower limbs feel heavy during exertion and during this period the plantar response becomes extensor. Rest makes the symptoms and signs disappear. Clearly, this phenomenon can affect also the cauda equina, e.g. by pressure from a disc protrusion. As a result the nerve-roots claudicate, resulting in root-pain and distal paraesthesia. Hence, in spinal claudication, walking causes backache and pain usually in both lower limbs, which ceases as soon as walking stops, but the pain is associated with pins and needles in both feet. Attention is thus drawn away from the vascular system and towards the nervous system, and this is reinforced when all the pulses are present on examination of the lower limbs. However, the symptoms, including the paraesthesia, come on only after walking a distance, and can be induced by exercising the limbs in bed. Evans (1964) attributes the disorder to anoxia of the nerve-roots, usually as the result of pressure from a disc protrusion. Laminectomy with removal of a small mid-line protrusion relieved three of his four patients.

12. Vertebral Hyperostosis

This rare disorder was first described by Forestier and Rotes-Querol in 1950. Elderly patients develop an ache in the entire trunk, with marked limitation of movement at every spinal joint. The radiological appearances are different from discogenic osteophytosis since the disc spaces are well-preserved and different again from ankylosing spondylitis in that ossification is confined to the anterior longitudinal ligament. Ott (1967) found that 21·8 of such patients have concomitant diabetes.

My youngest patient was 48 years old at his first visit, and had diffuse backache for fourteen years. Ossification of the anterior longitudinal ligament was confined to the first and second lumbar levels (plate 40).

13. Nutritional Osteomalacia

Female immigrants from Asia may live on a largely vegetarian diet, grossly deficient in lime salts. They lose a considerable amount of calcium if they bear a child, and more still by breast-feeding. Backache and bilateral sciatica then begin accompanied by complaints of lassitude. Since no physical signs are detectable on clinical examination, it is easy to dismiss the case as neurosis.

The early clinical sign—indeed often the only sign—is the characteristic waddle with which the patient walks. Even in the Punjab and West Pakistan where the disease is common, Vaishnava and Rizvi (1967) report that the condition is often missed. They see three or four cases a week, previously labelled psychogenic rheumatism, etc. One patient in five is pregnant and one in ten develops tetany as the first symptom.

The gait is diagnostic; the patient walks in with the feet turned outwards, dipping in the Trendelenberg way. Yet no abnormality of the lumbar spine, of the hip joints or of the muscles controlling them is found to account for this phenomenon. Radiography may not reveal rarefaction of bone at first, but the levels of calcium and phosphorus in the blood are low. In one such case of mine kindly investigated by Professor Prunty, the calcium level varied between 7·5 and 8·9 mg. while the plasma phosphorus varied between 2 and 3·1 mg.

Osteomalacia occurs in Europeans after gastrectomy.

14. 'Gonorrhoeal Fasciitis'

This is alleged to cause 'poker back' but is an entity copied from one text-book to another. I have never encountered such a case and, short of the fascia turning into bone, I do not believe that any such disorder could produce appreciable limitation of movement, in particular towards extension, which relaxes the fascia. Clearly, the idea of gonorrhoeal fasciitis depends on the co-existence in a single patient of gonorrhoea and ankylosing spondylitis—both diseases to which young men are prone. Moreover, spinal ankylosis is a well-known complication of Reiter's disease. Up to half of all cases of this disorder have radiological signs of sacro-iliac involvement, and in them there is an increased incidence of advancing spondylitis compared with the general population.

15. Pain Referred to the Back

When pain is referred to the back from an intra-abdominal or pelvic viscus, the outstanding finding is a full and painless range of movement at the lumbar spine. This finding focuses attention on the non-moving parts of the body, the kidney, colon, ovary, uterus and rectum. In cases of doubt, epidural local anaesthesia should be induced since it provides a clear, immediate answer.

Root-pain

A common cause of pain referred to the groin is misleading dural reference from a low lumbar disc lesion. Alternatively, third sacral root-pressure may be responsible. Far less often, it results from a lowest thoracic disc lesion. Pain in the groin was for a few months the only and, throughout, a prominent symptom in the case of fourth lumbar neuroma illustrated in Plate 52.

Osteo-arthritis of the hip, psoas bursitis and muscle strain may set up pain felt at first only in the groin. Intestinal and renal disorders, an ovarian cyst or a hernia may also cause pain felt chiefly in the groin. A gastric ulcer adherent to the lumbar spine sometimes causes puzzling symptoms there.

Second Lumbar Pain

Pain at the front of the thigh reaching as far as the knee occurs in lesions of structures developed from the second and third lumbar myotomes. These include the second and third lumbar nerve-roots, the hip joint, the psoas, adductor and quadriceps muscles, the psoas bursa, the femur and the bones about the acetabulum.

It must not be forgotten that obscure symptoms of numbness or weakness, not necessarily pain, felt in the anterior crural region after walking a short distance, may result from thrombosis of the lower aorta or external iliac artery. In the former case, both femoral pulses are lost; in the latter, only one. Although pain in the thigh brought on by walking naturally suggests a lesion in the moving parts, examination of the back and joints, muscles, etc., of the lower limb reveals no abnormality. This combination brings to mind the likelihood of claudication.

Pain at the front of the thigh which examination suggests has a local origin, but not in muscles, joints, etc., calls for radiography of the femur, which may disclose e.g. an osteoid osteoma.

Weakness of the Psoas Muscle

If the weakness is unilateral and is accompanied by lumbar pain on lumbar movements, a second lumbar disc lesion may be responsible. This is so rare, however, that the diagnosis should be unwillingly reached. If the weakness is considerable and pain felt in one iliac fossa is brought on when the muscle contracts, neoplasm invading the posterior abdominal wall should be suspected. If it is accompanied by increased pain in the thigh, metastatic invasion of the upper femur is likely, except in adolescents when avulsion of the epiphysis of the lesser femoral tuberosity occurs. Unilateral weakness is rarely the first sign of interference with the pyramidal tracts; if so, the resisted movement does not increase the pain.

Bilateral weakness characterizes neoplasm at the second lumbar level.

Meralgia Paraesthetica

This is an interesting condition (Figs. 76). The patient complains of pain and paraesthesia in the area of skin supplied by the lateral cutaneous

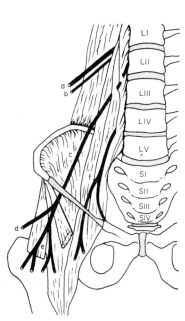

FIG. 76A. The second lumbar nerve root

(a) Greater abdomino-genital nerve
(b) Lesser abdomino-genital nerve
(c) Femoro-cutaneous nerve
(d) Gluteal branch
(e) Femoral branch
(f) Genito-crural branch

Note that the mid-point of the femoro-cutaneous nerve crosses the iliac crest and can suffer compression there in pregnancy.

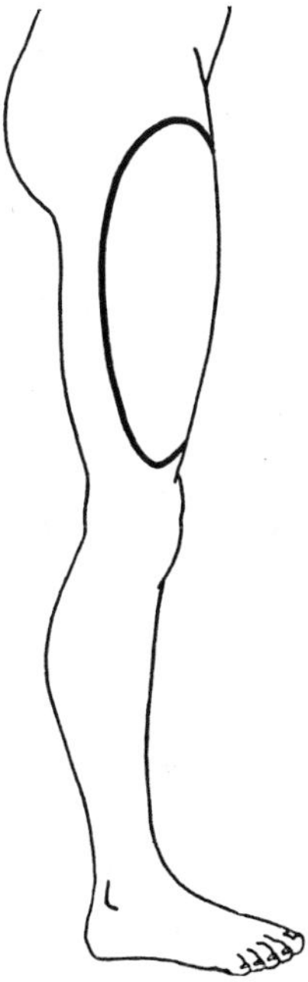

FIG. 76B. The area of skin supplied by the lateral cutaneous nerve of the thigh. The anterior edge does not reach to the mid-line of the thigh in front. Contrast the distribution of the second lumbar nerve-root (Fig. 17).

nerve of the thigh. This nerve emerges from the outer border of the psoas to cross the iliacus muscle. It passes under the lateral aspect of the inguinal ligament, and two inches below the anterior superior spine of the ilium pierces the fascia femoris. It emerges superficially two inches lower down, and it would seem that it can be irritated in any part of its course. The nerve may be nipped if, owing to congenital abnormality, it passes through the inguinal ligament instead of deeply. The difficult distinction between meralgia and a second lumbar root-lesion rests on: (1) A history of pain in the back or upper buttock preceding the appearance of the numbness. (2) Finding that one or more of the lumbar movements hurt in the trunk or provoke the pins and needles. (3) Careful delineation of the paraesthetic area. Comparison of Figs. 76 and 17 shows that the two areas correspond laterally, but only the second root supplies the front and inner aspect of the thigh. (4) The degree of analgesia. Since the second and third root territories overlap, the numbness is very slight in root-lesions, but may amount almost to anaesthesia with a clear-cut edge in pressure on the cutaneous nerve. (5) The induction of epidural local anaesthesia. Naturally this injection abolishes symptoms only in a root lesion.

In cases of friction at the fascial tunnel, injection of 10 ml. of 0·5 per cent procaine suffices. The difficulty is to find the right spot, since the position of the nerve varies considerably. A thin needle 5 cm. long is inserted superficially in line with the nerve and the point moved about until the prick induces the familiar paraesthesia. The whole injection is given here. If the nerve perforates the inguinal ligament, the deep fasciculus should be divided. If necessary, the nerve can be avulsed.

Meralgia during Pregnancy

Pain and numbness at the front of the thigh are a rare complication of pregnancy. At the fourth month, the mother begins to feel discomfort at the front of one thigh and a few days later the antero-lateral aspect of the thigh goes numb down to the patella. The symptoms disappear spontaneously in about three months. Since the symptoms are always unilateral, the cause would appear to be pressure from a small fibromyoma of the uterus, projecting postero-laterally. As the uterus enlarges, this impinges against the upper extent of the lateral cutaneous nerve close to its emergence at the lateral border of the psoas muscle where it can be caught against the iliac crest.

Haemophilic Meralgia

Haemorrhage into the ilio-psoas muscle may compress the lateral cutaneous nerve close to the inguinal ligament. In consequence, the outer thigh becomes analgesic.

Anterior Cutaneous Nerve

This emerges through the fascia of the thigh some three inches below the inguinal ligament. Here, it may be compressed by the edge of a corset pushed downwards when the patient sits, or by the clasp of a suspender when the patient leans, say, against the edge of a table.

The cutaneous analgesia occupies the whole of the front of the thigh as far as the knee, and has the characteristics of local pressure. There is a defined edge to the numb area which becomes almost anaesthetic at its centre. Examination reveals an absence of all other signs and enquiry elicits the cause. The patient has to await spontaneous recovery.

Obturator Nerve

An obturator hernia may compress this nerve and give rise to an area of cutaneous analgesia at the inner side of the thigh just above the knee.

Third Lumbar Pain

Apart from the nerve-root itself, the common cause of a third lumbar pain is osteo-arthritis of the hip joint, whose capsule is usually developed wholly within the third lumbar myotome. Indeed, it is a commonplace that, especially in children, pain at the knee may originate from the hip. Strain of the psoas muscle, psoas bursitis and a loose body in the hip joint also give rise to pain of third lumbar extent. Pain felt at the front of the thigh can, of course, originate from the femur itself. If a third lumbar pain is described and there are no signs of any lesion of muscles, joints, nerves, etc., the femur should be X-rayed. Osteoid osteoma, early sarcoma or osteitis deformans may be disclosed.

Long Saphenous Nerve

This may suffer irritation analogous to the lateral cutaneous nerve. It is exposed to friction at the foramen by which it pierces the fascia just below the inner side of the knee; alternatively, its sheath may be damaged by a direct blow or by kneeling. The pain may start at the knee, later spreading down the inner side of the leg to the medial aspect of the foot. In other cases it may begin at the inner side of the heel and then extend up to the knee. This is a most deceptive story, drawing attention away from the knee and suggesting that the pain originates at the foot. The symptoms seldom include paraesthesia and walking may increase the pain since the nerve is shifted in its foramen at each knee-flexion movement. Signs of loss of conduction are absent. The only physical sign is a small tender area situated at the inner side of the tibia an inch or so below the knee joint. This is present on the affected side only, at the foramen where the nerve emerges. Local anaesthesia here destroys the pain, which seldom returns appreciably.

Dissecting Aneurysm

Third lumbar pain, accompanied by severe backache, both left-sided, may result from a dissecting aneurysm of the aorta. Increasing pain accompanied by severe backache in an elderly patient should arouse suspicion. Epidural local anaesthesia affords no relief; myelography and laminectomy disclose no abnormality. Aortography reveals the lesion and should not be delayed.

Painless Weakness of the Quadriceps Muscles

When weakness is confined to the third lumbar myotome, without sensory changes, metastasis at the third vertebra are unlikely. Two other disorders have to be considered—localized myopathy and myositis. In either case, the weakness is bilateral and affects the quadriceps muscles only. By the time the patient has begun to notice that his legs are weak, very considerable loss of power is detectable clinically. Wasting is obvious, but the knee-jerks are preserved and paraesthesia absent.

Distinction is important, since myositis can be halted by steroid therapy whereas myopathy cannot. Biopsy should be undertaken at once, so that the cases capable of arrest can be singled out.

Fourth and Fifth Lumbar Pain

Sometimes the capsule of the hip joint is derived largely or wholly from the fourth lumbar segment; if so, arthritis gives rise to 'sciatic' pain. Acute lumbago, arthritis of both hips, spondylolisthesis, the mushroom phenomenon and malignant disease of the spine all set up bilateral pain in the limbs. Thrombosis of the external iliac artery may give rise to a cold foot and sciatic pain only after walking. This holds for out-patients only; for a day or two in bed restores equal warmth to the two extremities. A tight fascial compartment for the extensor group of muscles in the leg may mimic a root-lesion, especially if pins and needles are felt. A loose body at the back of the knee may compress the tibial nerve, causing pain at the back of the knee and pins and needles in the adjacent surfaces of the first and second toes. Spinal claudication causes bilateral root-pain with pins and needles in the feet, as do spondylolisthesis and the mushroom phenomenon.

Pressure on the peroneal nerve is usually postural; rarely is it caused by an osteoma at the head of the fibula. The patient habitually sits with his legs crossed, or with the outer aspect of his knee pressed against a hard edge. In due course, discomfort may be felt from the knee down the outer side of the leg to the foot. Distally, paraesthesia may be a prominent feature; as a rule weakness of the dorsiflex muscles and diminution in cutaneous sensibility are not marked. Spontaneous recovery begins as soon as the cause of the disorder is explained to the patient.

Peroneal Neuritis

This is the name given to sudden foot-drop, occurring unilaterally in elderly patients. The true nature of the condition is unknown; paralysis is the marked feature; the disorder is entirely painless. Careful examination usually reveals some weakness in the hamstring muscles and slight gluteal wasting as well. It is my belief that the lesion, whatever it is, lies not distally but at the sciatic nerve-roots or in the anterior horn cells. It may be the solitary example in the lower limb of the infectious neuritis that occurs at the scapula and upper limb. Spontaneous recovery, so common in the upper limb, does not usually take place. Peroneal atrophy is painless and leads to bilateral weakness of tibialis anterior and peroneal muscles.

Obstetric Palsy

This results from pressure exerted on the lumbo-sacral cord at the brim of the pelvis. Since the pressure is exerted on a nerve-trunk beyond its dural investment, local pain is absent and straight-leg raising neither painful nor limited. If full foot-drop occurs, the patient naturally reports the fact soon after confinement; but if only vague numbness and some weakness of the calf muscles are present, the paresis may pass unnoticed until she is up and about again. These cases are uncommon and recover spontaneously in a few months.

First Sacral and Second Sacral Pain

The sacro-iliac joints are derived from the first and second sacral segments, hence in early spondylitis ankylopoetica the ligamentous pain often radiates to the posterior thigh and calf. Intermittent claudication gives rise to pain in the calf and posterior thigh only on walking. Bilateral pain results from spondylolisthesis, the mushroom phenomenon, spinal claudication and secondary neoplasm. Gluteal bursitis, being a deep-seated lesion occurring at the upper extent of a low lumbar segment can give rise to pain radiating from buttock to ankle.

Neuromata are usually benign and sometimes multiple. Some are found lying superficial to the sciatic nerve-trunk in the thigh or lower buttock. Others are incorporated in the nerve, expanding it from within. Benign neuromata set up pressure effects when they form within the spinal canal. Hence the existence of multiple intraspinal neuromata can be inferred when they are found in the trunk or at a limb in conjunction with signs of impaired conduction at a higher level.

Deep phlebitis, osteitis deformans, neoplasm of the ilium or femur and various traumatic lesions of the muscles locally complete the list.

Fourth Sacral Pain

Rectal, penile, scrotal, testicular, vaginal and bladder disorders are by far the commonest causes, but a low lumbar disc lesion compressing the fourth sacral root is a possibility. If the diagnosis is in doubt, the induction of epidural local anaesthesia provides an immediate answer.

Multiple Root-palsy

Neuralgic Amyotrophy

This affects the lower limb only rarely. I have encountered only a few cases, all in men aged 50 to 70. There is no premonitory backache (in contradistinction to the neckache when the upper limb is affected). The pain is considerable for about three months, and then slowly eases in the course of another three months. Pins and needles or numbness are rare, and then only in the cutaneous area corresponding to the muscles most severely affected. The pain is usually unilateral, and third, fourth and fifth lumbar weakness is encountered. Alternatively the fourth and fifth lumbar and first and second sacral roots are all affected.

Examination discloses a complete absence of lumbar articular signs and a full and painless range of straight-leg raising. When muscle power is tested a triple or even quadruple motor-root palsy comes to light. Spinal metastases are of course suspected, but the patient though in pain feels well, his lumbar spine moves well, and the straight radiograph reveals nothing relevant. Moreover, the palsy is maximal from the first, does not increase nor spread to the other limb and there is little or no sensory loss. After six months muscle power begins to return and after a year recovery is complete.

Diagnosis is really retrospective. However, in any patient with a marked unilateral palsy of the third, fourth and fifth lumbar roots, or the fourth and fifth lumbar and first and second sacral roots, neuralgic amyotrophy should be suspected as soon as neoplasm has been excluded.

UNDIAGNOSED BACKACHE

There is at least one—there may be many—cause of backache yet to be discovered. In a review of a thousand cases seen in 1956 (Cyriax, 1965) with symptoms attributed to the lower back, 80·2 per cent were certainly disc lesions, but in 4·8 per cent no diagnosis was ever made. In nearly all, epidural anaesthesia had been induced diagnostically because of uncertainty and had shown that a disc lesion was not the cause of symptoms.

Three possibilities were: (1) That a variant of spondylitis ankylopoetica might exist starting at the lumbar joints without previous sacro-iliitis. Follow-up for ten years showed no extension of the symptoms or signs. (2) That a primary rheumatoid arthritis existed at the lower lumbar joints. Again, follow-up showed no tendency to the development of arthritis elsewhere as the years went by and cortisone had no beneficial effect. (3) That the osteopath had stumbled upon a correct ascription in shifting from his displaced vertebra to internal derangement at a lateral facet joint. In the former two instances, the pain would be central; in the third, unilateral.

These 48 patients were, therefore, carefully studied, but with very disappointing results. No common factor, no consistent pattern of pain or of physical signs emerged. The pain was as often in the lower limb as the back, and the backaches were neither all central nor all unilateral. One patient with unusual signs was seen only once, being asked to return next day for further examination. This he did not do, and he died a short time later of an unstated cause; he doubtless had spinal metastases.

Of the remaining 47 patients, 15 complained of central backache, one with numbness down the fronts of both thighs as well. Three patients had purely unilateral backache and four had pain in one buttock. In 16, the backache spread to one lower limb; in 6, to both limbs. Six patients had pain in one limb without backache, with no local cause discernible in the limb itself. Neurological signs were present in three cases. In three, marked limitation of movement at the lumbar joints suggested spondylitis, but the sacro-iliac joints were radiographically clear and cortisone brought no relief. Little change in symptoms or signs occurred as time went by, and they appeared not to suffer from undetected neurosis, nor could they have been missed neuromata, etc., or the lesions would have declared themselves by now. In none was the X-ray appearance then or later of any significance.

NEUROSIS

Since most people suffer slight backache on and off, it is to be expected that the neurotic patient, when searching—doubtless subconsciously—for an acceptable peg to hang symptoms on, should choose the back; for this is where his only suitable symptoms are felt. Depression causes patients to attribute their mood and their disinclination to activity to a somatic symptom in preference to an outright admission of misery. It seems to them more respectable, and it certainly engenders a more satisfactory attitude in family and friends. Admitted depression is apt to elicit exhortation—'pull yourself together'—whereas severe backache evokes a suitable degree of commiseration. In this way the patient, to his or her own disadvantage, misleads the doctor, and treatment directed to the actual disorder present is avoided.

Thus, it is common for neurotic patients with little or no backache to receive physiotherapy or osteopathy rather than the psychological assistance that they really need.

When a patient with backache is examined on the lines described— articular signs, dural signs, nerve-root signs, combined with tests for other joints and muscles—the patient who has no organic lesion answers at random and produces multiple inconsistencies and the self-contradictory pattern typical of neurosis emerges. It is not the absence of signs that enables a diagnosis of neurosis to be made; it is the presence of incongruity between what hurts and what does not hurt, and where; what is limited and what is not limited from one moment to another. In order that this pattern can emerge, a large number of movements, some relevant, some irrelevant, must be tested, consistency or inconsistency being noted throughout. This is important; for many depressed or nervous people have perfectly genuine backaches. The actual emotional state of the patient is not relevant in reaching a diagnosis, although it weighs considerably in reaching a decision on treatment. Clearly active measures are unsuited to patients too nervous to bear any discomfort, even in the presence of a slight organic lesion. Considerable care should be taken not to confuse genuine backache in a neurotic patient with neurasthenic pain; hence inquiries concerning the patient's domestic circumstances and attitude to life are made only *after* the physical examination. For the same reason, whether a compensation claim is pending is not asked until after the examination is completed, so as to avoid prejudice.

In the survey of a thousand consecutive patients, 5 per cent. were of slight organic lesion in a neurotic patient and in only a further 2·7 per cent were the symptoms wholly psychogenic. The clinical impression was that they were much commoner than that—a notion that clearly reflects the much greater time that such patients need to relate their history, and the concentration of the doctor's effort when they are examined, often several times, before a firm conclusion can be reached.

My psychological colleagues at St. Thomas's report that the type of case which reaches the orthopaedic physician because of somatic symptoms due to depression is particularly difficult to help. Although they confirm the diagnosis regularly enough, they find the prognosis poor.

COCCYGODYNIA

This may be referred or may arise locally.

Referred Coccygodynia

Coccygodynia can be referred from a lumbar disc lesion as a result of extra-segmental reference (Cyriax, 1954). This view was confirmed by Bohm, Franksson and Petersen in 1956, who found that stimulating the fourth sacral root gave rise to coccygeal pain. In 0·5 per cent of Fernström's cases, coccygeal pain was provoked at lumbar discography (1960) and adhesions about the dura mater at the fifth lumbar level were found by Gill *et al.* (1955) to be associated with coccygodynia.

Referred coccygodynia is distinguished from a local disorder firstly by the fact that it is present not only when the patient is seated, but also at other times. Moreover, it does not necessarily follow a fall seated, although this is a possible cause both of damage to the coccyx and to a low lumbar disc. Secondly, in referred coccygodynia coughing, some of the lumbar movements and, often, straight-leg raising, increase the pain. Trial of the relevant movements, coupled with those that detect psychogenic pain, provides the diagnostic criteria. A search for local tenderness affords no assistance; for this is to be expected whichever variety of coccygodynia is present (referred dural tenderness). This ascription must always be confirmed by epidural local anaesthesia, since this happens also to be the most reliable conservative treatment. Rarely, invasion of the sacrum by neoplasm of the prostate or rectum gives rise to coccygeal pain only, but the relentless increase in pain and early loss of ankle-jerks afford the clue.

Local Coccygodynia

This mysterious complaint is in reality perfectly simple. The common cause is a flexion injury or direct contusion of the coccyx, usually as the result of a fall in the sitting position; less often, childbirth causes an extension strain. In spondylitis ankylopoetica, fixation of the coccyx affords a minor additional discomfort.

Since the coccygeal segments occupy a restricted local area, the pain cannot spread in any direction and is felt at the coccyx only. Sitting, and the act of becoming seated, bring on the pain. Standing and lying do not hurt; walking causes pain only when the coccygeal fibres of the gluteus maximus muscle are involved. Defaecation sometimes hurts. In repeated subluxation, the patient experiences a painful click on getting up after sitting.

As the diagnosis rests on the subjective basis of the elicitation of tenderness, the elimination of psychogenic cases is a matter of importance. These are, however, much less common than is supposed. The history may help; the usual cause is aversion to coitus. Coccygeal pain of local provenance cannot spread; patients with neurotic symptoms are usually eager to describe radiation in various directions. Except in referred coccygodynia, the lumbar movements are painless. In all cases the tests for the sacro-iliac joints and lower limbs are negative; hence, psychogenic symptoms are not difficult to detect if the patient is given enough rope. When tenderness is sought, it is well to start at mid-sacrum.

Four varieties of coccygodynia occur:

1. Sprain of the posterior fibres of the sacro-coccygeal joint-capsule.

2. Contusion of the tip of the coccyx and the tissue immediately about it.

3. Contusion of the posterior intercoccygeal ligaments.

4. Strain of the coccygeal fibres of the gluteus maximus muscle. The patient states that the pain is perceptibly unilateral, and walking may set up discomfort.

Treatment

Massage is almost always quickly effective (see Vol. II). The alternative is the injection of hydrocortisone.

19

The Lumbar Region

PART IV: MANIPULATION AND TRACTION

All back troubles pose difficult problems, and it is often hard to decide on the best approach when, as may well happen, the various pointers conflict. Moreover, the arbiter of the result is the patient himself, and it is, therefore, useless to treat a lumbar lesion in a patient who is not going to admit he is better. *Since it is not the severity of the lesion but the amount of pain and disablement it causes that largely determines treatment,* it is vital that the examiner should provide himself with a clear idea of the course, situation and severity of symptoms, and with criteria adequate to judge not only the nature of the lesion but the patient's sensitivity and sincerity. This entails listening to his whole account of his troubles from the very beginning, and examining also parts of his body distant from the apparent lesion in order to ascertain his threshold for pain. This is a slow and painstaking process, requiring patience and humility.

It is doubtful if a more controversial subject exists in Medicine than the treatment of backache. Certainly, there is none in which a body of scientific men allow their judgment to be so strongly swayed by emotion. Some doctors would never allow a patient of theirs to be manipulated at all; others would themselves manipulate every case of lumbar pain. Obviously there must lie a rational way between these two extremes, which this book in the last twenty years has tried to express.

The main confusion that exists is on the conservative treatment of disc lesions. This diagnosis has left a therapeutic hiatus, largely filled today, alas, by lay manipulators. On the one hand, the realization that backache, fibrositis, lumbago, and sciatica result largely from disc lesions has deprived of the last vestige of theoretical justification the traditional measures: drugs (apart from analgesics), vitamins (particularly B_1), hormones, radiant heat, diathermy, massage, exercises, injection of myalgic spots and nodules, and 'taking the waters'. On the other hand, little has replaced these obsolete types of 'treatment'; and the distress of doctors and patients at the apparent absence of effective conservative measures is heightened when told that the only radical treatment is an operation, by no means always successful, and warranted only in extreme cases.

This therapeutic nihilism is quite unjustified; for there are a number of simple treatments, none a panacea, each with its due proportion of successes. Few patients remain wholly unrelieved if conservative means are intelligently employed, and it is only for some of these few that surgery need be contemplated at all. In order to show that the phrase 'therapeutic nihilism' is justified, the following quotation from the report of the October 1954 meeting of the Orthopaedic Association is appended. A panel of seven experts sat under the chairmanship of Professor McFarland. Q. 'One-third of all orthopaedic out-patients complain of low backache. Has the panel any suggestion for coping with this vast number?' A. 'The panel has none.'

TRADITIONAL TREATMENT

Myrin (1967) contrasted a series of cases of lumbar trouble treated by conventional methods (i.e. rest in bed, physiotherapy, corsetry) and by manipulation. His results were:

	Well (%)	Slight symptoms (%)	Moderate symptoms (%)	Unable to work (%)
Conventional treatment	4	21	49	26
Manipulation	23·5	23·5	53	0

Conservative treatment of the conventional type, will soon become obsolete. It comprises: (a) analgesics, (b) rest in bed, (c) heat and exercises, (d) less often, heat and massage, (e) muscle relaxants, (f) support, (g) embrocations. These measures depend on the hope that the patient will improve with the passage of time, and the endeavour is merely to keep him as comfortable as possible meanwhile. If playing for time fails, laminectomy is often advised.

Analgesics

These are necessary when immediate treatment directed to the lesion fails to relieve the pain adequately.

Rest in Bed

In lumbago, and minor sciatica, the compression strain on the joint exerted in the erect position ceases during recumbency, and this relief encourages reduction of the displaced fragment. It is often an adequate, but slow treatment. Again, in many cases of sciatica, lying down diminishes symptoms; hence, to stay in bed while awaiting spontaneous recovery passes the time more pleasantly for the patient.

Heat, Massage and Exercises

These treatments are anachronisms, left over from the time when back troubles were thought to be muscular (Gowers, 1904). But now that sciatica (Mixter and Barr, 1934) and lumbago (Cyriax, 1945) are widely accepted as articular lesions, it is to the joint and not to the muscles that treatment should be directed.

Originally, patients were given flexion exercises because it was thought that, if a patient could not bend forwards, mobility in this direction would be enhanced by constant endeavour. Had the lumbar joint been stiff from extra-articular causes, e.g., adhesions, this would have been reasonable, and in those days it was not realized that the limitation was caused by an intra-articular block. When disc lesions were accepted, extension exercises were substituted and are far less harmful, on the mistaken view that increasing muscle strength encourages reduction and diminishes the liability to internal derangement. One has only to consider who ruptures the meniscus in his knee—the footballer with superb muscles—to realise that vigorous use, such as fractures fibro-cartilage, is more, not less, likely to be performed by the individual with really strong muscles.

Heat is the treatment for sepsis and to afford temporary comfort in incurable disorders. In disc lesions, heat and massage though futile are quite harmless, but this does not apply to exercises, which are contra-indicated. If the displacement is in being, exercises grind the projection against sensitive tissues and increase pain. If it is no longer present, the main object of treatment must be to keep the joint motionless in a good position, so as to avoid recurrence. Exercises maintain mobility and are therefore harmful. By contrast, teaching the patient to keep his lumbar joints still by muscular effort is most helpful. This is how exercises should be used in cases of recurrent spinal internal derangement—the inculcation of a constant postural tone that keeps the joint still—and the important difference must be explained to physiotherapists, who have all learned to administer the very exercises that, for the above reasons, are so deplorable.

Support

A fracture, once reduced, is then often immobilized in plaster. The same should apply to a disc lesion. Reduction, followed by maintenance of the affected lumbar joint motionless in a good position, is logical treatment. After reduction, to keep the lumbar spine in lordosis by an effort of memory, a corset, a jacket of plastic or plaster is most reasonable.

Supports have a poor name with many patients, since they are often applied with the displacement still in being. This violates the orthopaedic principle of reduction, followed by the maintenance of reduction.

Muscle-relaxants

The idea still persists that the pain of lumbago is the result of muscle spasm; Capener held this view as lately as 1961. It follows from this notion that the treatment should be directed to relaxing muscle spasm. Unfortunately, one glance at a patient's back during lumbago will show that he is fixed bent forwards, not in extension as he would be if the sacrospinalis muscles were really in spasm. The muscles about a spinal joint with internal derangement contract to protect it, but it is the articular lesion, not the secondary muscle guarding, that hurts. No one considers that the treatment of displaced meniscus at the knee with a springy block on extension is a drug that relaxes the hamstring muscles. To give an ambulant patient a muscle relaxant diminishes his power to keep the joint voluntarily as still as possible and thus to avoid pain. Such drugs are, therefore, contra-indicated. By contrast, there is no harm in giving a relaxant to a patient in bed, when the compression strain is off the joint. It can then be hoped that he will be able to move the deranged joint more while recumbent as a result of the drug, and thus initiate reduction the sooner. A far more direct way of securing this mobility is to abolish the pain, and the secondary muscle guarding with it, by means of epidural local anaesthesia.

Embrocations

Lumbago is not a skin disease; hence rubbing something into the skin is as valueless as heating the skin. Nevertheless, various ointments are regularly prescribed. I have written to the vendors of various unguents, who maintain that their product relaxes muscle spasm, to explain that the flexed posture (immortalised in the picture for 'Doan's Backache and Kidney Pills') cannot be caused by spasm of the sacrospinalis muscles—the very muscles over which the embrocation is to be rubbed. In several cases the medical adviser to the company has had the illustration changed, but not the recommendation that the liniment should be applied.

ORTHOPAEDIC MEDICAL TREATMENT
OF DISC LESIONS

Conservative treatment as practised at St. Thomas's Hospital consists of: (1) postural prophylaxis; (2) manipulative reduction; (3) reduction by

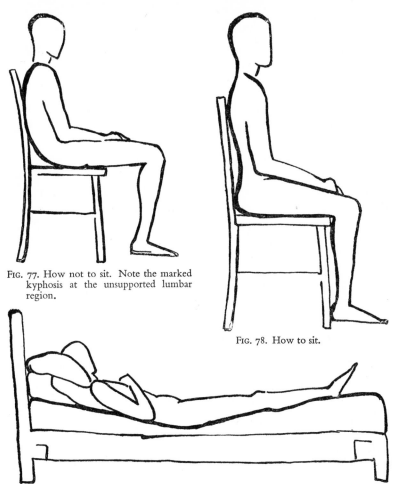

FIG. 77. How not to sit. Note the marked kyphosis at the unsupported lumbar region.

FIG. 78. How to sit.

FIG. 79. Bad posture in bed. So soft a mattress that the patient's lumbar region remains kyphotic all night often initiates a disc lesion or aggravates an existing defect.

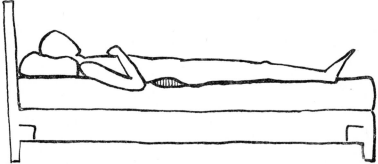

FIG. 80. Lumbago treated by recumbency. As soon as possible, a small pillow is introduced under the lumbar spine in order to maintain lordosis and encourage the intra-articular contents to move anteriorly.

traction; (4) the maintenance of reduction; (5) epidural local anaesthesia. These measures are set out below.

Prophylaxis

Realization that maintenance of the lumbar lordosis provides the main safeguard against disc protrusion is proceeding slowly. Aesthetic considerations have held the foreground for a century, and it is difficult even now to get gymnasts to realize that a reasonable degree of lordosis in children is a great advantage in later life. School medical officers can see to it that exercises towards trunk-flexion are carried out sparingly, and that, unless marked kypho-lordosis is present, no effort is made to flatten school-children's lumbar spine. If any individual cannot reach forwards far enough to touch his toes, he must not be encouraged to practise this useless range of movement. School-children should be taught to lift by using their knees with the back arched, in the hope that they will carry this on during work in adult life by force of habit.

Women's backache often dates from lying in bed in 'the nursing mother's position'—that is, many pillows propping the thorax and no proper support at the lumbar spine, which droops into kyphosis all day (Fig. 59). It is no wonder that the posterior longitudinal ligament finally stretches and the beginnings of disc protrusion are laid down. All recumbent patients, not only puerperal women, should lie flat when they have no reason to be sitting up, and as soon as their condition permits they should turn and lie prone for several periods daily.

Industrial medical officers can help by arranging that weights are presented to workers at a proper level and by showing them how to lift safely (Fig. 84). Since an attack of disc protrusion at work is clearly an industrial accident, they can also save their firms much money in time off work and claims for compensation. They should also arrange that immediate manipulative reduction is available to all their workmen, if an attack begins, as was done by Pringle (1956) in Dublin. They should find out—from me, if necessary—the name of the nearest manipulative physiotherapist.

Builders can put in sinks at a higher level than has hitherto been customary, and so on. The makers of car seats are among the worst offenders; these are often so shaped that it is all but impossible to maintain a lordosis while sitting in a front seat .

Explanation

Some patients state that they are usually free from symptoms but that various exertions, e.g. stooping, lifting or sitting sometimes bring on backache. When the cause of their pain and its mechanism is explained to them, they often devise a different way of doing the same work so as to render it harmless. Many patients perform daily exercises, even touching their toes, with the intention of keeping the joints of the trunk mobile. Alas, this endeavour is often successful. Mere explanation of the harmfulness of exercises in this disorder and the disadvantage of full mobility at the affected joint corrects the patient's attitude. The way I express it is to

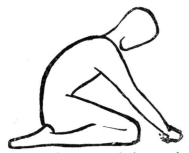

Fig. 81. Bad way to reach the ground. Note the lumbar kyphosis.

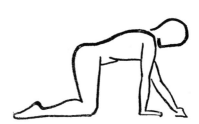

Fig. 82. Proper posture for reaching floor level.

say: 'When your disc is in place, if you never moved the joint again, you could not put it out again. Use your muscles, therefore to keep the joint still; this keeps the muscles strong without mobilizing the joint.'

It may be necessary for the patient to avoid some posture or exertion altogether, and the employer must be advised about this. When the patient is engaged in heavy work and has had several relapses, he should be sent to a rehabilitation centre to learn a lighter trade. The question of wearing a belt arises. In cases of recurrent trouble in labourers this is usually desirable; in sedentary workers the patient's age, sex, sport and personal inclinations combine to settle the matter.

On the one hand, the patient must not be turned into a neurasthenic, afraid to move his trunk at all; on the other, he must learn to treat his mechanically imperfect joint with respect. In my experience 'a piece of cartilage loose in the joint of the back' is not a frightening idea; it is a concrete, simple concept, and is as familiar as a harmless disorder in a footballer's knee. Moreover, stress may be laid on the frequency with which such fragments remain symptomless for years provided the patient is careful for a time and allows the disorder to subside. Many patients with disc lesions have been told, as a result of misinterpretation of radiographic appearances, that they are suffering from 'spinal arthritis'. This may suggest to them an incurable disease liable to spread and to end in paralysis or

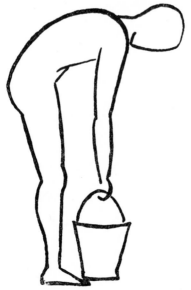

FIG. 83. Bad way to lift. Note the lumbar
kyphosis.

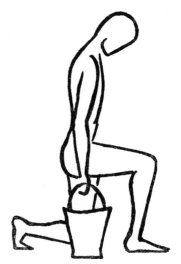

FIG. 84. A safe way to lift.

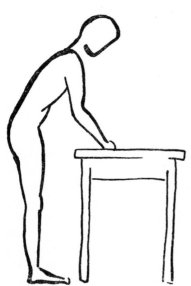

FIG. 85. Bad posture for work at a table.

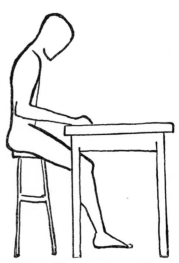

FIG. 86. How to work at a table.

crippledom. The purely local nature of the disorder should be explained, and the analogy with cartilage trouble at the knee, an obviously unprogressive condition, affords much reassurance.

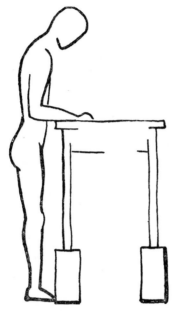

FIG. 87. How to stand at a bench

MANIPULATION

Naturally, if something is out of place the obvious treatment is to restore it to its proper position; it must then be maintained there. This is clinical orthodoxy throughout the body and applies also to the lumbar joints. Therefore, unless some good reason exists, manipulative reduction should be attempted as soon as the diagnosis of a disc lesion is made. This measure is universally adopted when a torn meniscus in the knee-joint has moved, but it has, till recently, been left largely to laymen to reduce cartilaginous subluxations at the spinal joints.

Indications for Manipulation

This is simply the diagnosis of a displacement and there are no contra-indications. *The positive indication is a cartilaginous displacement*, not too large and not placed too far laterally. Particularly suitable cases are subacute lumbago and patients in whom trunk-flexion, and/or extension, and/or side-flexion away from the painful side are found to hurt in the back. A painful arc is an encouraging sign. Two further desiderata are that the patient is not too neurotic to accept active treatment, and that he is anxious to get well. Thus, not only the type of displacement but the type of patient has to be assessed and each finding given due weight. It is unfortunate that, in this sort of work, the patient's uncorroborated (and controvertible only with difficulty) statement is paramount. If a patient who has been fully relieved of all his organic symptoms by, e.g. manipulation, alleges that he has been made worse, whether on account of neurosis or a compensation claim, it is difficult to refute the statement. Hence, all active treatment is contra-indicated unless there is a genuine intention on the patient's part to admit improvement.

Not all small disc displacements respond to manipulation. The reason is anatomical; the protrusion may be hard or soft, i.e. composed of fibro-cartilage or nuclear tissue. Naturally, the former respond to manipulation, and the latter to traction. My teaching is: 'You can hit a nail with a hammer, but treacle must be sucked.' R. H. Young, in an analysis of cases coming to laminectomy, showed that in 56 per cent of his cases the protrusion was cartilaginous, and in 44 per cent, nuclear. My impression is that in patients not requiring operation, the proportion is more like two cartilaginous protrusions to one nuclear. Manipulation can nearly always reduce a small cartilaginous displacement, but seldom affects a pulpy protrusion. Small and very recent nuclear herniations sometimes respond, provided that the technique of manipulation is changed from the jerk to sustained pressure.

Is Reduction a Possibility?

No one doubts, when a click is felt at the knee and the pain and limited movement caused by a displaced meniscus cease, that reduction has taken place. But many surgeons take the view that manipulative reduction is impossible in disc displacement. The opinion is in a way well founded; for it is based on operating on patients because this particular displacement *is* irreducible. Those in whom reduction can be achieved by manipulation do not require laminectomy and are not included in these surgeons' operative experience.

No one disputes that a click in the back, felt and heard by the patient and the manipulator, may afford instant relief. Something has moved in a therapeutically desirable way. It clicked and was, therefore, hard structure. The radiograph shows that the bone itself has not moved. The only alternative is a fragment of cartilage, which obviously can move inside an intervertebral joint. This fragment must, therefore, go back into place or move to a position right outside the joint. If it goes back into place it can, as at the knee, come out again and, in fact, lumbago is recognized as a very recurrent phenomenon. If it shifted farther outside the joint, lying at a point where it no longer compressed a sentient tissue, there would be no tendency to recurrence. Moreover, when a patient who had had twenty attacks of lumbago in twenty years finally came to laminectomy, twenty small extruded fragments of fibro-cartilage would have to be found lying at the edge of the joint or free in the neural canal. They are not. There can be no doubt that the click, which all sides admit heralds relief from symptoms and signs, results from reduction of the loose fragment of cartilage. R. H. Young, at laminectomy, has reduced protrusions under direct vision.

History

There is nothing new about manipulation, nor indeed about traction, nor even manipulation during traction. Hippocrates in the fifth century B.C. and Galen (131 to 202 A.D.) both practised it and wrote about it. About the year 1000, Avicenna in Bagdad used and taught Hippocrates's methods. Paré (1510–90) in France pointed out that severe backache could be brought on by heavy work with the spine held flexed, and included pictures on manipulative technique which have a very up-to-date flavour. Vidio (1500–69) advised and illustrated manipulation during traction. The authoritative account of the history of manipulation was written by E. Schiotz ('Tidsskift for den Norske Laege Forening', 1958), and the interested reader cannot do better than read his erudite and entertaining paper.

A book called *The Compleat Bone-Setter*, written by Friar Moulton, appeared in 1656, but it does not deal with bonesetting as it is understood today (i.e. the manipulation of joints). Wiseman in *Severall Chirurgical Treatises* (1676) states: '. . . I have had occasion to take notice of the inconvenience many people have fallen into through the wickedness of those who pretend to the reducing luxated joints by the peculiar name of bonesetter who that they may not want employment do usually represent every bone dislocated that they are called to look upon.' This was the very opinion that Paget deplored in his lecture 'Cases that Bonesetters Cure' (1866).

The first attempt to describe bonesetters' manipulations systematically was Hood's: a medical man who published a book *On Bonesetting* (1871) describing the methods of a bonesetter called Hutton. He makes a remark in the preface of his book that holds today as it did almost a hundred years ago. 'When I first knew Hutton, I often tried to argue the point with him, and to explain what it really was that he had done. I soon found, however, that, if I wished to learn from him, I must content myself with simply listening and observing. He had grown old in a faith, which it was impossible to overturn.' As recently as 1935, osteopaths showed the same obstinacy at the inquiry in the House of Lords, though it led them into a series of untenable positions. Even today, although osteopaths have changed the lesion that they are manipulating four times since Still (1874) first enunciated the hypothesis that a displaced vertebra compressing an artery was the cause of all disease—displaced vertebra pinching a nerve, displaced sacro-iliac joint, displaced disc, displaced facet—they hold fast to the hypothesis stated in the current edition of the 'Osteopathic Blue Book': 'Osteopaths maintain that the presence of spinal lesions exerts an influence upon the systems of the body through nerves and blood circulation, and it is held that removal of these lesions alleviates much physical disability and ill-health.' Hood goes on to say: 'If surgeons will only give proof of the knowledge of the good that bonesetters accomplish, the public would then be ready to listen to any reasonable warning about the harm.' So little notice was taken of this sensible advice that I wrote in 1947, 'Clearly nothing is easier than to dismiss osteopathic theory as pure fancy. Indeed, this negative attitude has governed doctors' views in the past. But this is not enough; for there remains on the postitive side the discovery of the real way in which manipulators achieve their undoubted results.' I might well have added that, if we want to obviate manipulation by laymen, this will be achieved not by denigrating the method, but by improving on these laymen. Doctors' informed selection of suitable cases and use of techniques more successful than osteopaths' will alone return manipulation to medical hands.

The reader is referred to five books other than my own. My two volumes set out the orthopaedic medical approach on diagnosis and manual treatment. The others derive largely from osteopathy and, therefore, treat diagnosis very sketchily but deal with manipulative techniques (mostly quite different from mine) in considerable detail.

Brodin, H. et al. (1966). *Manipulation av Ruggraden*. Scandinavian University Books: Stockholm.
Maigne, R. (1960). *Les Manipulations Vertébrales*. Expansion Scientifique Française: Paris.
Maitland, G. D. (1964). *Vertebral Manipulation*. Butterworth: London.
Niboyet, J. E. H. (1968). *La Practique de la Medicine Manuelle*. Maisonneuve: Paris.
Stoddard, A. (1959). *Manual of Osteopathic Techniques*. Hutchinson's Medical Publications: London.

Reducible or Irreducible?

History

This is often indicative. For example, a patient bends forwards and feels some aching in his back, which gets worse later in the day. Next morning he finds himself unable to get out of bed because of severe lumbago. This history indicates a protrusion that has gradually increased in size—that is, one consisting of nuclear material. By contrast, the patient who is subject to attacks, initiated by a click in the back followed by agonizing lumbar pain fixing him in flexion, has clearly suffered an abrupt cartilaginous displacement, suited to manipulation. Since the nucleus pulposus has ceased to exist by the age of sixty, nuclear protrusions do not occur in the elderly. Hence, the older the patient with a small displacement, the more certain that it is cartilaginous and will respond to manipulation, whether causing lumbar, gluteal or sciatic symptoms.

Primary postero-lateral protrusions causing sciatica are nearly always irreducible by manipulation. This is indicated when a patient with a low lumbar disc lesion states that his pain began in the calf or thigh without previous backache. Naturally, a central displacement impinges first against the dura mater, thus causing backache before it sets up sciatica; primary postero-lateral protrusions never touch the dura at all, hence premonitory backache is absent. By contrast, secondary postero-lateral protrusion (i.e. pain in the back followed by root-pain) is suited to manipulation unless gross lumbar deviation or neurological weakness has supervened.

The *self-reducing disc lesion* is characterized by a different history. The patient wakes comfortable but, as the day goes on, backache develops. This becomes worse, especially after exertion or stooping. A night's rest once more abolishes the pain. Naturally, if the posterior bulge at the joint recedes spontaneously as soon as the compression strain on the joint is released, only to recur when the joint bears weight again, the reduction brought about by manipulation is equally unstable and ephemeral. Alternatively, the patient may describe backache coming on after sitting some time, relieved by standing up. Many state that they have to get out of a car every half hour for a few minutes—an indictment of the shape of car seats. Clearly, if restoration of the lordosis results in the nuclear protrusion receding again, the problem is not reduction but its maintenance.

The *mushroom phenomenon* results from compression; it, too, is not amenable to manipulation, since no manoeuvre can relieve the affected joint of the compression due to body weight during standing. *Spondylolisthesis*

8

with a secondary disc lesion is treated in the same way as an uncomplicated disc lesion, but the tendency to recurrence is much enhanced.
When ligamentous stretch secondary to spondylolisthesis is the cause of
backache, manipulation is of course useless. *Recurrence after laminectomy* is
not a contra-indication to an attempt at manipulative reduction, but it
seldom succeeds if the lesion lies at the joint operated on, but often works
well if another joint contains the displacement.

Physical Signs

Manipulative reduction is so regularly successful in recent lumbago that
it should always be attempted unless the pain is so severe that the endeavour proves impossible to bear; if so, epidural local anaesthesia is
substituted. The appearance of the patient's back is most informative. If
no deviation is seen while he stands or during as much flexion of which he
is capable, one session of manipulation often suffices. If he stands symmetrically but deviates on trunk-flexion, reduction will probably take
two sessions. If he deviates considerably as he stands, the displacement is
large and two to four attempts may be required; some relapse between
sessions is to be expected. Displacements at the fourth level do best on
rotation strains, the ilium on the painful side being drawn forwards,
whereas at the fifth level the prone extension manoeuvres are usually the
most effective. Fifty per cent of all cases of lumbago get well in one
treatment.

Nuclear protrusion causing acute lumbago presents a difficult problem.
The patient wakes unable to get out of bed because of severe lumbar pain
the day after doing much stooping and lifting. However, effective
mechanical traction makes acute lumbago considerably worse, and no one
with twinging lumbago should ever be given strong traction. While he
lies stretched on the couch the pain ceases, but when the pull is abated he
suffers a series of agonizing pains. In consequence, the traction may have
to be released very slowly and it may take three or four hours to get the
patient off the couch, none the better for this ordeal. Hence the best must
be done with manipulation by maintained pressure followed by making
the patient lie deviating in the way that reverses his lateral deformity.
Alternatively the effect of epidural local anaesthesia must be tried and if
all else fails, pelvic traction in bed persevering until the symptoms have
abated considerably. Only then can traction on the couch be cautiously
begun.

In lumbago, the choice between manipulation and traction does not
arise. In backache, however, this is the constant problem. A sudden onset,
a click, or the existence of a painful arc, with or without momentary

deviation, suggests a small mobile fragment and augurs well for manipulation. If one of the lumbar movements other than flexion hurts in the thigh or calf rather than in the back or upper buttock, manipulation seldom succeeds. Reduction by manipulation may prove difficult or impossible in patients under sixty years old who have their greatest pain on pinching the lesion, i.e. on side-flexion towards the painful side.

Impaired condition along the relevant root shows the protrusion to be larger than the aperture whence it emerged. Hence this finding should be regarded as an indication of irreducibility, whether the lesion was originally of cartilage or nucleus. The only exception to this rule is in recurrent sciatica, when the weakness, etc., may have continued since a previous attack and be irrelevant to the present bout, which may well be caused by a small and recent protrusion, quite easy to reduce. In backache the sign that suggests that manipulation will succeed easily is the partial articular pattern, i.e., some lumbar movements hurting at their extreme, some not, the pain being felt in the centre or at one side of the lower lumbar region or upper buttock. A typical pattern would be trunk-flexion which hurts (it does not matter whether the pain is central or unilateral, limited or of full range); extension is merely uncomfortable; side-flexion towards the painful side does not hurt whereas away from that side does hurt. A painful arc exists. In sciatica, reduction seldom proves difficult if: (1) the backache continued when the root-pain came on; (2) the lumbar movements other than flexion hurt in the back rather than the limb; (3) there is no gross deviation or neurological weakness; (4) the root-pain is recent and straight-leg raising only moderately limited.

When, as may happen, the symptoms and signs point in opposite directions, the one suggesting traction the other manipulation, it is always worth while making one attempt. During the first session of manipulation, it usually becomes quickly clear whether reduction by this means will prove possible or not. By contrast, traction often has to be continued daily for a fortnight before its effectiveness can be ascertained.

If then neither the patient's age, nor history nor physical signs afford a pointer to the consistency of the displacement, manipulative reduction should be attempted forthwith. If it fails, traction is substituted from the next day. The reverse policy wastes a great deal of time.

Contra-indications to Manipulation

Manipulation is contra-indicated in all lumbar disorders not caused by a disc lesion.

Other contra-indications are:

1. Danger to the Fourth Sacral Root

A complaint of bladder weakness causing frequency of micturition without a strong urge affords an absolute bar to manipulation. Pain in the perineum, rectum, scrotum; impotence; paraesthesia in the genital area, saddle area or anus, all suggest that the third and fourth sacral roots are menaced by the protrusion and that the posterior ligament is bulging considerably and possibly partly ruptured. If so, manipulation may rupture it completely and allow massive extrusion of the entire disc. This has happened, but not (so far, I am happy to say) at our hands.

2. Hyperacute Lumbago

Ordinary patients with reasonably severe lumbago stand manipulation well, and most receive immediate relief. If the twinges of severe pain are such that no movement at the lumbar spine is possible, the patient holding himself quite rigid, manipulation is intolerable and the attempt unkind and unreasonable. In such cases: (a) when asked to turn to lie prone, it takes the patient some minutes to roll over; (b) when gentle pressure is applied to the patient's back, unbearable pain is set up. These patients should all be treated by the immediate induction of epidural anaesthesia.

Oscillatory Techniques

Manual vibrations (about ten a second) were given to patients immobilized by severe lumbago from the turn of the century by Edgar Cyriax, but they were altogether too gentle to have much effect. Osteopaths use a coarser oscillation which they describe (with cheerful disregard for English usage) as 'articulating'. Maitland (1964) also shakes the affected joint by a series of small thrusts, about two a second. This type of manoeuvre has to be carried on for a long time, e.g. half-an-hour, but persistence affords relief.

3. Pregnancy

During the first four months, the pregnancy can be disregarded. During the next four months, the supine and side-lying rotation manipulations can still be employed. During the last month, manipulation is impracticable, and rest in bed or epidural local anaesthesia should be substituted.

4. Spinal Claudication

In this disorder, the cauda equina is compressed sufficiently to impair circulation within the nerve-roots themselves. The existence of this syndrome must therefore imply considerable bulging of the posterior longitudinal ligament. Hence manipulation, though it has not been tried by us, must be regarded as contra-indicated.

5. Neurosis

It is very tempting to manipulate the back of a psychoneurotic patient when examination discloses a genuine minor disc displacement. The patient assures the physician that his or her nervous state is not as serious as all that and the treatment is given, the patient leaving the department happy and free. That evening, he or she has doubts about the consequences of the symptoms ceasing, and by midnight severe pain is alleged and the family doctor is called during the night to cope with an hysterical attack. Naturally, this does not endear him to manipulation.

The patient should be warned not to succumb to a 'post-manipulative nervous crisis' and the doctor warned that, if he is sent for on this account at night, he should not go. These precautions will usually prevent the family doctor being put to trouble for what is really the manipulator's fault; for he should have noticed the neurosis as well as the disc lesion and taken corresponding care.

Neurotic patients whose backache has no organic basis should not be treated by manipulation. It is useless; and if the patient's emotional state happens to get worse about this time, the treatment will be blamed. The family doctor should be apprised of the state of affairs and the almoner asked for a report on what can be done to help. Psychological referral may prove necessary. Quite apart from the fact that manipulation is treating a non-existent disorder, there are three further disadvantages: (1) Proper treatment to relieve the patient's depression is being withheld. Though he prefers treatment to the lesion not present than to the lesion present, it is the physician's duty not to offer a placebo when effective treatment may well exist. (2) It harms the reputation of manipulation when patients without an organic lesion report, as they so often do, years of futile manipulation by laymen. (3) At training schools for physiotherapists, manipulation, or, indeed, any other form of physical treatment given for psychological reasons has the unfortunate effect of bewildering the student and of fostering the pernicious notion that physiotherapy is a second-rate form of psychotherapy.

Compensation neurosis should not be treated by manipulation or physiotherapy. The patient has no desire to get better—indeed, he would be the poorer if he did; he attends hospital because his solicitor considers his case weakened if the client alleges severe symptoms and is not receiving hospital treatment. Alternatively, he wishes to be able to say that even treatment advised by an expert has failed or has aggravated the disorder. Such cases should be left until the suit is concluded; few bother to see the doctor again afterwards.

Manipulation is Useless

Manipulation is useless but not harmful and thus not exactly contra-indicated in the following types of disc lesion:

1. Too Large a Protrusion

This declares itself in three ways:

(a) *Neurological signs.* Signs of impaired conduction along the nerve root; i.e. muscle weakness, sluggish or absent reflex, cutaneous analgesia, indicate that the protrusion is larger than the aperture whence it emerged and that manipulation will fail.

(b) *Lumbar deformity with sciatica.* Patients with sciatica (i.e. root-pain with little or no backache, *not* backache with slight sciatic radiation) coupled with a considerable lateral deviation at the lumbar spine, nearly always prove irreducible whether they have neurological signs or not. Side-flexion in one direction barely reaches the vertical and shoots a pain down the lower limb.

(c) *Sciatica in flexion.* The pain is in the lower limb and the patient is reasonably comfortable sitting or standing slightly flexed. An attempt to stand erect shoots a severe pain down his leg and lumbar extension is markedly limited. Whether neurological signs coexist or not, manipula-tion fails.

In types (b) and (c) all conservative treatment is likely to fail, and the only successful measure is laminectomy.

2. Too Soft a Protrusion

Nuclear protrusions do not respond to manipulation but do well on traction. They identify themselves by a gradual onset, the pain slowly increasing after—not during—stooping or sitting, sometimes not till the next day. In these cases, side-flexion of the lumbar spine towards the painful side often hurts, and is a sign that manipulation is likely to fail.

Pulpy protrusions do not occur in the elderly, in whom the nucleus has degenerated and is no longer soft.

Primary postero-lateral protrusions (i.e. sciatica without immediately preceding backache) all appear to be nuclear; for manipulation always fails whereas, during the first few months, traction is regularly successful. However, recurrence soon after full reduction is a commonplace.

3. Too Long Duration

There is no limit in backache. However long the displacement has persisted, there is always some chance of successful reduction; my maximum to date is a constant displacement of 36 years' standing and my previous record was 22 years. In root-pain, without backache, six months is the limit, counting from when the pain in the limb became established, not from the onset of the preceding lumbar pain. After the age of sixty, there is no time limit, especially in those who retain some backache after the root-pain has appeared.

4. Compression Phenomena

The elderly patient who gets pain in the back or leg after standing for, say, ten minutes is suffering from the mushroom phenomenon: i.e. posterior bulging when the joint is compressed. This cannot be altered by manipulation. The patient with a pulpy self-reducing disc lesion awakes comfortable and is without pain for the first few hours. Then the ache comes on and continues for the rest of the day, but is once more abolished by the decompression of a night's rest. Since reduction takes place every night, manipulation, even if it secures reduction, proves equally transient.

5. Post-laminectomy

Manipulation seldom succeeds in recurrence after laminectomy, but there is no harm in trying, particularly if the signs suggest that this is a fresh protrusion at another joint. Traction is often successful in recurrence after operation. By contrast, mid or upper lumbar disc displacements secondary to a low lumbar arthrodesis often reduce quite easily.

6. Unfavourable Trunk-movements

In patients under the age of sixty, when trunk side-flexion hurts on the side towards which the patient leans, manipulation usually fails in backache, but not in lumbago. If any trunk movement other than flexion hurts in the lower limb instead of the back, manipulation is almost certain to fail. Over the age of sixty, these rules no longer apply. If pressure on the lumbar spine gives rise to root-pain in the lower limb while the patient lies prone, the manipulation is clearly pressing the protrusion harder against the nerve-root, and the attempt should be abandoned at once.

Dangers of Manipulation

I. Aggravation

As long as anaesthesia is avoided, this is a rare event since, if un-favourable signs show themselves, the examination which follows each manoeuvre discloses them. Manipulation is discontinued.

2. Fracture of a Transverse Process

When pressure to left or right of the lumbar spine is applied, a trans-verse process may snap. The click is felt much more sharply than that of a fragment of annulus shifting. This accident is of very little moment, since the pain is never severe and lasts only a week or two. The incidence is about one in ten thousand cases.

Technique of Manipulation

Manipulation should be carried out unless some contra-indication exists. In practice, it is found that about two-thirds of all cases of backache, and one third of all cases of sciatica, prove amenable to manipulative reduction. The patient lies prone on a low firm couch and the extension and rotation strains described in Vol. II are applied. The more the lumbar spine deviates, the more reliance should be placed on the rotatory man-oeuvres. After each attempt, the effect is estimated by, e.g. if coughing hurt originally, asking the patient to cough; if straight-leg raising was limited, ascertaining its range again; if one or more trunk-movements hurt, asking the patient to stand and try them again. Manipulation is successful quickly or not at all; hence one, two or three, or at the most four sessions are required. Each lasts about twenty minutes; for no patient, however willing, can relax adequately after this time and it is useless to go on.

If a patient needs manipulation and is to be treated by a physiotherapist, then she must learn to manipulate. It is, therefore, my practice to delegate almost all these treatments to physiotherapists trained—as is always the case at St. Thomas's—in manipulation. Most doctors in general practice clearly have not the time, inclination, assistants, or a proper couch for carrying out such manoeuvres themselves. It must, therefore, be made possible for them to send suitable cases to trained physiotherapists for this purpose.

Anaesthesia for Manipulation

For a *set* manipulation, anaesthesia is often an advantage. By 'set' is meant a manipulation during which the operator knows what he is proposing to do and requires no assistance from the patient. The reduction of a fracture, of a dislocation, and of the cartilage at the knee, affords examples of a set manipulation.

General anaesthesia must not be employed for disc lesions. The disc lesion that has previously been reduced under anaesthesia is, in my experience, at least as easily reduced on another occasion without. When manipulation under anaesthesia is attempted because it has failed without, renewed failure is to be expected; for it is not the manipulation that is at fault, but the protrusion which is irreducible.

When reduction is attempted at any spinal joint, the manipulation is *not set*. One manoeuvre is tried and its result on the physical signs assessed. If it has done good, it should be repeated. If it has not, another technique should be used, and the result assessed again, and so on. This is repeated until in successful cases the patient can move the affected joint in each direction painlessly. This can be determined only in the conscious patient, who co-operates throughout. Under anaesthesia, none of this knowledge is available to the operator, who has no means of knowing even whether he is making the patient better or worse. This deprivation is much more important than additional relaxation. Most orthopaedic surgeons warn about the dangers of spinal manipulation, and insofar as this relates to the practice of manipulating under anaesthesia, I fully agree with them. But these warnings do not apply when manipulation is performed with due safeguards on selected patients.

Lay manipulators seldom employ anaesthesia, and to that extent are reasonably safe, but their lack of medical knowledge prevents their exercising proper selection of cases. Hence they are forced to manipulate all comers, whatever the lesion present, and just await events.

SUSTAINED TRACTION

Just as the first approach to a displaced fragment of cartilage is manipulative reduction, so does a nuclear protrusion call for immediate reduction by traction, unless some contra-indication exists. Traction for the reduction of pulpy disc-protrusion was first suggested many years ago (Cyriax, 1950), but was used long before discs had ever been heard of. Guidi illustrates a traction table in his *Chirurgia*, 1544, and the photograph (Plate 42) shows one of his machines, now in the Wellcome Historical Museum.

Distraction at the affected joint has three effects: (1) Increase in the interval between the vertebral bodies, thus enlarging the space into which the protrusion must recede. (2) Tautening the posterior longitudinal

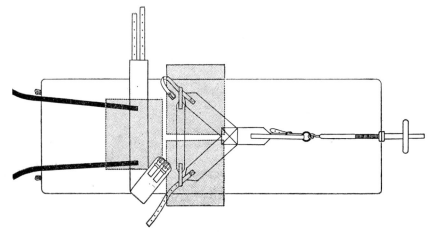

FIG. 88. The position of the straps before the patient lies down

ligament. Naturally, when the slack is taken up, the ligament joining the vertebral bodies tightens and exerts centripetal force at the back of the joint. (3) Suction. This draws the protrusion towards the centre of the joint.

Traction is likely to achieve positively what recumbency achieves in a neutral manner. In the erect position, the joint is compressed, and lying down avoids this squeeze. Traction affords positive decompression. It represents a way of achieving quickly, while the patient remains up and about, what would otherwise take perhaps weeks in bed. Since the intention is to bring about more reduction in half-an-hour than the ambulant patient can reverse by making his joint bear weight all the rest of the day, the distracting force must be (a) as strong as possible; (b) given daily; (c) continuous. Continuous traction fatigues the muscles; they relax and the strain now falls on the joint. For this reason, the rhythmic traction that so many osteopaths use is impressive rather than effective. It takes three minutes for electromyographic silence to be attained after traction begins;

hence, pulls of shorter duration than that merely elicit the stretch reflex and exercise the sacrospinalis muscles without distracting the joint surfaces.

Technique of Traction

The patient lies on the traction couch with a harness about his pelvis and another round his lower thorax. These belts are attached by bands to the hooks at each end of the couch. He may do best lying prone or supine, and there are four different ways of using the straps, each giving a slightly different tilt to the affected joint (see Vol. II). A good guide is that, if lumbar extension hurts, the patient should lie prone with both straps applied along the posterior aspect of his trunk. However, if a patient does not do well in one position or with the bands applied in any particular way, each of the eight different techniques must be tried until the right one is found. If, whatever alteration is made, no improvement follows, it becomes clear that traction will not help and the method is abandoned. This may well take a fortnight's daily sessions.

Traction must set up no discomfort; for the patient cannot relax his muscles unless this is so. If it hurts, something is wrong; there is either an unsuitable case or bad technique in applying the harness. A large man may need up to 85 kg. distracting force; the minimum for a small woman is 40 kg. Treatment lasts 30 to 45 minutes, and in cases of urgency may be given twice a day. The physiotherapist stays near the patient throughout treatment, adjusting the pull if the harness slips slightly. Plate 43 shows the amount of distraction obtainable at the lumbar spine; two X-ray photographs have been superimposed, one taken before, one during, traction; the iliac crests form the base line and have been made to coincide. If the amount of distraction possible at the lumbar is compared with that possible at the cervical joints (Plates 7 and 8), it will be seen why *manual* traction is such a great aid to manipulative reduction at the cervical spine and so little help at the lumbar spine. A few seconds' traction on the neck almost doubles the width of the joint space; several minutes' strong mechanical traction increases the width of a lumbar joint by only 2·5 mm. Hence, for lumbar disc lesions it is manipulation *or* traction, depending on the consistency of the protrusion. If manipulation is attempted during strong mechanical traction, it will be found that the lumbar region is so taut that an appreciable impression cannot be made on it manually. However, manipulation carried out immediately after traction, before the patient has risen from the couch, has an occasional success.

As soon as the traction is applied, most patients lose their pain, since the articular surfaces cease to exert their centrifugal pressure on the nuclear protrusion. However, it is not the posture that best eases the pain as he lies being stretched, nor the least amount of distracting force which stops the discomfort, that is the criterion of effective technique. It is the position and force that achieve reduction most quickly, as assessed by questioning and examination at each attendance. Hence the maximum stretch that the patient can tolerate without discomfort is always employed.

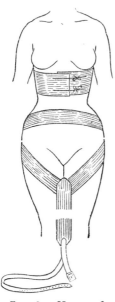

Fig. 89. Harness for traction. Anterior view

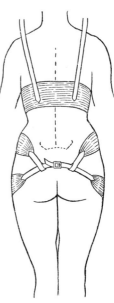

Fig. 90. Harness for traction. Posterior view

During traction a cough and a sneeze remain painful, and should be avoided during the stretching, otherwise the patient may feel sore for the rest of the day. The painfulness or not of the lumbar movements and of straight-leg raising is estimated at each attendance *before* treatment; for the physical signs present immediately after traction ceases are an unreliable guide to progress. When reduction is almost complete in a case of sciatica, this fact is often signalled by the appearance of a painful arc on straight-leg raising. Treatment must be given daily until reduction has been secured; this takes one to three weeks. If twelve adequate sessions have done no good, traction should be abandoned. The only exception to this rule is the long-standing backache of youngish persons in whom the lumbar movements other than flexion are of full range and painless, but straight-leg raising is markedly limited on both sides. Their only hope of avoiding permanent disability is sustained traction, which is justified for two to three months, since it is often only after the first month of daily traction that improvement begins.

Indications for Traction

At the lumbar joints, manipulation and traction are to some extent interchangeable. While it is true that some protrusions prove irreducible by traction yet reducible by manipulation and vice versa, others respond to both measures. However, since manipulation is so much the more quickly effective, if the choice is in real doubt, manipulation should be tried once. If it fails, no time is lost, and the patient feels assured that he is attending for the slower method of securing reduction with good reason. Sometimes, considerable improvement may be achieved by manipulation, the residual displacement not proving amenable to further attempt. Even so, such partial reduction saves the patient several sessions of traction.

The indications are:

1. *Nuclear Protrusion*
The history of gradual onset after exertion or stooping or remaining seated is coupled with signs of irreducibility by manipulation in a patient under sixty years of age. By contrast, the signs of total irreducibility are absent.

The signs suggesting that traction will succeed but manipulation fail are: trunk side-flexion towards the painful side increases pain; trunk movements, other than flexion, hurt down the lower limb; primary posterolateral protrusion.

2. *Indeterminate Protrusion*
The consistency of the protrusion is uncertain; manipulation has been tried and has failed or proved only partly successful.

It may happen that, although the protrusion consists of annular material, the adjacent vertebral surfaces have closed in behind it and the path for its return no longer exists. In such cases, the separation of the articular surfaces by traction restores the original width of the joint space and suction then induces reduction.

3. *Fourth Sacral Reference*
If reduction is to be attempted in cases with pain referred to the genital area or coccyx, traction must be attempted with caution at first. Even this measure is not entirely safe; for marked weakness of the bladder developed immediately after traction for sciatica in one patient (unhappily not seen

by myself, so I do not know if any contra-indications to traction were present or not). Laminectomy was performed the next day, and full control was restored.

4. *First and Second Lumbar Disc Lesion*

At these levels, in primary disc lesions, manipulation has always failed at my hands, whereas traction is regularly successful. In disc lesions secondary to lower lumbar arthrodesis, however, manipulation often succeeds.

5. *Recurrence after Laminectomy*

Manipulation is seldom successful, but can safely be attempted. Traction is more often effective, but the prognosis is, of course, less favourable in those who have, than in those who have not, had the operation.

Contra-indications to Traction

1. *Acute Lumbago*

This is *the* contra-indication to traction, and unwisely giving this treatment in such cases is responsible for most of the reports of severe unfavourable reactions. Lumbago with twinges is made much worse for several days by one session of traction. As soon as the force is applied pain ceases, straight-leg raising reaches full range and all seems to be going well, but as soon as the tension is diminished even slightly, the patient gets such agonizing twinges that the force cannot be reduced. It may take a patient three or four hours to get off the couch, and at the end of this ordeal he remains worse than before starting. Surprisingly enough, the twinges are abated but not abolished by the induction of epidural local anaesthesia, and are best treated by a rotation manipulation as the patient lies there. But he should never have been given traction in the first place.

2. *Cartilaginous Displacements*

Sustained traction is not suited to small annular displacements which should be reduced on the spot by manipulation.

3. *Certain Cases of Sciatica*

In patients with neurological signs, the attempt at reduction will fail whether manipulation or traction is tried, and for the same reason: the protrusion is larger than the path by which it emerged.

In patients with sciatica and gross lumbar deviation, or marked limitation of trunk extension which provokes the root-pain, it is seldom possible to give traction without increasing the pain as soon as the force is applied. Neither case responds, even if no neurological signs are present.

Sciatica in a patient aged under sixty years old which has persisted for six months has passed the time limit. It is too late for traction or manipulation.

4. *Fixation in Flexion*

Most patients fixed in flexion are suffering from acute lumbago and are therefore unsuited to traction. If fixation in flexion is present with more chronic pains in the back or lower limb, it is usually impossible to give traction, since no position can be found in which the pain is not increased as soon as the stretch is applied.

5. *Protrusion in Old Age*

In patients over 60, the disc has undergone degeneration and the nucleus has ceased to exist. Hence, manipulation, not traction, is the treatment of choice. Elderly patients, the emphysematous or those with impaired cardiac or respiratory function may find the thoracic harness an embarrassment.

6. *Long-standing Primary Postero-lateral Protrusions*

Primary postero-lateral protrusions all consist of nuclear material and respond very well to traction, whereas manipulation has no effect. Hence such a protrusion of a month or two's standing should be reduced by daily traction. However, in this type of lesion, the tendency to relapse after reduction is considerable. If then this is a second attack or the protrusion has continued for three or four months, it is sounder policy to leave it where it is, especially in a young patient with slight pain only—the common situation. Spontaneous recovery usually takes nine months from the onset of root-pain, and the strong tendency to recurrence is largely obviated by allowing the patient to get well himself. He should be kept under observation until the protrusion is stable at its maximum size, whereupon epidural local anaesthesia is induced. This secures recovery in a few weeks instead of some months. If the injection is unobtainable, it is best merely to wait.

7. *Manipulation has Failed*

Traction should not be given immediately afterwards, or it may make the pain worse. The patient should attend the next day.

Traction in Bed

Patients with acute lumbago, the result of a nuclear protrusion, set a very real problem. They cannot, as in nuclear backache or sciatica, be treated in the logical way, i.e. by daily traction, since this measure makes acute lumbago worse. An attempt at manipulative reduction does not achieve much and epidural local anaesthesia brings, let us say, some hours' relief only. Apart from leaving the patient in bed for as long as fortune dictates in the old-fashioned way, only one alternative exists—sustained traction during recumbency.

The foot of the bed is fitted with a pulley and raised 30 cm. on blocks. A pelvic belt is applied, to which a cord with a 20 kg. weight is attached. Traction is sustained continuously for up to a week—until a cough no longer hurts, straight-leg raising has become full and the constant ache has ceased. The patient is left free in bed for a day and then tries getting up for increasing periods daily. During the first few days up, he may stand or lie but not sit.

This method of traction works well in nuclear acute lumbago, getting the patient on his feet again in, say, a week instead of a month. It has nothing in common with traction in bed with adhesive plaster on one or both legs and, usually, 3 kg. weights. So small a distracting force does not overcome the frictional resistance of the leg on the bedclothes and is identical with lying in bed without traction. Moreover, this way of applying even a useless degree of traction carries with it an appreciable risk of venous thrombosis; hence, it should be abandoned.

Comment

There is a stage in the development of almost every disc lesion when it is reducible. The early cartilaginous displacement responds to manipulation, the nuclear to traction. If these two simple and logical measures were employed at once as a routine, the immense amount of invalidism caused by back-troubles would be reduced to a tiny fraction of today's figures. (This has already been proved in Germany and Norway.) Patients would benefit; so would industry; sickness insurance would be saved large sums.

20

The Lumbar Region

PART V : EPIDURAL LOCAL ANAESTHESIA

The three most effective treatments for low lumbar disc lesions are: manipulation, traction and epidural injection. Manipulation or traction is called for in a reducible displacement. The epidural injection is suitable to those cases in which the protrusion cannot be shifted, and the endeavour is then to deal with the dura matter and the nerve-root instead. It provides a most valuable method of dealing with lumbar disc lesions, with both diagnostic and therapeutic intentions. I have used this method since 1937 some 25,000 times on unprepared outpatients without disaster.

In France, Sicard and Catherine devised the technique of the injection separately in 1901; and by 1909, Caussade and Chauffard claimed cures of sciatica after one injection. There is thus nothing new about the method, except in its application. I first began to use epidural local anaesthesia thirty-two years ago, purely diagnostically, with the idea of finding out if the cause of backache and sciatica lay outside or inside the vertebral column. It was only when a proportion of patients came back after the diagnostic injection declaring themselves permanently improved that I realized I had stumbled on a method also with therapeutic applications.

Diagnostic Indications

It is chiefly in early cases with slight symptoms, and physical signs difficult to interpret, that epidural local anaesthesia is so helpful diagnostically. This often has medico-legal importance, too, since it may be alleged that the backache is muscular or ligamentous in origin and, therefore, likely to get well without sequelae, whereas injury to cartilage is permanent and the risks of recurrence must be taken into account when damages are assessed.

1. *Uncharacteristic Backache*

Cases are quite frequent in which neither the history nor the physical signs clearly define any one lesion. There have been no frank attacks of internal derangement; the symptoms do not vary according to posture or exertion in the discish manner; the lumbar movements cause aching in a way not much like disc-trouble; there is no painful arc. To make matters worse, other tests prove contradictorily positive, e.g. of the sacro-iliac joints, when the lumbar movements have already indicated that the lesion, though indeterminate, is lumbar.

2. *Referred Pain*

There may be no backache at all, the question being whether a pain, say, in the groin has a low lumbar origin or results from perhaps chronic appendicitis or an ovarian cyst. Since extra-segmental reference from the dura mater is not widely appreciated, when a pain felt in the twelfth thoracic or first lumbar dermatome is attributed to a low lumbar disc lesion, the orthopaedic physician may well be met with incredulity, which it may need an epidural injection to dispel. Or a pain in the buttock, thigh or calf may have an undetectable origin, no lumbar movement hurting, but no abnormality being detectable in the limb itself either. This is particularly apt to happen in slight but persistent bilateral sciatica, the question in each case being whether the symptoms have a local source or are referred from the back.

3. *Contradictory Opinions*

Various medical men, perhaps in a medico-legal case, have stated that a disc lesion is present, and others have disagreed. There is no point in taking sides in this argument since judge, patient and family doctor alike are not going to be impressed by words, of which they have already had a surfeit. The matter is resolved and confidence restored when the patient himself is made the arbiter of the diagnosis. He is kept in the dark on the same lines as for psychoneurosis (see below).

4. *Psychoneurosis*

Then there is the patient with psychoneurosis in whom it is uncertain whether a small underlying organic lesion is present or not. In such cases, when the injection is given diagnostically, no mention is made of the nature of the fluid to be injected. After the induction, it is well to wait for at least ten minutes (since 0·5 per cent procaine works rather slowly to achieve its full effect) and the patient must in any case be given time to recover from any giddiness caused. The question is then put misleadingly: 'I am afraid this injection may have made you a bit sore; how is your back (or limb) now?' If the patient, after so broad a hint of what to expect, nevertheless maintains that his pain has gone, and when he later stands and the lumbar movements are tested these are now painless, he clearly has a minor disc lesion.

Diagnostic Response

The fluid runs up the neural canal and along the external aspect of the lower lumbar nerve-roots (Plates 47 and 48). It does not enter any joint. This is indeed theoretically impossible; for Nackemson (1963) has shown that even in excised specimens of the lumbar spine the ligaments exert a pressure of 0·7 kg. per square cm.: a far greater force than that at which the solution drips into the sacrum. Moreover, the radiographs show that it does not. Nor can the solution bathe the anterior aspect of the posterior longitudinal ligament, where pressure from a protruded disc would be exerted. If 0·5 per cent procaine is employed, it does not penetrate the dural membrane nor the sheath of the nerve-root; no lower motor neurone lesion results. The lumbar muscles and those of the lower limbs are unaffected, and the skin (except rarely over the sacrum) retains its sensitivity. The only structures rendered anaesthetic are the exterior surface of the dura mater and nerve-roots. Presumably the posterior surface of the posterior longitudinal ligament and the anterior surface of the ligamentum flavum are numbed too, but the effect of 0·5 per cent procaine does not penetrate to the substance of such tissues. If, then, a patient has a lesion of the moving parts of the back and epidural local anaesthesia affords one to two hours' relief, the cause must be pressure on the dura mater or dural root-sleeve without adherence. The solution can pass between two adjacent surfaces if they are merely pressed together, but cannot percolate to the point of impact if adherence or invasion has occurred. Cessation of symptoms after the injection shows that the solution has been able to pass between two surfaces and there is only one tissue apt to protrude posteriorly without invasion: a disc lesion.

In conditions like sacro-iliac strain or arthritis, ankylosing spondylitis, afebrile osteomyelitis, neuroma, secondary neoplasm, claudication in the buttock, gluteal bursitis, spondylolisthesis without a disc lesion, the injection makes no difference to the pain for the time being. The response is also negative in some 5 per cent of patients with backache whose cause remains obscure to me; these may be instances of ligamentous strain. Hackett's sclerosis is particularly suitable for many such cases.

Therapeutic Indications

It is fortunate that epidural local anaesthesia is often an effective treatment for just those cases unsuited to manipulation or traction. The way that permanent benefit results appears different in different disorders.

1. Hyperacute Lumbago

If the patient has such a large protrusion impinging *via* the ligament against the dura mater that he experiences severe twinges on the slightest movement, an attempt at manipulative reduction is unthinkable and even rhythmic oscillations cannot be borne. A long period in bed is then often thought to provide the only hope of eventual relief. But there is one— only one—rapidly effective treatment: epidural local anaesthesia. Failing the injection, agonizing twinges force the patient to lie motionless, his muscles guarding and compressing the joint. Hence the immobility and muscle-tension are such that the gradual reduction in the degree of displacement, that relief from weight-bearing is intended to secure, begins very slowly. By contrast, the injection affords immediate, complete relief and not much pain returns when the anaesthesia has worn off. It would seem that, as the patient lies prone, during absence of compression, the free movement rendered practicable for ninety minutes by the anaesthesia allows spontaneous reduction to begin days or weeks before it would otherwise have become possible. By next morning, he is usually able to get up, still fairly sore, and to travel up for manipulative reduction of any residual displacement.

It follows that a patient treated for severe lumbago by this injection should not be permitted to get up from the couch and walk home. He should return, as he came, by ambulance; alternatively, the injection should be given in bed at home. The patient stays recumbent till next day.

It is interesting to note that immediately after the induction of local anaesthesia, all pain ceases, but, if marked lateral deviation has been present before the injection, it often continues for a while, the patient averring that painless stiffness restricts the movement. This is theoretically correct, since the displacement is still in being, limiting joint movement, but impinging against a now insensitive structure. By contrast, as is also to be expected, all the dural manifestations cease completely; a cough and neck-flexion no longer hurt and straight-leg raising on each side becomes of full range and painless.

2. Intractable Backache

When backache, the result of a low lumbar disc lesion, proves refractory to both manipulation and traction, it must be regarded as caused by an irreducible displacement. The only approach is then to attempt desensitization of the dural tube, in the hope that symptoms will thus be mitigated. They often are; the constant ache may be lastingly abolished, leaving only the momentary pain on certain movements which the patient learns to avoid, or can wear a corset to prevent.

3. Chronic Backache

There is a type of chronic ache in middle-aged or elderly patients in which articular signs are virtually absent. The ache is constant, little altered by posture or exertion. Examination reveals that perhaps only one lumbar movement increases it slightly; sometimes no movement makes any difference. Such a symptom can often be permanently abolished by one induction of epidural local anaesthesia. If this should fail, ligamentous sclerosis offers the only other chance of relief.

4. Matutinal or Nocturnal Backache

The patient can do everything, even heavy work, by day but is regularly woken in the small hours by backache severe enough to force him out of bed to walk round the room. After half an hour or so the ache subsides and he can then sleep on. Other patients wake in the same sort of pain at, say, 7 a.m., which ceases after they have been up for about an hour, and are pain free for the rest of the twenty-four hours. Examination during the day reveals nothing, but the patient may make one revealing statement: that during the time his back is hurting, a cough causes pain—not otherwise. This suggests dural compression of some sort and gives the injection its theoretical justification. Often one epidural injection is curative. One patient who had had to get out of bed nightly for 27 years, had two months' relief, but then relapsed after a day's digging. Failure is encountered, of course; if so, ligamentous sclerosis is indicated.

5. Pregnancy

During the last month of pregnancy, backache or sciatica caused by a disc lesion is best treated by either rest in bed or epidural local anaesthesia.

6. Root-pain with Neurological Signs

Signs of interference with conduction show that the protrusion has reached a size that makes reduction impossible; the bulge is larger than the aperture whence it emerged and cannot return. Desensitization of the nerve-root at the point of impact is then strongly indicated by epidural local anaesthesia. It might well have been supposed that adding hydrocortisone to the solution would enhance the desensitizing effect, but this was not so when tried out originally (Cyriax, 1957); and in two recent cases, epidural local anaesthesia afforded immediate lasting relief some days after hydrocortisone by the lumbar route had had no effect.

The relative value of recumbency and epidural local anaesthesia was estimated in a series of 50 patients (Coomes and Groggono, 1963). All the patients had sciatica with severe pain and signs of impaired conduction along the nerve-root. Half the patients were admitted to hospital for bed rest; the other half received one or two epidural injections and rested at home. The conclusion was that the injected patients had largely recovered in ten days, whereas the recumbent took 30 days to reach the same degree of comfort. The injection thus saves the patient almost three weeks' pain, and the Health Service about £200 per patient.

The injection then is the main weapon for treating root-pain with absent or sluggish reflex, one or more weak muscles, analgesic skin (not mere pins and needles). Indeed, there is no other treatment possible, unless, exceptionally, laminectomy is indicated. In hospitals where a surgeon exists who removes protruded discs but there is no physician skilled in inducing epidural local anaesthesia, numbers of avoidable laminectomies are inevitable. If laminectomy were always successful and left the patient with a strong back afterwards, this would not matter much; it would merely represent a waste of money and hospital beds. However, after operation, the patient must be permanently careful of his back, whereas those who get well with the epidural injection can go back to reasonably heavy work. Moreover, if laminectomy fails, subsequent epidural local anaesthesia is seldom effective, whereas if the injection fails, laminectomy is in no way embarrassed.

Patients in whom lumbar extension is markedly limited by pain shooting down the limb, and patients with marked lumbar deviation in whom attempted side-flexion in the limited direction is restricted by severe root-pain, are often refractory to epidural local anaesthesia. Indeed, it is these two types of case that often end with operation. Prognosis is not so bad when the patient stands in a symmetrical posture and merely deviates on trunk-flexion. It is my practice, when the issue is uncertain, to give the injection and wait a week. If there has been no improvement, laminectomy is indicated.

Patients with severe neurological weakness usually lose their pain fairly quickly as the result of root-atrophy. Occasionally, the pressure of the protrusion falls just short of producing the requisite degree of ischaemia, and in spite of marked signs they continue to have root-pain. Most such patients are permanently relieved by the epidural injection. If this does not succeed, and the root-pain has continued for some months, it is no good waiting further, laminectomy being indicated at once.

Patients with sciatica who are over 60 do not respond as favourably to epidural injections as do younger people, but this is not universal, and an occasional good result is seen in patients even over 80. In third lumbar disc lesions with root-pain, the injection works less well than in lesions at the fourth or fifth levels. The immediate relief is often not quite complete; a greater number of injections is required, and the failure rate is higher.

The number of injections usually required is two or three. If the pain is severe, the next is given four or five days later; if not so bad, seven or ten days later suffices. If, some weeks after the second injection, an ache remains, a third is indicated. In less severe sciatica, one or two injections often suffice. Since the infiltration has a marked result or none at all, there is seldom any doubt when the patient attends a second time. There is no theoretical limit to the number that can be given, and cases do present themselves in which each injection affords a little improvement only; if so, they are continued until adequate relief has been achieved, which very seldom requires more than six. If the first injection does no lasting good, merely relieving the pain for an hour or two, there is no point in repeating it.

One type of sciatica often requires more than the usual number of epidural injections, up to, say, five. The patient has had unilateral root-pain for, say, six months and on examination does not deviate, has slight or no neurological signs but straight-leg raising is limited to 20 degrees on the painful side and 45 degrees on the painless side, both bringing on the unilateral sciatic pain. Immediately after the first epidural injection, the good leg rises to 90 degrees but the range of straight-leg raising on the painful side is only slightly increased. At the second visit, the range of straight-leg raising on the good side is found to have remained full. After the second injection, the leg on the bad side rises a little farther and progress is gradual thenceforward.

7. Root-pain without Neurological Signs

There are four conditions that strongly indicate the injection.

Root-pain that has Continued for too Long

Root-pain caused by a disc lesion at the third, fourth or fifth level should recover spontaneously in a year at the most if there is no neurological deficit; and more quickly if impaired conduction is present. Cases occur in which spontaneous recovery is delayed, the pain and often limitation of straight-leg raising continuing. In these cases, the pain is not very severe but has persisted for so long that laminectomy is contemplated. These cases respond excellently to the injection, with only few exceptions. (These are the patients already mentioned with limited trunk-extension causing pain in the lower limb, and those with sciatica and gross lumbar deviation while standing.) The patient has, say, 45 degrees limitation of straight-leg raising; after the injection, full range is restored (if not, an adherent root is present). At his next visit ten days later, he states that his pain has been much less and straight-leg raising is now found only 20 degrees limited. The injection is repeated and when seen a fortnight later, the patient has lost his symptoms and full straight-leg raising is at most slightly uncomfortable. No more need be done. The result appears to be achieved by mobilization of the nerve-root during local anaesthesia, which may afford lasting desensitization there as well. The injection is very often entirely effective, and restores the patient's capacity for quite heavy work; hence, in these cases, laminectomy is strongly contra-indicated until the injection has had an adequate trial.

Full Evolution of the Root Syndrome

This applies chiefly to young people with primary postero-lateral disc protrusions at the fourth or fifth level. The patient may attend complaining of increasing pain in the calf and/or thigh after sitting which, in a month or two, becomes a constant ache. The range of straight-leg raising is diminishing and the discomfort in the limb—there is none in the back— is becoming more persistent. Epidural local anaesthesia affords no benefit in a case that is still evolving, and the choice lies between reduction by traction, or awaiting stabilization of the protrusion in the position of maximum displacement and then giving the injection. In the very early case, reduction by traction may well be preferred, but the recurrence rate is high and reduction seldom lasts a year. Since the patient is never in severe pain, it is better practice to wait and to examine him each few weeks until his range of straight-leg raising becomes stable (usually 30 degrees to 45 degrees range); and once this point has been reached to give the epidural injection. If this is done, he is likely to recover in six months instead of spontaneously in twelve, and, having come out of his sciatica on the far side, as it were, he is much less likely to suffer recurrence. This is all explained to the patient and the choice left to him. Sometimes, there is a compromise; reduction by traction is carried out with agreement that, if the root-pain recurs soon, it will then be left to evolve on the second occasion.

Recurrent Sciatica after a Root-palsy

Recurrence at the same level from sciatica with neurological signs is uncommon following recovery, whether spontaneous or after an epidural injection. However, it can happen that a patient who lost all his pain after a couple of epidural injections gets another attack of sciatica within a year. It might well be argued that this is a small recent protrusion and should, therefore, be treated by manipulation or traction. This is logical, but both these measures are apt to fail, whereas epidural local anaesthesia usually succeeds. This does not apply if a patient gets sciatica again many years later or at a new level.

Root-pain without Physical Signs

Sometimes a patient has root-pain, with or without backache, and the history suggests a disc lesion. Examination reveals a full range of painless lumbar movements, full painless straight-leg raising; no alternative cause for the pain is detected in the lower limbs either. Such root-pain may be unilateral or bilateral (if bilateral, spondylolisthesis should be considered). Epidural local anaesthesia is necessary diagnostically. If the injection is successful in abolishing the pain for the time being, it is not uncommon for the relief to continue.

In these cases, one can only suppose that persistent bruising of dura mater or nerve-root(s) has resulted from a past disc lesion, which has undergone sufficient reduction or shrinkage no longer to interfere with joint or root mobility. The local anaesthesia appears permanently to desensitize the tender tissue at the point of past impact.

8. Recovering Sciatica

If there is sciatic pain without backache, even though neurological signs are absent and the case seems otherwise suitable, manipulation and traction are best avoided if reasonably intense root-symptoms are subsiding. The patient has spent some days or weeks in bed and is over the worst, but still has a considerable ache in the limb and limited straight-leg raising. The treatment of choice is epidural local anaesthesia.

9. Nocturnal Cramp

Severe cramp coming on each night may continue to wake a patient long after a sciatica has become well. It occurs in the calf of the affected leg only.

Epidural local anaesthesia serves to desensitize the nerve-root whence the stimulus to the cramp presumably originates, and gives the patient comfortable nights. The injection may need repetition about six months later. This approach often succeeds when muscle-relaxants have failed.

10. Coccygodynia

It is often difficult to know whether pain in the coccyx is local or referred, since the bone may be tender on sitting and on palpation (as a referred dural phenomenon) in either case.

Epidural local anaesthesia, followed by asking the patient to sit again determines the issue at once; moreover, in referred cases it may prove curative.

TECHNIQUE OF EPIDURAL INJECTION

This is a simple procedure, suitable for out-patient use. It is best to say that an injection will be given which passes between the disc and the compressed tissue (dura mater in backache, nerve-root in sciatica), and will merely cause some aching. Patients who have heard alarming tales about lumbar puncture are informed that this is a different manoeuvre; that it is intrasacral, that the needle does not penetrate to the spinal fluid, and that no one has to rest in bed for 24 hours afterwards. Enquiry should be made about sensitivity to local anaesthesia. Since almost everyone has at one time or another had a local anaesthetic injection into the gum for dentistry, it suffices to ask if untoward symptoms were caused thereby. If apparent sensitivity is reported, it is more often due to adrenalin than to the anaesthetic agent itself, especially if the patient is taking an anti-depressant drug. The patient is then given a test dose of 10 cc. 0·5 per cent procaine without adrenalin into, say, the buttock. If nothing happens, the epidural injection is given next day.

Palpation

The patient lies prone and an assistant stretches the skin (see Plate 45). If much hair is present, the lower sacrum is shaved. He must relax the gluteal muscles since, during contraction, they lift the palpating finger off the posterior aspect of the sacrum. The cornua are identified as two bony prominences just to either side of the midline at the fourth sacral level (Fig. 91). The gap between the cornua indicates the position of the sacral hiatus, the lower extremity of the sacral canal. This is continuous with the neural canal at the lumbar, thoracic and cervical regions of the spine. The canal is closed above by the dural attachment round the foramen magnum of the skull which experiments on cadavers have shown is reached by 400 ml. of fluid. The physician should stand on the patient's left side, palpating the cornua with his left thumb and keeping his right hand free for

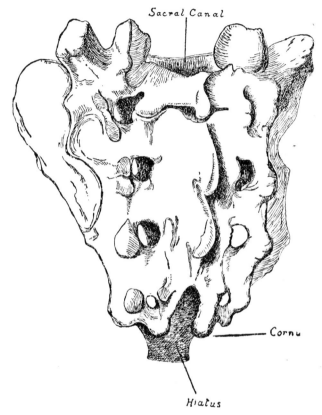

Sacral Canal

Cornu

Hiatus

FIG. 91. Anatomy of the sacrum. The needle is inserted into the sacrum via the hiatus between the cornua.

inserting the needle. After superficial sterilization locally (e.g. with acriflavine in water 1:1000), the skin and subcutaneous tissue over the hiatus are rendered anaesthetic with a 2 per cent solution of procaine without adrenalin (since monoamine-oxidase inhibitor drugs are so widely prescribed nowadays), injected from a small syringe with a fine needle. Not more than 1 cc. should be used, for too much solution obscures the bony landmarks. Note is taken of the angle at which this little needle has to be held to penetrate the intercornual ligament. The physician grasps an ordinary lumbar-puncture needle, equipped with a stylet, and thrusts it through the spot in the skin already anaesthetized, just below the hiatus. He must now consider the direction the needle must take, first to reach the intercornual space and then to pass within the sacrum. For the first target, he aims at the bone his left thumb can feel; then he tilts the needle to conform with the obliquity of the sacral surface, as determined by the plane palpable from the sacro-coccygial junction to where the cornua begin. The needle is advanced until it reaches bone; or it may slip intra-sacrally without further ado. If it meets bone, the angle of the needle must be altered to conform with the shape of the mid-sacrum, assessed by palpation of the lowest two sacral spinous processes. This is the difficult part of the procedure. To get the point to lie between the cornua is only occasionally awkward; then to judge the angle of further insertion may need considerable experience (see Plate 46). A very curved sacrum may demand a skin puncture low down with the needle aimed at the patient's occiput; a flat sacrum with prominent cornua may call for aim at the umbilicus. A bifid over-curved sacrum has to be approached by puncture at the third sacral level, otherwise the needle will slide along the floor of the sacrum and emerge at the second level through the bony defect; alterna-tively, the tip of the needle may become lost in the fibrous tissue closing the defect and lie in the roof, not in the canal. If so, when the attempt is made to begin injecting, it is found impossible to force the fluid in. The physician is helped in finding this angle of thrust by remembering the tilt his first needle took at the preliminary probe for anaesthetizing the skin and intercornual area. There are occasional difficulties. Many women have a thick layer of subcutaneous fat over the sacrum, obscuring the cornua. Some people appear not to possess cornua. If these cannot be felt at all, the needle instead of the thumb is used for palpation. It is inserted at the correct level strictly in the midline, and the sacrum tested fan-wise until the soft spot—the intercornual ligament—is found. In my experience it is impossible to insert the needle correctly in less than one per cent of cases.

Those interested in studying the great variations in curve, surface and bifidity of individual sacra should visit the basilica of the church in Evora (Portugal) where there is a huge column encrusted with several hundred human sacra and the Ossuary at Kutna Hora (Czechoslovakia), where the remains of thirty thousand victims of plague have been turned into orna-ments.

The Injection

In most patients, the theca ends at the lower level of the first sacral vertebra, and the needle must stop short of this line. Hence, the needle is passed to a depth of 5–7 cm. from the skin, unless the puncture is high up because of a bifid hiatus, when the distance is correspondingly less. If it catches against an intrasacral bony projection, it must be withdrawn a short distance and thrust in again with a slightly different tilt. If necessary, the needle may be rotated through 180 degrees, so as to alter the direction of the bevel on its point. The stylet is withdrawn as soon as the needle is in far enough (Fig. 92) and care is taken that neither cerebrospinal fluid nor blood escapes. A 50 ml. syringe, full of 0·5 per cent procaine in normal saline *without adrenalin*, is attached to the needle. A stronger solution must

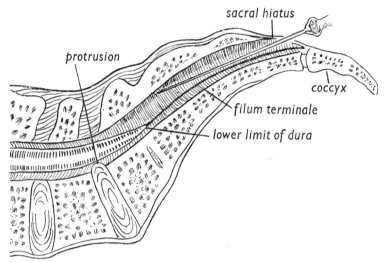

FIG. 92. Epidural injection. The needle in position.

not be used lest the anaesthesia penetrate the dural sleeve of the nerve-root and temporarily paralyse the lower limbs and sphincters. Pure water must not be used for the solution, or really severe pain for about 24 hours is to be expected as soon as the anaesthetic effect wears off.

Suction is applied, to make sure that the tip of the needle has not pierced the theca or a vein during this manoeuvre. Aspiration is attempted after each 10 ml. to ensure that the end of the needle has not shifted unnoticeably. If all is well, the solution is run in at the rate of 5 or 10 ml. a minute, depending on the patient's sensations. If he feels no appreciable local discomfort, or dizziness, or headache, the solution is put in at a fair rate; if it proves uncomfortable or engenders any of these symptoms, there is a pause until they have passed off before introducing any more solution. The patient should be engaged in quiet conversation during the injection, since the earliest warning of adverse effect is usually a faltering voice. No more should then be run in until the patient feels better.

With these precautions, the injection is only vaguely unpleasant. This is important: for the injection often has to be repeated and must, therefore, be so given that the patient does not dread it on a future occasion.

The physician does not hold on to the butt of the needle with his left hand, once the syringe is affixed. He places this palm flat on the patient's sacrum, where it is ready to feel a projection mounting on one or other side. This is his main safeguard against a misplaced needle. Since there is no test to prove that the needle lies intrasacrally, and the needle cannot penetrate the solid floor of the sacrum, a faulty insertion can lead only to the needle lying superficial to the sacrum, in the substance of the sacro-spinalis muscle. After about 10 ml. the hand begins to feel hardening and swelling of the muscle to one or other side of the upper sacrum. If so, the needle is withdrawn and the insertion attempted again. Another difficulty arises when the tip of the needle, lying correctly intrasacral, has passed subperiosteally and the fluid cannot be forced in. Merely rotating the needle through two right angles so that the bevel lies the other way may suffice. If that fails, the needle may be withdrawn a millimetre or two. If it has to be advanced, suction must be reapplied before injection, to ensure that neither theca nor a vein has been punctured. An extrasacral injection does no harm; the disadvantages are purely negative. It is, however, essential to know that the mistake has been made, so that a false diagnostic conclusion or an unjustified ascription of therapeutic failure is avoided.

As the solution runs in, most patients feel some lower sacral aching, sometimes referred to the back of both thighs. A sufferer from sciatica nearly always states that the pain in the limb is reproduced first in the buttock, then in the thigh and leg. Although the solution bathes the nerve-roots on each side equally, it is only the sheath already irritated by pressure that is tender enough to set up further pain as the acid solution reaches it. This finding was confirmed by Lindahl (1966), who gave epidural injections at various spinal levels, so as rapidly to increase the pressure on the nerve-roots. He found that, whatever the level of the injection, the nerve-root was sensitive to increased hydraulic pressure, the root-pain being reproduced in patients with sciatica but not in other patients.

Occasionally, the dura mater ends at an abnormally low level; if so, the needle pierces it and comes to lie intrathecally. When the stylet is withdrawn, cerebrospinal fluid escapes. If so, the needle is slowly withdrawn until the flow ceases; this indicates the level beyond which the needle must not be thrust when the second attempt is made a few days later. The injection of 50 cc. of even 0·5 per cent procaine into the cerebrospinal fluid would surely prove fatal; but it is an error easily avoided. Sometimes a patient moves during the injection. If so, aspiration is repeated to make sure that no fluid emerges. If the theca has been pierced the needle should be taken right out; it must not merely be withdrawn a little until it lies extradurally and the injection then continued. Enough of the solution is apt to ooze through the hole to give rise to a sacral-root block. The patient cannot therefore walk and may become incontinent, and is unable to leave for several hours. It is curious that after such an unintentional lumbar puncture the patient gets up quite happily and walks home at once without any symptoms or a headache developing later. Since it is widely held that the headache, so often experienced after lumbar puncture and avoided by 24 hours' recumbency, is caused by cerebrospinal fluid leaking out through the puncture hole, it is most surprising that puncture from below instead of from behind should have no sequelae, especially since the fluid pressure is at its greatest at the lower extremity of the tube.

If blood issues when the stylet is withdrawn, the attempt should be made to manoeuvre the tip of the needle into a harmless position. If this succeeds, aspiration showing the needle to lie extravenously, the injection can safely be given. If the point remains in the vein or in the haematoma (there is no telling which), the injection is postponed for a couple of days. An intrasacral haematoma causes no inconvenience to the patient, who walks home quite unaware of its existence.

Study of Plates 47 and 48 will show that the central part of the infiltration, running up the extradural canal, reaches the third lumbar level after 20 ml. This is different from the clinical effect as assessed by the reproduction of root-pain. In fifth lumbar disc lesions, the pain in the limb is usually provoked or augmented after 10 to 15 ml. have been injected; at the fourth lumbar level it usually takes 20 to 25 ml. In third lumbar lesions, the crural pain is seldom reproduced before 40 ml. have been injected, and often nothing is felt in the thigh at all. Yet the root has been reached; for a few minutes later the root-pain ceases. Fifty millilitres suffices for any patient, however large; to a very small woman I give a minimum of 35 ml. Rarely, the feet become warm. This indicates that sympathetic tone has been abolished, i.e. that the solution has reached the second lumbar level. There is no advantage in introducing more than 50 ml.; for the solution merely passes farther down the nerve-trunks and farther up the spine, where no lesion exists.

Ryder (1953) showed that quickly raising the pressure in the CSF causes an abrupt drop in venous pressure in the sagittal sinus. Since, on epidural injection, fluid is introduced into a closed space, the pressure in the fluid must rise and be transmitted upwards. For this reason, the injection is given slowly and restricted to 50 ml. A few minutes' headache may occur, and nearly all patients feel giddy if allowed to get up too soon, before a new equilibrium has become established. In the elderly, the cerebral circulation is less easily altered, and after 70 most patients can rise as soon as the infiltration is concluded. Nearly all patients are fit to get up after ten minutes prone, and another five minutes supine. After twenty minutes they can walk out. Driving a car home is quite safe. Half per cent procaine does not soak through the dura mater nor the root-sleeve, and thus there is no interference with conduction; only the external surface of the theca and the nerve-roots has been rendered insensitive. Very occasionally, temporary numbness in the third and fourth sacral areas results; after the injection, when the patient sits down, he does not feel the impact of the chair. Bladder control is retained.

If a patient feels really odd after only 20 ml. have been injected, and this continues for five minutes, the attempt should be abandoned. An occasional patient feels very faint, usually a few minutes after the injection is over; if so, he lies with his legs raised. Since it is possible (though improbable) that any patient who has had an epidural injection may need to lie there for an hour, it is unwise to attempt it unless there is time enough, or a skilled assistant to remain with the patient, who must on no account be left alone for the first 15 minutes.

Hydrocortisone added to the anaesthetic solution does not enhance the effect, although in cases of unexpectedly poor response to the normal injection, 10 ml. pure hydrocortisone suspension, or 5 cc. of suspension in 20 ml. of 0·5 per cent of procaine solution may well be given. Epidural injection with saline solution only, i.e. without procaine, is without effect, and it seems that it is the desensitizing rather than the hydraulic effect which is required. Two interesting cases are worth recording. One was a young footballer who had had some months' sciatica, not very severe, with 30 degrees limitation of straight-leg raising without neurological signs. Several attempts had been made to induce epidural local anaesthesia via the sacral hiatus; this was awkwardly shaped and it was not possible to introduce the needle correctly. An extradural anaesthetic injection via the lumbar route was therefore given, and must have been correctly sited; for the patient felt his sciatic pain reproduced by the injection and found his leg numb for some hours afterwards; no lasting good accrued. A week later an ordinary epidural injection by the sacral hiatus made him perfectly well in a few days and he has played ever since (five years). It seems, therefore, that even the route matters. The other, reported to me by Y. MacKenzie (1966), was a case of severe sciatica in which an extradural injection of hydrocortisone via the lumbar route had had no effect. Epidural local anaesthesia carried out a few days later gave immediate lasting relief. In this comparison of two techniques it seems

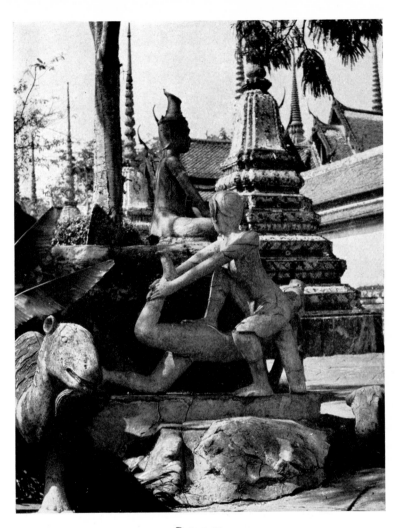

PLATE 41

Reduction of lumbar disc lesion by manipulation. Photograph taken by Dr K. L. Mah at an ancient Buddhist temple at Bangkok, Siam and regarded as 2000 years old. (By courtesy of *Doctors Only*.)

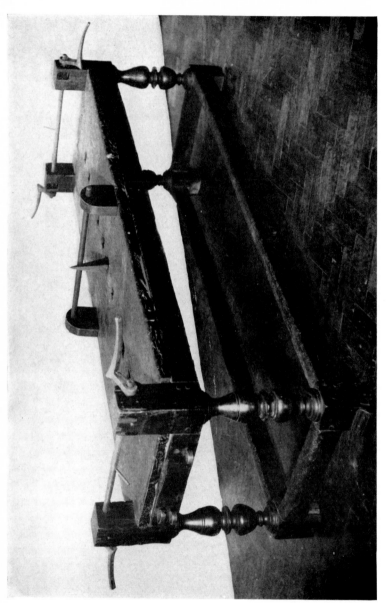

PLATE 42

Mediaeval traction couch. As used by Hippocrates and illustrated in Guidi's *Chirurgia*, 1544. Discovered in 1923 near Urbino, Italy and now in the Wellcome Historical Museum. (By courtesy of the Curator.)

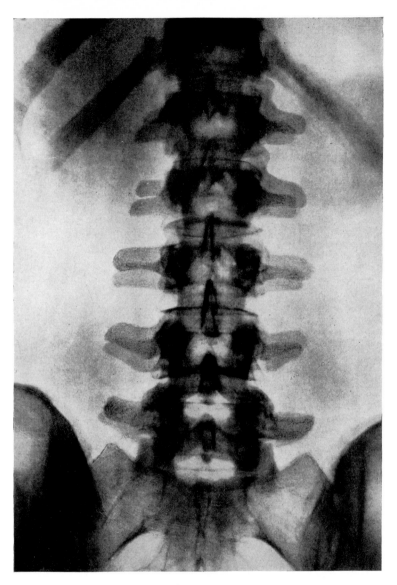

PLATE 43

Traction on lumbar spine. Two photographs have been superimposed, corresponding at the sacrum and iliac crests. The first was taken as the subject lay prone, the second after ten minutes' traction by 100 lb. The amount of distraction obtained is visible, and can be seen to be less than that secured so easily at the cervical spinal joints (see Plate 8).

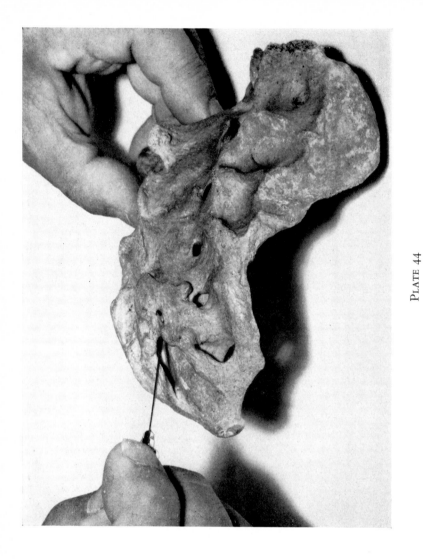

PLATE 44

Epidural local anaesthesia I. The needle lies in position between the two cornua with its point within the sacrum.

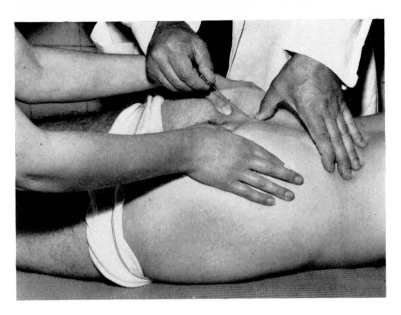

PLATE 45

Epidural local anaesthesia II. The physician's left thumb identifies the cornua and the needle is thrust between them to lie intrasacrally. An assistant stretches the skin.

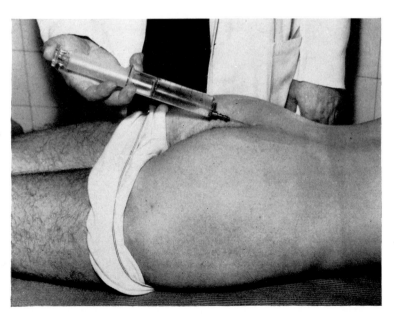

PLATE 46

Epidural local anaesthesia III. The injection is begun.

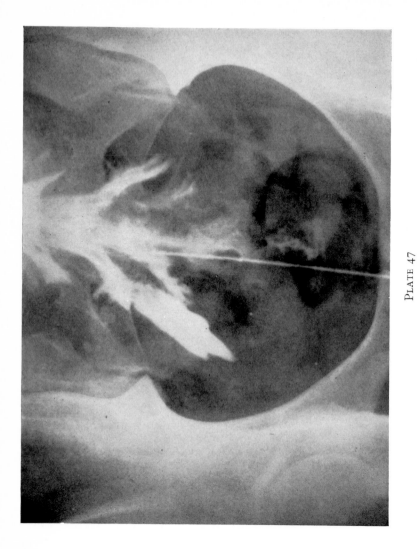

PLATE 47

Epidural local anaesthesia IV. Ten ml of a half-and-half mixture of 1:200 procaine and urographin have been injected. Needle *in situ*. The contrast medium is spreading down the sciatic nerve-roots.

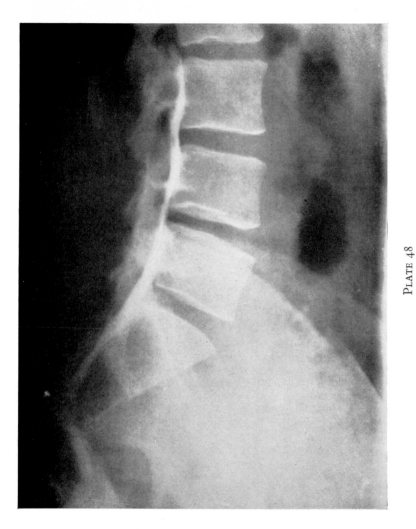

PLATE 48

Epidural local anaesthesia V. Twenty ml have been injected. The opaque solution has travelled extra-durally as far as the third lumbar level.

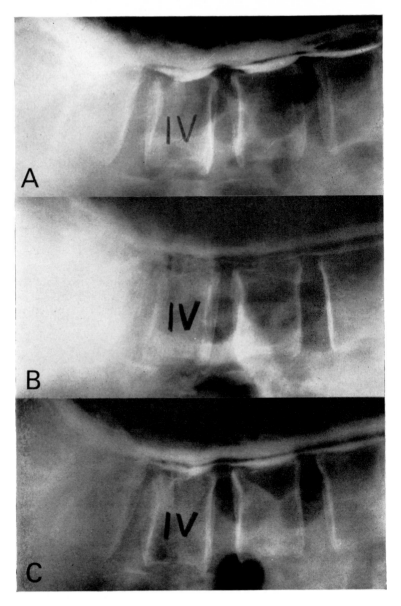

PLATE 49

Epidural local anaesthesia VI. Contrast radiography by J. A. Mathews (St Thomas's Hospital) before, during and after traction. A man of 67 with root-pain due to prolapse of disc-material at the third lumbar level. A. Appearances before traction. B. After twenty minutes' traction of 65 kg. C. Ten minutes after traction ceased. The prolapse between the third and fourth vertebrae is seen to become less prominent during traction but partly to return after its release.

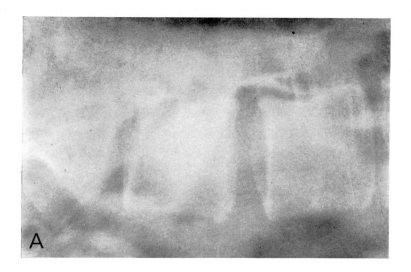

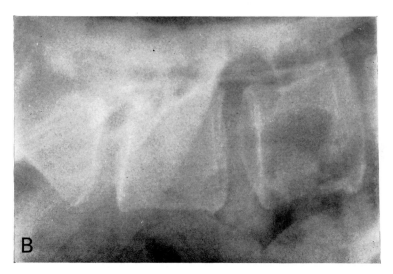

PLATE 50

Epidurogram. Patient with acute lumbago. A. Contrast radiograph showing posterior longitudinal ligament at the fourth lumbar level bulging posteriorly on account of the central protrusion. B. Second radiograph taken thirty minutes later, after manipulative reduction had succeeded. Note that the posterior ligament now follows a straight line. (By courtesy of J. A. Mathews, St Thomas's Hospital.)

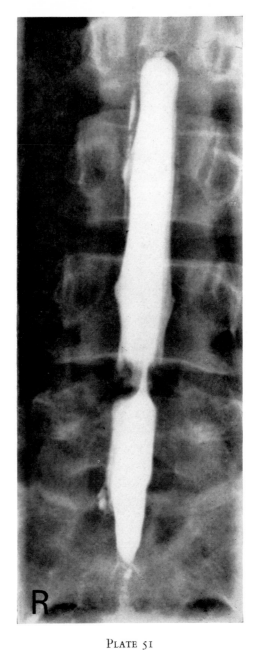

PLATE 51

Myelogram. A fourth lumbar protrusion is shown. The patient was fixed in flexion by right-sided sciatica.

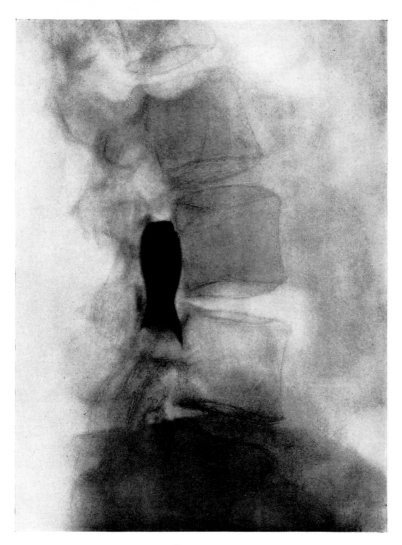

PLATE 52

Lumbar myelogram. Spinal tumour at the fourth lumbar level. The patient had had nine months' pain in the right groin and six months' sciatica. Straight-leg raising was limited on the right; no alteration of muscle power or reflex was detectable, but the patient's flexed posture aroused immediate suspicion.

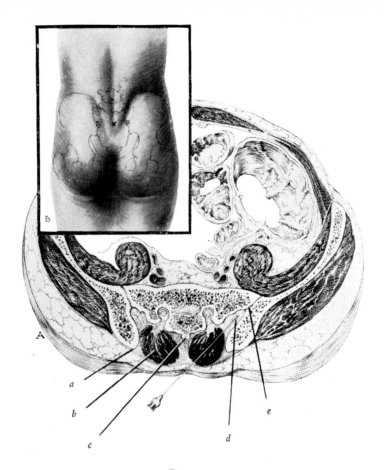

Plate 53

Relations of sacro-iliac joint. Note the impossibility of eliciting tenderness of the posterior ligament by digital pressure. (*a*) Posterior superior spine. (*b*) Sacrospinalis muscle. (*c*) Spinous process of first sacral vertebra. (*d*) Interosseous sacro-iliac ligament. (*e*) Sacro-iliac joint. (From *J. Bone Jt. Surg.*, 1938.)

that Sicard's method is the more beneficial and certainly the one to try first.

Patients with severe pain, especially those with sciatica and signs of interference with conduction, should be seen again four or five days later for another injection. Patients with long-standing root-pain should wait a fortnight. A week should elapse before assessing the result of the injection; *the immediate result is very variable.* Some patients have increased pain for a day or two, then improve rapidly. Others lose their symptoms for a couple of days, then relapse. Hence, during the first few days neither symptoms nor clinical examination are positively helpful. Unless severe pain makes it necessary to see the patient sooner, a week is the minimum interval for a clear-cut result to emerge. Usually, diminution in symptoms and signs runs parallel; if not, the pain lessens before the signs decrease. In assessing the result of the induction, subjective as much as objective improvement must be considered, and a change for the better in either warrants a second injection. A second injection is indicated in a patient whose pain is not diminished but whose straight-leg raising has considerably increased. However, if there has been no lasting change in pain or signs, repetition is vain (regardless of the result immediately after the induction). In sciatica, the immediate result of the local anaesthesia has some prognostic value. If full painless straight-leg raising is restored, one more injection should be enough; if it is full but remains uncomfortable, two; if it is still a little limited and remains quite uncomfortable, several. Very rarely, two or three injections restore full, painless straight-leg raising in a case of marked limitation, but the patient insists that the pain is as severe as ever; if so, laminectomy is indicated.

Contra-indications

These are few, since local anaesthesia cannot itself do lasting harm.

General Anaesthesia

It is dangerous to give the injection while the patient is unconscious; for he cannot then report that e.g. it is making him feel faint, etc. Moreover, the diagnostic action is lost, since he has only ninety minutes in which to report the effect on the pain and, even after a short-acting barbiturate, not all patients are composed enough to be sure. Moreover, it unduly complicates and makes inconvenient what is a simple measure.

Local Sepsis

Since the introduction of bacteria into the neural canal is a disaster, the risk must not be taken. Injection must be postponed if the neighbouring

T

skin is not clear from sepsis. If a needle has to be reinserted, a fresh one should be used.

Previous Sepsis

Old septic adhesions at the lower end of the theca may be disturbed by the infiltration, which in one case temporarily reactivated an undiagnosed febrile neurological infection from which recovery had been complete six years before.

Previous Laminectomy

Sterile gloves used to be packed in talcum powder, and enough came off their exterior surface to set up diffuse fibrosis wherever it fell. In consequence, the whole neural canal became filled with white fibrous tissue adherent to the dura mater and the nerve-roots and indistinguishable from them. A second laminectomy therefore became extremely difficult and time-consuming. The cause of this dense fibrosis was discovered in 1952 and is now avoided.

In patients operated on since then there is a reasonable chance that the epidural anaesthetic solution will reach the correct level, and there is some chance of benefit, though the likelihood of lasting relief is much diminished. In a difficult case, the attempt is worth making.

Recent Myelogram

It is probably best to wait a few days before epidural local anaesthesia is induced.

Sensitivity

Patients may state that they are sensitive to procaine. This is a very rare event; they are sensitive instead to adrenalin. However, in order to be certain, 10 ml. of 0·5 per cent procaine are injected into, say, the buttock. If nothing untoward happens, the epidural injection is given the next day.

Excessive Volume of Fluid

Clark and Whitwell (1961) injected two patients suffering from sciatica with 120 cc. of isotonic saline epidurally under general anaesthesia. Blurred vision caused by intraocular haemorrhage resulted. Hoffman (1950) had already reported two cases. These events provide no contra-indication to the slow injection of a reasonable volume of fluid without anaesthesia, using the correct technique.

Dangers of Epidural Injection

These have been grossly exaggerated, Provided the precautions outlined here are conscientiously observed, little trouble is to be expected. My experience includes four misfortunes, but no disaster, i.e. less than one per 6,000 injections. No sepsis has resulted.

Hypersensitivity

One patient was highly sensitive to procaine and had, in fact, fainted after dental injection: a fact that, when interrogated before the induction, he neglected to mention. He took 20 minutes to become unconscious, which excludes an intrathecal injection, which would have taken less than a minute. He had to be given artificial respiration for two hours before he recovered perfectly.

Semipermeable Dura Mater

One patient developed a paraplegia to the mid-thorax, which took a quarter of an hour to appear. Diaphragmatic breathing was retained, and in two hours he recovered, but the injection was a therapeutic failure.

Chemical Meningitis

Two other patients possessed a semi-permeable dura mater and developed a paraplegia from the lower thorax downwards; they had to lie for two hours until muscle power returned. Some hours later, each patient complained of headache, nausea, and neck-rigidity. Meningism was present, next day there was fever. Lumbar puncture showed 400 mgm. of protein and 4,000 white cells per cubic mm. Culture was sterile. As a precaution, both patients were treated with penicillin and recovered in a week, without sequelae.

Both these cases occurred before central sterilization, when syringes were boiled before use. The dural inflammation was probably caused by some chemical, possibly an antiseptic, polluting the water in which the instruments lay. There has been no case in recent years.

Extradural Hydrocortisone

Hydrocortisone added to the local anaesthetic solution and introduced by the sacral route was not found to help (Cyriax, 1957). Using the same approach, injection of 10 ml. of the suspension undiluted did not help either. However, hydrocortisone introduced extrathecally at a lumbar level has since been advocated by Barry and Kendall (1962). Harley (1966) has made an interesting film of the technique and its results.

21

The Lumbar Region

PART VI : OTHER TREATMENTS

The three mainstays in treatment are manipulation, traction and epidural local anaesthesia. In this chapter other methods are discussed.

REST IN BED

Browse (1965) states that 'the bed is often a sign of our therapeutic inadequacy, rather than a therapeutic measure deserving of praise. The bed is the non-specific treatment of our time, the great placebo'. This is certainly so in low lumbar disc lesions. Yet rest in bed, the traditional management for lumbago and sciatica is still universally practised. In lumbago, though tedious and time-consuming, it nearly always succeeds in the end, but this is not always so in sciatica. Recumbency admits failure and should be the doctor's last thought, not his first. In fact, it is seldom called for, to be contemplated only when adequate conservative methods do not succeed.

It has been alleged that gradual reduction by rest in bed, by causing less trauma to the joint and to the disc, results in a 'better' reduction than that secured by manipulation. This is merely an excuse for inactivity; for once the loose fragment is back in place, the agency is immaterial, except that the more quickly this is achieved, the shorter the time during which the posterior longitudinal ligament remains stretched. The idea that rest in bed allows the disc to heal is a chimera; cartilage is avascular and cannot unite.

Rest in bed in lumbago serves a double purpose; reduction and relief from pain; but in sciatica, there are two different situations; one, reduction and consequent relief; the other, relief without reduction.

Relief from Pain by Reduction

Lumbago

As soon as the body-weight is off the joint, the centrifugal force on the disc eases greatly; hence, in lumbago the protrusion recedes to some extent and the pain is correspondingly lessened as soon as the patient lies down. The marked difference between the range of trunk-flexion and of straight-leg raising illustrates this point well. The patient with lumbago may scarcely be able to bend forwards at all whereas, if the attack is not too severe, when compression on the joint stops, he may regain a full range of straight-leg raising. The same applies to cough, which may hurt standing and sitting, not lying. Staying supine in bed, therefore, has two immediate effects: (1) the cessation of centrifugal force acting on the protrusion and (2) relief from pain. Hence the stress bulging the disc out backwards diminishes at the same time as relief from pain enables the patient to move more easily, and thus assist reduction.

The patient stays in bed as long as is necessary, usually one to four weeks, and is fit to get up when the attempt ceases to be unduly painful and remaining up does not cause the symptoms to return. So long as coughing hurts and straight-leg raising remains limited, recumbency continues.

That recumbency will effect reduction is by no means certain after the age of sixty; for by then osteophyte formation and ligamentous contracture often combine to prevent the vertebral bodies moving apart when the compression of weight-bearing ceases. Hence, the older the patient is, the more his lumbar movements are limited, and the more osteophytes the radiograph shows, the more he needs manipulation rather than rest in bed for his lumbago—the reverse of what would be expected and indeed of what is commonly believed. The warm regard for lay manipulators expressed by some elderly members of the House of Lords in 1935 at the inquiry into osteopathy clearly stems partly from this fact.

Recurrence after Recumbency

It has been argued that rest in bed allows the disc to heal—an impossibility in an avascular structure—and that patients treated by recumbency achieve a more stable reduction than those treated by manipulation. The opposite is to be expected since immediate reduction spares the posterior longitudinal ligament prolonged stretching and thus should obviate instability due to ligamentous laxity. In fact, the figures for recurrence after either treatment are very similar and it would seem that recovery allowed to proceed gradually carries an identical prognosis with swift reduction.

A personal series (1957), followed up for three years had a recurrence rate of 44 per cent for lumbar pain and 40 per cent for sciatica. Pearce and Moll (1967) describe 43 per cent recurrences and Dillane, Fry and Kalten (1966), who treated all their lumbagos by rest in bed, also reported a 44·6 per cent recurrence rate in four years.

Comment

Before lightly putting a patient with lumbago to bed, one should pause to ponder the harm that results to the patient, to the community and to the doctor. The patient has a displacement that can be reduced by one manipulation in 50 per cent of cases. Alternatively, if the pain is too severe for that, epidural local anaesthesia can be relied on largely to abort the attack. Mere recumbency thus often condemns the patient to days or weeks of avoidable pain. Moreover, during the time that, mentally active, he lies there deploring his plight and the absence of effective treatment, ideas of industrial compensation begin to take root, as would never have happened if brisk treatment had returned him to his work in a few days. There is also the financial loss to the community, the cost of avoidable time off work being borne by either the patient or sickness insurance. Finally, there is the loss to the doctor himself in esteem and time. If the patient consults a lay manipulator who makes him more comfortable, the medical profession is regarded the less. If the doctor pays two visits the first week and one a week after that for a month (five minutes' journey there, five minutes back and ten at the bedside), this adds up to 100 minutes. Adequate examination, followed by a manipulative session, cannot take less than half this period. Hence recumbency wastes the doctor's time too.

Sciatica

In minor sciatica, the patient is put to bed in the hope that relieving the compression stress on the joint will result in gradual reduction, the signs and symptoms ceasing together. The mechanism is the same as in lumbago. But if reduction is going to take place gradually during relief from weight-bearing, why not actively decompress the joint by traction? It was this argument that originally made me contemplate traction as an ambulant treatment (Cyriax, 1950).

Relief from Pain without Reduction

In major sciatica, the question of reduction does not arise. The patient gets well eventually by shrinkage of the disc, by vertebral erosion or by root-atrophy; hence, the object is relief from pain during the process.

Most patients suffer less pain while in bed, and should thus be kept there until the root-pain has largely abated and getting up does not return the pain appreciably. Some patients cannot lie in bed, being obliged to walk the room at night; they need morphia. Since the protrusion is fixed and maximal, getting out of bed will not increase its size, but merely cause additional pain. When the worst symptoms are over, it is for the patient to decide which he dislikes more—not doing what he wants or getting increased pain if he does. There is no point, therefore, in keeping a patient of this sort in bed any longer than he wishes, or making him wear a corset.

The treatment of choice in most major sciatica is epidural local anaesthesia. This is agreed by Coomes and Groggono (1963) who found that the injection reduced the period of recumbency by two-thirds and often obviated the need for complete bed-rest altogether.

Rest in bed should not be continued for too long. If six weeks' recumbency and epidural local anaesthesia both fail, laminectomy is nearly always indicated, unless there is a large neurotic element in the symptoms.

AWAITING SPONTANEOUS RECOVERY

Shrunken Protrusion or Vertebral Erosion

Backache shows little tendency to spontaneous cure. A possible reason is that a central protrusion remains intra-articular, covered as it is by the posterior longitudinal ligament. Postero-lateral protrusion, since no ligament confines it, becomes extra-articular. In consequence the fibro-cartilage loses its nutrient synovial fluid and slowly shrinks.

Backache eases only in the very long run. Between the ages of fifty and sixty, the spinal joints tend to lose their range of movement owing to ligamentous contracture; moreover, at this age, osteophytes, both cupping the disc and further limiting articular movement, make their welcome appearance. Hence intermittent backache or attacks of lumbago often cease at this time of life. By analogy with lumbago, which does regularly recover spontaneously, patients are often told that their backache will soon go. Any backache may recover, it is true; but it often does not, and intermittent or constant aching over several decades is a commonplace. To await spontaneous recovery in lumbago is, therefore, reasonable but in backache, or in backache with a minor degree of root-pain, the main symptoms remaining lumbar, it is fraught with disappointment.

In root-pain the position is quite different, and spontaneous recovery is to be expected, *provided that the backache ceases when the pain shifts to the limb.* Time is counted from the appearance of the root-pain, not from the onset of lumbar symptoms, which may have continued for months or years.

Shrinkage of the protrusion or its accommodation in a neutral position by vertebral erosion takes from eight to twelve months. As at the cervical spine, the larger the displacement, the sooner the patient recovers. This is understandable in erosion, when it can be argued that, the larger the protrusion, the more pressure it exerts and the sooner it nests itself in; but it applies also to recovery by shrinkage. Sciatica of three months' standing with, say, 45 degrees of straight-leg raising and no neurological signs, is unlikely to become well in less than another nine months, unless epidural local anaesthesia is induced. The same situation, but with some neurological deficit, may well indicate recovery in another three or four months, assuming that an epidural injection is not given. Spontaneous recovery is rather quicker at the third level than at the fourth and fifth.

These rules do not apply once the patient has reached sixty years of age. In sciatica in the elderly, the backache is seldom lost and no limit can be placed on the natural history of the pain. Even if the backache does cease when the root-pain comes on, the older the patient is, the less certain it is that it will not continue indefinitely.

By contrast, root-atrophy may come on in the course of seconds or weeks. A patient may awake with an excruciating pain in one lower limb that lasts for a few seconds; then his foot goes numb, his pain ceases and he falls asleep again. Next morning his foot feels weak and examination shows a disc lesion without limitation of straight-leg raising but a complete root-palsy. Another patient may lie in bed with increasing root-pain for days or weeks and then suffer several days' agony before the numbness and the relief appear.

Patients who have recovered with the passage of time, by shrinkage, erosion or root-atrophy, do not need to be particularly careful afterwards. The displacement has not been reduced with the restoration of the status quo; hence the likelihood that what has moved once may move again does not arise. They are, of course, neither more nor less likely to develop a disc-lesion at a fresh level than any other individual, and disc-lesions are so common that everyone should always maintain his lordosis during lifting whether he has had trouble in the past or not. But they need not wear a belt or avoid reasonably strenuous work.

Recovery from Palsy

Recovery is the rule, especially in those patients who get well slowly by shrinkage or erosion. If it has not begun after a year, time is unlikely to bring recovery; after two years, no further change is to be expected. Usually, after some months, often before the root-pain has wholly ceased, the muscles begin to strengthen and the skin to regain its sensitivity. The ankle-jerk is permanently lost in about half of all cases; the knee-jerk returns more often. Root-atrophy may lead to a little permanent weakness, especially when two roots are compressed, when the muscle common to both roots may never recover, e.g., the extensor hallucis in a combined fourth and fifth lumbar root paresis. In general, weakness confined to one root recovers; affecting two roots, largely so. However, if disc-protrusion gives rise to complete paralysis of a muscle—this is most uncommon—the loss of power is apt to be permanent. If a root-palsy is developing or has just occurred, laminectomy would doubtless lead to swift restoration of conduction, but patients are well advised to risk the minor disability of a weak muscle rather than operation. A professional footballer may insist that his foot must not be allowed to weaken, but after laminectomy, he is permanently unfit for football. There is no guarantee that laminectomy will restore muscle power if carried out late, since actual pressure necrosis of some nerve fibres may lead to permanent paresis.

Recovery does not necessarily occur at the nerve-root itself; for Woolf and Till's muscle biopsies (1955), based on van Bogaert's findings, show that reinnervating fibres wander out from the intact nerves within the muscle; hence, such recovery occurs as the result of this distal mechanism. Excellent microphotographs are contained in Coomes's (1959) paper showing the branching out of new terminal neurones to supply several adjacent non-innervated muscle fibres. He regards this as brought about by terminal branching within 1 mm. of the motor end-plate of healthy nerve-fibres derived from another root supplying the same muscle. They grew down the empty endoneural tubes of the fibres that had lost their central connection and new end-plates were formed. Yates (1964) studied 48 patients with radicular weakness due to disc protrusion. In only one out of eight multiradicular cases did full recovery ensue, but he found that in all 40 patients in whom one root was only involved, full recovery was completed in an average of seven months.

The speed of recovery is very variable. Sometimes a root-palsy recovers inexplicably in a month or two, even before the pain has ceased, and cutaneous analgesia may begin to diminish after only a few weeks. Since regrowth of nerve is at the rate of 1·5 mm. a day, this cannot be the mechanism. Normally a root-palsy recovers slowly in six to twelve months, i.e. at the expected rate of nerve-regeneration, and improvement goes on for two years in all. When patients with a palsy involving even two roots are seen again for some other disorder years later, it is remarkable how few have any muscle weakness or appreciable cutaneous analgesia. If an ankle-jerk was lost, it often remains absent, but the knee-jerk nearly always returns within a year. Estimates based on short follow-up periods tend to excessive pessimism.

It is well to realize that muscle weakness is a sign that is detected rather than a phenomenon apparent to the patient. In fourth lumbar paresis, he may notice the foot flopping after he has walked some distance; in fifth lumbar paresis he is apt to turn his ankle over easily; in first or second sacral paresis he cannot rise on tiptoe on the affected leg. But he notes rather than minds, and certainly—and rightly—prefers this slight and temporary inconvenience to laminectomy. In fact, most patients with weakness are quite unaware of it.

Aggravation of the Palsy

This is rare. Past compression has induced root-atrophy which time has not improved. Laminectomy has sometimes been performed in vain. There is no change for years; then the patient suddenly notices increased painless weakness in the foot. Examination confirms that further loss of power has taken place, sometimes to the point of complete paralysis. This finding clearly implies that the protrusion has become even larger but, pressing as it does against the dural sleeve rendered insensitive by ischaemia, the phenomenon evokes no pain.

The condition is best left untreated except, perhaps, by an orthopaedic boot.

LAMINECTOMY

This should not be lightly undertaken, but should not, on the other hand, be unreasonably withheld. It is apt to be recommended far too readily, without giving sufficient weight to the effectiveness of conservative treatment and also of the passage of time. There is also a smaller group of patients who do require laminectomy but for the same reasons are denied it.

Even in the best hands, the results of laminectomy in sciatica are not perfect; immediate relief is secured in about 90 per cent of patients but recurrences bring this figure down to 80 per cent within five years. This tendency to recurrence—which may, of course, result from disc-displacement at another level—should prohibit patients from ever resuming heavy work.

Laminectomy in the presence of lumbar symptoms alone carries only half the cure-rate obtained when root-pain is present. Hence, in such a case, if there is nothing for it but operation, the patient is asked to exert himself, e.g. dig, in an endeavour to induce root-pain and to have the operation at a time when this is present. If he cannot bring on any sciatica, the chances of a successful result are diminished.

Laminectomy is seldom required in young adults. My youngest patient was seventeen and was found at operation to have a large protrusion at both fourth and fifth levels. Laminectomy is also seldom required at the third lumbar level. The pain when this root is affected may be fairly severe for some weeks, but scarcely ever reaches the agonizing pitch that raises the question of operation. Out of 913 patients operated on by Young (1951), only seven had the third disc removed. Twenty per cent of Young's patients had a double protrusion.

Patients who have not severe root-pain, but after, say six months are getting weary of their symptoms should be told that spontaneous recovery will take another three months at the third level and another six months at the fourth or fifth level. A patient who believes that he will be in discomfort for life—this is not an unreasonable idea after six months—will accept laminectomy unless the non-operative prognosis is explained to him. Laminectomy—even more, laminectomy without even trying the effect of epidural local anaesthesia first—is not an easy way out and does the patient real disservice. He stands a 90 per cent chance of immediate relief it is true, but the cure-rate of merely waiting another six months is higher. When he gets well without operation, he can return to heavy work; after the operation he must be permanently careful of his back. It is worth recalling that the patients who had sciatica in pre-laminectomy days were not operated on and nearly all recovered notwithstanding. Time healed all but a few. If, then, a patient suffering from tolerable root-pain does not respond to conservative treatment, especially epidural local anaesthesia, he should be advised to wait till a year has elapsed since the root-pain began. Only the very few who are not well by then need surgery.

Laminectomy has one important disadvantage: it abolishes the tendency to spontaneous recovery in sciatica and third lumbar root-pain. Hence, if the operation proves unsuccessful, the normal recovery from root-pain with the passage of time can no longer be counted upon; the same applies to recurrence after laminectomy.

After laminectomy, no patient should be allowed to do heavy work again. Recurrence takes place (not necessarily at the same level) in at least 10 per cent even of those who are careful of their lumbar joints. Renewed root-pain after laminectomy is difficult to treat and shows little tendency to spontaneous cure with the passage of time. It may prove intractable, and a second laminectomy is a formidable operation. Hence, a patient who proposes putting his back in jeopardy again must be given a strong warning. All patients should be warned not to do exercises while in bed after the operation, nor afterwards at home.

Indications

1. Severe Intractable Root-pain

It is not the severity of the lesion but the severity of the pain that matters
Identical disc-protrusions and identical signs may be present in patients
with severe root-pain or merely slight aching in the limb. Hence, the
problem must be approached subjectively. The simple idea that sciatica
with neurological signs warrants operation, and without such signs does
not, must be entirely abandoned; nothing could be more fallacious. First,
the size and level of the protrusion must be estimated, then the amount
of pain alleged must be set against the patient's sincerity and sensitivity to
pain; then the likelihood of time bringing relief (and, if so, how long a
time) and the possibilities of conservative treatment must be assessed.
This is not the work of a few minutes, and requires experience if errors
are to be avoided. Care is taken to ensure that the physical signs are
consistent with each other and compatible with allegations of severe pain.

Intractable pain may mean that part of the annulus has protruded
postero-laterally upwards or downwards and has come to lie on the
posterior surface of the vertebral body; in such a case, conservative
treatment, however prolonged, is bound to fail. It is also possible for more
and more of the nucleus to escape past an intact annulus and form a large
bulge with a thin neck; then, as the joint space in consequence narrows,
the herniation is trapped by contact between annulus and vertebral body—
the collar-stud phenomenon. Unless erosion of the vertebral body allows
the protrusion to nest itself away, lasting root-pain results.

The worse the symptoms and signs, the better the results of the operation. A history of previous attacks also augurs well, for it implies that the
lesion is as mature as possible. In particular, by operating late, ample
opportunity is given for protrusion at both levels to develop. If so, both
discs are dealt with and the likelihood of recurrence is correspondingly
diminished.

The cases in which laminectomy most often proves necessary are those
of sciatica, with or without neurological signs, in which either trunk-
extension is markedly restricted by pain felt in the lower limb, or there is
a considerable lateral tilt of the lumbar spine, with side-flexion in the
limited direction inhibited by severe root-pain.

2. Gross Lumbar Deformity

Sciatica with gross lumbar side-flexion deformity visible as the patient
stands, often proves refractory to conservative treatment, although the

pain may cease spontaneously after a year or two. However, it often leaves the back permanently deviated and, in a young woman, operation to avoid lasting disfigurement may be required.

3. Incipient Drop-foot

A patient who develops weakness of all the muscles controlled by two adjacent roots must be warned of the possibility of permanent weakness of the muscle common to both roots. Moreover any completely paralysed muscles (e.g. the peronei) usually remain permanently so. But, the athlete or ballet-dancer who insists on the importance of a strong foot cannot return to heavy sport or dancing after laminectomy, whereas this is possible in recovery without operation. Hence, it is better to wait, relying on the considerable probability that the muscles will recover. Though seldom indicated on the grounds of muscle weakness alone, immediate laminectomy does afford the best hope of rapid restoration of muscle power. It is not however a certainty; for necrosis of the root fibres may have supervened; if so, nothing will restore strength, and even peripheral reinervation is no longer probable.

When pressure atrophy causes complete insensitivity of the nerve-root, pain is abolished and straight-leg raising quickly reaches full range at the same time as the palsy becomes complete. The patient is apt mistakenly to believe himself to be improving; so he is, subjectively; but the true position must be explained to him. Extreme weakness or full paralysis of two or three muscles is apt to prove permanent: whereas considerable weakness usually disappears to the point where it is no longer perceived by the patient in six to twelve months.

4. Third and Fourth Sacral Root-palsy

Weakness of the bladder with incontinence or retention of urine (usually the former) during an attack of lumbago or sciatica calls for immediate laminectomy. Since the impact of the protruded disc is applied in a pre-ganglionic position, severe maintained pressure on the third and fourth sacral roots may well lead to permanent incontinence. Moreover, late laminectomy usually fails (4 in 25 cases in Jowitt's series) to restore vesical control. Hence, operation is urgent. In twelve cases, all early, post-operative recovery was complete.

If a patient with lumbago is improving and power is returning to the bladder or rectum, or his sacrum is becoming less analgesic or the impotence is waning, there is no urgency. Nevertheless, prophylactic laminectomy is indicated; for there can be no guarantee that the next time he gets lumbago his protrusion will not transect the fourth sacral root, and this may happen in a country where urgent laminectomy is unobtainable; alternatively the importance of acting quickly in this type of lumbago may be overlooked, since it is after all very seldom a dangerous disease. All my patients have accepted prophylactic laminectomy and, so far, all have remained free from further trouble.

5. Adherent Root

If the symptoms warrant, the adhesions must be divided at laminectomy. In fact, after about two years the discomfort becomes slight or even ceases entirely, and the patient's only disability is that he cannot stand up and bend forwards. He is well advised to put up with this minor disability.

6. Buckled End-plate

This is a rarity. The end-plate covering the vertebral body may become detached and finally double over on itself, forming a block at the back of the joint. When the patient attempts to bend backwards, he cannot, and when he tries he squeezes the cartilaginous displacement and is seen to recoil forward again in a characteristic manner suggesting the springy block of a meniscal displacement at the knee. Only laminectomy discloses the state of affairs, and there is no other cure.

7. Arterial Obstruction to the Cauda Equina

Spinal claudication leading to bilateral root-pain with paraesthetic feet has not in my experience responded to traction; manipulation is clearly contra-indicated. Hence laminectomy provides the only answer.

8. Arterial Obstruction to the Cord

A lumbar disc-protrusion may interfere with the arterial flow at the lower segment of the spinal cord. If the branch running upwards from the low lumbar or the ilio-lumbar artery is compressed, sciatica accompanied by spasticity of the lower limb on the painful side results, together with an extensor plantar response. The mechanism is explained in Fig. 93.

Should this phenomenon supervene in a case of sciatica, laminectomy should be considered, in order to preserve the blood supply in the spinal cord.

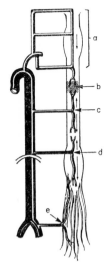

(a) Cervical and upper thoracic cord supplied by branches of vertebral,
    ascending cervical and superior intercostal arteries
(b) 'Watershed' at level of fourth thoracic segment
(c) Mid-thoracic cord supplied from a single intercostal artery
(d) Thoraco-lumbar region supplied by a large vessel near the diaphragm
    (arteria magna)
(e) Cauda equina supplied from lower lumbar, ilio-lumbar, and lateral
    sacral arteries, which occasionally supply the distal part of the cord
    also
Note that pressure at a low lumbar level may interfere with the artery as
    it passes upwards to the lowest segment of the spinal cord.
    (By kind permission of R. A. Henson and the Editor of the Quarterly
    Journal of Medicine, 1967)

FIG. 93. The arterial supply of the spinal cord

9. Repeated Crippling Attacks

These may occur so often and be so severe while they last, that the
patient's life is a misery. Even if reduction is easily achieved, whether
spontaneously or as a result of treatment, another attack follows in spite of
adequate precautions for the maintenance of reduction.

In such cases, laminectomy may be indicated. If it is decided upon,
the operation should be carried out at a time when maximum displacement is present, even if this has to be purposely induced just before the
operation.

Contra-indications to Laminectomy

Relievable by Conservative Means

If a patient can be got well by conservative means, or will clearly
recover with the passage of a reasonable length of time, no operation is
required.

Neurosis

As has already been pointed out, it is not so much the severity of the
lesion as the amount of pain experienced that provides the main indication

for laminectomy. Moreover, the criterion of cure is largely the patient's own statement afterwards. It is thus essential to provide the surgeon with cooperative patients; for a patient anxious to make the worst of his disorder will not allow himself to be deprived of it by surgery, nor after an operation is it any longer feasible to convince the patient that the organic part of his trouble has ceased. Individual sensitivity to pain is gauged in two ways. First, by the assessment of personality afforded by listening carefully to the patient's account of his troubles, together with his digressions. Secondly, by noting the responses when irrelevant as well as relevant movements are performed. Since minor symptoms due to a low lumbar disc lesion are all but universal, it is not difficult for a patient credibly to describe and to exaggerate backache or sciatica, severe disablement being alleged to obtain sympathy or compensation or pension, or escape from some domestic situation. Such symptoms may appear confirmed when a narrow disc-space (such as many middle-aged patients symptomlessly possess) is visible on the radiograph. These patients may welcome operation and, once it has been performed, it becomes very difficult to estimate how much of the patient's disablement has an organic origin, and impossible to get the patient to agree to the assessment.

It must be remembered that, when a complaint of backache is made, it is seldom wholly groundless. Some discomfort may well exist and careful examination may disclose signs of a past or present minor organic disorder. Purely psychogenic symptoms are easily detected; a slight organic disorder complicated by a large psychogenic overlay is more difficult to separate accurately into its two components. Prolonged disability after operation is to be expected in such patients, even if such organic trouble as was found was adequately dealt with. After all, any laminectomy, however successful, may be followed by some intermittent backache. Ordinary patients are so vastly improved that they ignore this slight symptom, but it is gladly grasped by the psychoneurotic. Unrecognized psychoneurosis is becoming, in my experience, increasingly treated by measures designed to affect a disc-lesion, especially manipulation, immobilization in plaster and laminectomy. Hence, the operation should be avoided if the patient's character precludes the achievement of a good result.

ARTHRODESIS

By comparison with laminectomy, spinal grafting is a minor operation; for it is performed outside the spine without removing bone or exposing dura mater or nerve-roots. An incision is made; the muscles on each side are separated from bone down to the bases of the spinous processes where periosteum is stripped up locally. Two grafts are laid in place and secured here. It is the fact that the patient has to await fusion by lying for three months on a plaster bed and then remains immobilized in plaster for a further three months that gives the operation its formidable character. However, R. H. Young has developed a technique whereby the grafts are held in position by strips of aluminium foil; this method involves only one month in bed post-operatively. Transabdominal anterior arthrodesis has its advocates, but the reported results are on the whole less satisfactory and the rate of complications higher. Freebody keeps his patients in bed only three weeks, since the erect posture and any movement towards flexion squeeze the uniting surfaces more strongly together.

There is one great disadvantage to arthrodesis. The joint immediately above the fusion now takes double strain when the patient moves. After the operation many patients can still bend to reach their ankles, which must involve considerable stress at the other lumbar joints. Hence, some years later a fresh disc lesion is apt to appear at the joint just above the graft. Indeed, the few disc lesions that are encountered at the first or second lumbar levels are mostly the result of lower lumbar arthrodesis.

The indications are: (1) Spondylolisthesis causing ligamentous lumbar pain or bilateral sciatica. (2) Anterior protrusion (the mushroom phenomenon). The backache comes on after standing and ceases within a minute of sitting down or lying. (3) Nuclear self-reducing protrusions. The patient wakes comfortable and can do everything soon after getting up. By noon, backache begins which gets slowly worse as the day goes on but is abolished again by a night's rest. The pain is not severe, but persists for years, until finally the patient, understandably enough, insists on the only effective treatment, i.e. arthrodesis. (4) Unsuccessful laminectomy. (5) Intractable severe backache, absent on lying. If this is so, the operation stops the compression strain on the joint otherwise present when the body-weight falls on the joint. (6) Frequent severe attacks.

One important point must be observed before spinal fusion is undertaken—namely, that no displacement exists at the time when the operation is performed. This precaution is sometimes neglected, especially in spondylolisthesis with a secondary disc lesion, with the result that the symptoms continue and later the graft has to be removed and laminectomy carried out.

PREVENTION OF RECURRENCE

Once the displacement is reduced, or the protrusion has been removed at laminectomy, the question of preventing recurrence arises.

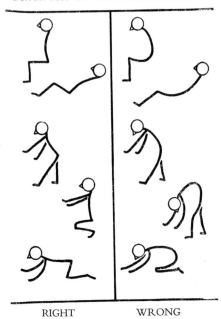

RIGHT   WRONG

Fig. 94. Posture chart. This card, showing how to avoid re-displacement in low lumbar disc lesion, is given to patients

Advice to the Patient

The mechanics of lumbar disc protrusion must be explained to the patient. He must be told that, so long as his lumbar spine is held in lordosis, movement backwards of the loose part of the disc is virtually impossible (Figs. 61 and 94). He must be shown how to stand, sit not crossing his legs, bend, and lift, using his knees rather than his back. His car-seat and his chair at home and at the office must be corrected so that the hollow in his back is maintained while he is seated. He must go on all fours if he wants to do things on the ground, e.g., weeding. Neurosis is prevented by explaining that the disorder is purely mechanical, and not the precursor of a crippling disease. With the exception of digging, he can go on doing whatever he did before; it is merely the way of doing it that has to be changed. Tennis and similar games must be avoided by patients with a fragment of cartilage loose in the joint; but in patients with a tendency to nuclear protrusion, the quick up and down of tennis does not matter.

Avoidance of Exercises

Exercises that maintain or enhance lumbar mobility are contra-indicated after a disc lesion. It is by keeping the joint still, not by moving it, that further intra-articular displacement is best prevented. Patients should be taught how to use their sacrospinalis muscles to keep the lumbar joints motionless in extension and to flex the trunk at hips and thorax. The inculcation of a permanent postural tone in the sacrospinalis muscles is taught as soon as the patient is seen, and he must grasp the idea of how preventing movement at a joint when forces act on it, is itself a muscular exertion.

Avoidance of Compression

Those who have to lift and carry heavy objects should take a tip from the Turkish furniture-remover. He straps a saddle round his waist and bends forwards until his trunk is horizontal. The saddle now bears directly on his sacrum and lowest lumbar vertebrae. The lordosis is maintained and the lower lumbar vertebrae are forced forwards by the load. But not compressed. The weight of the burden now passed directly from sacrum to pelvis to hip joints. Those who balance the weight they are carrying against one iliac crest are doing the same thing.

Support

A Plaster Jacket

This is usually employed wrongly—in the hope of securing reduction rather than of maintaining it. It is a mistaken policy to put a patient with an annular protrusion into plaster, for such displacements have been reduced by one manipulation, after as long as six months' vain immobilization. By contrast, pulpy herniations often do reduce themselves slowly in plaster, but these are the simple ones that do so much more quickly when treated by sustained traction or recumbency. Plaster acquires a spurious reputation when a patient with sciatica, who will get well of himself in the course of, say, eight months, is kept in plaster until he has all but recovered. He has, in fact, had a rather more uncomfortable time than necessary, but naturally attributes his relief to the 'treatment' imposed. One untenable reason for immobilization has been expressed (Crisp, 1948): that rest in plaster allows the broken cartilage to unite. Intra-articular cartilage has no blood-supply, therefore it cannot heal.

Patients are sometimes put into plaster to enable them to get about with the displacement *in situ*, and the endeavour may succeed. However, though it may stop the back from moving and thus prevent the severe twinges, it does so at the expense of the posterior longitudinal ligament. Weight-bearing with a displacement bulging out backwards is apt to cause permanent stretching and enhance the likelihood of recurrence.

The real indication for a plaster jacket is—as for a fracture—the maintenance of reduction. If reduction proves unstable, support must be supplied. A plaster jacket may thus be worn for a few days until a more suitable appliance is ready. Since a plaster cannot be made really tight or the patient's breathing is restricted after meals, and weighs twelve to twenty pounds, it should be abandoned as soon as the alternative is to hand.

A Plastic Jacket

This is far more effective than any plaster jacket and weighs only three to four pounds. It takes only two days to make and is hygienic; moreover, it can be worn for an indefinite period, whereas sooner or later a plaster must be removed. It can be taken off at night and can be tightened to any fit required, thus allowing changes in the volume of the trunk after meals. For any of the purposes to which a plaster jacket is put, a perforated plastic corset is better. It is pleasanter, lighter, non-absorbent and washable, and can be worn for months or years, if necessary, without renewal or getting out of shape.

A Corset

As a rule, neither a plaster nor a plastic jacket is needed. In the ordinary case, a surgical corset made of cloth with two posterior steels, or two anterior, or both, answers the purpose excellently. Whereas a plaster jacket cannot be worn for longer than some months, and thus cannot provide lasting protection against recurrence, corsets, renewed each year or two, can be worn indefinitely. If the two steels are accurately moulded to the lumbar curve, lordosis is maintained and the joints held steady in a good posture. Moreover, if the patient bends too far forwards or sags as he sits, the front of the corset presses unpleasantly against his lower ribs—a salutary reminder. Many patients fear that wearing a corset will weaken their sacrospinalis muscles. This apprehension can be allayed by explaining that these muscles extend as far as the neck and must still work to maintain the thorax erect. It should be explained that the corset acts as a postural educator. Every time the patient flexes his lumbar spine, the upper edge of the corset impinges against the lower ribs in front. Once the patient has learnt to avoid postures causing this recurrent discomfort, he can leave off the corset. Forgetful or impulsive patients may need to wear it indefinitely.

The essential features of a corset intended to support the lower lumbar spine are:

Stiffness

There must be two posterior steels accurately moulded to the sides of the sacrum and to the lumbar lordosis, and their tendency must be to hold the thorax slightly backwards; they must on no account press it forwards. If the curve of the steels is less than that of the patient's lordosis as he stands upright, the effect is to force the thorax forwards—the exact posture the corset ought to prevent. This is a common failing, making an otherwise acceptable corset worse than useless. These two steels must avoid pressing on the posterior superior spine of each ilium, to which they should pass laterally. The anterior whalebones must reach high enough to engage against the patient's lower ribs if he bends forwards too far. They must not indent the abdominal wall just under the ribs, as they will if they are too short, or they will erode the skin. A stiffener must not lie directly against the anterior superior spine of the ilium; it must pass medial or lateral to this. Some patients prefer anterior steels; if so, the posterior ones can be omitted or included, depending on how severe is the instability.

Balance

The centre of the posterior aspect of the corset must lie at the level of the lesion, so that there is the same extent of corset above and below the point requiring support.

Contra-indications to Corsetry

A corset is useless in lesions caused by compression, e.g., the mushroom phenomenon. It stabilizes the lumbar joints but cannot alter the compression of weight-bearing. A corset is contra-indicated in lumbar disc lesions secondary to unilateral osteoarthritis of the hip joint. As he walks, the patient, since he cannot extend at the hip, has to bring his thigh backwards by extension at his lumbar joints. Such excessive use leads to hypermobility and, later on, to a low lumbar disc lesion. If an attempt is made to control this by a corset, it is secured only at the expense of further hindrance to walking. Patients with heart disease or liable to indigestion or asthma often cannot tolerate a corset.

A Proper Seat

Nachemson (1963) has shown that the pressure on the disc while seated is 30 per cent more than standing and 50 per cent more than lying. Hence, it is not surprising that one of the commonest symptoms in lumbar disc lesions is pain in the back after sitting for some time. People remain seated for long periods in cars, trains, aeroplanes, theatres and in their own armchairs at home. They may also sit continuously in offices, where the whole staff may spend nearly the whole working day in chairs. The complaints that patients make about car seats far transcend, in number and degree, all the others put together. A person can move about in his chair and change his posture from time to time, but in a car his attention is focused on driving and he is fixed in the position that the car designers select for him. The defects of today's designs are so glaring that various devices to correct the shape of car-seats are available and their popularity is an index of the prevalence of disregard of anatomy. Yet it costs no more to make a proper seat than a poor one.

The essence of the design is, of course, that it maintains the driver's lordosis while he is seated. This obviates the wanton encouragement of backward stress on the disc in those who, as yet, have no lesion, no less than keeping in place the already damaged disc.

The requisities for comfort while sitting are:

1. *High Enough Chair*

Excessive flexion at the hip tilts the lower part of the pelvis forwards, thus obliterating the lumbar concavity from below. Hence the seat of a chair must be high enough off the floor to prevent flexion of the thigh on the trunk to more than a right-angle. To this end, the height of the front of the seat should be the same as the distance from the flexure at the back of the knee to the bottom of the sitter's shod heel.

2. *High Enough Car Seat*

In a car, the legs are more outstretched and the height should be such that the thighs are well supported when the feet rest on the controls. I.e. height equals the vertical dropped to the floor from the back of the knee when the driver is in position. The knee must not be held too straight or the hamstrings will pull the lower pelvis round; the minimum angle of the thigh on the leg is 45 degrees.

3. *Tilt for a Chair*

The upper surface of the seat of an ordinary chair is horizontal. Normally, there is nothing to bring the patient's lumbar region against the back of the chair and seek support there. This must be provided, and takes the shape of a plane, inclined downwards, occupying the posterior third of the seat. Naturally, in order to make the inclined plane effective in bringing the sitter's body backwards, the surface of the seat must be made of slippery material.

4. *Tilt for a Car Seat*

The whole seat can be tilted backwards. If so, the further angulation of

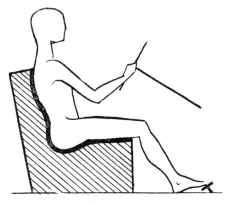

FIG. 95A. Tilted car seat with *further inclination* to accommodate buttocks

the posterior third of the seat surface can be made less marked. Again, the surface of the seat must be of glossy material to make sure that the driver slides backwards on the inclined surface.

5. *The Lumbar Support*

Some eight inches above the seat, a rounded support about four inches wide is provided to fill the lumbar concavity. This should not be too soft, and is two inches thick at the centre. It must be placed so as entirely to clear the sacrum, but to support the lumbar spine in lordosis from the fifth to the second level. It comes exactly where an individual's forearm rests when he puts it horizontally behind his back.

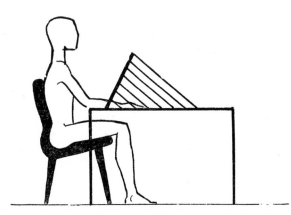

FIG. 95B. The extra tilt at the back of the seat brings the buttocks backwards; in consequence the lumbar region is applied to the back of the chair. The triangle on the desk makes the patient bend backwards, once more against the back of the chair.

6. *The Gluteal Concavity*

Below this lumbar support, the back of the seat is made slightly concave to accommodate the convexity of the driver's buttocks.

Stand for Office Workers

There is a further desideratum for those who sit at a desk for long periods. Naturally, however well designed the chair, it is no help unless the worker can keep his back in contact with it. He must not bend forwards all the time to look at, or write on, papers lying horizontally on the desk. This posture is avoided by presenting his work to him almost at eye level and slightly too close, so that he has to lean back away from it, as if he were long-sighted. To this end, the desk is fitted with a large triangle—merely an adaption of the old-fashioned music-stand. Papers put on this surface force the reader to lean away from them against the back of his chair, and writing is by no means impossible on such an inclined surface. Reading in this position has the further merit of avoiding prolonged flexion of the neck, a common cause of neckache in typists and headache in the elderly. Typists must have their machine in front of them. They should, therefore, be given a similar stand at eye level above their typewriter so as to prevent their necks being inclined downwards and to one side.

Inducing Posterior Contracture

Permanent shortening of the supraspinous, the adjacent part of the interspinous ligament and the ligaments that allow sliding at the facet joints would clearly prove beneficial in disc lesions by limiting the range of flexion at the affected joint. Two different ways of provoking posterior contracture present themselves.

Division of the Supraspinous Ligament

If the ligament is divided longitudinally and allowed to heal without lengthening, the scar will contract, like any other.

The overlying skin and the ligament are infiltrated with a local anaesthetic and the ligament divided by vertical cuts to a depth of 1 cm. in several places by a tenotomy knife. A plastic corset is then applied, maintaining lumbar extension for a month. This ensures that no lengthening takes place during healing. Thereupon the support is discarded and the patient awaits events.

Sclerosing Injections

This treatment was instituted by Hackett (1956). As a young surgeon, when operating on patients for hernia who had been treated years previously by sclerosing injections into the inguinal canal, he noticed hard lumps of fibrous tissue difficult to cut with a scalpel. Years later he applied this finding to the idea of ligamentous sclerosis. His original solution consisted of zinc sulphate and carbolic acid. R. Ongley of New Zealand, decided to try these injections out on a large scale. He varied his method and his solution until he found the most effective; Barbor and I profited by his extensive experience. Barbor (1964) described the method in detail, giving indications, methods and results. In 74 per cent of his patients satisfactory relief ensued.

The solution is available as P25G and was originally intended to sclerosing varicose veins. I use 8 ml. of the sclerosant mixed in the syringe before use with 2 ml. of 2 per cent procaine, without adrenalin (to avoid monoamine-oxidase inhibitor reactions); this amounts to a 0·5 per cent solution of procaine.

The patient lies prone.
One cc. is then injected into:

1. The fifth lumbar supra- and inter-spinous
   ligaments,   1 ml.
2. The fourth lumbar supra- and inter-spinous
   ligaments,   1 ml.
3. Each facet joint at the fourth level,   1 ml. each = 2
4. Each facet joint at the fifth level,   1 ml. each = 2
5. The iliac extremity of the ilio-lumbar
   ligament on each side.   1 ml. each = 2
                                                        ―
                                                      8 ml.
                                                        ―

This involves eight insertions altogether, but with a needle 7 or 8 cm. long tissues 1, 2, 4 and 5 can be reached by one puncture of the skin in the midline at the fifth level. The only ligaments difficult to inject are those of the facet joints. By a fresh skin-puncture, the needle is thrust in vertically. At about 5 cm. from the surface, the needle hits bone—the lamina or the base of the transverse process. It must then be manœuvred, about 2·5 cm. from the midline at the fifth level, and 1·5 cm. at the fourth level, until the point impinges not against unyielding bone, but penetrates a soft structure hitting bone a millimetre beyond. This is the ligament at the lateral joint, and the injection is given here at each of the four joints.

It is only fair to add that both Ongley and Barbor, the leading exponents of sclerosant therapy, take the view that secondary strain of the sacro-iliac ligaments complicates low lumbar disc lesions and they proceed to in-filtrate the posterior sacro-iliac ligaments as well, but I am too much of a purist to follow their example. A more detailed account of Barbor's experience and method of sclerosant infections, including infiltration of the sacro-iliac ligaments, follows on p. 588.

A chemical irritant is being forced into tough ligaments; this hurts. Then the local anaesthesia takes effect; hence, the discomfort ceases in a few minutes; soreness returns an hour later, of course, and the back aches for the next twenty-four hours. Three such infiltrations are given at seven- to ten-day intervals; after the last, the patient waits three weeks for the inflammatory response to resolve with fibrosis, and finally for contracture of the scar-tissue. During this time he must not bend forwards. By maintaining his lordosis at all times, he avoids stretching the intended contracture. He then tries out his back, carefully at first, and sees how much it will now take. If there is clear improvement, a further course may be considered some months later.

DISC LESIONS IN THE ELDERLY

After the age of sixty, most disc lesions are small and cartilaginous; therefore, they are nearly always reducible by manipulation. Moreover, they lie within joints at which movement, and therefore distraction, is very limited by osteophyte formation and ligamentous contracture. Hence, several months in bed, with or without traction, usually prove equally ineffective; for neither method achieves enough separation of the joint surfaces to let the displaced fragment slip back. Owing partly to the small size of the fragment of annulus and partly to sclerosis of bone at the joint margins, the young person's mechanism for spontaneous cure of root-pain does not operate; hence, not only backache but also sciatica can go on indefinitely.

The history is distinctive in sciatica; for the backache seldom ceases when the root-pain comes on. Examination shows some of the lumbar movements to elicit the backache in the expected way; trunk-flexion and straight-leg raising are seldom restricted and may not even set up pain in the limb. Muscular weakness is uncommon, and the ankle-jerk is apt to become sluggish only after many months; if so, it is even then worth while trying manipulation once.

In cases of this type, the orthopaedic physician's hand is forced. How-ever unwilling he may be, however old and frail the patient, however fearful both may be, the choice lies between leaving the patient in pain, perhaps for life, and manipulation. If they agree, manipulation must be attempted with adequate care but also with enough firmness to give the patient a chance of being helped.

Manipulative technique should be restricted to the prone-lying extension pressures and the rotation movements that are carried out with one hand on the buttock and the other on the thorax, since applying a rotation strain using the thigh as a lever might easily fracture the femoral neck.

DISC LESIONS IN PREGNANCY

Some women make room for the enlarging uterus by bending forwards over it, losing their lumbar lordosis. Others counterbalance the forward shift of their centre of gravity by bending backwards, increasing their lordosis. The former alteration in posture may result in backache. In contrast, these women with low lumbar disc lesions who adopt extension, find to their surprise that they are more comfortable when pregnant than at any other time.

A young woman with a lumbar disc lesion can be assured that pregnancy will not harm her back, and that labour itself will not be affected. It is the stooping involved in looking after the baby after the puerperium that is apt to make the backache worse. An expanding lumbar corset may be prescribed. She should, however, be warned that her posture in bed during the puerperium is important. Proper support for her lordosis must be forthcoming throughout the period of rest in bed (Figs. 59 and 80).

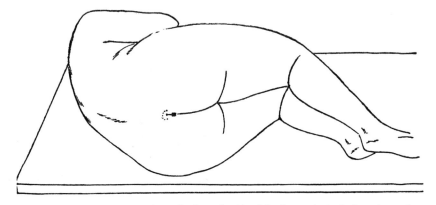

FIG. 96. Position of patient for induction of epidural local anaesthesia during advanced pregnancy. The patient lies on the affected side.

She should turn to lie prone for several periods each day as soon as her condition permits.

During the first four months of pregnancy a disc lesion can be treated by manipulation or traction in the same way as if the woman were not pregnant. During the next four months, traction and the prone-lying manipulations cannot be employed, but side-lying and supine rotations are still practicable. During the last month, epidural local anaesthesia remains quite safe and is often effective. The injection must be given with the patient lying on her side (Fig. 96). Since the fluid injected tends to gravitate downwards, she must lie on the affected side during the induction.

If the epidural injection fails, rest in bed is indicated.

DISC LESIONS IN ADOLESCENCE

If patients in their twenties with lumbar disc lesions are asked when their trouble began, they often recall an attack of lumbago while at school, or describe recurrent minor backache beginning at ten or twelve years old. During the early teens, though disc lesions are uncommon and usually dismissed as 'growing pains' or 'muscle strain', they certainly occur. Sciatica with limited straight-leg raising begins at twelve and, at this age, is much commoner in girls. The ankle-jerk may be lost alone. My youngest patients with a root-palsy so far are a boy of twelve with considerable fifth root weakness, and a girl of sixteen with a first sacral sensory and motor root paresis. In the latter, the muscles recovered full strength in three months. An X-ray photograph must be taken, to make sure that no bony disorder is present.

Diagnosis is always difficult; for young people are just as likely as adults to use an ache to avoid a disagreeable situation, such as an overbearing parent who wishes all sorts of things done. But it is hard to be sure that the inconsistencies such children show on examination are not just the product of a child's willingness to say what he thinks is expected of him, merely from a wish to please. Nevertheless, when the examination discloses the same pattern of inconsistencies as for psychoneurosis in adults, attention should be directed to the parent. If over-solicitude or domination is a factor, reference to a Child Guidance Clinic often has a good result.

When one of the normal patterns for a disc lesion is found on examination, the diagnosis should not be shunned merely because of the patient's youth.

In backache, manipulative reduction is the therapeutic standby, repeated as often as necessary, followed by the prevention of recurrence by postural training. When wedging of the vertebral body from osteo-chondritis is present, manipulative reduction will require frequent repetition at first. It is useless merely to tell a youngster that he must not bend forwards; he forgets; his life must be so arranged for him that he does not have to do so, i.e. no gym or games; but swimming and running are encouraged. Unless it is absolutely necessary, a corset should not be advised, particularly for boys during their time at boarding school; it is a great embarrassment.

Traction is seldom required, but is quite successful. One boy of twelve proved to have a protrusion irreducible by manipulation but recovered with traction and, by the age of nineteen, had had no further trouble. Rarely, a week in bed is indicated; this succeeded in a boy of ten with backache referred to the back of one thigh, in whom manipulation failedt By the age of seventeen he had had no recurrence. Nevertheless, most disc lesions in children do recur, although the fact that growth con-tinues enables articular changes to occur that may prevent further trouble.

Treatment in disc lesions causing root-pain is expectant. They are nearly always of the primary postero-lateral type and it suffices to explain that the disorder will pass off in about nine months from the onset, leav-ing the child well and able to do everything. Since the pain is never severe, however marked the physical signs, this period of waiting is not particularly disagreeable. Once the disc protrusion has reached its maximum size and is stable, epidural local anaesthesia is indicated, and I have given it from the age of fifteen upwards with consistent benefit. The last measure that should be considered in these young people is laminec-tomy; indeed, I have so far never found it necessary under the age of seventeen. This boy had had two months' unilateral sciatica and had 10 degrees range of straight-leg raising on each side. He was found to have huge protrusions at both the fourth and fifth lumbar levels.

There is one very curious type of backache without sciatica that begins only between the ages of fifteen and twenty-five. The pain is persistent and central and continues unchanged for years. The only sign is limitation of trunk-flexion and a corresponding *bilateral* limitation of straight-leg raising. It can be shown by epidural local anaesthesia to be caused by a low lumbar disc protrusion but, although a full range of straight-leg raising is restored for the time being, no lasting improvement follows. Only one such case of mine has come to laminectomy (D. H. Urquhart); a central disc protrusion at the fourth lumbar level was removed with excellent result.

Since the protrusion is central, its duration cannot be forecast; although straight-leg raising is limited, there is no root-pain and thus no tendency to spontaneous cure, at any rate within five years. Manipulation is quite useless; the only effective conservative treatment is traction, which has to be continued daily for at least two or three months. Neither doctor nor patient must lose heart if there is no improvement after the first month; persistence is essential and seldom fails to bring eventual reward.

BACKACHE IN CHILDREN

Under the age of ten, the likelihood of backache being due to a disc lesion is remote. However, Young's earliest case of sciatica was a girl of seven who had two years' sciatica with limited straight-leg raising, and he has described a case of lumbago in a boy of eighteen months. Fernström found postmortem a partly ruptured fifth lumbar disc in a boy of six. My youngest patient with lumbago was the daughter, aged $6\frac{3}{4}$ years, of one of my physiotherapy graduates; she recognized the disorder at once. The pain had lasted for five days after a fall; coughing hurt. Lumbar flexion and extension and full straight-leg raising hurt at the centre of the lower back and all my tests for psychogenic trouble proved negative. Manipulative reduction succeeded.

Backache in children is rare, and must be investigated thoroughly. If limitation of lumbar movement is present, the fact that the patient is afebrile does not rule out osteomyelitis or an extradural abscess, and the first X-ray photograph does not always disclose tuberculosis. Previous lumbar puncture should give rise to suspicion of an epidermoid implant.

Backache in children is very seldom due to neurosis; at that age such symptoms affect a limb.

DISC LESIONS AND SPORT

The emphasis throughout is on the fact that the patient can do much of what he did before, but must do it differently. He must flex his knees rather than his lumbar spine.

Swimming is the only actively beneficial sport. While in the water, the swimmer keeps his trunk extended in order to raise his head to breathe; moreover, he is suspended in a fluid medium and all compression on the lumbar spinal joints ceases. Diving is dangerous, since patients liable to lumbago have been known not only to become fixed in flexion in mid-air, but also to experience great difficulty in reaching land again.

Tennis can be permitted to patients with pulpy herniations, for the quick movements of down and up do not allow enough time for the nucleus to ooze. Patients with an annular fragment, on the other hand, play at their own risk.

Riding is harmless as long as the patient does not tire. While he is fresh, he maintains his lordosis—the correct posture for riding. If he continues to the point of fatigue, he may slump, thus losing his lordosis. Hence, he must work up to a day's hunting by degrees.

A schoolboy can usually play rugby football if he is kept out of the scrum.

INTRACTABLE BACKACHE

Originally I believed that backache arose from the muscles and ligaments of the lumbo-sacral region. In consequence, I spent much time in trying to single out these spots, and in infiltrating them with a local anaesthetic solution in an endeavour to confirm or disprove these tentative localizations. It is clear, of course, that I was treating secondary phenomena, but by infiltrating what I now realize were normal tissues at the site of pain and of referred tenderness, dramatic relief was occasionally secured without the solution reaching the lesion. The wheel has now turned the full circle, and Ritchie Russell (1959) points out the increasing evidence that pain can sometimes be relieved by treatment to the area where it is felt, ignoring the lesion. Hackaday and Whitty confirm this view (1967). He puts forward two hypotheses to explain this unlikely fact:

(1) Raising peripheral thresholds reduces afferent impulses, or
(2) The introduction of a competing system of afferent stimuli causes physiological interference with the passage of the noxious afferent impulses.

Since treatment of the site of pain, regardless of the site of the lesion, often consists in the local injection of anaesthetic solutions, my own view is somewhat different. After the induction, the subliminal impulses that normally reach the cerebral layers below the cortex cease for the time being. The patient, therefore, loses his subconscious awareness of possessing that part of his body, and is thus inhibited from feeling pain in it. The difficulty is to understand how this relief persists, as it may, long after the anaesthetic effect has worn off.

There is no doubt in my mind that backache does not arise from such points in the lumbar region as are found the site of localized tenderness.

For example, patients with a third or fourth lumbar disc lesion (as demonstrated by such unequivocal signs as a root-palsy) are all found more tender on the fifth lumbar supraspinous ligament than on the third or fourth. Localized tenderness on palpation found at a point inconsistent with the physical signs is common and must be ignored. Local tenderness does not indicate any lesion; it is the familiar phenomenon of referred tenderness resulting from pressure on the dura mater. In fact, apart from lesions caused by local contusion, backache arises from tissues beyond fingers' reach; hence palpation for tenderness is futile and can only mislead. However, when all rational methods have failed, neurosis is absent, no operative method appears applicable, rest by recumbency or support does not help, and the passage of time brings no relief, the time for science and logic is past.

Local Anaesthesia

In these cases, the induction of local anaesthesia at some spot, ligamentous or muscular, where marked tenderness has been found is worth trying, at least once. Sturniols (1966) in the Argentine pointed out that local anaesthesia induced at the tip of the third lumbar vertebra is an effective treatment for some lumbar lesions. (He calls it the apico-transverse syndrome.) It is, in fact, usually just about there that patients with unilateral pain are tender, and I too have had an occasional good result from local anaesthesia induced here.

Sclerosant Injections

There remains a hard core of cases—4·8 per cent in a series of a thousand cases (Cyriax, 1965)—undiagnosable today, in which the absence of relief for the duration of epidural local anaesthesia shows that a disc lesion is not responsible, and repeated clinical examination and radiography reveal nothing comprehensible. The ache is as often central as unilateral and may spread to one or both limbs. It is in these cases that empirical infiltration of tender spots, using Hackett's sclerosant method, is indicated and may succeed. He infiltrates ligaments not muscles, and his book contains a chart of where to inject according to whither the pain is referred (Fig. 97). The sacro-iliac ligaments are infiltrated if the pain radiates to the lower limb and it is regarded as a good sign if the referred pain that the patient recognizes is provoked by the injection (whereas I should regard it as evidence that a tissue derived from the correct segment was being infiltrated). His book contains a number of remarkable statements, one of which is that disc lesions do not occur. There exists at present no alter-

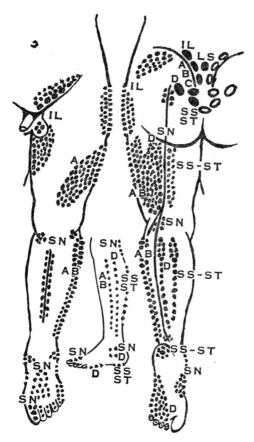

FIG. 97. The diagram in Hackett's book indicating where the injection is made, depending on the area to which pain is referred. *(By kind permission of the author and Messrs. Blackwell Scientific Publications.)*

native, and, though I have not been vouchsafed the consistent successes that Hackett achieves (82 per cent), some patients have been relieved when all else had proved fruitless. Previous laminectomy, arthrodesis or cordotomy are no bar to success in his view, and I can confirm that pain persisting or recurring after laminectomy has proved amenable to this treatment.

Indications

A good prognosis is afforded by the following criteria (Barbor, 1966):
1. Pain on standing or sitting some time. If the pain is brought on thus,

U

and is absent lying and walking, the likelihood of the injections succeeding is enhanced.

2. Adduction of the flexed thigh hurts. The patient lies on his back and the hip on the painful side is flexed to a right-angle. The examiner grasps the knee and forces the thigh into adduction, towards the other groin. If this hurts, especially if in unilateral pain it evokes discomfort only when that side is stretched, the prognosis is good.

In many of these patients, there is a history of past attacks of lumbago, and it is clear that initially the trouble was a disc lesion. Barbor considers that this may in the long run lead to ligamentous strain, not only of the posterior spinal ligaments but also secondarily of the ilio-lumbar and sacro-iliac ligaments. He therefore infiltrates each of these structures on both sides of the body, even when the pain is wholly unilateral, as well as the supra- and interspinous ligaments. In this type of case, the injections may well be regarded as desensitizing rather than sclerosant.

At St Thomas's Sanford is carrying out a double-blind trial of sclerosant therapy, and ligamentous infiltration with normal saline and with a local anaesthetic solution. The results are not yet to hand.

Pathological Investigations in Sclerosant Therapy

There can be no doubt that the fibrous tissue Hackett found in the inguinal canal was formed in response to sclerosant injections. Anderson and Duke (1924) described the histological picture produced by injecting haemorrhoids with phenol in 10 per cent solution of glycerine and water.

'Carbolic acid, being a powerful irritant to the tissues, initiates an aseptic inflammation, characterized by dilation of the vessels, emigration of leucocytes and transudation of lymph.

By these means the alien liquid is diluted and removed; thereafter, the inflammation quickly subsides.'

Troisier (1961) reported to me that visible ligamentous fibrosis could be provoked. A patient of his, who was to have his lateral meniscus removed, received three injections at weekly intervals of sclerosant solution into the coronary ligament at the knee two months before the operation. At meniscectomy, it was authoritatively agreed that the ligament had developed marked localized thickening, up to four times the normal, at the extent infiltrated.

In order to ascertain the sclerosing effect of the injection, a series of experiments were kindly carried out for me by M. Sarias, under Prof.

Trueta's direction. Unfortunately, the results were entirely negative. Twenty-two adult rabbits were used, aged about four months. He reports as follows:

Before injection the animal was given a general anaesthetic. The site of injection of the anaesthetic proliferent solution (1 ml.) in each animal was the interspinous ligament between L 5 and L 4. In half the animals 1 ml. of saline was injected in the interspinous ligament between L 3 and L 2, and in the other half 1 ml. of alcohol was injected. Nothing was injected between L 4 and L 3 in any of the rabbits, so a normal interspinous ligament could be compared with the injected one above and below.

4 rabbits killed 1 week(s) after injections

3	2
4	5
1	8
5	12
5	13

After being killed, each animal was injected through the upper abdominal aorta with a solution of 50 per cent micropaque and 50 per cent solution of 2 per cent Blue Berlin, so as to visualize radiogically and histologically the blood vessels. The whole of the lumbar spine was removed, fixed in formaline, decalcified, fine grain X-rayed, and sectioned and stained with haematoxylin eosin for histological examination.

Results

Fine grain radiography. No change was seen. *Histology.* The slides were examined under the light microscope at a low powered view. Attention was focused on the insertion of the ligament into bone, in the anaesthetic proliferent solution injected area, in the control area, and in the alcohol or saline injected area.

In the transitional zone into fibro-cartilage, no gross changes were seen in any of the three examined areas.

The proportion of collagenic fibres and amorphus intercellular substance in the two injected areas was like that of the non-injected area, as was the proportion of encapsulated fibroblasts and Sharpey's fibres. This picture remained constant, irrespective of the time after injection in which the animals were killed. The dark areas seen in the fine grain X-rays proved, when examined under the microscope, to be a free extravasation of the micropaque Blue Berlin injection with no tissue reaction around them, and they have the same characteristics in the anaesthetic proliferent zone, as they have in the alcohol or saline zone.

OBSOLESCENT TREATMENTS

Two measures have been universally employed in the treatment of backache in spite of their manifest lack of success. They are mobilization under anaesthesia and postural exercises.

Mobilization under Anaesthesia

The justification for this method of treatment rests on a misapprehension of the lesion present. Mobilization under anaesthesia—i.e. putting the joint through its full range of movement during complete muscular relaxation—is suited to rupturing adhesions. But in backache and sciatica no adhesions are present; a displacement exists requiring reduction. Admittedly, it can be reduced under anaesthesia, but only by good fortune and with difficulties and dangers that are avoided if the patient remains conscious. Reduction is not a set manipulation; each manœuvre depends on what effect previous steps have had. Deprived by anaesthesia of the patient's active cooperation, the manipulator has no idea whether to go on or stop, whether to repeat a manipulation or avoid it. Moreover, incontinence may result from the manipulation (it has been described) as the result of pressure on the fourth sacral root. Another hazard under anaesthesia is death from rupture of an arteriosclerotic aorta during forced hyperextension.

Even worse is forcing a full range of straight-leg raising under anaesthesia. However haphazard a lumbar manipulation *can* secure reduction, to treat the limb for a lesion in the back is unjustifiable. The only way benefit appears to follow 'stretching the sciatic nerve' is when the root is so tautened over the projection that an immediate pressure palsy results. Patients are encountered who lost their pain but acquired the weak numb foot of rootatrophy; they form a moderately pleased minority.

Postural Exercises

It is widely believed that postural exercises are an excellent remedy for backache. This belief is so ingrained that doctors tend to dismiss as fanciful or prompted by laziness, patients' complaints that the exercises make the backache worse. Nevertheless, the patients are right. Postural exercises are harmful in backache; they are suited only to children with postural deformity without backache. Even then they are of doubtful efficacy. There is all the difference in the world between teaching the patient to hold a certain posture and giving postural exercises. Strengthening the sacrospinalis muscles does not increase the stability of the lumbar joints, which is dependent on ligaments and the interlocking facet joints. The huge strength of a footballer's quadriceps does not hinder a rotation strain on the joint from breaking the meniscus. If a joint subject to internal derangement is exercised, it is moved to its extremes of range; as a result mobility is maintained and, with it, the liability to intra-articular displacements. If a joint is kept still in a position unfavourable to the development of internal derangement, obvious benefit follows. Postural instruction in the use of the sacrospinalis muscles to immobilize the lumbar joint, yes; postural exercises, no.

FUTURE TREATMENTS

Suggestions, not altogether fanciful, are as follows:

A New Disc

The restoration of the disc and its space is not a theoretical impossibility. A plastic substance in solution could be injected into the affected joint while traction kept the vertebral bodies apart. This would then set, enclosing the fragments of disc, during the time that the tautened capsule of the joint exerted centripetal force. The disc would then become one solid mass again, the hitherto loose pieces lying embedded in the plastic material.

This idea was put forward in the 1954 edition of this book and a year later Cleveland was filling the emptied joint at laminectomy with methyl-acrylic. This paste becomes solid by polymerization in about ten minutes, producing heat up to 180° F. Hamby and Glaser also introduced the paste at laminectomy and compared fourteen patients with and without acrylic implant. They detected no difference between the two groups in post-operative course or in the width of the joint spaces determined radiographically a year later. Then Fernström began replacing the nucleus pulposus with a stainless-steel ball-bearing in 1962. His published results of 191 such insertions by 1966 show the considerable advantages of the prothesis, and the retention of a good range of movement, visible radiographically. His figures were:

Post-laminectomy	Ball bearing (%)	No ball bearing (%)
Backache continued	40	88
Sciatica continued (protrusion found)	14	50
Sciatica continued (negative exploration)	47	80

Chemical Arthrodesis

An alternative is chemically induced arthrodesis. If a substance were discovered that promotes the formation of new bone and was introduced into the intervertebral joint, permanent fixation would be achieved without operation. Since capsular ossification occurs after bacterial arthritis, in ankylosing spondylitis and in fluorine poisoning, stimuli with this effect clearly exist. Animal experiments on the effect on joints of injecting various concentrations of fluorides in solution might well prove the starting-point for discovering a safe method suited to human joints. Giving fluoride by mouth is not advisable. It was given in dosage of 100 mgr. daily by Cohen (1966) for myelomatosis. Unfortunately, nausea, vomiting and optic atrophy were apt to result. Matin's research on implants of vesical mucosa in guinea-pigs offers another approach on these lines. At the site of implantation a cyst formed containing a glairy fluid which, on escape into adjoining tissues, stimulated bone-formation there. Should a similar phenomenon be reproducible in humans, a means of fixing the joint without operation in backache and arthritis at the hip may at last be in sight.

Simplified Arthrodesis

In the meanwhile, simplified techniques of arthrodesis not requring appreciable post-operative rest in bed ought to be investigated. The adjacent surfaces of two spinous processes might be stripped of periosteum and the interspinous ligament excised. A wedge of bone could then be introduced between the spinous processes. The two spinous processes would now be tightly wired together squeezing the graft. The patient should be allowed up in a plastic corset, holding the lumbar spine extended so as further to pinch the wedge, within a few days. It is difficult to believe that an operation on these lines could not become successful and remove the important disadvantage of arthrodesis: the long immobilization afterwards.

A Lasting Anaesthetic Agent

Epidural local anaesthesia abolishes backache and sciatica due to a disc protrusion for an hour or two; then the pain often returns. If a local anaesthetic agent could be devised that lasted for several months, it would be well worth while for those patients who have an intractable constant backache due to a minor disc lesion to attend at whatever intervals proved necessary for repeated epidural injections. It is very galling that, although a remedy for chronic backache and root-pain exists in theory, the agent appears no closer to discovery now than at the turn of the century.

Erosion of the Disc

L. Smith (1964) introduced an enzyme into the intervertebral joint. Apparently chymopapain disrupts polysaccharide-protein complexes, and can thus destroy the disc, without attacking bone or ligament. This treatment is clearly an arresting novelty.

TREATMENT OF OTHER LUMBAR DISORDERS

These are treated on standard lines.

Simple Wedge-fracture

Contrary to general belief, uncomplicated wedge-fracture of a vertebral body does not require immobilization in plaster. Indeed, many such fractures are discovered years later on a radiograph taken for some other reason.

A fortnight in bed, during which prone-lying trunk-extension exercises are prescribed, suffices. The patient must not, of course, lie with pillows in flexion. For a further month, he is up and about, but is not allowed to bend forwards. At the end of three months the fracture is consolidated. After that, however the vertebral body may appear on the radiograph, the presence or absence of symptoms depends on what has happened to the adjacent discs and to the patient's state of mind.

Fracture-dislocation

This is an entirely different matter. The spinal cord and cauda equina are in grave danger and surgery is usually required.

Fractured Transverse Process

A fractured transverse process is really a muscle-injury; it gives rise to muscle-signs and strictly unilateral pain. Hence the diagnosis becomes clear if the patient, after a blow on his back, is found to have pain on resisted movement when the joints and muscles are tested separately.

It is an unimportant injury, spontaneous recovery without treatment taking at most a fortnight. Whether eventual union by fibrous tissue or by bone takes place is insignificant. If the patient is anxious for exceptionally speedy recovery, he can be got well in less than a week by local anaesthesia induced between the bone ends; then deep massage is given to the lateral aspect of the scarospinalis muscle in the vicinity of the transverse process, followed by gentle exercises. Rest in bed, plaster and so on are all contra-indicated.

Force sufficient to break bone may damage the disc. Hence pain persisting longer than two weeks almost certainly arises from a lesion other than the fracture visible on the radiograph.

Adolescent Osteochondritis

If this causes symptoms, these appear due to a disc lesion secondary to the kyphosis at the affected joint that results from the wedging. Manipu-lative reduction should be carried out as required.

The wedging never becomes extreme and wearing a plaster jacket or rest in bed is not required.

Tuberculous Caries

For years, treatment has consisted of immobilization followed by arthrodesis. But Konstam and Blesovsky (1962), working on unpromising patients in Nigeria, achieved results quite as satisfactory by giving ambul-ant patients para-amino-salicylic acid and isoniazid for at least a year. Abscesses were drained and only those who could not walk were put to bed for an average period of three weeks while costectomy was carried out (28 out of 56 paraplegics). The result in patients without paraplegia were: 199 healed, 5 not healed, died, 3. In the 56 with paraplegia, 51 made a complete recovery; 2 others became able to walk; there were two operative deaths and no improvement in one case.

Senile Osteoporosis

This does not itself cause symptoms and care must be taken that elderly women with a disc lesion complicating symptomless osteoporosis are not regarded as suffering from the condition shown on the radiograph. If pathological fracture results, this causes bone pain for up to three monhs.

Calcium gluconate by mouth and anabolic steroids are said to arrest the disorder. Calcitonin, one of the hormones elaborated by the thyroid gland, diminishes the plasma-level of calcium and may prove a suitable treatment for osteoporosis.

Spondylolisthesis

If this causes lumbar pain of ligamentous origin, sclerosing injections may help. If not, and in bilateral sciatica, arthrodesis is required unless a corset affords adequate relief. A secondary disc lesion is treated on standard lines, disregarding the spondylolisthesis, but of course the liability to recurrence is much enhanced.

Chronic Osteomyelitis

Immobilization on a plaster-bed is instituted at once and maintained until ankylosis is well advanced. This usually takes three or four months from the time that it becomes possible to make the diagnosis with certainty. Antibiotics are administered, but as these patients often remain afebrile throughout, the best criterion of when to stop is return of the sedimentation rate to normal. If pain continues, surgical evacuation of the abscess in the vertebral body is indicated as soon as it becomes radiologically visible.

Osteitis Deformans

No known treatment has any effect on the disease as such, but if only one vertebra has collapsed and is causing symptoms, arthrodesis locally prevents increased pain and deformity. Butazolidine is often helpful.

Anterior Longitudinal Ligament

Since this suffers when the abdominal and sacrospinalis muscles are weakened as the result of myopathy or anterior poliomyelitis, a stiff corset or a brace is indicated according to circumstances. In spondylitis and vertebral hyperostosis, butazolidine is indicated.

Facet Joint in Spondylitis

Unilateral upper lumbar pain may result from invasion by the spondylitic process of one lateral articulation. Curiously enough, movement of the lumbar spine does not evoke or increase the constant discomfort and only the fact that the patient has sacral or lumbar spondylitis ankylopoetica brings the disorder to mind. The level must be ascertained as accurately as possible by palpation for tenderness.

One injection of 1 ml. hydrocortisone suspension affords many months' relief, but several endeavours may have to be made before the exact spot is reached.

PAIN ARISING FROM THE LIGAMENTS
OF THE LOWER BACK

by R. Barbor B.A., M.B., Chir., M.R.C.S., L.R.C.P.

Ligaments are fibrous bands, connecting one bone to another. Muscles move a joint; ligaments stabilize it. They are made of tough inelastic fibrous tissue which is capable of withstanding considerable force without tearing or stretching. Ligaments are connected at both ends to periosteum: some obliquely, allowing for a strong attachment; some at right-angles, making a weaker attachment more susceptible to minor ruptures.

A weakness occurs at the ligamento-periosteal junction when the fibrous tissue is strained by an accident or by continuous excessive tension. The latter results in what I call ligamentous fatigue; in my opinion such prolonged overstrain is the cause of much backache. Ligamentous fatigue may pass undetected, because the strain put on the ligament by clinical examination does not last long enough to set up the fatigue in the ligament that causes the symptoms. Mengert, in his paper on referred pelvic pain (1943), referred to such fatigue, as did Magnuson in 1944.

A ligament is weakest at its attachment to bone where the greatest number of nerve-endings and blood vessels are found, and it is here that it is apt to give way and later develop a painful scar. This can heal, but it is reasonable to assume that if normal healing does not take place the process can be restarted chemically by a substance which will produce a proliferation of fibroblasts. This was first advocated by Hackett in the U.S.A. many years ago, but the chemicals he used (phenol and zinc sulphate) produced such a painful reaction that we could not use it. I had previously used a dextrose sclerosant solution to obliterate varicose veins by proliferation of fibrous tissue, so Ongley of New Zealand and I substituted this preparation for Hackett's solution.

Applied Anatomy

1. *Supraspinous ligaments.* These run vertically between the spinous processes of the vertebrae to prevent hyperflexion of the spine.

2. *Ilio-lumbar ligaments.* These run horizontally from the fifth lumbar transverse process to the crest of the ilium and limit side-flexion of the fifth lumbar vertebra on the sacrum.

3. *Interosseous sacro-iliac ligaments.* These are short powerful fibrous strands adjacent to the articular surface of the joint, immediately above and posteriorly.

4. *Posterior sacro-iliac ligaments.* (*a*) The upper fibres run almost hori-

zontally from the posterior superior iliac spine to the upper four transverse tubercles of the sacrum. (b) The lower fibres run obliquely from the posterior superior iliac spine and blend with the sacro-tuberous ligament.

5. *Sacro-tuberous ligaments.* These are attached by a broad base to the third, fourth and fifth transverse tubercles, and to the outer border of the lower part of the sacrum and the upper part of the coccyx. The fibres run obliquely downwards, laterally and forwards, to be fixed to the medial margin of the ischial tuberosity, where some of them blend with the tendon of the long head of biceps femoris. This anatomical fact has a bearing on the straight-leg raising test, as considerable tension exerted on the hamstrings will be transmitted to the sacro-tuberous ligament.

6. *Sacro-spinous ligaments.* These are attached medially to the outer border of the lower part of the sacrum and upper coccyx, and run almost horizontally forwards and laterally to be attached to the spine of the ischia. The sacro-tuberous and sacro-spinous ligaments prevent the lower part of the sacrum from rotating backwards and upwards in relation to the pelvis.

Aetiology

Indirect trauma. A ligamentous lesion results from an accident straining the joint more than the stabilizing ligaments can withstand.

Shearing strain. This happens when the ilium is stabilized and the sacrum is forced forward as in a car crash, or downwards as when one falls on to one or both ischial tuberosities in a sitting position. The same strain results when the trunk is rotated while bent forwards, especially if a weight in the hands is swung from one side of the body to the other.

Lumbar hyperflexion. This can cause a strain of the supraspinous and/or the interspinous ligaments by sudden or repeated stretching.

Hyperextension of the lumbar spine. Although this movement relaxes the supraspinous ligaments, it can damage them by the 'kissing' of the spinous processes. It can also rotate the sacrum backwards on a fixed ilium, thus causing strain of the posterior sacro-iliac ligaments.

Puerperium. During the latter weeks of pregnancy the sacro-iliac ligaments soften and may be further stretched during delivery. Commonly, restitution occurs, but this may be prevented by a flexed posture during the puerperium. Persistent pain may result.

Fair wear and tear. Just as some people have not the muscular physique of others, so others have not the ligamentous strength. This is, of course, not measurable or visible, but the result is that the normal repetitive actions of everyday life produce ligamentous fatigue in some people.

Intervertebral disc protrusion. Just as a fragment of displaced cartilage in the knee sets up ligamentous strain, so can a displacement of disc-substance cause secondary ligamentous strain, especially of the supra- and inter-spinous ligaments. At the fifth lumbar level, the ilio-lumbar ligaments may suffer too. Over-stretching of these ligaments causes excessive strain on the sacro-iliac and, later, sacro-tuberous ligaments. This is an import-ant sequence of events. If the progression is not noted, a correct initial diagnosis will be made but an incorrect final assessment. In my experience this is a common event.

Symptoms of Lumbar Ligamentous Lesions

Response to Posture and Activity

The symptom is pain brought on when the ligament is stretched. The less the damage to the ligament, the longer the stretch must continue be-fore the ache begins. This fact must be accepted, since clinical examination may prove negative if tension is applied too briefly. Ligamentous pain is worse after immobility than during activity. Since the pain is not caused by a momentary stretch but by maintained tension, it is the maintenance of a posture that causes the ache. During activity, e.g. walking or playing games, the ligaments are under intermittent tension, whereas standing still or sitting sets up a continuous stretch in the posterior sacro-iliac ligaments that eventually brings on pain. The greater the ligamentous damage the more quickly the pain will start. The back feels stiff on waking and lean-ing over the wash-hand basin hurts at first. Any prolonged leaning for-wards, as in washing up or ironing, brings on pain, but bending down and up again produces no discomfort. By contrast, the patient will be able to play golf or tennis or even football without ill effect. A common com-plaint is of inability to stand for long, as at a cocktail party, or sit long, as in a theatre or a car, and the patient has to change his position frequently to keep comfortable. When the sacro-iliac ligaments are damaged, a violent cough or a sneeze may cause pain owing to the sudden pull of the trunk muscles on the sacrum and ilium. Patients often complain of a tingling sensation, sometimes described as a numb feeling, in the lower limb. Neurological examination reveals no alteration in sensation, but after the injection of a local anaesthetic agent into the affected ligaments, the paraesthesiae cease.

Reference of Pain as an Aid to Diagnosis

Ligaments, like most other structures, refer pain felt within the relevant dermatome. The ilio-lumbar ligament forms part of the second lumbar segment, hence pain from this ligament is felt in the second lumbar dermatome, namely over the greater trochanter and in the groin. An accurate idea of the situation of a pain greatly assists the discovery of which structure is at fault. Therefore, the patient must be led to describe where the pain started and where it has spread to, since this information indicates which dermatome contains the pain and narrows the search to the appropriate segment.

Areas of reference

(1) Low back centrally radiating to one or both sides: *supraspinous ligament.*

(2) Upper buttock, greater trochanter, groin and occasionally scrotum: *ilio-lumbar ligament.* (The ilio-lumbar ligament is often said to be derived from the fourth or fifth lumbar segment; if so, pain would be referred from it to the fourth or fifth dermatome, but in fact the area of reference is the second lumbar dermatome. In 1966 Duckworth, Professor of Anatomy at Toronto University, verified the surprising fact that it is innervated from the second lumbar level.)

(3) Lower buttock and outer and posterior surfaces of thigh and outer side of calf: *upper posterior and interosseous sacro-iliac ligaments.*

(4) Back of thigh, lateral side of back of calf and outer side of foot: *lower posterior sacro-iliac ligaments.*

(5) Back of thigh, back of calf and under heel: *sacro-tuberous and sacro-spinous ligaments. Note:* Pain felt in the second sacral dermatome, i.e. at the back of the thigh, is more likely to be referred from a ligament forming part of the second sacral segment than from pressure on the second sacral nerve-root.

These areas of pain reference were worked out by Hackett (1958), and agree closely with the segmental reference of pain described by Kellgren (1939) and with the shape of the dermatomes described by Foerster (1933). They have been confirmed by me by the use of local anaesthesia.

Summary

Ligamentous Strain	Disc Protrusion
1. Stiffness on waking	1. Rest eases condition
2. Prolonged sitting causes pain	2. Sitting may ease, but pain is increased on getting up
3. Prolonged standing causes pain	3. Prolonged standing may increase or decrease pain
4. Activity eases pain	4. Activity increases pain
5 Pain is nagging	5. Pain may be acute

Examination

Standing with Feet Together

Inspection
Ligament injury *per se* causes no asymmetry, but it will be noted, if there is a concomitant lumbar disc protrusion, or a sacro-iliac subluxation, or a short leg.

Lumbar Movements
Flexion: this movement rotates the sacrum forwards on the ilium, and therefore stretches the posterior sacro-iliac ligaments. As long as there is no low lumbar disc-displacement flexion is of full range, unless there is a subluxation of the sacro-iliac joint accompanied by a strain of the sacro-tuberous ligament. *Extension:* at its extreme this movement pinches the supraspinous ligaments and also exerts a backward rotary force of the sacrum on the ilium. In sacro-iliac strain it commonly causes pain but no limitation of range. *Side-flexion:* this movement tenses the ilio-lumbar ligament on the opposite side and the posterior sacro-iliac ligament on the same side becomes taut. The range is seldom limited in ligamentous strain unless there is also an acute sacro-iliac subluxation.

Lying on his Back

Straight-leg Raise
This movement is generally thought of as testing the mobility of the lower lumbar and upper sacral nerve-roots, but it does more than that. Clearly, full straight-leg raising also stretches the hamstrings, whose origin lies at the ischial tuberosity. Continuous with the tendon at the tuberosity is the lower attachment of the sacro-tuberous ligament to which tension is transmitted. Straight-leg raising may thus evoke pain from lesions of the sacro-tuberous ligament. Three signs are useful in differentiation from nerve-root irritation.

(1) When the leg is raised and pain has begun the examiner can raise the leg farther, in spite of pain, to full range in ligamentous trouble, whereas in the case of nerve-root irritation such spasm of the hamstrings is evoked as prevents any further raising of the leg.

(2) The straight leg is raised as far as possible until pain starts. The patient is then asked to bend his head forwards. Stretching the dura mater thus clearly has no effect on the lumbar ligaments and indicates that the nerve-root is at fault.

(3) When pain is produced on raising the leg, dorsiflexion of the foot further stretches the lower part of the sciatic nerve and increases the pain in root but not in ligamentous lesions.

Sacro-iliac Tests

(1) 'Springing' test. The patient lies supine and the examiner exerts a downward and outward pressure on both anterior iliac spines thus stretching the anterior ligaments. It is my experience that the anterior ligaments do not suffer from strain and that this test is positive only in sacro-iliac arthritis, which is the initial stage of ankylosing spondylitis. This test may well be positive months or even years before X-ray examination of the sacro-iliac joints shows the typical sclerosis (Cyriax, p. 607).

(2) The patient lies on his side and the examiner exerts pressure downwards on the upper iliac crest. This stretches all the posterior ligaments and is positive in sacro-iliac arthritis and in gross ligamentous lesions.

(3) The patient lies prone and pressure is exerted downwards on the sacrum, thus straining both sacro-iliac joints.

(4) A more specific manoeuvre tests each individual ligament. The patient lies supine. The hip-joint is fully flexed and then hyperflexed. This action tilts the pelvis forwards on the sacrum and also pulls on the ischial tuberosity via the hamstrings, thus tautening the sacro-tuberous and sacro-spinous ligaments. The test can be varied slightly; instead of full flexion of the hip, the hip can be fully adducted during 90 degrees of hip-flexion. This force stretches the posterior and interosseous ligaments of the sacro-iliac joint and the ilio-lumbar ligament on the side of the test. The hip is then flexed farther with less adduction and the thigh pushed obliquely on to the abdomen. This stretches the posterior ligaments and the sacro-tuberous and sacro-spinous ligaments. The offending ligament can thus be singled out.

Precaution. As the leverage of these tests involves the hip-joint, care must be taken not to confuse pain arising from the hip-joint with that from the sacro-iliac ligaments. Pain originating from the hip is felt in the third lumbar dermatome, i.e. at the front of the thigh, whereas these ligaments provoke pain referred to the buttock and back of the thigh. Moreover, the examination is not complete until the power of the lumbar muscles and the reflexes have been tested to exclude nerve-root damage or neurological disease.

Cutaneous Sensation

This should be tested especially at the extremity of the dermatome in which the pain is felt. The patient may complain of altered sensation, but in ligamentous lesions this is not demonstrable.

Palpation

Once the offending ligament has been identified, pressure should be applied to the structure in which the lesion probably lies, thus adding accuracy to the diagnosis.

Radiology

This is useful only to exclude bony abnormalities.

Summary

The following list may assist in the differential diagnosis between ligamentous injury and lumbar-disc protrusion.

Ligamentous strain	*Disc protrusion*
1. Trunk movements are of full range with or without pain; if limited by pain, they can be pushed to full range.	1. Trunk movements are limited in one or more directions by a block in the joint
2. Straight-leg raise is full, perhaps painful, or may appear limited at first but can be pushed to full range, sometimes with tilting of the pelvis.	2. Straight-leg raise is usually limited and cannot be pushed farther, because of spasm of the hamstrings.
3. Hip-flexion hurts unilaterally.	3. Hip-flexion is painless.
4. Hip-adduction in flexion hurts.	4. Hip adduction in flexion does not hurt.
5. No neurological signs, unless a disc lesion co-exists.	5. Often, signs of nerve-root pressure.
6. Palpation; the affected ligament is tender and pressure on it may set up the referred pain.	6. Palpation; there may be tenderness confined to the supraspinous ligament of the affected joint.
7. X-ray examination may show tilting of the sacrum.	7. X-ray examination excludes bony disease and may show a diminished disc space.

Table I: Causative Lesions

Low back pain			Thigh pain with or without back pain		
Disc protrusion	235	50%	Disc protrusion	148	39%
Ligaments including sacro-iliac	225	48%	Ligaments including sacro-iliac	223	59%
Other causes	9	2%	Other causes	7	2%
Total cases	469		Total cases	378	

Table I gives an analysis of 847 patients seen in my practice. The source of pain was deduced from the symptoms and examination on the lines set out above. Especial note should be taken of how many 'sciaticas' are due to ligamentous strain. My practice is highly specialized, hence these figures may well differ from those derived from general orthopaedic practice.

Treatment

Object of Treatment

The object is to increase the amount of fibrous tissue in the ligament at its attachment to bone, and minutely to shorten the ligament when organization of scar-tissue leads to the usual contraction. The intention is a stouter and shorter ligament. Such cellular proliferation is provoked by local infiltration with dextrose solution.

Precaution. Before treatment starts, the physician must make sure that no displacement persists at the joint whose ligaments are to be treated. Any subluxation at a sacro-iliac joint must be corrected by manipulation. If a fragment of disc is protruding at a lumbar intervertebral joint, this too must be reduced by, e.g. bed rest, manipulation or spinal traction. It must be remembered that the treatment to be described not only provides sound ligaments but also produces a tightening of those infiltrated. It is therefore unwise to tighten a joint while the displacement persists. However, after reduction of the protrusion, ligamentous sclerosis stabilizes the joint and lessens the liability to recurrence. Treatment is concentrated at the ligamento-periosteal junction.

Requirements

(1) Dextrose sclerosant solution (20–25 per cent dextrose, 20–25 per cent glycerine, 2 per cent phenol, pyrogen-free water to 100 per cent and $\frac{1}{2}$–2 per cent procaine in normal saline. These solutions are used in the ratio of two of dextrose to three of procaine solution. The aim is to inject half to 1 ml. of the mixture into the ligamento-periosteal attachments of all the affected ligaments.

(2) 10 ml. Luer-Lock syringe.

(3) six cm. 20 gauge Luer-Lock needle. Such a needle is long enough to reach all ligaments, except in very obese patients.

Technique

This may vary. Each ligament can be infiltrated via a separate insertion of the needle. Better, they can all be reached through one insertion in the manner now described.

Supraspinous ligaments. The skin is punctured between the fifth lumbar and first sacral spinous processes. The needle is aimed at the former, then

is withdrawn partially and aimed at the latter. If the supraspinous ligaments between the fourth and fifth lumbar spinous processes requires infiltration too, the fourth lumbar spinous process can be reached by again
partially withdrawing the needle and pulling the skin, and the needle with
it, upwards.

Ilio-lumbar ligaments. The lumbar attachment of the ilio-lumbar ligaments is reached by partially withdrawing the needle and then pointing
it at an angle of 45 degrees to the skin, aiming laterally at the tip of the
fifth lumbar transverse process. To reach the iliac end of this ligament,
the thumb of the free hand is placed on the iliac crest. The needle is now
partly withdrawn and the syringe brought down almost level with the
skin. The needle is now aimed deep to the tip of the thumb.

Interosseous sacro-iliac ligaments. The needle is partly withdrawn again
and directed laterally at 45 degrees to the skin, it is then thrust outwards
about two inches until it hits bone.

Posterior sacro-iliac ligaments. The slope of the needle is changed in the
direction of the posterior superior iliac spine. Infiltration here is performed at several adjacent spots since the ligamentous attachment at this
area is extensive.

Sacro-tuberous and sacro-spinous ligaments. The needle is partly withdrawn.
The skin is pulled downwards as far as possible, and the needle aimed at the
lateral border of the sacrum at about 30 degrees from the line of the spinal
column. These ligaments may be difficult to hit by this approach, in
which case the needle is withdrawn and the skin punctured lateral to the
border of the sacrum and the needle directed at the sacral ligamentous insertion. Occasionally the ischial attachment of the sacro-tuberous ligament requires sclerosis; if so, the upper and medial surface of the ischial
tuberosity is injected directly.

The injection

At each of these sites the plunger should be pressed *only* when the needle
is touching bone, for two reasons. First, because it is then in contact with
the ligamento-periosteal junction: second, this makes the injection
absolutely safe, avoiding accidental infiltration of, for example, a nerve or
blood vessel. Moreover, this precaution prevents perforation of the
ligamentum flavum or dura mater. At each site 0·5 to 1 ml. of the mixture
is injected. The whole process is repeated on the contra-lateral side, as this
is usually affected to a lesser degree. In all, twelve sites are infiltrated with
10 ml. of solution. All the ligaments are infiltrated again a week, and then
another week, later. Some patients require more than three treatments,
and many require 'booster' treatments at varying intervals.

Immediate Results

In cases of pure ligamentous strain, a common sequence follows the first infiltration. Patients usually report that the back was sore and tender at the site of the injection for up to 48 hours; after that there was an improvement for two days or even two days' freedom from pain; on the fifth or sixth day the pain returned, but with less intensity. When questioned on the seventh day they frequently say they are no better because they have forgotten the one or two days' improvement! On re-examination their physical signs should have diminished; indeed they have frequently disappeared, even though the pain has returned. During the week after the second injection the pattern is roughly the same but less discomfort returns at the end of that week. Before the third injection, testing the lumbar and sacro-iliac ligaments no longer causes pain in the majority of cases. About fourteen to twenty days after the third injection all pain should have ceased. In very long-standing chronic cases, success may be achieved only after six weeks.

Rehabilitation

By the time the sclerosant has taken effect, i.e. three or four weeks after the last injection, it is essential that the back should be used normally. A full range of movement should be obtained and retained. To this end trunk side-flexion exercises are prescribed. Rhythmic games such as golf and swimming are excellent, so is walking. I find the most difficult aspect of this treatment is to give the patient sufficient confidence once more to use his back normally, especially those who have in the past been instructed not to move it at all. Failures due to refusal of active movement are encountered, but many of these patients recover without further ado after they have agreed to increase activity.

Table II: Ordinary Results

Relieved to the patient's satisfaction	111	74%
Of these, 'booster' injections required for maintained relief	31	21%
Failed	17	11%
'Lost'	25	16%

This first series contained 153 patients complaining of chronic backache with or without limb pain. They had symptoms of ligamentous strain, verified by examination. The duration of the complaint varied from six months to twenty years. All patients had previously had many forms of treatment. The results were obtained from the answers to a letter of inquiry sent one year after treatment had been completed. It will be noted that 74 per cent of the patients were relieved, but of these, 21 per cent equired a fourth injection within the year.

Table III: Exceptional Results

Relieved to patient's satisfaction	37	57%
Improved	5	8%
Psychogenic	3	5%
No improvement	11	17% 28%
Laminectomy	4	6%
'Lost'	5	8%
Total cases	65	

This was a carefully selected series of formidable cases, intended to put sclerosis to the most searching test possible. These sixty-five patients were all seen by Cyriax in the course of a year and were regarded by him as entirely intractable, unless sclerosis were to succeed. All had had every imaginable sort of treatment, and some were hypersensitive, though in none were the symptoms wholly psychogenic. All but five answered a letter sent to them six to twelve months after treatment had been completed. That 57 per cent of patients should have experienced full relief is regarded by both of us as very satisfactory; indeed, in Cyriax's view a good result in only one case would have provided cause for congratulation. Of the 28 per cent who showed no improvement, 5 per cent required psychiatric treatment, 6 per cent required surgical interference, and 17 per cent had to learn to live with their discomfort.

22

The Sacro-iliac Joint

Lesions of the sacro-iliac joint are as rare as pain at the inner aspect of the buttock is common.

NOMENCLATURE

The uncertainty that surrounds the vexed question of 'sacro-iliac strain' is almost wholly caused by loose nomenclature. This term may be used for any pain felt at the medial part of the buttock, implying merely pain felt in the sacro-iliac region; alternatively it is used to designate pain arising from the sacro-iliac ligaments. The former usage is to be deplored; for a better word in such cases is 'gluteal pain'; the term 'sacro-iliac strain' should be reserved for pain originating in the sacro-iliac ligaments. The disagreement between the views of those who hold sacro-iliac strain to be a common cause for low backache and sciatica and those who doubt its very existence is based on differences in the interpretation of physical signs.

Great individual variations exist in the criteria held to justify a diagnosis of sacro-iliac strain. When pain felt in the sacro-iliac area with local tenderness suffices, strain is found to have occurred in a fair proportion of all patients with gluteal pain, but when the diagnosis is restricted to those showing a positive response to one or more of the sacro-iliac tests set out below, the incidence is only 1 in 230 in my experience.

The term 'sacro-iliac strain' should be reserved for cases of pain arising from the sacro-iliac ligaments in the absence of arthritis. This creates a difficulty; for in 14 per cent of cases of early sacro-iliitis the pain and clinical signs precede the appearance of radiographic sclerosis. Sacro-iliac strain never alternates, whereas in one-third of all cases of arthritis this is mentioned. Unless, therefore, the pain has lasted for some years, negative X-ray appearances do not preclude arthritis.

SACRO-ILIAC MOBILITY

Whether or not movement occurs at the sacro-iliac joint has long been a vexed question. If it can move, then the fixed subluxation so dear to lay-manipulators is at least a possibility. In fact, a small range of rotation does exist between the sacrum and ilium, elicited at the extremes of flexion and extension of trunk on pelvis. The axis is horizontal and transverse, and lies about a third of the way down the auricular surface, where a small prominence on the ilium fits into a corresponding depression on the sacrum. This rotation enables the individual to bend a little farther forwards and backwards than would otherwise have been possible. When the patient stands and bends forwards, contraction of the psoas and rectus abdominis muscles draws the upper part of the sacrum forwards as far as the sacro-tuberous and sacro-spinous ligaments will allow. Mobility at the sacro-iliac joint, therefore, relieves part of the flexion strain on the lumbar spine by providing rotation elsewhere; this is clearly beneficial and no endeavour should be made to diminish it, particularly if a lumbar lesion is already present.

Mobility doubtless decreases with age; for elderly patients often possess osteophytes at the lower margin of the sacro-iliac joints. Clearly such ligamentous ossification must diminish the range of movement and may eventually fix the joint, as does ultimate fusion in advanced ankylosing spondylitis.

The possibility of a fixed sacro-iliac subluxation causing symptoms is very dubious; no evidence for it exists. It is hard to grasp how the displacement could be maintained if it did occur; for no muscles span the joint that, by their contraction, could keep it displaced. The joint contains no intra-articular meniscus; hence, it cannot suffer the type of internal derangement that is so common at the spinal joints and the knee, where muscle guarding does militate against reduction. It is not to be denied that pain can arise in the sacro-iliac ligaments from strain in cases of excessive ligamentous laxity or from spondylitic inflammation, but I find no evidence for the concept of pain arising from fixed subluxation.

Stimulated by a conversation with Barbor in 1965 on tests for sacro-iliac mobility, Professor Duckworth of Toronto carried out a series of postmortem studies on fresh specimens, and has kindly sent me a summary of his findings (1967).

'*Movement at the Sacro-iliac Joints.* The normal movements that occur at the sacro-iliac joints are determined by the direction of the auricular surfaces, the ligaments, the muscles acting on the joint, and the symphysis pubis.

The movement that occurs is a rotation of the sacrum (or ilia) around the axis of the shortest and strongest part of the posterior interosseous sacro-iliac ligament, which is situated in the angle between the postero-superior and postero-inferior limbs of the auricular surfaces. When rotation of the upper end of the sacrum occurs in a forward direction the promontary of the sacrum will move in an anteroinferior direction, narrowing the antero-posterior diameter of the pelvic inlet, widening the antero-posterior diameter of the pelvic outlet and tightening the sacro-tuberous and sacro-spinous ligaments. On backward rotation of the upper end of the sacrum, the reverse movements will occur together with a widening of the antero-posterior diameter of the pelvic inlet, a narrowing of the antero-posterior

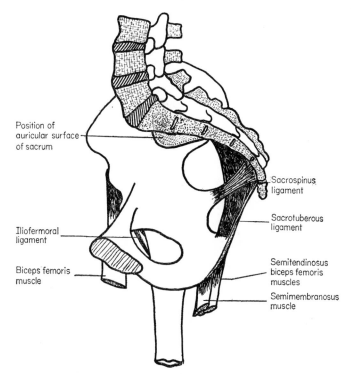

Position of
auricular surface
of sacrum

Iliofermoral
ligament

Biceps femoris
muscle

Sacrospinus
ligament

Sacrotuberous
ligament

Semitendinosus
biceps femoris
muscles

Semimembranosus
muscle

Fig. 98a. Median section of bony pelvis showing ligaments and muscles acting on sacro-iliac joint.

diameter of the pelvic outlet and a relaxing of the sacro-tuberous and sacro-spinous ligaments. During the above movement the long posterior sacro-iliac ligaments will tighten and restrict this backward rotation of the sacrum on the ilia.

In addition because the auricular surfaces of the sacrum are nearer the median plane inferiorly than they are superiorly, forward rotation of the sacrum will result in a slight widening of the symphysis pubis, while backward rotation of the sacrum will result in the symphysis pubis being compressed.

When a rotation force is applied to the hip bones in opposite directions such as in extending one thigh while flexing the other thigh, e.g. in stepping up on to a high stool, the extended thigh anchors the hip bone on that side through the ilio-femoral and ischio-femoral ligaments and the rectus femoris muscle, while the flexed thigh through the pull of the hamstring muscles rotates the ilium in a backward direction. In addition, the sacrum will move with the ilium on the flexed side because the pull of the hamstring muscles is transmitted to it via the sacro-tuberous and sacro-spinous ligaments. The result above of the facts will be that rotation of the sacrum in a backward direction will occur at the sacro-iliac joint on the extended side only.

While these movements at the sacro-iliac joints are small in extent, especially in males, they are quite definite. They are increased when jumping from a height, and in females especially towards the end of pregnancy and for up to three months after pregnancy, owing to the action of the hormone relaxin.'

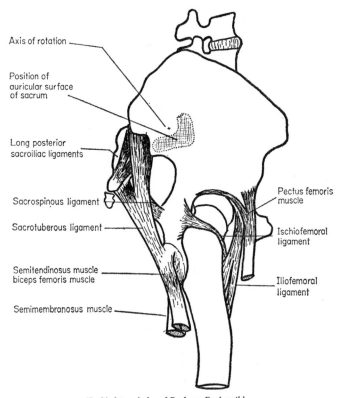

Axis of rotation

Position of
auricular surface
of sacrum

Long posterior
sacroiliac ligaments

Sacrospinous ligament

Sacrotuberous ligament

Semitendinosus muscle
biceps femoris muscle

Semimembranosus muscle

Pectus femoris
muscle

Ischiofemoral
ligament

Iliofemoral
ligament

(By kind permission of Professor Duckworth)

FIG. 98B. Lateral view of pelvis showing ligaments and muscles acting on sacro-iliac joint. The position of the axis of rotation is also defined.

TESTING THE SACRO-ILIAC JOINT

The finding that directs immediate attention to the sacro-iliac joint as a possible cause of pain in the buttock and/or thigh is the unusual discovery that no lumbar movement affects the gluteal symptoms. Rarely, in acute arthritis, the lumbar movements do increase the pain a little, since at the extreme of any lumbar movement an added stress falls on the sacro-iliac ligaments. This does not confuse; for, if such an indirect strain on the joints hurts, much more severe pain is set up as soon as the sacro-iliac joints are directly tested.

Three methods exist whereby tension can be exerted on sacro-iliac ligaments without affecting the lumbar spine. These are:

1. Stretching the Anterior Sacro-iliac Ligaments

The patient lies on his back. The examiner places his hands on the anterior superior spine of each ilium and presses downwards and laterally. Crossing the arms increases the lateral component of the strain on the ligaments. Such pressure applies the patient's sacrum to the couch, of

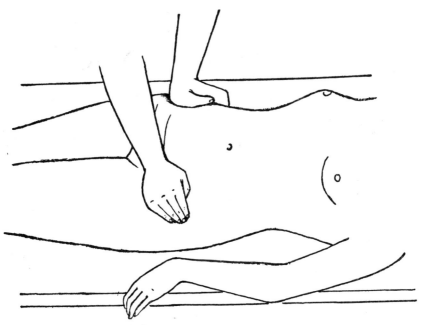

Fig. 99. Stretching the anterior sacro-iliac ligaments. The patient lies supine and the examiner applies increasing pressure to the anterior superior spines of the ilia in a downward and outward direction. The pressure must be exerted evenly so that the lumbar region does not move

course, and may prove uncomfortable centrally. This the patient can identify as due to pressure on the skin, and is quite different from his deep-seated unilateral ache. The pelvis must not be allowed to rock, since the lumbar spine then moves. The examiner's hands cause discomfort anteriorly, and it must be made quite clear to the patient that what is sought is not local pain but aggravation of the gluteal symptom. The response to this test is positive *only if it is stated to evoke unilateral gluteal or posterior crural pain.*

Stretching the anterior ligaments in the manner described is the most delicate test for the sacro-iliac joint. It is interesting to note that patients recovering from a flare may say that all pain ceased some days before. They walk and bend about painlessly; yet for a week or ten days after subjective recovery, straining the joint in this way still evokes the remembered discomfort. It is thus clear that this test applies more stress to the sacro-iliac ligaments than do ordinary daily activities. Hence, if a patient has symptoms referable to the joint, this manœuvre will elicit them.

Two other ways exist of stretching the anterior ligaments indirectly: forcing lateral rotation at the hip joint and resisted adduction of the thighs. The patient, by squeezing the examiner's hand between his knees, exerts an equally strong distraction force at the sacro-iliac joints.

When ankylosing spondylitis is more advanced and reaches the lumbar spine, testing the sacro-iliac joints ceases to hurt. They are by now painlessly fixed. In, say, acute lumbago, this test is sure to appear positive; for the slightest movement transmitted to the lumbar spinal joints must prove most painful; hence, the support of a cushion or of the patient's forearm under the back may be required to stabilize the lumbar joints. In any case, in lumbago far greater pain is elicited when the lumbar movements are examined.

2. Stretching the Posterior Sacro-iliac Ligaments

The patient lies on his side and the uppermost part of the iliac crest is pressed towards the floor. If the pressure is applied well forward along the bone, the posterior ligaments bear the greater stress (Fig. 100). This test is much less delicate and gives rise to pain only in severe cases; indeed, in half of all patients, no discomfort is caused thus. Its advantage lies in the fact that the sacrum is not in contact with the couch, thereby obviating confusion between pain due to pressure of the couch on the skin and that due to stretching the ligaments.

Two other ways exist of indirectly stretching the posterior sacro-iliac ligaments: forcing full medial rotation at the hip and adducting the flexed thigh across to the other side of the body. The latter clearly does apply tension there, but also stretches the gluteal muscles and hip joint and is thus not very specific. Nevertheless, Barbor finds it a useful prognostic test: if it sets up the pain in the buttock, sclerosing injections at the posterior sacro-iliac ligaments are likely to prove beneficial.

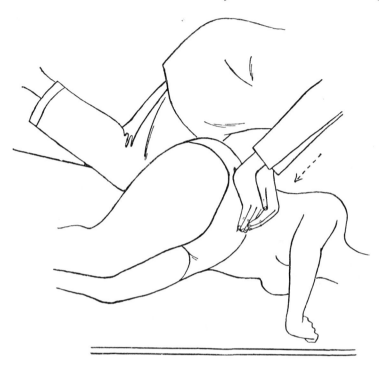

FIG. 100. Stretching the posterior sacro-iliac ligaments. The patient lies on the painless side while the examiner exerts pressure towards the floor on the antero-lateral part of the iliac crest.

3. Forward Pressure on the Sacrum

This is a repetition in reverse of the first test for the sacro-iliac ligaments (Fig. 101). The patient lies prone and the sacrum is pressed smartly forwards while the pelvis stays motionless, supported on the couch. It has the advantage that the examiner can compare the amount of pain—felt in the buttock, not where his hand rests—produced when passive extension of the lumbar spine and forward luxation of the sacrum are attempted in turn. If a lumbar lesion is causing pain in the buttock, this will be evoked only by an extension strain applied to the lumbar spine. If the lesion is sacro-iliac, although transmitted stress usually results in slight gluteal aching when the lumbar spine is pushed towards the couch, much more severe pain is set up when the sacrum is pressed upon. Illouz (1964) confirms the value of this method of eliciting pain from the sacro-iliac ligaments; he calls it 'the sign of the tripod'.

During any of these movements, a slight local click may be felt in adolescent boys and in women of childbearing age; it does not hurt. If, instead of a click, a snap is felt as if an adhesion had parted, the radiograph nearly always shows 'sacro-iliitis condensans'.

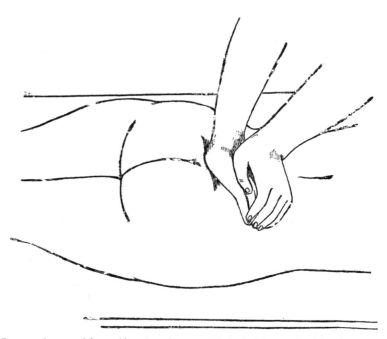

FIG. 101. Attempted forward luxation of sacrum. The heel of the examiner's hand presses on the centre of the patient's sacrum.

CONFIRMATION

1. *Negative Component*

Examination of the lumbar spine and lower limbs reveals no disorder contradicting the ascription of the symptoms to the sacro-iliac joint. Straight-leg raising is not limited; there are no neurological signs; the arteries are patent; there is no palpable mass in the buttock; and so on. Each rotation of the hip may prove painful *at full range*; this is a consistent finding, since forcing this movement stretches the sacro-iliac ligaments. In psychoneurosis, strong pressure on bony points is often strongly resented; hence the examination must include the lower limb in order to reveal the inconsistencies that indicate the presence of pain caused emotionally.

2. Tenderness 'Over the Joint'

Tenderness 'over the sacro-iliac joint' usually implies tenderness of the upper sacral extent of the sacrospinalis muscle. A glance at Plate 53, which shows the relations of the sacro-iliac joint, should finally dispose of the idea that tenderness of any structure within reach of the human finger denotes tenderness of the sacro-iliac ligaments; for they lie covered by the overhang of the ilium and the sacral extent of the sacrospinalis muscle. Hence, even if the joint is at fault, tenderness will not be found. By contrast, since referred tenderness is a common finding in lumbar-disc lesions, the discovery of tenderness somewhere in the region of the sacro-iliac joint is then a likelihood—a positively misleading sign.

3. Local Anaesthesia

This cannot be induced at the anterior sacro-iliac ligaments, and injecting the whole of the posterior mass of ligaments would prove a huge task. Hence, positive confirmation by local anaesthesia is impracticable. In a sincere patient with an uninformative radiograph, it is my practice to carry out negative confirmation by inducing epidural local anaesthesia, in case, after all, a lumbar-disc lesion should be responsible, especially in those cases where both the lumbar and the sacro-iliac tests are stated to hurt. If, when the sacro-iliac joints are tested, say, a quarter of an hour later after the injection has been completed they still hurt, a lumbar-disc lesion with false sacro-iliac signs has been excluded.

4. Radiography

This may help. In sacro-iliac strain nothing is revealed. This is in keeping with the results of radiography of a skeleton pelvis (J. Young, 1940). X-ray photographs taken with the symphysis pubis closed and forced wide open showed no detectable change at the sacro-iliac joints. In the sacro-iliac arthritis of early spondylitis, the radiograph shows the typical sclerosis in 86 per cent of cases. Sclerosis also occurs in Reiter's disease, chronic rheumatoid arthritis, psoriasis, ulcerative colitis and sarcoidosis, but pain in the buttock is then a rarity, the sclerotic process being painles. I have met only one patient with Reiter's disease and one after colectomy for colitis, who had attacks of pain in the buttock arising from the sacro-iliac joint.

In spondylitis, the iliac side of the lower part of the joint shows the sclerosis first, with blurring of the articular margin. It is often bilateral in cases of purely unilateral pain; when unilateral, it is usually on the same side as the symptoms, but not always. After many years, the joint disappears and sacrum and ilia fuse, obliterating the joint (Plate 55).

It is widely believed that a diagnosis of spondylitis ankylopoetica can be made only by inspecting the radiograph, and that a normal appearance of the sacro-iliac joints excludes this disease. This is not so. Clinical signs at the sacro-iliac joints may precede by months or years the appearance of early sclerosis. Spondylitis spreading up the vertebral column without sclerosis ever appearing on the radiograph of the sacro-iliac joints is a rarity; I have met four instances only. In one patient, whose first symptom was increasing stiffness of the neck, one sacro-iliac joint was normal, the other fused.

5. *Sedimentation Rate.*

This too may help, but much cannot be expected in the difficult cases. When the disease is obvious, the erythrocyte sedimentation rate is greatly raised, perhaps to 50 mm. or even 100 mm. in the first hour. However, in a doubtful case, the sedimentation rate is apt to be in the region of 5 to 10 mm. and thus prove of no assistance.

Lay Manipulators and the Sacro-iliac Joint

They describe a number of other tests for the sacro-iliac joints, some direct, some straining the joint from a distance. I have compared the specificity of some of these tests with the three advocated above, on patients with pain arising from the sacro-iliac ligaments, confirmed radiographically, in early spondylitis. The upshot has been that springing the pelvis and pressing the sacrum forwards on the iliac bones have proved the most delicate and reliable tests.

Much controversy exists among lay manipulators on what signs are and are not compatible with a sacro-iliac subluxation. Some maintain that a sacro-iliac subluxation can cause such and such limitation of straight-leg raising, but that greater restriction indicates a disc lesion. I have therefore been at pains to test these movements on patients with severe degrees of spondylitic arthritis, some bad enough hardly to be able to walk. Presumably, such arthritis would produce more advanced physical signs than a mere minor subluxation.

The signs were those to be logically expected. Any movement straining the joint proved painful but was not limited. In addition to a positive result from the three tests advocated above, full trunk-flexion puts a rotational strain on the joint, as does full straight-leg raising. Trunk side-flexion towards the painful side increases the shearing stress on the joint. At their extremes, all passive movements of the hip stretch the joint and resisted adduction of the thighs distracts the articular surfaces. All these movements hurt at the buttock, but none was limited in range. In particular, straight-leg-raising has never been found limited and no muscle spasm could ever be detected.

Sacro-iliac Arthritis

Although it is well-recognized that ankylosing spondylitis begins radiologically at the sacro-iliac joints, it is not widely appreciated that this can also be established by clinical examination. Spondylitis may begin as a pain in one or other buttock or thigh; if so, clinical examination shows one sacro-iliac joint to be at fault. Radiography usually confirms this, but clinical signs may precede the radiological evidence by some years.

Pathology

The ligamentous ossification in the advanced case is well-known. The periphery of each intervertebral is ossified and the facet joints are also the site of bony ankylosis. The ilia and sacrum fuse. Postmortem studies of early cases are few but Bywaters (1968) reports that the disease starts by invasion of articular cartilage, and its localized replacement, by granulation tissue. About these areas the bone is sclerotic. Pannus can be seen at the facet joints causing marginal erosion of cartilage; His conclusion on the aetiology of spondylitis is 'some change in cartilage, or some change in the body's reactions to cartilage, whereby the latter becomes an active auto-immune target, so that it gets invaded either at the margins where it joins normal connective tissue, or where the normal bony layer protecting it from marrow blood vessels becomes deficient'.

Frequency

Between 1950 and 1965, 18,629 patients with pain in the lower back, buttock or thigh were seen by me at St. Thomas's Hospital. Of these, 255 were suffering from ankylosing spondylitis, and 81 of them were in the stage of early sacro-iliac involvement only (52 men and 29 women). This is probably a higher proportion than in the general run of spondylitics; for St. Thomas's is known to attract the problem of obscure back trouble. In consequence, I doubtless see an undue preponderance of patients suffering from hitherto intractable sciatica.

These patients were singled out because in every case the sacro-iliac joints were tested clinically as part of the routine examination of the lower back. It is true that most spondylitis begins as a diffuse lumbar ache; sometimes the earliest symptoms are thoracic; in a few, painless inability to turn the neck first draws attention to the disorder. In these cases, although radiography of the sacro-iliac joints shows gross sclerosis or even fusion, testing the joint clinically provokes no discomfort, since this can be elicited only in the early stage of active inflammation in the sacro-iliac ligaments.

It is interesting to note that in these 81 cases, no less than 70 showed sclerosis on the first radiograph, and in the rest it appeared on skiagrams taken later, but in two cases it took five years for this to happen. Clinical testing of the joint is, therefore, a very accurate means of deciding whether it is affected or not, more so indeed than radiography, although the two seldom fail to tally.

Age

The age at onset of the pain in the buttock and thigh is shown in the accompanying table. The figures for men and women are virtually the

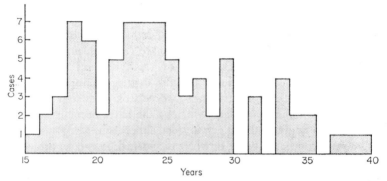

FIG. 102. Age at onset of sacro-iliac arthritis

same; the disorder is merely twice as common in men. Clinical arthritis can begin any time between the age of 15 and 39 and has its maximum incidence between the ages of 18 and 29. In this series, no case of sacro-iliac arthritis began at, or over the age of forty, but I have encountered two cases, confirmed radiologically, in a man of 48 who had pain in the buttock after some years of recurrent iritis; and in a woman of 47.

Symptoms

The usual complaint is pain in one buttock radiating perhaps to the back of the thigh and calf. The pain never reaches the foot and there is, of course, no paraesthesia. By the time that lumbar invasion has followed involvement of sacro-iliac joints, the buttock-ache has largely ceased.

Since the sacro-iliac ligaments are developed at the proximal extent of the first and second sacral segments, pain is referred from them in exactly the same way as it is referred from the first and second sacral nerve-roots.

There is therefore nothing in the nature or extent of the pain to distinguish sacro-iliac arthritis from a disc protrusion compressing either of these nerve-roots. Moreover, a cough usually jars the buttock or thigh in sacro-iliac arthritis. Just as a momentary increase in intradural pressure jolts the nerve-root, so does the same sudden increase in intra-abdominal pressure distract the ilium from the sacrum. When the ligaments joining the two bones are inflamed, this naturally hurts. This deceptive feature had led to nearly every patient being treated on the assumption that a disc lesion was present. Many had had osteopathy, which might well have been expected to cause lasting harm; in fact, it did not. Surprisingly enough, many patients experienced some hours' relief after manipulation, then the pain returned to its previous intensity. Only in the rare hyperacute case did osteopathy cause immediate aggravation, and even then for only a few days.

The characteristic of the pain is that it comes and goes irrespective of posture and exertion. This is the reverse of the history in disc lesions, where pain follows certain activities and subsides after their avoidance. When present, the pain can be increased by such exertion as strained the joint, but when absent the hardest work is powerless to provoke it. The pain often changes sides; it alternates and is scarcely ever bilateral, except rarely for a day or two at the changeover. The pain was recorded as alternating in 28 cases, right-sided only in 27 and left-sided only in 17. These flares are unprovoked and indeed unprovokable, and can last days, months, exceptionally years. One joint is often the main source of pain, the flares on the other side being infrequent, mild and transitory.

The appearance of these patients bears no resemblance to the accepted picture of advanced spondylitis. They are cheerful, often well covered, agile in their movements and, on examination, possess a full and painless range at every spinal joint. Anaemia, iritis and trouble in the peripheral joints is so far noticeably absent, and the clinical arthritis was found secondary to Reiter's disease and to ulcerative colitis in only one case each.

Symptoms in Pregnancy

By analogy with rheumatoid arthritis, it was to be expected that pregnancy would temporarily stop the symptoms, and, in fact, 5 out of 29 female patients reported freedom from ache in the buttock for the period of the pregnancy and a month or two afterwards. However, in three others, the original attack of pain in the buttock was during pregnancy, and two other patients experienced such a severe flare during pregnancy that they could scarcely walk, though the pre-pregnancy attacks had been quite minor.

Prognosis in Sacro-iliac Arthritis

In most cases of sacro-iliac arthritis, extension of the spondylitic process to the spinal joints takes place within a few years, especially in younger patients. A few patients, however, experience flares less frequently, they become less painful and last a shorter time; after five or ten years the disease appears to have burnt itself out. The sedimentation rate is of no prognostic value, nor is the presence or absence of sclerosis visible on the first film. My impression is that women do better than men, and that the course of sacro-iliitis starting in the late twenties, certainly in the thirties, follows a benign course.

Since most patients eventually develop spinal arthritis but a few do not, it is unwise, when only the sacro-iliac joints are affected, to draw too pessimistic a conclusion about extension to the spinal joints with final ankylosis. Naturally, a guarded long-term prognosis must be given. It is not possible to avoid extension to the spine in those in whom it is going to happen. A sound policy is to make no prognosis at all, but merely to state that the pain arises from the sacro-iliac joint, which will flare on and off for at least some years; and that the patient can be kept comfortable.

Treatment of Sacro-iliac Arthritis

There are a number of very effective remedies, all of which stop pain but none affects the liability to extension to the spinal joints.

1. *Butazolidine*

Quite small doses suffice. Dosage of 200 mg. twice a day as soon as a flare starts, followed by 100 mg. once or twice a day for the next week was often all that is needed.

2. *Indomethacin*

Twenty-five mg. two or three times a day for a few days abates a flare quickly.

3. *Prednisone*

A few days on 5 mg. twice a day followed by one tablet a day for another few days is usually enough.

4. *Intra-articular injection of hydrocortisone*

It is not easy to get the needle into the right spot on account of the large sacral foramina into which the tip is apt to pass; the suspension then passes intrasacrally or even intrapelvically. A needle 8 cm. long is introduced at the midline at the first sacral level and thrust in at an angle of 45 degrees. It strikes bone and the point must then be manœuvred until it is felt to hit cartilage. Once the needle point penetrates cartilage nothing can be forced out of the syringe. The needle is then withdrawn during pressure on the piston until the suspension just begins to flow. Five ml. of the suspension are now injected between the posterior ligament and the articular cartilage, and must therefore reach the right spot. After a day's soreness the pain ceases, often for months.

5. X-ray therapy

If, rarely, systemic steroids, butazolidine, indomethacin and topical hydrocortisone all fail, X-ray therapy should be considered. Subsidence of the pain after the third or fourth exposure takes place in four out of five cases. Exposure of 200 r. three times a week for a fortnight (i.e. 1,200 r. in all) is average dosage. Return of pain is to be expected, in six to twelve months if the patient is young, not for some years if the patient is over thirty. In a woman, the sacro-iliac joints cannot be irradiated without some damage to the ovaries. A woman over, say, thirty may choose, if she already has several children, to accept the slight chance of sterilization for the relief of pain. The husband should be a party to this decision. The Medical Defence Union holds the opinion that the risks inherent in this treatment should be explained to the patient in the presence of a witness, and that she should sign a statement that she consents to the treatment knowing and accepting the risks; the witness should also sign the document. This procedure, in the Union's view, adequately safeguards the medical man concerned. The Medical Research Council's report on the hazards to man of nuclear radiation (1956) points out that the incidence of leukaemia is ten times greater in spondylitics who have received radiation than in those who have not; even so, the incidence is only 3:1,000. The report is based on about 13,500 cases and the mean latent period between first exposure to X-rays and the development of leukaemia was six years. This fact must be kept in mind and irradiation avoided during pregnancy for fear of harming the foetus. In fact, pregnancy sometimes abolishes the pain temporarily.

Claims have been made that X-ray treatment arrests the disease. This is not so. It abates the pain of ankylosing spondylitis but has no influence on its eventual evolution. The speed of evolution at different ages, however, is so different that the patient may have to be followed up for some years before it becomes clear that the effect of radiotherapy wears off in the end.

6. Compression

When a patient is seen scarcely able to walk because each step jars the severely inflamed ligaments, a tight binder must be applied at once and a strong compression strain maintained for a week or two. This enables the patient to walk comfortably until drug treatment becomes effective. Some women understandably refuse all drugs during pregnancy; if so, this is the only possible measure.

Prostatitis and Sacro-iliitis

Kelly's historical research has disclosed that Rolleston quotes Musgrave as having described arthritis after non-venereal urethritis as early as 1703. He also found that Lorimer (1884) mentioned this occurrence, and that Coulson (1858) stated that arthritis can follow urethral suppuration from any cause. In fact, there appears to be some connection between sacro-iliac arthritis and non-specific prostatitis; for Csodka (1958) noted that 8·6 per cent of his patients with Reiter's syndrome suffered from sacro-iliitis and 10·8 per cent from iritis; Oates and Young's (1959) figures were 45 and 24 per cent; and 32 per cent of Mason's (1964) cases had sacro-iliitis; 42 out of 234 of Wright and Watkinson's cases (1965). Bywaters and Ansdell (1958) found that 6 out of 37 patients with arthritis secondary to ulcerative colitis had radiological changes in the sacro-iliac joints indistinguishable from those of ankylosing spondylitis. Mason et al. (1958) found evidence of prostatitis in 33 per cent of cases of rheumatoid arthritis, in 83 per cent of ankylosing spondylitis and in 95 per cent of Reiter's disease. However, this is clearly not the whole story, since women also suffer from sacro-iliac arthritis. Golding, Baker and Thompson (1963) found sclerosis at the sacro-iliac joints in 15 out of 60 patients with gross psoriatic arthritis. Indeed, it looks as if a number of different stimuli can provoke sacro-iliac sclerosis. But there are two important differences. First, except rarely in Reiter's disease and ulcerative colitis, the patient does not suffer pain in his buttock arising from his sacro-iliac joint; it is a radiological finding without a clinical counterpart. Secondly, the existence of the sacro-iliac sclerosis does not then imply that the disease is ankylosing spondylitis which will spread relentlessly up the spine.

PROGRESS OF ANKYLOSING SPONDYLITIS

The Usual Course

Sclerosing sacro-iliac arthritis usually takes place silently, for less than 10 per cent of patients with advanced disease can ever recollect having had pain in the buttock of sciatica.

The first complaint is often vague discomfort and stiffness in the lower back, usually worst on waking and eased by exercise. This comes and goes, irrespective of exertion, in bouts lasting weeks or months, often with symptom-free intervals of similar length. Then the pain spreads to the thorax, tending to leave the lower lumbar levels. The patient notices that breathing has become restricted, owing to stiffness at the costo-vertebral joints; in the end, his respiration becomes purely diaphragmatic. Finally, the neck is involved in the ossifying process, becoming increasingly rigid. The two upper joints are affected late; hence, hyperextension here contrasts with the flattening out of the lumbar lordosis and the marked thoraco-cervical rounded kyphosis. The patient's face becomes pinched and haggard, the eyes hollow and the body loses its fatty covering. Microcytic anaemia is a common, and iritis an uncommon, complication. When bony ankylosis is complete, pain ceases; the pain in the trunk therefore travels upwards and comes to an end after many years.

Then the hips become affected. Until then, the patient, curved and fixed though his back is, has been able to look up by extending at the hip joints. Now this ceases to be possible and some patients are reduced to a pitiable state of crippledom. The knees, shoulders and other joints are seldom affected; indeed, spondylitis is more likely to *present* as arthritis at the knee or tarsus than to lead to involvement of these joints as a late manifestation.

Happily, this sequence of events is not a certainty. The speed and extent of spread depend partly on the patient's sex and age. A few patients now aged thirty-five to forty have been followed up for ten years; radiographic evidence of sacro-iliac sclerosis has appeared during this time, but the disorder has not yet spread to the lumbar spine. The younger the patient is at the onset, the worse the prognosis, and men do worse than women. When spondylitis appears before the age of twenty, in either sex, severe disablement soon is very probable. Evolution of the spinal component will probably take two to seven years; the hips will be affected within another five years, treatment or no treatment. By contrast, sacro-iliac arthritis coming on after the age of twenty-five may, even in men, go on flaring and subsiding for, say, five years before the lower lumbar joints become involved, and in women the joints may flare alternately for ten or fifteen years on end. Spread upwards may be very slow, and the thoracic spine only becomes affected by the time the patient reaches forty or fifty. The cervical spine may never fix at all; the hips usually retain full mobility indefinitely. Sclerosing sacro-iliac arthritis coming on after the age of thirty is quite unimportant, except that the patient may be led mistakenly to believe that he will soon be a cripple.

Occasionally, the lumbar spine fixes, not in flexion but with its ordinary lordosis. Inspection of the patient's back then yields no information, but, directly he is asked to perform trunk movements, the fixation becomes evident and is particularly obvious on attempted side-flexion. Rarely, the constitutional signs are absent; the patient is cheerful, looks well, and is amply covered. Nothing then in the patient's appearance suggests the diagnosis, but once more, side-flexion of the lumbar, and probably thoracic, spine is much restricted.

TREATMENT OF ANKYLOSING SPONDYLITIS

Explanation

When a patient aged over twenty-five is seen at the stage of sacro-iliac arthritis, little need be said to him about future disablement. Unless his job involves very heavy work, he may never become appreciably incapacitated. On the other hand, when spondylitis has already reached the lumbar spine in a man aged, say, twenty-five, it is important to steer him towards a suitable career (unless chance has already led him to do so). It is best to state that the spine is sure ultimately to stiffen in a way that does not interfere with sedentary work; that the pain is controllable and that the disorder very seldom spreads, e.g., to the hands, thus impeding manual tasks.

When the spinal column is already stiffening, it is wise to explain that the stiffness is permanent but unimportant to a sedentary worker, whereas the pain responds to treatment, eventually disappearing altogether. The patient must be persuaded to view his disability in as cheerful a light as possible, to resign himself to avoid some pursuits, and to adopt work suited to his capacity. The question of spread to other joints, can only be answered evasively in young patients, but quite a strong negative is justified to a patient in the thirties in whom only the sacro-iliac or lower lumbar joints are as yet affected.

The capacity for sedentary work is often not appreciably impaired for years. It is not deformity so much as pain keeping the patient awake and rendering his daily life miserable that upsets him. A rigid lumbo-thoracic spine is remarkably little inconvenience to a sedentary worker. When the disease spreads to the hip joints, however, the position is very different. Fixed flexion deformity of the thigh combined with a rigid kyphosis of the lumbar spine is a great disability.

The Prevention of Further Deformity

This is aided by the following routine. The patient should sleep on one mattress on fracture boards, with only one pillow, and should avoid lying curled up on his side. He should lie face downwards on an unyielding couch for an hour—even for less is of some value—in the middle of his working day. If he has to sit bent over a desk for any length of time, he should make a conscious effort to pull himself up straight as often as he can remember, not less than once an hour. For the prevention of deformity this regimen is more valuable than any physiotherapy. However, this is indicated from time to time, if deformity appears to be increasing. The physiotherapist should force extension at the lumbo-thoracic spine and, if necessary, stretch out both hip joints towards extension.

Osteotomy at the lower thoracic level can straighten out a gross flexion deformity of the spine.

Recumbency is no longer regarded as useful in spondylitis ankylopoetica.

Treatment of Ligamentous Pain

Butazolidine is very effective and should be tried first. A mere 100 mg. taken last thing at night will often abolish the severe ache waking the patient each morning. So small a dose can be continued indefinitely, but there is no need for medication during pain-free periods. The next most useful drug is indomethacin, 25 mg. once to three times a day. During a flare, it quickly abates the pain, and need be taken for a week or so as a rule. If this fails, prednisone 5 mg. twice a day should be prescribed. This dose satisfies the body's daily requirement of hydrocortisone. Hence, it should not be given for too long and, when a flare subsides, it should not be dropped abruptly, but tailed off.

The patient should be informed that the pain disappears when the ankylosing process is completed.

Sharp and Purser (1957) described ten cases of spontaneous atlanto-axial dislocation in patients with advanced spondylitis, causing pressure on the spinal cord. Skull traction followed by occipito-cervical arthrodesis relieved pain and caused regression in the neurological signs. Bowie and Glasgow (1961) described cauda equina lesions in spondylitis ankylopoetica leading to numbness in both lower limbs, absent ankle-jerks and urinary incontinence. How these symptoms are produced is unknown. Laminectomy disclosed no abnormality and afforded no benefit. I have encountered two cases in which straight-leg raising was so limited in lumbar spondylitis that the patient could scarcely walk; in the worse instance, the range of straight-leg raising was 5 degrees on one side and 15 degrees on the other.

Stretching either leg up caused no pain; it was merely impossible. Presumably, the dura mater or the dural sleeve of the lower lumbar roots had become inflamed as the result of the spondylitic process. Certainly, it is not a purely superficial lesion; for epidural local anaesthesia did not increase the range of straight-leg raising then or afterwards, whereas a few weeks of indomethacin increased range by 30 degrees on each side. On two patients laminectomy had been performed before the radiograph showed the sclerosis. In both cases each surgeon on enquiry reported that inspection showed the dura mater and nerve-roots macroscopically normal.

Treatment at the Peripheral Joints

Hydrocortisone, injected into the joint at whatever intervals prove necessary, is strongly indicated during a flare of arthritis at hip, knee, shoulder or elbow. Two large joints can be dealt with at one sitting and the injections are repeated as soon as discomfort returns. During the chronic phase, this may prove effective for many months, even years. The range of movement in joints affected for a long time does not return. Intra-articular injections at such long intervals do not provoke steriod arthropathy.

Treatment at Costo-vertebral Joints

Sometimes one lower costs-vertebral joint becomes painfully included in the spondylitic process. The pattern that one would have expected in this disorder would be unilateral posterior pain on thoracic movements, on breathing and on passively springing the ribs. This occasionally proves so; surprisingly enough, more often no movement whatever affects the constant ache. Hydrocortisone injected at the affected joint is most effective.

'LUMBAGO' IN SPONDYLITIS

A deceptive phenomenon is occasionally encountered. The patient, usually aged thirty to thirty-five, complains that he may feel a sudden jar in his back on bending to lift a heavy weight, after which his back is painful for some weeks. He recovers, but further exertion brings on the same pain again. Naturally, a diagnosis of lumbago is made and the presence of a disc lesion appears confirmed when the X-ray appearances of his lumbar spine reveal no other cause for his symptoms. In fact, he is straining his stiffening lumbar joints, the site of the spondylitic process, having perhaps fracturing an ossifying ligament. When this occurs at a low lumbar joint, nothing arouses suspicion until the range of lumbar movement is found grossly restricted for a man of his age. If, however, he identifies the site of his pain as upper lumbar, this sequence of events comes to mind at once; for he is indicating the 'forbidden area' where disc lesions are most uncommon. It is, of course, the radiograph of the sacro-iliac joints, not the lumbar joints, that confirms the diagnosis.

Another possibility is the presence of a lumbar disc lesion in a patient whose disc has become invaded by the spondylitic process. Granulomatous penetration of cartilage naturally weakens it and a disc lesion may result. Alternatively a disc lesion may be caused by trauma in the ordinary way. In either of these two events there is no restriction of side-flexion of the lumbar spine such as is found in a patient whose sudden pain arises from severe strain of an ossifying ligament. Lumbago in a patient with sacro-iliac spondylitis causes the same attacks of fixation, with pain on coughing, that occur in ordinary people, and the treatment is similar. Eventually, lumbar ankylosis cures the disc-trouble.

OSTEITIS CONDENSANS ILII

This is a purely radiological finding, important only because the appearance of spondylitic arthritis may be closely mimicked. Osteitis condensans occurs only in women, some of whom give a history of past minor abdominal sepsis. It is non-progressive and is essentially a sclerosis of bone without blurring of the joint margins. In the more obvious cases, the sclerosis occupies the mid-part of the joint, and is seldom confined to the lower aspect of the ilium, being more extensive upwards. Osteitis condensans bears no connection with spondylitis nor does it cause pain in the buttock. It was tempting to regard the sclerosis as a manifestation of past low-grade infection, but Gillespie and Lloyd-Roberts (1953) consider it an aseptic necrosis caused by vascular occlusion. They detected osteitis in 2·2 per cent of 760 routine radiographs of the lumbo-sacral area and removed a specimen for biopsy. This showed non-inflammatory deposition of extra bone.

SACRO-ILIAC OSTEOARTHRITIS

Radiological evidence of osteophytosis at the edges of the joint shows that the ligaments are ossifying. This entails complete stabilization of the joint. Hence, the discovery that osteoarthritis is present at the sacro-iliac joint positively excludes the joint as the source of whatever symptoms the patient may have. Taken as a disease, osteoarthritis of the sacro-iliac joints is an imaginary disorder.

SACRO-ILIAC GOUT

This occurs in the late stages of gout in about 10 per cent of patients (Malawista *et al.*, 1965). The patient, amongst his other accesses of pain, suffers recurrent discomfort at one side of his sacrum. He has had gout in his peripheral joints for years, and the X-ray photograph shows juxta-articular cysts, which Lipson and Slocumb (1965) have shown by biopsy to contain encapulated deposits of urate.

SPECIFIC SACRO-ILIAC ARTHRITIS

This may be tuberculous or septic. In tuberculosis the first symptom is the swelling in the buttock; the patient does not experience appreciable pain. Fluctuation shows that a cold abscess is present and aspiration followed by inoculation of a guinea-pig shows it to be tuberculous. Testing the joint does not elicit pain, on account of the fibrous ankylosis produced by the infection.

Septic arthritis is dealt with on p. 625.

SACRO-ILIAC STRAIN

This occurs only in women, between the ages of fifteen and thirty-five. It is rare, and always unilateral, never alternating. It differs from the arthritis of spondylitis in that, far from coming and going for no reason, the pain in one buttock is evoked by exertion and avoided by resting the joint. It may be associated with pregnancy but as often is not. Though it is true that, as can be shown by radiography, slight relaxation of the sacro-iliac ligaments occurs in some pregnant women, this is physiological. In consequence, symptoms do not arise and testing the sacro-iliac joint does not set up any pain. The existence of a hormone named 'relaxin' is responsible for the ligamentous change. Luckily, no appreciable in-stability of the joints results and even pre-natal exercises intended to increase the mobility at the sacro-iliac joints prove harmless; however, they are best avoided for the sake of the lumbar spine, as nearly all of them involve trunk-flexion.

Examination of women whose backache dates from pregnancy shows that the cause is very seldom sacro-iliac strain but an early disc lesion—the result of ten days in bed in 'the nursing mother's position' (Fig. 59, p. 387). The facile assumption that, merely because a woman's backache started during pregnancy or the puerperium, it must be due to sacro-iliac strain, is not borne out by clinical examination.

Treatment of Sacro-iliac Strain

The sacro-iliac is like the acromio-clavicular joint in that no muscle controls movement at the joint, which relies for its stability solely on its ligaments. Hence, movement plays no part in the treatment of sacro-iliac strain. Mobilization of the joint, as might be expected, leads to further over-stretching and increased pain; indeed, the stresses put upon the joint merely by clinical examination temporarily aggravate the symptoms. Exercises are also harmful.

The joint requires protection. In fact, the wearing of a suitable belt for

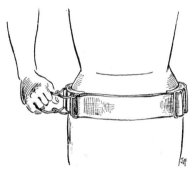

FIG. 103. Corrugator belt for sacro-iliac strain
(Austlid, Stockholm)

a month or two usually abolishes the symptoms, often permanently. The most suitable is the 'corrugator' (Fig. 103). Should this fail, sclerosing injections into the posterior sacro-iliac ligaments are indicated.

Sclerosing Injections

Many are now returning to the concept of sacro-iliac strain, influenced by osteopathic ideas. Before the role of the disc in lumbo-gluteal pain was put forward (Cyriax, 1945), most backache was attributed to the sacro-iliac strain. This notion is now being revived in a slightly different form, and the argument runs something like this: There has been recurrent lumbar pain and the radiograph shows marked narrowing and osteophytosis at, say, the fifth lumbar level. Diminished movement at this joint must throw excessive strain on adjacent joints, i.e., the fourth lumbar joint and the sacro-iliac ligaments. Hence, sacro-iliac strain follows and complicates what was originally a fifth lumbar disc lesion or (as the osteopaths prefer it) a facet-joint lesion.

This is not an unreasonable hypothesis, but there is considerable evidence against it. In the first place, if limited movement caused by erosion of disc-substance causes sacro-iliac strain, then all patients with a fifth lumbar joint fixed by sacralization would suffer much more and much earlier in life. Moreover, examination shows that (a) one or more lumbar movements hurt, (b) testing the sacro-iliac joint does not hurt, and (c) epidural local anaesthesia (which does not deprive the sacro-iliac joints of sensibility) abolishes the pain for the time being.

For these reasons, such gluteal pain ought to be regarded as referred from the lumbar spine, and if sclerosing injections are to be given, they should be used to infiltrate the lumbar ligaments not the sacro-iliac. If the sacro-iliac joint were to lose mobility, additional strain would be transmitted to the affected lumbar joint. Sacro-iliac mobility spares the lumbar joints and must be advantageous to them, the more so if a lumbar lesion already exists.

23

The Buttock and Hip

Most pain in the buttock has a lumbar origin. Lesions in the buttock itself, although uncommon, are often serious, some requiring urgent treatment. Their immediate clinical recognition is therefore important.

All ideas of 'gluteal fibrositis' must be discarded. Just as pressure on the dura mater in the neck sets up pain accompanied by characteristic tenderness in the upper thorax, so does the same phenomenon occur in the buttock, where pain and tenderness often result from pressure of a disc lesion on the dura mater. The lumbar spine, sacro-iliac joints, buttock and hip all require examination to reach a diagnosis. If trunk-extension elicits the gluteal ache, it cannot have a muscular origin. This movement relaxes the sacrospinalis and gluteal muscles, but extends the lumbar and hip-joints, and puts a rotation strain on the sacro-iliac joint. Gluteal pain evoked by trunk-extension must, therefore, have an articular origin. It is only when gluteal pain is evoked on resisted extension of the hip that a lesion of a muscle in the buttock—a great rarity—need be considered at all.

Symmetrical collections of fat may form in the superficial tissue of the buttocks and on the outer aspect of each thigh in middle-aged women. Clinical examination shows that they do not interfere with muscle function, but their presence has misled those who rely chiefly on palpation for diagnosis, into creating a disease called 'panniculitis'. It is a myth.

Segmentation of the Buttock

Many dermatomes meet at the buttock. The skin of the whole outer buttock is derived from the first lumbar segment, but at the inner upper quadrant the second and third dermatomes overlap the first. These two areas are separate from the second and third dermatomes along the front of the thigh. The first and second sacral segments start at mid-buttock and continue down the back of the thigh.

The muscles of the buttock are all of fourth and fifth lumbar and first sacral provenance. The gluteus medius is weak in a fifth lumbar root-palsy, whereas wasted glutei accompany only a sacral root-palsy. Hence, this appears to be the way the myotomes are composed.

In theory, pain in the buttock can result from any lesion situated in a tissue derived from the first, second or third lumbar or upper two sacral segments. In fact, pain is referred to the buttock and the front of the thigh chiefly in third lumbar disc lesions and osteoarthritis of the hip.

The only common cause of pain in the buttock spreading down the outer aspect of the thigh is pressure from a disc-protrusion on the fourth or fifth lumbar nerve-root. If the pain runs to the back of the thigh, the first or second sacral nerve-root is probably affected. Sacro-iliac arthritis and gluteal bursitis refer in a similar way but are both uncommon.

Major Lesions in the Buttock

These possess in common an arresting pattern of physical signs that draws immediate attention to the buttock. Passive hip-flexion with the knee held extended (i.e. straight-leg raising) is limited and painful. Passive hip-flexion, this time with the knee more flexed, is also limited and painful. Further examination reveals a non-capsular pattern of limitation of movement at the hip-joint. The deductions to be drawn are as follows: Straight-leg raising is limited; the lesion is, therefore, connected with the tissues lying behind the hip-joint. Hip-flexion with the knee bent is also limited; hence, neither the sciatic nerve and its roots, nor the hamstring muscles, are at fault. Were the hip-joint itself affected, straight-leg raising would not be limited (except in such gross arthritis that less than 90 degrees flexion range had resulted). The only structure left is the buttock. Thus, when passing from testing straight-leg raising to testing the passive movements at the hip-joint, the *sign of the buttock* emerges at once.

There is nothing characteristic about the pain. It is felt in the buttock and spreads down the back of the thigh to the knee or calf; naturally, a disc lesion is suspected. Trunk-flexion is limited, since the patient has pain when tension falls on the tissues of the buttock; the other lumbar movements are of full range. It is only when the patient is examined supine on the couch that the typical combination of signs emerges. This naturally leads to careful examination of the passive and resisted hip-movements. A non-capsular pattern emerges on passive testing, medial rotation nearly always proving of full range. Moreover, the characteristic feel of a hip-joint at its extreme of range is replaced by the patient's asking the examiner, because of increasing pain, not to force a movement which the latter can clearly feel not yet to have reached its full amplitude. The resisted movements often hurt, since they too alter tensions in the buttock. Palpation may disclose a tumour.

The patient's temperature is noted; a rectal examination is performed and a radiograph secured without delay.

The Sign of the Buttock

When the sign of the buttock emerges on examination, the various possibilities are:

Osteomyolitis of the Upper Femur

The symptoms and signs are very marked and the sign of the buttock obtrudes. Straight-leg raising and hip-flexion are both considerably limited and cause intense pain. Rotation at the hip is restricted by pain with the characteristic empty end-feel.

Fulminating infection with high fever is correctly attributed at once; it is only cases with a gradual onset that are mistaken for a disc lesion and reach the orthopaedic physician. Sciatic pain is indeed present, but the patient walks in, often supported by a relative, with a far worse limp than is ever seen in a disc lesion; it resembles that of iliac metastases or advanced arthritis at the hip. Sooner or later fever appears and the upper part of the shaft of the femur becomes very tender. The radiograph is negative at this stage. Antibiotics are given at once, and the patient transferred to surgical care.

Septic Sacro-iliac Arthritis

The symptoms and signs are very like those of osteomyelitis of the upper femur. In addition to 'the sign of the buttock', testing the sacro-iliac joint is most painful. The femur is not tender. It is only some months later, when local new bone formation begins to show that the exact position of the abscess becomes clear. Rest and antibiotic therapy are indicated at once.

Ischio-rectal Abscess

Occasionally, an ischio-rectal abscess points towards the buttock instead of pointing towards the rectum. The patient limps badly, preferring not to put his foot to the ground at all. The hip is fixed in considerable flexion; further flexion is limited; so is straight-leg raising. Fever is present and rectal examination reveals the cause.

Septic Bursitis

Septic bursitis gives rise to the characteristic 'sign of the buttock'. When the patient is first seen his pain at rest may not be severe and he may not yet feel ill; but either he hobbles in with a gait suggesting an arthritic hip, or he lies in bed unable to put that leg to the ground or rest that buttock on the mattress. Such major disablement contrasts with the minor degree of discomfort; much greater pain would have been required to secure such disablement had a disc lesion, for example, been present. The temperature is between 99° and 100° F.; the next day it is a little higher. Rectal examination and the radiograph reveal no abnormality. Palpation may reveal a vague area of tenderness just behind and above the greater trochanter. Rarely, a swelling is encountered lying postero-laterally at the upper end of the femoral shaft, level with the lesser trochanter. Rest in bed and antibiotics are required. Recurrence some years later is not uncommon.

Very occasionally the swelling results from acute, often haemorrhagic, bursitis due to a fall on the outer side of the hip. Pain is slight; the patient walks well. Aspiration suffices.

Rheumatic Fever with Bursitis

In adults, recrudescence of rheumatic fever may lead to pain in the buttock and thigh; examination shows the characteristic 'sign of the buttock'. Fever is present and the patient dyspnoeic at rest. Admission to hospital for the cardiac condition is called for in any case, and the lesion in the buttock, presumably a rheumatic bursitis, clears up in the course of three or four weeks, as the result of the rest in bed.

Neoplasm at Upper Femur

Metastases at upper femur give rise to a very similar picture, but without fever. If, as is common, the erosion of bone lies close to the lesser trochanter, resisted flexion of the hip is very weak and also painful. The patient cannot bear weight on the affected limb and often attends in a wheel-chair.

Iliac Neoplasm

Primary and secondary neoplasm occur at the ilium deep to the gluteal muscles. The patient can scarcely hobble with assistance. The 'sign of the buttock' is present. Marked wasting of the quadriceps and hamstring muscles contrasts with an almost full range of movement at the hip-joint. If movement is limited, the capsular pattern and the capsular feel are both absent and the intensity of the pain quite out of keeping with the minor limitation of movement. The radiograph is diagnostic.

Fractured Sacrum

The history is of a fall on the buttocks. Sacral pain results which the patient ascribes to local bruising; he often continues to get about. The symptoms continue, tending at first to become worse. During the first week or so, when the lower limbs are examined, the 'sign of the buttock' is found on both sides. The sacrum is swollen and tender superficially (which might be due to soft tissue bruising) but equally tender when the anterior aspect of the bone is palpated per rectum. A sacral haematoma often forms.

The radiograph confirms the diagnosis. Although the patient will be more comfortable in bed, bony union without deformity takes place whether he rests or not. It is thus reasonable to leave it to the patient to make his own choice. Subsidence of symptoms takes about two months. A haematoma may be aspirated.

MINOR LESIONS ABOUT THE HIP

These do not give rise to the 'sign of the buttock', straight-leg raising being of full range and very seldom even uncomfortable.

A minor lesion at the hip is suggested when a patient complains of pain in the buttock and testing the lumbar and sacro-iliac joints draw a blank. If so, the main symptom should be pain brought on or increased by walking. The passive movements reveal a full range of movement at the hip, but some are found to hurt, others not, in a non-capsular manner, e.g. full lateral rotation hurts, full medial does not: the reverse of the situation in arthritis. This finding strongly suggests bursitis. Very early arthritis is usually symptomless, but, if it does set up pain at the extreme of range, the capsular pattern is retained. The end-feel in arthritis is hard, in bursitis soft; hence, the sensation imparted to the hand is most helpful in diagnosis.

Unfortunately, the significance of the passive hip movements is often ambiguous: for full flexion may squeeze the psoas bursa painfully, as well as stretch the hip-joint and the structures lying behind it. Again full passive abduction may squeeze tissues lying between the greater trochanter and the blade of the ilium.

If then, the pattern for bursitis emerges, the main diagnostic aid is the position of the pain and its area of reference. If these are felt at the front of the thigh, the psoas bursa is incriminated; if postero-laterally, one of the gluteal bursae.

To make matters yet more complicated, one or two resisted movements usually hurt in bursitis. In the buttock, pain on a resisted movement should not be taken as suggesting a muscle lesion; it indicates instead tenderness of a bursa, painfully squeezed when an adjacent muscle contracts. The buttock is the only area in the body where this situation obtains, and in fact muscle lesions in the buttock are almost unknown. Indeed, the only

(?)

two resisted movements which imply trouble in the muscle itself are: (a) flexion, in psoas muscle strain, and (b) lateral rotation, when the tendon of the quadratus femoris is affected. In neither of these lesions do any of the passive hip movements hurt.

Since the passive movements often have an equivocal significance, and the common cause of pain on a resisted movement is not a muscle lesion but compression of a near-by tender bursa, diagnosis at the buttock is extremely difficult. It is the most awkward area in the whole body. The situation is aggravated by the fact that the tissues apt to become painful all lie so deeply that palpation for tenderness is futile.

Psoas Bursitis

The psoas bursa is developed from the second and third lumbar segments. The pain is therefore felt in the groin or within the upper thigh anteriorly, and is referred along the front of the thigh to the patellar area.

The passive hip movements reproduce the pain, and adduction in flexion, by squeezing the bursa, is usually the most painful movement. Passive lateral rotation usually hurts; medial does not, and the capsular-end-feel is absent. The resisted hip movements do not hurt, nor does resisted extension of the knee as the patient lies prone, thus showing that the tendon of the rectus femoris muscle is not strained. In psoas bursitis, resisted flexion of the hip does not hurt; this hurts in a lesion of the psoas muscle, of the tendon of the rectus femoris and in obturator hernia.

The main diagnostic difficulty lies between psoas bursitis and a loose body in the hip-joint without osteoarthritis. In the latter case, intermittent pain and sudden twinges are a prominent feature.

The diagnosis is always uncertain, and is not established until local anaesthesia has been induced at the front of the hip-joint and found to abolish the signs for the time being. It is often curative as well. If not, hydrocortisone is injected in the spot indentified by the local anaesthesia.

It should be remembered that painful weakness of the psoas muscle is present in malignant invasion of the belly itself retroperitoneally, and in metastases at the upper femur. In the latter case, marked restriction of range at the hip-joint is also found, with an empty end-feel.

Weakness and pain when the psoas muscles are tested are a common complaint in psychoneurosis, in combination then with all sorts of other inconsistencies.

Gluteal Bursitis

The condition is uncommon. It shows little tendency to spontaneous resolution and most cases are of many years' standing. Diagnosis is complicated. The pain is felt at the lateral or posterior trochanteric area and is referred to the outer thigh and, sometimes, outer leg. Some of the passive hip movements hurt in a non-capsular way, and the arthritic end-feel is absent. The twinges typical of a loose body in the hip are not mentioned. This combination of signs suggests gluteal bursitis.

Further localization now depends on finding which accessory movements affect the pain. For example, full passive abduction squeezes a tender structure lying between the greater trochanter and the blade of the ilium. A tender bursa is often painfully squeezed when an adjacent muscle contracts. Indeed, the common cause of pain on a resisted hip movement is not a lesion of the muscle itself but compression of a nearby bursa. Hence, it is the responses to the resisted movements that help to indicate in relation to which muscle the affected bursa lies; for palpation affords little assistance.

Diagnosis and treatment are pursued together. The likeliest spot is chosen, usually above the trochanter, and infiltrated with 50 ml. 0·5 per cent procaine solution. After some minutes, whichever movements had been found painful are tested again. If relief is not secured, a further diagnostic injection is given at each attendance until the right area is finally reached. If, as is usual, one or two correctly placed injections of procaine prove curative, this is all that need be done, although the patient may have had several injections before the necessary accuracy in siting the fluid has been achieved. If the immediate result of the injection shows that it has been correctly placed, but no lasting benefit is reported at the patient's next attendance, 5 cc. hydrocortisone suspension must be injected into the area already identified by the local anaesthesia.

Intractable cases are rare, and operative exploration of the buttock seldom reveals anything definite or effects a cure. Hence, if conservative treatment fails, it is usually best, since the symptoms are never severe, to admit defeat.

Ischial Bursitis

Weaver's bottom is uncommon nowadays. Indeed, gluteal pain coming on after sitting for some time, especially in a soft chair, and easing soon after the patient is upright again, is much more often due to a nuclear self-reducing protrusion at a low lumbar level. However, in bursitis the pain comes on as soon as the ischium touches the chair, especially if this is hard, and ceases the moment the patient stands up.

Ischial bursitis is brought to mind when the history indicates that a tender tissue lies between the ischium and the chair, and testing the lumbar and sacro-iliac joints, the hip-joint and the tissues about it is completely negative. The only finding is tenderness at, or just above, the ischial tuberosity. Local anaesthesia is induced here and the patient asked to sit once more. If there is now no discomfort, the diagnosis is confirmed, but it is not usual for the injection to give continuing benefit. At his next attendance, the tender spot is infiltrated with 5 ml. hydrocortisone suspension. Should this fail, excision is indicated.

Haemorrhagic Psoas Bursitis

This is an interesting rarity. The patient states that he jarred his thigh, slipping. Within a minute, the front of the upper thigh became painful and he found he could not flex the hip-joint. Examination shows 90 degree limitation of passive flexion at the hip-joint, all the other movements being of full range. There is no pain or weakness on any resisted movement. It is clear that a space-occupying lesion has suddenly appeared at the front of the hip-joint, i.e. the psoas bursa is tensely filled with blood. These patients may be suspected of malingering; for under anaesthesia, a full range of flexion may well be obtained, the limitation returning as soon as the patient recovers.

Aspiration confirms the diagnosis and cures the patient; failing that, spontaneous cure takes three or four months, no treatment availing.

Claudication in the Buttock

This is a rare condition, the original description of which was given in the 1954 edition of this book. Unless the suggestion contained in the history is noted, the disorder may be most puzzling; for the pain is felt at mid-buttock just where symptoms due to a low lumbar disc lesion are so often experienced.

History

The patient states that after walking for fifty or a hundred yards he gets such pain in his buttock that he has to stop. Occasionally, he complains that the limb goes numb rather than hurts, thus suggesting some neurological disorder. He stands still and the pain (or numbness) goes. After a minute or two, he walks on and can cover the same distance before the symptom comes on again.

Examination

This is essentially negative. The movements of the lumbar spine, the hip-joint, and testing the buttock and thigh muscles against resistance— none of them hurts. Pulsation in the arterial tree of the limb is adequate, unless the block has occurred in the common iliac as opposed to the internal iliac artery. Then the diagnosis is less likely to be missed, since all the arteries of the limb are pulseless and, in lesions of the external iliac artery, after walking the leg and foot go objectively cold. If an epidural injection is given it does not affect the symptom.

When this condition is suspected, the patient should be asked to lie prone. His hip on the affected side is passively extended; this proves painless. He should then be told fully to extend his hip, and actively to keep his lower limb off the couch for several minutes. The result of this sustained gluteal contraction is the recognized pain in the buttock. When maintenance of active extension at the hip-joint hurts, but passive extension does not, the cause must be muscular ischaemia. Bonney (1956) confirmed these views and described ten cases of gluteal claudication, in some of which prolonged fruitless treatment had been directed to the lumbar spine.

This diagnosis can sometimes be confirmed by radiography, which may show a dense unilateral calcification of the internal iliac artery.

No treatment is effective except operative recanalization of the artery.

Tuberculous Abscess

A cold abscess may form in the buttock in tuberculosis of the fifth lumbar vertebra or the sacro-iliac joint. A painless fluctuant swelling forms, which should be aspirated and the fluid examined for tuberculosis. When the lumbar vertebra is affected, marked limitation of range is present on lumbar movements, together with a small kyphos. When the sacro-iliac joint is at fault, testing the joint causes no pain; for fibrosis takes place as fast as does erosion. Nor does the abscess cause limitation of, or pain on, hip movements, passive or resisted.

Psychogenic Pain

It so happens that 90 degrees limitation of flexion at the hip-joints is a common finding in psychoneurotic patients complaining of pain in the lower back or thigh. If such a finding is combined with the discovery of a full range of rotation at the joint, one gross inconsistency has been detected. Another sign may be fixation of the hip in medial rotation; in arthritis fixation in lateral rotation is invariable. However in view of the matter set out in the first paragraph (bursitis) above, minor unusual signs at the hip-joint should be ascribed to psychological causes only with caution. Most such patients oblige by offering a multiplicity of signs indicating, as it were, that the lumbar region, the sacro-iliac and knee-joints and the muscles in the thigh are affected as well. It is important to test all muscles and joints in detail, and to perform a number of movements twice—e.g. first standing and then lying down; or first lying supine, then lying prone—to see if the responses tally.

THE HIP-JOINT

Referred Pain

The hip-joint is formed largely from the third lumbar segment. Hence, pain is referred from the groin, down the front of the thigh to the knee, and thence down the front of the leg to just above the ankle (Figs. 16 and 18.) Since the upper inner quadrant of the buttock represents part of the third lumbar dermatome, arthritis at the hip often also hurts here; rarely, the only pain is there and the patient very deceptively complains only of unilateral backache. At times the crural component is absent, the patient complaining solely of an anterior pain at the knee, spreading perhaps along the front of the tibia. Rarely, the hip-joint is developed chiefly within the fourth lumbar segment; if so, the pain spreads along the fourth dermatome to the outer side of the mid-thigh and of the leg. In such cases, the fourth lumbar pain of sciatica is reproduced.

Pain felt only at the front of the thigh occupies the area of the second and third dermatomes; hence, its source should be sought at these levels of the lumbar spine, at the hip-joint, at the anterior and inner muscles of the thigh, and at the knee. If the pain spreads down the front of the tibia as well, only the structures forming part of the third lumbar segment need be considered.

Examination

Since most pains in the buttock stem from the lumbar spine, and pain in the thigh is as often referred thither as of local origin, the lumbar spine and sacro-iliac joints must be examined before the hip. Moreover, it is when the patient stands for the lumbar examination that the best moment arises for noting any fixation of the thigh in adduction and flexion. Now too, it is appropriate to inquire whether raising the heel on the affected side alters the pain.

Bending backwards while standing extends both the lumbar spine and

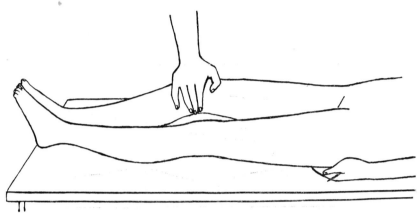

FIG. 104. Resisted flexion at hip. The patient presses his knee towards the examiner's hand.

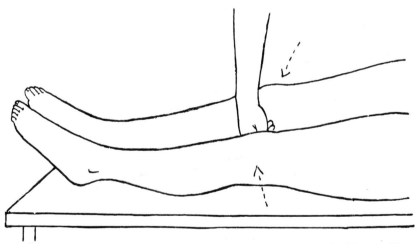

FIG. 105. Resisted adduction at hips. The patient squeezes the examiner's hand between his knees.

the hip-joint. Hence pain in the thigh brought on by this movement cannot be ascribed to a lumbar structure unless full extension of the hip is later shown to be painless as the patient lies prone. Care must then be taken to press on the buttock with one hand when the other extends the thigh, so as to exclude the lumbar spine from the test.

Examination of the hip-joint begins by noting the range, painfulness or not, and end-feel of flexion, lateral rotation and medial rotation while the patient lies supine, and extension (and medial rotation again) while the patient lies prone. If, as in bursitis, it is important to know whether full

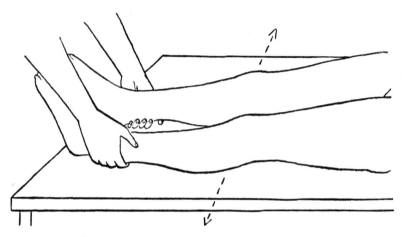

Fig. 106. Resisted abduction at hips. The examiner faces the patient and resists the abduction movement by holding his ankles together.

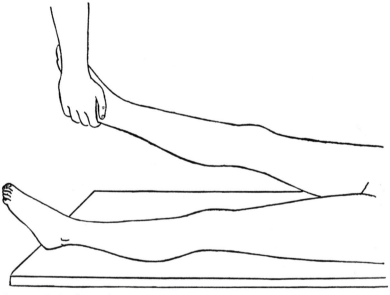

Fig. 107. Resisted extension at hip. The examiner resists the downward pressure at the patient's heel.

passive abduction is painful or not, an assistant abducts the other leg first. Passive adduction is tested after raising up the good leg so as to get it out of the way.

The resisted movements follow. Supine: flexion, extension, adduction and abduction at the hip; prone: both rotations (with the knee flexed to a right-angle); flexion and extension at the knee. In fact, muscle lesions at

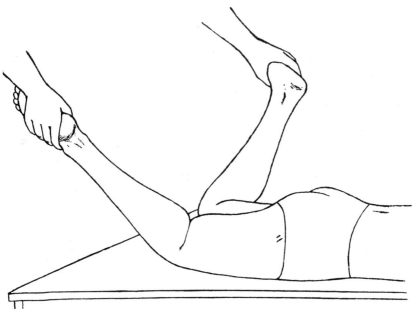

FIG. 108. Passive medial rotation at the hips. The patient lies face downwards, his knees together. The examiner rotates the thighs by pressing the feet apart. The buttocks must be kept level. A small amount of limitation of medial rotation can now be ascertained. Detection is often important for this is the movement first to become restricted at the onset of arthritis.

the upper thigh are far outnumbered in the middle-aged by lesions of the hip-joint; in children, this tendency is even more pronounced and nearly all pain felt to spread down from the front of the thigh towards the knee originates from the hip-joint itself. It is chiefly young adults who during sport or athletics sprain a muscle in the thigh.

The end-feel is a great help in diagnosis at the hip, particularly when bursitis or a loose body in a normal hip-joint is a possibility. The extreme of passive flexion and both rotations has a very hard feel in arthritis, quite different from the soft end-feel of bursitis or an impacted loose body in a joint not yet arthritic. In these two disorders, the capsular pattern is absent, lateral rotation usually hurting, medial rotation not, so that two clear findings—non-capsular pattern, soft end-feel—combine to inform the examiner that, although pain is elicited at the extremes of range, arthritis is absent.

The range of movement at most individuals' hip joint is: flexion until the thigh touches the trunk (although the last 45 to 60 degrees of this apparent hip movement take place by the pelvis flexing on the lumbar joints); extension 15 to 30 degrees beyond the anatomical position; 60 degrees of medial rotation, 90 degrees of lateral rotation, 45 degrees of abduction and 30 degrees of adduction. The typical pattern of capsular limitation of movement in gross arthritis is as follows: (1) fixed in slight adduction (i.e. 50 to 55 degrees limitation of abduction); (2) no range of medial rotation; (3) 90 degrees limitation of flexion; (4) 10 to 30 degrees limitation of extension; (5) full lateral rotation. In very early arthritis, medial rotation is the first movement to become measurably restricted; slight limitation of flexion soon follows. In arthritis, medial rotation is the most painful passive movement.

LESIONS OF THE HIP-JOINT

Children

These are nearly all serious and differential diagnosis rests largely on the radiographic appearances. Hence any child found limping or complaining of even a slight ache in the thigh or knee, who shows the slightest limitation of movement at the hip-joint, should be put to bed immediately and not allowed up until the result of the X-ray examination is known. This is vital; otherwise, for example, a slipping epiphysis may slip completely and life-long deformity result.

1. Pseudo-coxalgia (Perthes)

This may be unilateral or bilateral and affects boys aged four to twelve. It is a manifestation of osteochondritis—a disorder of unknown aetiology. The symptoms are trivial, perhaps an ache in the knee, but the parents have noticed a limp. Examination reveals marked limitation of movement at the hip-joint. The radiograph shows flattening of the upper surface of the femoral head and a widening of the epiphyseal line. As a result, the femoral head no longer fits the acetabulum, and although prolonged recumbency leads to resolution of the arthritis and a good range of movement for the time being, osteoarthritis is very apt to supervene during the patient's late twenties or early thirties. The prognosis is good if the disorder starts at say, four years old, but poor if it starts at or after the age of eight, with or without treatment.

2. Tuberculosis of the Hip

This may be difficult to distinguish from pseudo-coxalgia. Clinically, the hip is found fixed in flexion, adduction and lateral rotation; muscle wasting is considerable. The patient is seldom over ten years of age. Generalized rarefaction and a diminished joint space seen on the radiograph suggest infection.

3. Slipped Epiphysis

Since this may be bilateral, but more advanced on one side, the X-ray photograph should include the whole pelvis. For unknown reasons, the epiphyseal junction softens, whereupon weight-bearing results in a gradual downward slipping of the head on the neck of the femur. The disorder arises between the ages of twelve and seventeen, and examination merely reveals the capsular pattern at the hip-joint with pain on passive movement, but not against resistance. The radiograph reveals the condition.

4. Transitory Arthritis

Occasionally the radiograph reveals nothing; yet limitation of movement has been found at the hip joint. The child should be kept in bed for a fortnight. Such rest may result in speedy return of a full range of movement to the joint. He is allowed up and examined again a few days later; full range remains. The condition is thought merely to result from overuse and has no evil significance for the future. G. F. Mayall (1965) states that in acute synovitis of the hip, good quality films often show increased density of the soft-tissues about the joint.

5. Coxa Vara

This is usually bilateral and results from any disorder causing softening of bone. Alternatively, coxa vara may follow pseudo-coxalgia. Rarely, the deformity is congenital. The range of abduction is markedly limited; the other movements may be of full range. The radiograph is diagnostic.

6. Haemophilia

The hip is a very uncommon site for intra-articular bleeding, but after several episodes thinning of cartilage with juxta-articular cysts form, and by his teens the boy may have developed permanent limitation of movement at the joint.

7. Congenital Dislocation

In Great Britain, the incidence is twelve in 10,000 girls and two in 10,000 boys, and is ten times commoner in breech presentation. It is bilateral in

10 to 25 per cent of cases and there is then no shortening of one leg or asymmetry of the folds in the thigh to draw attention to the dislocation. There is about 5 per cent chance of a second child being affected. Since early treatment (i.e. begun well before the child begins to walk) is so successful and avoids the later supervention of osteoarthritis, it is important to make the diagnosis as soon after birth as possible. To this end the baby is examined as follows (Ortolani, 1937). The baby lies on her back with the knees flexed and the thighs at right-angles to the trunk. The examiner's thumbs are placed at the inner aspect of her knees; his fingers along the outer thigh. The knees are now pushed apart, and on the dislocated side resistance to abduction is felt at 45 degrees. If this resistance is overcome by continued pressure towards abduction and lateral rotation, a sudden thud is felt as the head of the femur rides over the edge of the acetabulum and comes to lie in its socket. Full abduction is now free. If the thighs are now brought back to adduction again, during slight posteriorly-directed pressure on the upper part of the femur, the hip redislocates.

Barlow (1962) tests the baby's hip by grasping the uppermost femur between fingers and thumb. Pressure directed anteriorly then posteriorly can then be felt to move the head of the femur in and out of the acetabulum if the joint is unstable.

These tests afford the diagnosis before the X-ray picture reveals the displacement. In due course, the epiphysis is shown radiologically to lie above the acetabulum and to be about half the size of the one on the normal side.

ARTHRITIS IN ADULTS

The capsular pattern is present; the resisted movements do not hurt. The following conditions occur:

1. Osteoarthritis

This is revealed by osteophyte formation and a diminished joint space, especially superiorly, visible on the radiograph. If it comes on before the age of forty, it is usually the result of a severe sprain, fracture or previous disease of the hip, usually pseudo-coxalgia. Limitation of movement is often quite considerable before appreciable symptoms begin.

The careful studies of Harrison, Schajowicz and Trueta (1953) have shown that degeneration of cartilage at the femoral head is already present by the age of fourteen. It usually begins in the area of articular cartilage not subjected to pressure. Ossification of cartilage at points of instability then supervenes and increased vascularity is noted at these non-pressure areas. In due course, the whole head of the femur becomes riddled with new, dilated blood vessels. Cysts appear in the bone formed by fibrous masses with vascular walls. The head of the bone tends to flatten. It is their view that the trouble in osteoarthritis is 'not the degeneration of the cartilage, but the vigorous and persistent attempts to repair: attempts which aggravate the already disordered function of the joint, not only by osteophyte formation but also by hypervascularity which weakens the structure of the bone beyond the point where it can carry its load'. In their view daily use is desirable; this preserves rather than erodes cartilage.

There is a favourable and an unfavourable type of osteoarthritis at the hip. The very slowly progressive type is often bilateral and is characterized by the formation of a large collar of osteophytes all round the lateral edge of the femoral head, making it U-shaped instead of round (Plate 58). Cartilage between acetabulum and femoral head is reasonably well preserved. In more progressive osteoarthritis, there is no joint space at the upper surface of the femoral head, and the adjacent part of the acetabulum; sclerosis of bone is seen there. The erosion is confined to the weight-bearing aspect and osteophyte formation is inconspicuous. This is the type that may well come to operation.

It is remarkable how little index to the severity of the symptoms is afforded by the radiographic appearances. Erosion of cartilage and osteophyte formation of equal degrees may be accompanied by a good deal of movement and little pain, a good deal of movement and much pain, little movement and little pain, and little movement and much pain. Outward subluxation of the head of the femur with localized erosion of cartilage superiorly is often accompanied by an almost full range of movement and much pain.

Limitation of extension at the hip leads to low backache. No longer being able to extend at the hip, the patient moves his whole pelvis instead, hyperextending the lower lumbar joints at every step. It is no use treating this backache with a corset, for the movement is essential to the patient's gait.

2. Loose Body in the Hip-joint

There are three types, but it is a diagnosis which is seldom made since it is very exceptional for the loose body to contain an osseous nucleus which is X-ray opaque. The condition is not rare, merely unsuspected and, therefore, unrecognized (Plate 59).

The symptoms are clearly indicative of momentary subluxation of a loose body. The patient complains that, as he walks, he is suddenly halted by a severe twinge felt shooting down the front of the thigh from the groin to the knee. The leg tends to let him down at this moment. The twinge may be repeated at each step or at many weeks' intervals. The painful twinge that makes the leg momentarily give way under the patient is quite different from the painless weakness, again causing the leg to let him down, of the patient with a weak quadriceps, usually the result of a third lumbar disc lesion causing a root-palsy.

(a) *Osteochondritis Dessicans*

I have met with only one case. Vague symptoms began at the age of thirteen, when slight articular signs led to X-ray examination which showed bilateral osteo-chondritis at the medial aspect of the femoral head by the epiphyseal line. By the time the patient was twenty, he had for a year suffered from recurrent attacks of internal derangement at the right hip. They lasted up to two days and made walking impossible. During an attack, slight limitation of movement was present; between attacks, the joint was clinically normal.

The mechanism of this type of internal derangement was obscure to me until R. H. Young, who had operated on such a case, explained that it was a question of the loose fragment becoming tilted within its cave and suddenly forming a projection against the acetabulum.

Manipulation proved of little help, but a day or two in bed has so far brought about reduction.

(b) *Loose Fragments without Osteoarthritis*

This condition is rare. A small piece, presumably of exfoliated articular cartilage, becomes loose in the joint, presumably as the result of past trauma. It would seem to lie harmlessly inside the capsule about the neck of the femur for long periods at a time, but then to move and become nipped at the acetabular edge. When this happens, a severe twinge is felt with giving way of the limb. The patient has to stand on only the good leg for some moments; he then puts weight on his bad leg and finds it sound again. The twinge may be repeated a few steps later, or not again for some months. Those who suffer many twinges a day are severely dis-abled and, since at any moment they may become rooted to the spot, become understandably afraid of crossing the road.

Examination shows a full range of movement at the hip-joint, with some discomfort on, as a rule, full flexion and full lateral rotation. This would correspond with psoas bursitis, but in this disorder there are never any twinges. It is thus the history that supplies the differential diagnosis.

(c) *Loose Fragment with Osteoarthritis.*

A loose body may form secondarily to osteoarthritis; alternatively, a loose body that keeps subluxating may set up osteoarthritis later.

These are the commonest cases, and since the radiograph shows the osteoarthritis and not the loose body, the condition is missed. This is an important error; for the loose body can often be shifted to a position within the joint whence it no longer subluxates. If so, the patient, instead of suffering repeated twinges which make walking very difficult, merely suffers some discomfort after a long walk. In such cases, manipulative reduction affords several years' great relief.

3. Rheumatoid Arthritis

Monarticular rheumatoid arthritis at the hip is very uncommon. Considerable aching in the thigh on exertion with slight limitation of movement of the capsular pattern results. In the early case, X-ray shows no abnormality at the hip or the sacro-iliac joint. Later on, the loss of joint space is not, as in osteoarthritis, localized at the upper part of the joint, but generalized, often more marked at the medial part of the joint line. The acetabulum may begin to protrude, with simultaneous erosion of the femoral head.

4. Spondylitic Arthritis

In ankylosing spondylitis after the spine has stiffened, arthritis spreads to the hip-joints. This progresses, by flares and subsidences, until the joints become almost or quite fixed in flexion. Although the radiograph of the hip-joints reveals nothing at first, sacro-iliac arthritis, later fusion, is clearly visible.

5. Osteitis Deformans

If the hip-joints are affected early in the disease, there may as yet be no palpable thickening of the femora or tibiae, nor increase in the size of the skull. In such cases, only the radiograph of the pelvis discloses the true state of affairs.

6. Acetabular Protrusion

The signs are the same as in bilateral osteoarthritis but all abduction is lost early, and, in contrast to other forms of non-specific arthritis, adduction is also limited.

7. Arthritis

Rare cases are encountered in middle-aged persons who experience aching in the upper thigh on exertion, associated with *slight* limitation of movement at the hip-joint. It continues unchanged for months. The radiograph reveals nothing. Treatment by stretching out the capsule of the joint is quickly curative and there is no tendency to recurrence within five years. The nature of this type of arthritis is obscure.

8. Other Lesions

Pain felt only on full passive rotation occurs in lesions of the psoas muscle, tendinitis of the rectus femoris, gluteal and psoas bursitis, obturator hernia and invasion of the pubic bone by a neoplasm.

9. Hysteria

The hip shares with the shoulder and intervertebral joints an enhanced liability to fixation for psychological reasons. The patient walks in with a marked limp, often leaning on a thick stick. Inspection of gait reveals the limb fixed in medial rotation instead of the lateral rotation of organic disease. Examination begins at the lumbar spine and goes on to the toes; it reveals multiple inconsistencies. The commonest are: inability to use the psoas muscle when it is tested with the patient supine; 90 degrees limitation of passive hip flexion accompanied by a full range of passive rotations.

Treatment

1. Osteoarthritis

Osteoarthritis at the hip-joint is very difficult to alleviate. Full relief from symptoms is seldom attained even temporarily. Cure, even prevention of further aggravation, is impossible.

In the early stage, capsular stretching by the physiotherapist under heat analgesia is indicated. The joint is heated by short-wave diathermy and movement gradually forced (see Vol. II). A month's treatment twice a week is often followed by many months' ease. In particular, pain at night can often be abolished. In the end, however, stretching ceases to be effective. Hydrocortisone or silicone injected into the joint then becomes the treatment of choice (see below).

Later, a raised heel (to compensate for the apparent shortening) and a walking-stick are required.

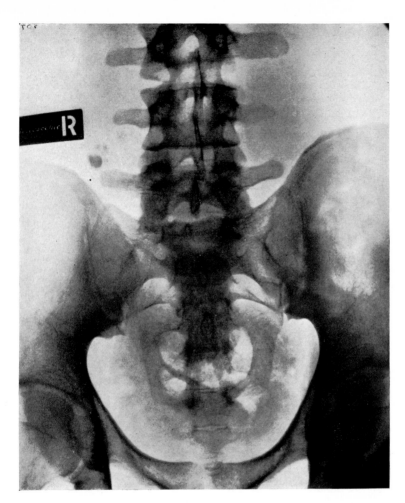

PLATE 54

Early spondylitis deformans. Sclerosis at the iliac side of the lower part of the left sacro-iliac joint is beginning. The patient was aged 19 and had had bouts of pain in one or other buttock for a year and a half. Previous radiographs had revealed nothing.

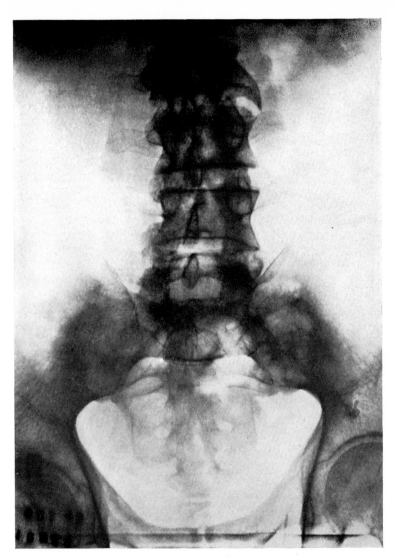

PLATE 55

Sacro-iliac fusion. The sacro-iliac joints have disappeared as the result of spondylitis deformans of thirty years' standing. Note the ossification of the left side of the second lumbar vertebra.

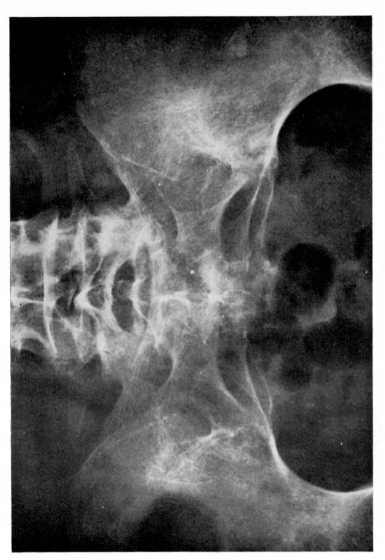

PLATE 56

Aborted spondylitis. A woman of 65 reported intermittent sciatica from the age of 17 to 27. She had had no subsequent symptoms and a good range of painless movement was present at her lumbar and thoracic joints.

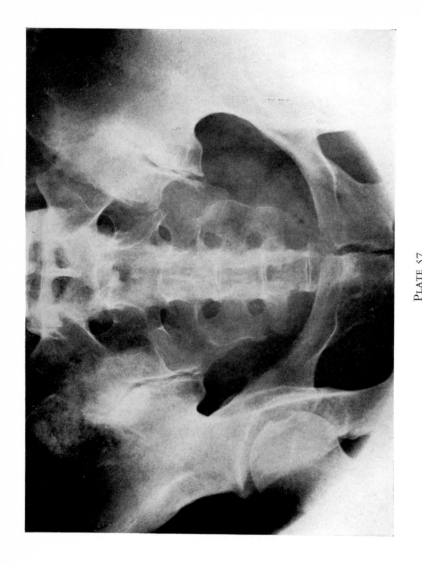

PLATE 57

Osteitis condensans ilii. The sclerosis occupies the central part of the joint whose margins are not blurred.

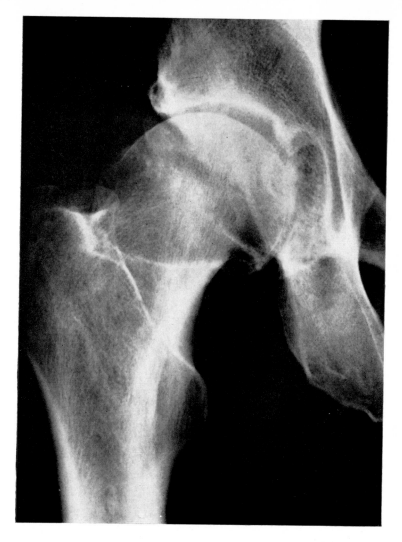

PLATE 58

Osteo-arthritis of hip. This is the type that carries a good prognosis.

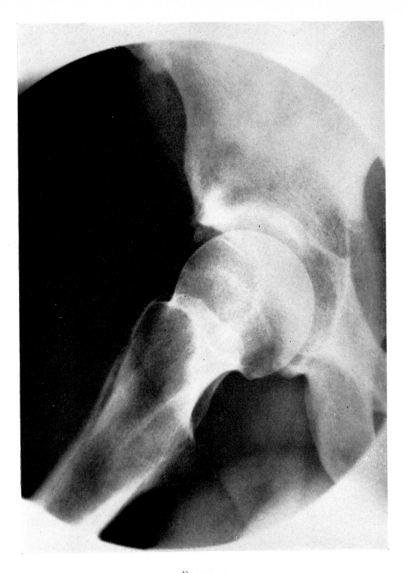

PLATE 59

Loose body in normal hip-joint. The patient, aged 38, had suffered three weeks' twinges.

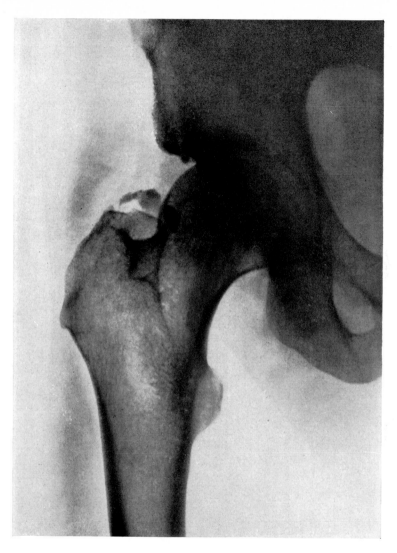

PLATE 60

Calcification in the gluteal bursa.

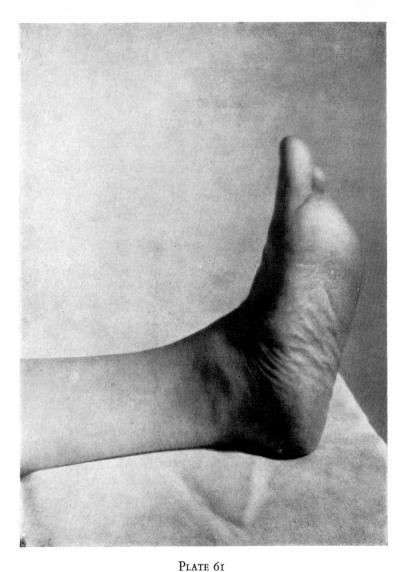

PLATE 61

Metatarsus inversus. Note the medial rotation deformity of the forefoot on the hindfoot.

If the pain is severe, and also disturbs sleep, operation is indicated, unless the patient is unwilling or too aged, in which case he must use a crutch. Arthrodesis is the operation of choice in unilateral cases; arthrodesis on one side and arthroplasty on the other when both hips are affected. When unilateral osteoarthritis comes on in early middle age, the sooner arthrodesis is performed the better; for fusion sooner or later is clearly inevitable, and there is no point in allowing the patient to suffer years of pain. In general, however, the time to operate is when pain compels the patient to ask for surgical interference.

A number of other treatments have been tried; none are fully successful. They are:

Intra-articular Hydrocortisone or Silicone Oil

In so far as there is often an element of overuse as the cause of pain in osteoarthritis, hydrocortisone can be employed to abate such traumatic inflammation. At the hip, hydrocortisone often succeeds in relieving pain, although it does not increase the range of movement.

The patient lies on his good side with the lower hip flexed. The painful hip is extended and the thigh allowed to adduct until the knee touches the couch. The edge of the trochanter is identified and a needle 12 cm. long introduced just above it and pointing vertically downwards. The needle clears the upper surface of the trochanter and is aimed at the junction of the head and the neck of the femur. After the needle has traversed the muscles, the resistance offered by the thick capsule can be felt; the point then strikes bone. Five cc. of hydrocortisone are injected. If the ensuing relief lasts several months, the injection can be repeated, say, twice a year. If it lasts a few weeks only, further injections should be avoided for fear of inducing a steroid arthropathy. The longest period of success to date is two years.

Chandler *et al.* (1959) reported a case of osteoarthritis of the hip given a monthly injection of only 50 mgr. hydrocortisone on eighteen occasions. As a result, the joint became painless but completely disorganized, the head of the femur disappearing with the development of 5 cm. shortening. The authors liken the condition to a Charcot's arthropathy. So far, this has not occurred in any of my cases, but it is clear that repeated injections at short intervals may prove dangerous. Sweetnam (1960) reported a case of cortisone arthropathy at the hip in a patient in whom the drug had been taken orally only. Views on the dangers of steroid therapy were challenged by Isdale (1962). He surveyed 600 patients who had their hips X-rayed, and found 27 with bone absorption. One of three with marked destructions and eight out of twelve with moderate absorption had never had any steroid treatment. He concluded that little statistical evidence existed of harm from steroid therapy, and to discontinue it would be a mistake. Sutton (1963) considered that steroid therapy enhanced the likelihood of arthropathy and described cases in which the joints become affected, though the disease being treated was non-articular, e.g. eczema.

Silicone oil is a bland, inert stable fluid 200 times as viscous as water. It lubricates roughened surfaces and is very suitable for osteoarthritis of the hip (Helal and Karadi, 1968). Ongley (1969) uses a far more viscid oil: dinethyl polysiloxane.

Intrathecal Alcohol

Since the capsule of the hip joint is so largely developed from the third lumbar segment, it seemed probable that, if the posterior root of the third lumbar nerve were destroyed by an intrathecal injection of alcohol, the pain of osteoarthritis of the hip might cease. Cases with clear third lumbar reference were chosen; J. D. Laycock kindly performed the injection. The patient lay on the unaffected side with a cushion so arranged at the loin that the third lumbar vertebra formed the top of a lumbar convexity. Alcohol (0·5 ml.) was introduced at the third lumbar inter-space. Numbness and tingling along the front of the thigh were noted by the patient. However, no improvement followed in six cases thus treated.

Denervation

The obturator nerve and the nerve to the quadratus femoris muscle carry most of the sensory fibres to the hip-joint. These can be removed. This operation is more favoured on the continent of Europe than in England. The result is usually disappointing. Herfort and Nickerson (1959) reported excellent results continuing for up to four years in fifteen patients with advanced arthritis of hip or knee in whom they carried out an extensive sympathetic denervation.

Operation

McMurray's intertrochanteric osteotomy has the advantage of diminishing pain while maintaining a useful range of movement at the hip-joint, and thus preventing the lumbar pain that so often complicates fixation of the hip in considerable flexion. It is indicated in the painful hip with good mobility. The period of rest in bed is seldom more than a month and weight-bearing is possible after three months. The altered angulation of the neck on the shaft of the femur presents a new area of uneroded cartilage to the acetabulum. Charnley's operation offers an interesting alternative; the floor of the acetabulum is bored away and the hip displaced medialwards. Adduction deformity is automatically corrected.

Six weeks in bed are required. Nailing the hip by forcing a Smith-Petersen pin through the head of the femur into the floor of the acetabulum fixes the joint but the pin may work loose. Pauwel's (1959) method of subtrochanteric angulation appears to offer hope. His operation causes rotation of the femoral head, such that the eroded area at the uppermost part of the femoral head is shifted medially, and a new area of cartilage bears against the acetabulum. Smith-Petersen's vitallium cup arthroplasty has the advantage of requiring only a month in bed and walking is possible after two months. The same period applies to Moore's prosthesis.

Some surgeons are now veering towards total replacement, a new acetabulum being fitted as well as a new head of femur. This multiplicity of operations discloses dissatisfaction with today's treatment, and no operation so far devised (except arthrodesis) appears to give better than a 50 per cent good result after five years.

A Future Treatment

It is clear that the answer to osteoarthritis of the hip-joint has not yet been found. A most promising approach would be the discovery of a substance that, when injected into the hip joint, would lead to ankylosis—in other words, a chemically induced arthrodesis.

Capsular ossification accompanies fluorine poisoning; hence, intra-articular injection of a fluorine salt in suitable dilution might have a good result. Naturally, animal experiments would have to be carried out first to find out whether a therapeutic dose can be achieved without general toxic manifestations. Alternatively, it is well-established that vesical mucosa, implanted into tissues free from bone, engenders ossification. In rats, at first a cyst forms, which shows osteogenesis round it three weeks later. The cyst contains a mucous fluid which promotes ossification when it spreads elsewhere after the cyst has been punctured. It is by no means impossible that this fluid, injected into or round the hip joint, would set up capsular ossification.

2. Loose Body in the Hip-joint

Manipulative reduction should be attempted at once. It does not always succeed, but if the loose fragment of cartilage can be moved to a position within the joint whence it stops subluxating, great benefit results, and many patients have been afforded up to several years' relief. If the symptoms return, the manipulation should be repeated (see Vol. II).

Removal is possible only if the loose fragment contains an osseous nucleus and its position is visible.

3. Other Disorders

In monarticular rheumatoid arthritis, hydrocortisone injected into the joint is effective. Forcing movement is contra-indicated. *Spondylitic arthritis* is also best treated during a flare-up by intra-articular injection of hydrocortisone. When the arthritis is subsiding, gentle stretching out by the physiotherapist is indicated. Fixation is best treated by arthroplasty. The joint nearly always fixes again in the end. Nothing can be done for *osteitis deformans* except to prescribe butazolidine. *Acetabular protrusion* is treated on lines similar to osteoarthritis; i.e. by stretching the joints out in the early stage and operation, if necessary, later on. The pain originating from the posterior aspect of the capsule of the pseudarthrosis resulting from long-standing *congenital dislocation* can, surprisingly enough, often be permanently relieved by one or two local anaesthetic infiltrations.

Mobilization of the Hip under Anaesthesia. This is not to be undertaken lightly. Though relief lasting for some time may be obtained in younger patients with deformity due to a past psuedo-coxalgia or protrusion acetabuli, in elderly patients with osteoarthritis the neck of the femur may break. At best, only evanescent relief follows. Rheumatoid arthritis is aggravated by forced movement.

MUSCLE LESIONS ABOUT THE HIP

These are all uncommon. It must be remembered that, when several resisted hip movements hurt, the likely cause is gluteal bursitis.

The Adductor Muscles

The patient is asked to lie supine and to squeeze the physician's closed fist between his knees. If resisted adduction hurts at the inner upper thigh, the upper extent of the adductor muscle is strained, most often at the musculo-tendinous junction, sometimes at the teno-periosteal junction. Tenderness identifies the exact site of the lesion. This is known as *rider's sprain*, and is uncommon except in athletes. Massage is curative at either site; hydrocortisone is effective at the tendon and local anaesthesia helps, especially in recent cases, at the upper belly.

Pain on resisted adduction is also elicited in fracture or neoplastic invasion of the os pubis. Fracture may follow a fall, or may be a stress fracture coming on without injury. If, therefore, no tenderness of the adductor muscles can be found in a case of pain on resisted adduction, an X-ray photograph should be taken of the pubic bone. Union is established in six to eight weeks. If resisted adduction of the thigh hurts in the buttock, the examiner must remember that this movement distracts the ilium from the sacrum and is painful in lesions of the sacro-iliac joint.

The Psoas Muscle

Strain here is uncommon, but a pleasure to meet; for it responds well to massage, but continues for years otherwise.

Pain arising from the psoas muscle may not be elicited when flexion is resisted as the patient lies with his thigh flat on the couch, since the upper part of the quadriceps muscle then shares the work with the psoas. Weakness is also obscured for the same reason. The hip must be bent to a right-angle before the movement is tested. Even if a hip is already osteoarthritic, psoas strain may complicate the joint lesion; hence, the resisted movements must be examined. In difficult cases, the induction of local anaesthesia diagnostically is indicated. It may of itself afford some degree of relief, but the consistently effective treatment is deep massage. Luckily, it seems that it is always the lower part of the muscle that becomes strained; the affected fibres lie immediately below the inguinal ligament, just medial to the inner edge of sartorius, where they are accessible to the physiotherapist's finger on deep palpation.

An obdurator hernia interferes with the pelvic course of the psoas muscle, pressing on it from behind. Resisted flexion, therefore, hurts in the iliac fossa. If the patient lies in the Trendelenburg position for ten minutes, the pain on resisted flexion ceases. This test appears to be pathognomonic.

Slight discomfort on resisted flexion may be felt in tendinitis of the rectus femoris or in partial rupture at the upper extent of the quadriceps muscle. If so, resisted extension of the knee, tested with the patient prone so as to maintain extension at the hip, evokes the pain more readily. For this reason, resisted flexion and extension at the knee are always included in the examination of the muscles about the hip.

Painful Weakness

Weakness accompanied by increased pain when the psoas muscle contracts is found in three conditions: (1) Traction-fracture of the lesser trochanter. This occurs in schoolboys. The onset is not sudden. Weakness *and* pain are elicited when the resisted flexion movement is tested. The patient is put to bed in a half-sitting position for two or three weeks. When walking no longer hurts, he can be allowed up. (2) Abdominal neoplasm infiltrating the psoas muscle. (3) Metastases at the upper femur. The weakness may be gross, and is associated with pain, and with marked limitation of movement at the hip-joint.

Painless Weakness

Weakness, without increased pain when the muscle is tested, occurs in two other conditions. (1) Paresis of the psoas muscle forms the less obvious part of a third lumbar root-palsy. (2) Neoplasm, benign or malignant, at the second lumbar level naturally leads to weakness.

Sartorius Muscle

'Cricket-leg' was thought to be caused by rupture of the sartorius muscle, but in fact some fibres of the quadriceps have ruptured at mid-thigh.

The only lesion of the sartorius muscle is traction-fracture of the anterior superior spine of the ilium. The boy is aged fifteen to eighteen and, while running, feels a painful click in his groin and uppermost thigh. He now finds walking painful and running impossible.

A full range of painless passive movement is present at the hip-joint, but resisted flexion and lateral rotation hurt. Resisted extension at the knee also causes some discomfort. Tenderness is localized to the anterior superior spine of the ilium and the uppermost inch of the sartorius muscle, and radiography shows the separation at the iliac spine. Spontaneous recovery takes two or three weeks. If the youngster wants to run, local anaesthesia can be induced just before the race.

Gluteal Muscle

Lesions of these muscles appear not to occur, apart from direct bruising. In such cases, spontaneous recovery seldom takes longer than some days. Obstruction of the internal iliac artery leads to claudicational pain, re-produced by maintained contraction of the gluteal muscles.

Weakness of abduction accompanied by pain in a schoolboy suggests a traction-fracture of the greater trochanter. Painless weakness occurs in congenital dislocation of the hip, when the greater trochanter has risen so high that contraction of the gluteus medius muscle has become ineffective. As the patient walks, the result is a characteristic dipping of the pelvis towards the leg that is off the ground—the Trendelenburg gait. The gluteus medius weakens in a fifth lumbar, and the gluteus maximus in a first sacral, root-palsy.

The Ilio-tibial Band

'Contracture' of the ilio-tibial band is no longer regarded as causing symptoms.

Sprain occurs only in dancers and athletes, and causes pain in the trochanteric region. Bursitis underlying the ilio-tibial band gives rise to identical symptoms but there is no trauma. If the band has become strained the characteristic signs are: (1) Pain on trunk side-flexion towards the painless side, increased if the patient stands with his legs crossed before he bends sideways. (2) Pain on full passive adduction at the hip. (3) No pain on any other passive hip movement. (4) No pain on resisted abduction at the hip, or when the other resisted movements are tested. If the diagnosis is in doubt, local anaesthesia should be induced at the painful spot just behind and above the greater trochanter. A few sessions of massage are curative. In bursitis, local anaesthesia is usually effective alone; if it is not, hydrocortisone must be injected.

Quadriceps and Hamstring Muscles

Partial rupture from indirect violence with, often, the formation of a haematoma is common in athletes. During some strenuous movement the patient feels something give way; he supplies the diagnosis correctly himself. Although the pain is not severe at the time, that evening and next morning the pain and disablement are considerable. Direct trauma, e.g. a kick on the thigh, may be responsible.

Resisted flexion and extension of the knee are examined with the patient lying prone, the hip being thus kept extended. Pain felt in the groin on resisted extension shows some part of the upper quadriceps muscle to be at fault. This used to be termed 'cricket-leg' and mistakenly ascribed to rupture of the sartorius muscle. If the rupture is at all extensive and a haematoma is present, passive knee-flexion is limited so long as the patient stays prone. When he is turned to lie supine, a full range of knee-flexion is revealed. This is due to the quadriceps muscle being released above as fast as it is tautened below when the hip-joint and knee-joint are flexed simultaneously. Tenderness, distension of the muscle by effused blood and, sometimes, fluctuation demonstrates the site of the lesion. A third lumbar disc lesion is the only other condition in which the range of knee-flexion alters according to whether the hip is kept extended or flexed. Both are instances of extra-articular limitation of movement with the sign dependent on the constant length phenomenon. By contrast, if the quadriceps muscle has become adherent to the mid-shaft of a fractured femur, the amount of flexion at the knee does not alter with the position of the hip.

Tendinitis of the rectus femoris shows itself by pain felt at the groin on resisted extension at the knee coupled with pain on full passive flexion of the hip, especially flexion in adduction. This implies that the lesion in the muscle lies in a position where it can be pinched.

When resisted flexion at the knee hurts at the back of the thigh, the hamstring muscles are at fault. If the sprain is tendinous and lies at the ischium, straight-leg raising is of full range. If a haematoma is present after a rupture in the belly, straight-leg raising is limited, though hip-flexion with the knee bent is of full range—the constant length phenomenon again.

Treatment

In either case, this consists of aspiration of the haematoma; the immediate induction of local anaesthesia (at least 50 ml.); prolonged deep massage to the whole area of the tear and to the hardish swelling on either side due to infiltration of the belly with blood. Voluntary movement without weight-bearing is encouraged from the outset and faradism is of real value. It should be given with the knee kept passively fully flexed (for the hamstrings) or the knee held passively fully extended and the hip flexed (for the quadriceps). Full broadening of the muscles is then attained without pull on the healing breach. Progress is slow after a fair-sized rupture, especially towards the end. In sprinters, a recurrence is quite common unless too early a return to racing is prevented by continuing treatment for a fortnight after the patient has recovered clinically.

Painless Weakness

If this is unilateral, a lesion of the third lumbar nerve-root is present. If the weakness is bilateral, localized myopathy or myositis should be suspected. Painful weakness characterizes a partial muscle rupture or a fractured patella.

Painless weakness of the hamstring muscles characterizes lesions of the first and second sacral roots, usually due to a disc lesion.

24

The Knee

Although a large variety of conditions arise in the knee, an exact diagnosis can be made with greater certainty than at any other joint. This is because different symptoms characterize different lesions, and because the greater part of the joint with its ligaments and tendons is accessible to direct palpation.

EXAMINATION OF THE KNEE

Examination of the knee has to be conducted in the light of the history; for, by itself, the clinical state of the knee is often not characteristic of any one disorder. When diagnosis at the knee proves impossible, it is well to remember that a small cartilaginous loose body is commonplace at and after middle-age, and may cause symptoms and signs that defy interpretation. Minor articular signs, particularly when associated with pain localized to one part of the knee, should suggest this probability.

Pain Referred to the Knee

Lesions of the knee-joint give rise to pain felt accurately at the knee, often at some particular part of the joint. An impacted loose body complicating osteoarthritis is the only disorder of the knee that is apt to cause pain referred up the thigh and down the leg; even so, it is usually quite clear to the patient that the symptoms stem from the knee.

The front of the knee represents the second and third lumbar segments. Hence, the origin of pain referred to this area should be sought within these segments. The diagnostic point in the history, when pain is referred to the knee, is the indefinite area of which the patient complains. He may point to the whole suprapatellar area, and may have noted an ache running up the front or inner thigh towards the groin. The two principal structures apt to give rise to referred anterior crural pain are the hip-joint and the third lumbar nerve-root. In a third lumbar disc lesion the pain usually begins in the buttock, later affecting the front of the thigh; it is not aggravated by exertion or walking but a cough often hurts. Such a history exculpates the knee. When the hip-joint is at fault, the pain is diffuse, although often worst at the knee; it is aggravated by walking and the patient may describe twinges which make the knee suddenly let him down. Only the extent of the pain then makes the examiner cautious, but later discovery of a normal knee on clinical examination naturally focuses attention on the hip: a joint also subject to internal derangement. A common error is to have an X-ray photograph taken of an elderly person's knee because pain is felt there; to find it osteoarthritic (a fair certainty) and regard this as diagnostic. Many osteoarthritic hips are missed this way.

The back of the knee is developed from the first and second sacral segments. Disorders of the knee itself very seldom cause posterior pain only. Hence the source of pain felt there is most often pressure on the first sacral nerve-root as the result of a fifth lumbar disc lesion. Primary postero-lateral pulpy protrusions at this level occasionally begin with pain only at the back of the knee, nothing being felt in the buttock at first. However, the patient may notice that sitting or coughing hurts his knee, whereas walking does not. A lesion of the lower part of the hamstring muscles or the upper part of the calf, whether ischaemic or due to a minor rupture, causes pain correctly attributed by the patient to the back of his knee.

History

A detailed history is essential. A short list follows of the more important points that must be ascertained.

What is the age and occupation of the patient? What was he doing when the pain first appeared? In what position was his body and his leg, and what forces were acting on his knee at the time? Alternatively, did the pain come on for no apparent reason? Did the knee give way; if so, did the knee lock; if so, did it lock in extension or flexion; if so, how did it become unlocked? On which side of the knee was the pain or was it right inside, or was it all over? Did the pain change from one side of the knee to the other? Did it spread; if so, where to? Was the patient able to walk? Did the joint swell; if so, how quickly? For how long was he disabled? Were there recurrences; if so, what brought them on? How did they progress? What is the effect of going up and down stairs; is going down more troublesome than up? Are there sudden twinges? Does the knee click? Does it grate? Does it feel as if it might give way; if so, does the patient actually fall? What treatment has he had, and with what effect? Enquiry is made of the existence of arthritis elsewhere.

Inspection

Diffuse swelling and the adoption of a flexed position of the knee suggest advanced arthritis, with fluid in the joint or synovial thickening, sometimes both. Limitation of extension coming on suddenly suggests displacement of part of a meniscus. The speed with which an effusion appears after an injury is significant: if it appears in a few minutes, it is haemorrhagic; if in some hours, it is probably serous. Localized swellings are usually caused by a cyst of the lateral meniscus or by bursae, especially the pre-patellar and the semi-membranosus.

Muscular wasting is noted, but has no great diagnostic value unless it is extreme, when it suggests severe arthritis. Reddening of the skin suggests sepsis or gout.

The alignment of the tibia on the femur is noted. A genu valgum deformity in a child may be due to rickets or to a valgus position of the heel from inversion of the fore-foot, but it often comes on apparently without cause and disappears with growth. Some degree of genu varum is normal in babies. Its development in an elderly patient suggests osteitis deformans. A tiny pattela characterises the nail-knee syndrome.

Palpation of the Stationary Joint

Site of Tenderness

Since nearly all the tissues at the knee lie superficially, palpation lends great accuracy to diagnosis, and follows the clinical examination. Tenderness is always sought along the structure thus identified, provided that history and physical signs indicate that it lies within finger's reach.

Heat

Heat means that the lesion, whatever it may be, is in the active stage; localized heat naturally has a strong diagnostic value. The joint should be palpated again at the end of the examination of movements, for it may have been rendered warm merely by the minor stresses entailed. The discovery of heat indicates: (a) recent injury or operation, (b) blood in the joint, (c) bacterial, rheumatoid, spondylitic, gonorrhoeal or Reiter's arthritis, (d) a loose body impacted with an osteoarthritis joint, (e) gout, (f) fracture, (g) osteitis deformans.

Fluid

Testing for fluid in the knee-joint can be done in two ways.

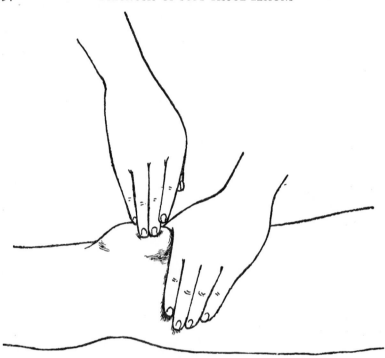

FIG. 109A. Test for fluid in the knee-joint: patellar tap. If the patella is raised from the femur by fluid, it can be felt to tap against the bone when jerked dowards by the examiner's finger. Unless the joint contains a good deal of fluid, the suprapatellar pouch must first be emptied by the pressure of the examiner's other hand.

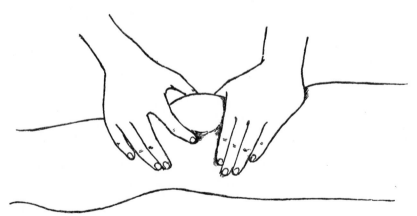

FIG. 109B. Test for fluid in the knee-joint: eliciting fluctuation. The examiner lays one hand flat on the suprapatellar pouch. Pressure here forces fluid into the lower part of the joint. If fluid is present, the fingers of his other hand, lying to each side of the patella, are forced apart as the pressure is applied.

Patellar Tap

Unless the joint is very full, the suprapatellar pouch is first emptied by manual pressure with the palm of the hand. Fluid, if present, is thus forced downwards, lifting the patella off the femur. The patella can be felt to hit the femur with a palpable tap as it is pushed smartly backwards by the examiner's hand. In the normal knee, the cartilaginous surfaces of patella and femur are already in contact and thus cannot be made to click against each other.

Eliciting Fluctuation

This is a more delicate test and should therefore always be preferred to the above manœuvre. The examiner places his thumb to one side of the patella, and one of his fingers to the other. With the palm of his other hand over the whole suprapatellar pouch, he presses backwards. If fluid lies in the suprapatellar pouch, it is made to run towards the lower part of the joint and thus will push apart the fingers of the examiner's other hand. Even the presence of only a little fluid can be detected in this way. By this method—but not by eliciting patellar tap—experience enables the examiner to tell blood from clear fluid. Blood fluctuates *en bloc* like a jelly moving, whereas a clear effusion runs up and down piecemeal.

Whenever the question arises of blood in the knee-joint—common after direct trauma—diagnostic aspiration is immediately indicated. If blood is present, it is all aspirated, since this is the important therapeutic measure. If the fluid turns out to be clear, there is no point in emptying the joint, since the treatment of a clear effusion is to deal with the cause.

If an effusion has developed without adequate trauma in a boy, and aspiration proves that it consists of blood, the cooperation of the pathologist should be sought and anti-haemophilic globulin administered at once. This prevents the knee filling again.

Synovial Thickening

Whether the synovial membrane is thickened or not is difficult to estimate at times; yet it may be a vital clinical finding. The examiner's finger should seek the reflexion of the membrane, where it overlies each condyle of the femur (Fig. 110), about 2 cm. posterior to the medial and lateral edges of the patella. He rolls this edge under his finger, carefully comparing the two knees. Synovial swelling indicates a bacterial, rheumatoid or inflammatory arthritis (e.g. gout, tuberculosis, gonorrhoea, Reiter's disease, ulcerative colitis, ankylosing spondylitis). Warmth and fluid without synovial swelling suggest traumatic arthritis (including that secondary to impaction of a small loose body), recent injury, fracture or operation, or blood in the joint. Localized warmth felt after the examination of the joint, not present at first, characterizes an impacted loose body complicating osteoarthritis.

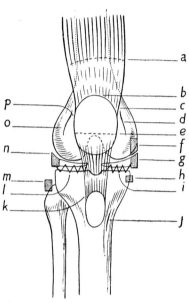

(a) Musculo-tendinous junction.
(b) Insertion of suprapatellar tendon.
(c) Quadriceps expansion.
(d) Capsular attachment to the femur.
(e) Usual site of transverse patellar fracture.
(f) Medial collateral ligament: upper end.
(g) Medial collateral ligament: at the joint line.
(h) Semimembranosus tendon.

(i) Medial coronary ligament.
(j) Insertion of semitendinosus muscle.
(k) Infrapatellar tendon.
(l) Lateral coronary ligament.
(m) Biceps tendon.
(n) Lateral collateral ligament.
(o) Capsular attachment to the femur.
(p) Quadriceps expansion.

FIG. 110. Knee: points of tenderness

Other Findings

Palpation clearly reveals osteophytes of any size. Bony deformity may be seen and felt, e.g. upper tibial fracture, or the enlargement of the patella that results from the old stellate fracture or osteitis deformans. The bony expansion caused by neoplasm or chronic osteomyelitis can be palpated. When osteitis deformans affects the tibia, the sharp anterior edge is eventually lost and the front of the leg may be warm. Prominence of the tibial tuberosity left after Schlatter's disease has no significance in adult life. Syphilitic periostitis is very rare; traumatic periostitis not uncommon. A prepatellar bursa is most easily felt when the tissues at the front of the patella are pinched up. Calcified areas in the suprapatellar pouch may form palpable thickening.

Intra-articular loose bodies should be sought if the patient mentions severe momentary twinges or locking. The patient or the doctor may feel the loose body move; hence the German name 'gelenkenmaus'.

A cyst of the lateral meniscus can be felt by palpation along the joint-line during extension. When the knee is flexed, the small projection disappears.

Palpation of the Moving Joint

This discloses the state of the opposed surfaces of articular cartilage. It may reveal fine crepitus, some degree of which is normal in all middle-aged individuals. Coarse crepitus indicates marked fragmentation of the surface of articular cartilage. If bone is felt creaking against bone, cartilage has been completely eroded.

In patellar-femoral osteoarthritis, when the patient is examined lying down, the patella is not kept strongly enough applied to the front of the femur by muscular action for the marked crepitus characteristic of this condition to be felt. Hence the knee must be palpated while the patient stands, squats and comes up again, by the examiner's hand applied to the front of the knee. A number of other manoeuvres are appropriate if evidence of a ruptured meniscus is sought.

Diagnostic Movements at the Knee

Passive Movements

The primary movements are four: flexion, extension and rotation each way during flexion. If limitation of movement in all directions is found, severe arthritis is present. The *capsular pattern* is great limitation of flexion and slight limitation of extension. For example, 5 or 10 degrees limitation of extension corresponds with 60 to 90 degrees limitation of flexion. Rotation is little restricted, except in gross arthritis. A painful arc should be noted; it occurs in impaction of a loose body, patellar irregularity, patellar-femoral osteoarthritis, and, rarely, torn meniscus.

The secondary movements, picking out particular ligaments, are also four: varus and valgus strain (for the collateral ligaments); anterior and posterior pressure on the tibia while the knee is held bent to a right-angle (stretching each cruciate ligament); applying a shearing strain to the joint when it is held bent to a right-angle, the femur and tibia being pressed sideways in opposite directions. This may evoke pain when a loose body or a torn meniscus is present, and forcing the tibia laterally on the femur often elicits pain from a painful posterior cruciate ligament. The discovery that pain is provoked is just as important as that the range is excessive, i.e. the ligament has become overstretched.

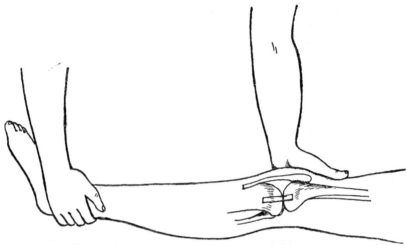

FIG. 111. Application of valgus strain. The knee is forced medially and the ankle laterally; as a result the inner aspect of the knee is stretched.

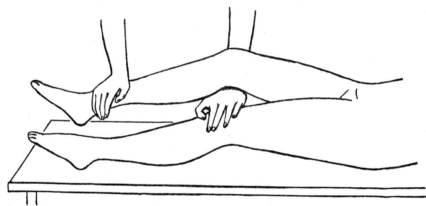

FIG. 112. Resisted extension of knee. The examiner passes his forearm under the knee and supports his hand on the other knee. The patient's flexed knee rests on his lower forearm. The extension movement is resisted by the examiner's other hand at the ankle.

Resisted Movements

These are best examined as the patient lies prone (Fig. 73) but may for convenience be tested supine (Fig. 112). The primary movements are two: flexion and extension. Pain on a resisted muscular contraction is noted, likewise weakness, likewise the two together. If extension is painful, a lesion of the quadriceps muscle is present; if it is painful and weak, a fractured patella or a major rupture of the belly is the cause; if it is weak but the muscular contraction does not hurt, a third lumbar root-palsy is suggested. If flexion is painful, medial and lateral rotation are tested against resistance while the knee is held passively flexed; this test distinguishes between the biceps (lateral rotator) and the other members of the hamstring group (all medial rotators).

Summary

For the proper examination of the knee, twelve tests are carried out while the patient lies supine on the couch.

The Joint

Four passive movements. Flexion, extension, medial and lateral rotation. Painful, painless; full range, limited range. Capsular or noncapsular pattern.

The Ligaments

Four passive movements. Valgus strain for the medial ligament; varus strain for the lateral ligament; pulling the tibia forwards for the anterior cruciate ligament; pushing the tibia backwards for the posterior cruciate ligament. Painful, painless; full range, excessive range.

The Muscles

Two resisted movements. Resisted extension for the patella, its tendons and the quadriceps muscle. Resisted flexion for the hamstring muscles.

Palpation

For heat, fluid or synovial thickening. For tenderness.

DISORDERS OF THE KNEE JOINT

The following conditions occur at the knee; the history taken together with the physical sign forms a series of characteristic patterns, though neither taken alone may be of itself diagnostic.

Ligamentous Sprain

(a) Medial Collateral Ligament

History

The patient falls awkwardly while skiing or strains the inner side of his knee on the football field. A strong valgus strain is imposed on his knee;

he feels a sudden pain or crack at the inner side of the knee. At first he can walk, but he becomes increasingly disabled and half-an-hour later is hobbling only with assistance. Some hours later, the knee is swollen and the pain worse. He has to spend some days in bed. He limps about in great discomfort for several weeks. Then the pain and swelling slowly subside; after two or three months he has largely recovered.

Signs

In the acute stage, which lasts up to a fortnight, the knee is full of fluid, hot to the touch, and extension is about 5 degrees limited, flexion 90 degrees limited. An acute traumatic arthritis is present, obscuring all other signs. But the patient knows that he sprained the inner side of the joint and localized tenderness is easily found at some point along the ligament.

In the subacute stage, which lasts four to six weeks in the untreated case, the limitation of movement at the knee slowly diminishes. The knee remains warm, more so at the inner side. Testing the ligament by applying valgus strain is now possible and elicits pain, whereas varus strain does not. If the ligament was over-stretched and is now permanently lengthened, an excessive range of valgus movement exists when the two knees are compared. If adhesions consolidate themselves because healing is allowed to take place without adequate movement at the knee, the chronic stage is reached.

Localization

The medial collateral ligament is nearly always damaged at the point where it crosses the joint-line and is attached to the medial meniscus. Nevertheless, its whole extent must be palpated. The lower part of the tibial attachment is scarcely ever affected; the lesion lies, in order of frequency: (1) at the joint-line; (2) at the femoral origin; (3) at the edge of the tibial condyle. Puzzling signs are found when the lesion lies high up on the femoral condyle. When this motionless part of the ligament suffers contusion, there may be little or no restriction of movement, yet the knee hurts and is warm, contains fluid and valgus strain is painful. Palpation reveals the reason for the small degree of limitation.

(b) Lateral Collateral Ligament

This is very seldom sprained. If it is, the articular signs are less severe, owing to the less intimate attachment of this ligament to the joint compared with the medial ligament. Hence the knee is warm, contains fluid, but the range of movement is almost full from the outset. The patient knows that he sprained the outer side of his knee and varus strain hurts. Palpation of the ligament discloses the site of the lesion.

(c) Coronary Ligament

History

The patient describes a rotation strain, usually at football. He stands on one foot and, wishing to kick to one side, twists his body on this leg. He feels an immediate pain in his knee, localized to the inner or the outer side. He may fall to the ground but gets up again almost at once and may even be able to go on playing. That evening the knee is painful and swollen; the next day he hobbles with difficulty. The sprain resolves very slowly, usually (unless treated) taking at least three months to recover.

Signs

The coronary ligament attaches the meniscus to the edge of the tibial condyle. In extension at the knee, the menisci are forced forwards, thus stretching the ligament. Whatever the degree of flexion, the semilunar cartilages lie in neutral position, undisturbed. Hence extension is characteristically the really painful movement in coronary sprain.

Medial rotation tends to stretch the lateral coronary ligament; lateral rotation the medial coronary ligament; hence one or other of these passive movements is painful but not limited.

Examination soon after the accident shows the knee to be warm and filling with fluid, extension being 5 degrees limited whereas flexion is merely full and painful. By next day traumatic arthritis has supervened, and the capsular pattern, now with marked limitation of flexion, appears. The passive rotation movements remain of full range, the one towards the painless side hurting.

The history of a rotation sprain is clear, and the pain is at one side of the knee only. Applying varus and valgus strains does not hurt; this excludes the collateral ligaments. It follows that one or other of the coronary ligaments has been strained. Tenderness is sought with the knee well bent and the appropriate coronary ligament is tender, the collateral ligament is not.

After a time, the traumatic arthritis subsides; later full extension returns, but the warmth and fluid persist for several months in the absence of adequate treatment.

(d) Cruciate Ligaments

Recent Injury

The history is of a sprain but not in any characteristic direction. During extension, a small degree of lateral rotation of the tibia on the femur takes place, relaxing the anterior cruciate ligament enough to allow full extension to be reached. Hence a sprain of the anterior ligament may be caused by a hyperextension strain combined with force towards medial rotation. Examination shows a warm and swollen knee containing fluid, with a full range of movement in each direction, all extremes hurting; for the cruciate ligaments limit rotation as well as extension (the anterior is

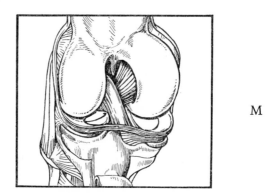

L   M

FIG. 113. The cruciate ligaments at the knee. The best approach to the anterior end of the posterior cruciate ligament is obliquely under the patella from its lateral aspect with the knee held bent to a right-angle.

then taut) and flexion (the posterior is taut). Valgus and varus strains cause no pain, but when the tibia is rocked backwards (stretching the posterior cruciate ligament) and forwards (stretching the anterior ligament) one or other of these movements is painful (Fig. 114).

When the posterior cruciate ligament is affected, forcing the tibia laterally on the femur with the joint at a right-angle stretches it painfully. After a severe injury, permanent lengthening is common; if so, an excessive range of antero-posterior movement of the tibia on the femur is detected when the two sides are compared. No tenderness can be elicited; for no part of either ligament is within finger's reach. Adhesions cannot form about the cruciate ligaments; the trouble is that the range of movement becomes too great. Manipulation is therefore futile.

Spontaneous recovery is very slow; it often takes six to twelve months. An occasional patient fails to recover at all and, say a year later, is still unable to run, let alone play football. In such chronic strain, if the posterior cruciate ligament is affected, the lesion usually lies at the attachment to the posterior edge of the tibia.

Permanent Lengthening

The history is now most misleading; for it simulates closely that of a ruptured meniscus.

The patient states that he suffered a severe injury to his knee a year or more ago; ever since, he has had to be careful of his knee. If he twists on it, the knee appears to him to 'go out' with a click and he has to stand on the other leg and give his leg a shake; there is another click and all is well.

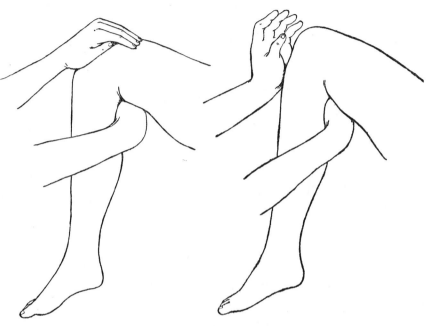

FIG. 114A. Stretching anterior cruciate ligament. The patient relaxes his muscles and the tibia is pulled forwards on the femur, while the knee is held at a right-angle.

FIG. 114B. Stretching posterior cruciate ligament. The knee is held passively at a right-angle and the tibia pushed backwards on the femur.

Actual subluxation of the tibia on the femur by rotation during weight-bearing is being described. Only when the cruciate ligaments are tested during examination of the knee does the nature of the disorder become obvious.

Post-traumatic Adhesions

History

A common history is that of a sprain of some part of the knee, followed by swelling, which has been treated by a few days', possibly weeks', rest in bed and then by gradually increasing use. After a time the knee has become quite adequate for ordinary walking, but hurts at one small spot when the patient takes vigorous exercise, and is apt to become stiff after he has kept it still for any length of time, e.g. sitting. It is clear that abnormally adherent scars have been allowed to form about the torn structure during the period of healing. Quiet use of the knee does not pull at these adhesions; exertion does. Thus vigorous exercise of the knee each time sprains anew the ligament whose mobility is impaired. Each time, after a few days, the pain and swelling subside and the knee gives no more trouble until exerted again.

Signs

As a rule the adhesions lie at the mid-part of the medial collateral ligament. The signs are: full extension hurts at the inner side; flexion is 5 or 10 degrees limited; full lateral rotation hurts; full medial rotation is painless. The knee is not warm and there is no fluid in the joint unless the patient is seen on the day of, or after, some exertion. The resisted movements are painless. Valgus strain hurts; testing the lateral ligament causes no pain and stretching the cruciate ligaments sets up no discomfort either. Tenderness is sought and found at some part of the medial ligament, usually at the joint line.

If a full range of movement is found, and localized discomfort together with a history of a former sprain nevertheless suggest adhesions about a ligament, tenderness should be sought at the femoral origin of the medial collateral ligament if valgus strain hurts, but at the coronary ligament if valgus strain is painless.

Stieda-Pellegrini's Disease

After an apparently ordinary sprain of the inner side of the knee, in due course the range of movement is found not to be increasing but actually to have diminished. Examination reveals the lesion to lie at the medial collateral ligament at its upper extent. By a month after the injury, radiography shows a linear shadow along the whole inner side of the medial femoral condyle. The periosteum has been torn up by the ligamentous pull at the time of the accident, and bone grows until it reaches the periosteum once more. Recovery in slight cases takes six months, in more severe cases up to a year. Treatment is useless.

Torn Meniscus

History

The characteristic features are (a) locking *in flexion*, and (b) manipulative *unlocking*. The first injury leading to rupture of the meniscus nearly always takes place between the ages of sixteen and thirty. If a child, nearly always a girl, say, aged twelve has signs of cartilage trouble, the condition to be suspected is a congenital discoid meniscus, more often the lateral. Cartilage trouble at the knee occurs at any age; the earliest age at which Young has performed excision and found a ruptured meniscus is nine months. If a patient is aged over thirty when he first fractures his meniscus, the crack is sometimes posterior or horizontal. Indeed, Hadfield (1966) explored twenty-one knees in patients over forty who had persistent symptoms and found that fourteen had a meniscus split horizontally forming a sliding tear.

During flexion-extension, the menisci move with the tibia, but when the femur is rotated on the tibia with the knee flexed, they move with the femur. It is therefore this movement that most strongly strains the coronary ligaments and the tissue of the meniscus itself. Hence tearing of a meniscus is caused by a strong rotation strain with the knee slightly bent. Thus, in the course of violent exertion, very often a game of football, the knee is severely twisted, usually in an attempt by the player to kick sideways, turning his whole body while the knee is fixed by the foot on the ground. It is this rotation strain of body on leg that fractures the intra-articular meniscus of the knee on which the player is standing. He feels a click and a sudden agonizing pain in the joint, which gives way under him, making him fall to the ground. A minute later when, recovering, he tries to move his knee, he finds that he can bend it a little but not straighten it. Then, or later, either he or the trainer forces it, and, with a click, full extension is regained. Then the knee swells and is painful for a few days. Later still when the patient has recovered, he finds that he is apt, if twisting on his knee once more, to feel something 'go out' painfully in his joint; whereupon the leg gives way under him and he falls with the knee locked again in a semi-flexed position. He then kicks his leg straight or has it manipulated and suddenly the obstruction slips away and his knee becomes serviceable once more. Occasionally, the layman's attempt at immediate reduction proves too painful; if so medical attention and general anaesthesia are required.

The side of the knee on which the patient felt the pain indicates which meniscus was torn; the medial meniscus is much the more commonly torn of the two (various surgeons give the proportion as three, five or seven to one). If a lesion of the lateral meniscus is present, it should be recalled that rupture is only twice as common as cyst formation. Cyst at the medial meniscus is a great rarity.

In posterior meniscal cracks occurring for the first time between the ages of thirty and forty-five the history is less dramatic. The patient states that if he twists on his knee quickly he occasionally feels something go out at the back of the joint with a click; he kicks his knee out straight, the knee clicks again and is at once fit for use. In these cases, locking of sufficient degree to require reduction by another person or eventual excision is uncommon. Middle-aged patients describe an even slighter disorder when the crack merely causes a bifid posterior extremity to the meniscus. The patient says that rotation in flexion during weight-bearing (i.e. movement while squatting) gives rise to an uncomfortable click, remedied as he stands up by another click.

In middle-age and later, the meniscus may crack horizontally. The tag that forms can then become displaced and form a visible and palpable projection at the joint-line. Digital pressure often suffices for reduction. If the tag gets twisted round the edge of the meniscus, the free end lying on the superior surface, reduction by manipulation becomes impossible; excision is then the only remedy.

Calcification of the meniscus occurs in pseudo-gout as the result of deposition of crystals of calcium pyrophosphate, but does not itself cause symptoms.

Signs

As the knee straightens, the fact that the curve of the femoral condyles follows a spiral comes into play. In extension, the anterior cruciate, the collateral and the posterior aspect of the joint capsule all become taut. When all the slack in the ligaments has been taken up, the femur and tibia are strongly approximated, extension beyond 180 degrees being prevented. At this point, there is no room for a displacement lying between the two bones. Extension of the knee must therefore be limited if a fragment of meniscus intervenes at the joint surfaces.

The coronary ligament holds the meniscus in place; force sufficient to rupture the cartilage must sprain the ligament first. Indeed, coronary strain leading to rupture of the meniscus is analogous to sprain of the fibular collateral ligament leading to Pott's fracture. When the meniscus splits, the coronary ligament holds the rim in place—the handle of the bucket—but the rest of the meniscus slips across the dome of the femoral condyle to rest on the other side, i.e. displaced towards the centre of the joint (see Fig. 114). Here the displaced portion gets in the way and prevents the painless approximation of the articular surfaces that accompanies extension, but it does not interfere with flexion, since in this position the ligaments are relaxed.

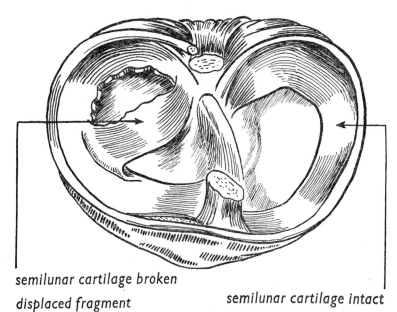

semilunar cartilage broken

displaced fragment   *semilunar cartilage intact*

FIG. 115. Torn cartilage at the knee. View from above showing tear with displacement of part of the medial meniscus. The lateral meniscus is intact.

Rupture with Displacement

The patient's gait is characteristic. He hops into the room on one leg, the knee on the affected side held flexed and the limb medially rotated, the foot plantiflexed with the toes just touching the ground.

On examination the knee is warm, full of fluid, and when extension is attempted a springy block is felt limiting this movement by 5 or 10 degrees. Flexion is somewhat limited by the traumatic arthritis, rotation away from the affected side hurts but towards it does not. However much the joint is cajoled, the springy block prevents full extension. A posterior tear with displacement in middle-age may just allow full, but very painful, extension.

The patient knows which side of his knee he has hurt, thus indicating which meniscus has been torn. Cartilage possesses no nerves; hence it cannot itself be tender. The tenderness on the joint-line in meniscal tears is dependent on the coincident sprain of the coronary ligament. It is best sought by pressure from above downwards on the edge of the tibial condyle while the knee is kept flexed—the same position as for massage to the coronary ligament (see Vol. II). In posterior cracks, no tenderness can be elicited. Intra-articular cartilage has no access to blood; hence the fracture cannot unite, however long the broken surfaces remain in apposition. Thus, once the meniscus has ruptured and the loose part has shifted, recurrence is the rule.

Rupture without Displacement

If the patient is seen some time after reduction of internal derangement at the knee, this may appear normal. The history is often strongly suggestive, and the following tests can be used to elicit signs of a ruptured meniscus. (1) The knee is fully flexed and the knee rotated quickly to and fro. A tell-tale click may be felt as the examiner's thumb presses first to one side of the infra-patellar ligament then the other, on the joint-line. (2) The knee is flexed and fully rotated, first in one direction, then the other. It is then slowly extended while the pressure maintaining rotation continues. As extension proceeds, the possible range of rotation diminishes and a click may be felt as the leg approaches the neutral position at almost full extension. (3) The knee is held at a right-angle. The examiner interlocks his fingers and places the heel of one hand on one side of the upper tibia, the heel of the other hand on the other side of the lower femur (Fig. 116). He then applies a strong shearing strain, as if to move the femur sideways on the tibia. He tries first one way, then the other. This manœuvre may displace the loose part of the meniscus to the other side of the femoral dome, with a loud click; simultaneously, the full range of passive extension at the knee is lost. Manipulative reduction follows. (4) The knee is held well flexed. The examiner passes his flexed finger-tip from above downwards over the joint-line. He may be able to hook the rim of the meniscus and pull it downwards; then it jumps back into place again with a click. (5) When the meniscus is split horizontally, a tag of cartilage may protrude at the joint-line. It can be pushed back into place by the examiner with a palpable click; the patient has often learnt to do this himself. Pain on full extension and the painful arc that is often present in such cases then cease.

These tests, particularly the last two, are repeatable at will. Hence in doubtful cases, they are most useful since they can be demonstrated to a surgeon undecided about operation. If all these tests are negative, the patient should be sent back to full athletics, to ascertain if recurrence is thus provoked or not. If it is, the patient is asked to return at once, so that his knee can be examined again during the acute phase.

It is unwise to let the knee of a young person suffer repeated attacks of internal derangement owing to a torn meniscus. These frequent traumata set up an intractable osteoarthritis which becomes troublesome by middle-age.

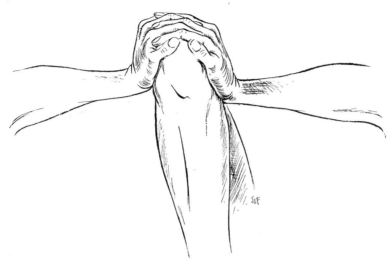

FIG. 116. Side-pressure at the knee. A strong shearing stress is applied, first in one direction, then the other. As the femur and tibia move against each other, a torn cartilage may subluxate. This is an accessory test for a meniscal tear.

Cyst of the Meniscus

The patient complains of intermittent pain at the joint-line, almost always at the lateral aspect, since a cyst of the medial meniscus is very rare. Alternatively, he may complain of attacks of frank internal derangement, the cystic meniscus being also torn.

There is often a history of injury some months previously, which may merely bring to light a previously existing weakness. The alternative theory is that trauma may result in the implantation of synovial cells between the meniscus and the capsule of the joint, where the ectopic focus secretes and enlarges.

The history suggests attack of internal derangement and, when the joint-line is palpated during full extension, the cyst is felt there as a small, hard swelling. If the knee is now bent, the little tumour disappears. Had the cyst been outside the joint, unconnected with the meniscus, it would still have been palpable with the knee flexed.

Since cartilage is avascular and cannot heal, a puncture hole made in the mensicus forms a permanent vent, and is curative unless the cartilage is also fractured. If so, excision is required.

Torsion of the Infrapatellar Pad of Fat

This mimics a cyst of the meniscus. I have encountered only one case—a man of fifty-two who had had a painful knee for two months. Examination showed a small projection at the antero-lateral aspect of the joint line. Exploration unexpectedly showed a pedunculated offshoot from the infrapatellar pad of fat instead of meniscal cyst.

Loose Body in Young Persons

History

Loose bodies, often multiple, form in the knee-joint of young people as the result of osteochondritis dessicans, chondromalacia patellae or chip-fractures. The loose bodies have an osseous nucleus and thus show on the radiograph. In osteochondritis dessicans, the gap at the inner femoral condyle whence the loose body arose is also revealed.

The history is that of momentary locking *in extension*. The knee neither gives way nor does it have to be manipulatively unlocked after the attack; hence there is little resemblance to the sequence of events in meniscal tears. The patient says that, from time to time as he walks along, the knee suddenly locks and tends to pitch him forwards on to his face, since it is fixed straight just when he expects to bend it. He is halted in mid-stride; he may fall. When he tries to move his knee again, he finds he can move it quite well, and walks on. The knee aches and swells a little for a few days. The pain may vary in position if, as often happens, the loose body moves to another part of the joint. Pain shifting from one side of the knee to the other can only be due to a loose body. Rarely the loose fragment is a foreign body.

Signs

For a week or two after an attack of internal derangement, the knee is warm and contains fluid, and clinical examination reveals no localized lesion, merely a subsiding traumatic arthritis. Occasionally, a loose body can be felt moving about in the suprapatellar pouch. If the patella is pushed to one side and its posterior aspect palpated, the gap whence the loose body arose may be felt. Radiography is diagnostic.

Loose Body Pressing on the Tibial Nerve

On rare occasions a loose body lying at the back of the knee-joint impinges against the tibial nerve. The patient complains of attacks suggesting internal derangement at the knee and also of intermittent numbness of the posterior two-thirds of the sole of the foot and the adjacent surfaces of the big and second toes. Vague aching may be felt in the thigh.

The symptoms are abolished by manipulative reduction at the knee.

Loose Body Complicating Osteoarthritis

History

Whereas minor degrees of osteoarthritis of the knee cause no symptoms, the fact that crepitating osteoarthritis is present means that articular cartilage is roughened. A small piece may flake off; it would be interesting to know if the loose body originates from a meniscus or the articular cartilage itself. Such a loose fragment usually occupies a harmless position at the back of the joint; however, it may move and come to lie impacted between the articular surfaces. The history is typical.

A middle-aged or elderly patient states that for no apparent reason swelling and *localized* pain has arisen at one knee. He may wake up with it, or as he is walking along suddenly find that each step hurts. The essential point is the absence of injury; for examination later gives rise to signs strongly suggesting a sprained knee. In fact, each time the patient bears weight on the knee, the presence of the impacted loose body does sprain it. Thus the diagnosis is suggested by the discovery of a traumatic arthritis without apparent trauma. This view has since been corroborated by Helfet (1963) who states that 'most traumatic arthritis of the knee in middle-aged and elderly people is due to minor derangements of the menisci . . . .'

The pain is usually at the inner side of the joint, sometimes at the outer side, sometimes felt 'right inside'—never all over. If it moves from one side of the joint to the other, the diagnosis is obvious. Sometimes the pain spreads up the outer side of the thigh and down the leg in a way suggesting a sciatic distribution. The patient is afraid to go downstairs and does so a step at a time for fear of a sudden twinge which makes the knee suddenly give way. Such twinges and the same feeling of instability are experienced less often during ordinary walking; they indicate momentary subluxations of the loose body.

Signs

These vary with the position of the loose fragment and may be difficult to interpret. The knee is often warm to the touch, and warmer on the painful aspect of the joint than elsewhere. Osteoarthritis is a cold de-generation of a joint; the mere presence of warmth proves that un-complicated osteoarthritis is not a sufficient diagnosis. If the joint is not warm, the examination proceeds. At the end, the palpation is repeated and it is often then noted that the minor stresses imposed on the joint by examining its range of movement have given rise to local warmth, lasting only a minute or two. Fluid is often present in the joint, whether it is warm or not. The following possible findings suggest an impacted cartilaginous body. (1) Non-capsular pattern. Naturally if extension is, say, 5 degrees limited but flexion of full range, a block and not arthritis is present in the joint. Again, if extension is full and painless, but flexion markedly limited by an articular lesion, internal derangement is suspected at once. Such obvious non-capsular findings are uncommon, but were the signs that originally drew attention to this hitherto undescribed condition. (2) Flexion at the knee is slightly limited, but it is localized pain, not the supervention of muscle spasm that limits range. In other words, the movement does not come to a characteristic hard stop; it feels as if it will go farther; the limiting factor is pain. (3) Varus strain hurts at the inner side of the joint. A space-occupying lesion lies medially. (4) A sprained knee that has not been sprained. Localized pain at the extreme of range, warmth, fluid in the joint, no synovial thickening—these are the signs of a sprained knee. But the middle-aged or elderly patient, when questioned afresh, denies having strained his knee in any way. In addition to these signs of a sprain, the medial collateral ligament is usually very tender at the joint line. In such a case, the conclusion is that this ligament is being strained. It is; but if the cause is not external violence, it must lie within the joint. This inference is correct; a small cartilaginous body has suddenly displaced itself towards the inner side of the joint and, every time the endeavour is made to extend the knee, the ligament is strained by the existence of a space-occupying lesion between tibia and femur.

At this age, some X-ray evidence of osteoarthritis is bound to be seen at both knees; and the loose body, being usually composed entirely of cartilage, does not show. If it has an osseous nucleus, the correct diagnosis is, of course, made. The most elementary error is thus to ignore the sudden onset, the fluid, warmth and localized pain and tenderness, and regard the patient as suffering from osteoarthritis of the knee. A more reasonable error is to make a diagnosis of medial ligament strain com-plicating osteoarthritis. This is factually correct, but omits to specify the cause and leads to futile treatment of the secondary phenomenon—the ligamentous strain.

Some authorities describe 'acute episodes' punctuating the progress of what they call 'osteoarthritis'. The actual cause, be it at the knee or the lumbar spine, is this type of minor recurrent internal derangement. The loose body sets up no symptoms as long as it lies at the back of the joint, not interfering with movement. It is only when it engages between the articular surfaces that pain results. It is sound to regard any patient over fifty who has á sprained knee but has not sprained his knee, as suffering from this type of minor chronic internal derangement. It may continue for several years and yet be susceptible to reduction by manipulation in one session.

Monarticular Rheumatoid Arthritis

History

The patient complains of the gradual onset of unprovoked swelling in one or both knees, at first painless. Then the knee begins to ache all over. If the patient is under forty, the diagnosis suggests itself. A Brodie's abscess close to the joint may simulate this type of arthritis but is excluded by radiography.

Signs

Palpation of the joint reveals diffuse warmth, fluid and, sooner or later, synovial thickening. In the early case, these marked local signs contrast strongly with the discovery of a full and virtually painless range of movement at the knee. Later on, limitation of movement of the capsular pattern supervenes. If the presence of fluid interferes with palpation of the synovial edge, the joint should be aspirated and palpated again.

Inflammatory arthritis may complicate subacute gonorrhoea, gout, ankylosing spondylitis, ulcerative colitis or Reiter's disease (non-specific urethritis) and is the first joint affected as a rule in pseudo-gout.

If the arthritis attacks one or more toes as well, and the knee is not improved by intra-articular hydrocortisone, Reiter's disease is very probably present. If a middle-aged woman is found to have arthritis in both knees together with swelling of the hands and ankles, sarcoidosis should be suspected. Far more often, however, the arthritis is not secondary to any other disease, thus belonging to the rheumatoid group. *Villous arthritis* is merely another name for advanced arthritis with great synovial thickening.

Differential Diagnosis

In middle-aged patients, the distinction between monarticular rheumatoid arthritis and osteoarthritis with an impacted loose body may prove very difficult. In either case, the joint is warm and contains fluid, but in rheumatoid arthritis the pain and warmth are equal all over the joint. The radiograph naturally shows osteophyte formation, as in any patient of that age, and is thus actively misleading. In rheumatoid arthritis affecting one large joint, the sedimentation rate is seldom raised—another misleading finding. Rheumatoid arthritis does not cause sudden twinges, but secondary wasting of the quadriceps muscle may make the patient complain that the knee feels weak, and that stairs are difficult for him. However, in a loose body, the onset is sudden, and twinges a prominent feature. Both disorders are apt to recur.

The only certain criterion is synovial thickening, a slight degree of which is most difficult to be sure about, particularly when the patient is a middle-aged woman whose subcutaneous tissues are already somewhat thickened. Since treatment is on entirely different lines in the two cases, the distinction is vital.

Haemarthrosis

History

Occasionally, the patient is an adolescent youth, with a minor tendency to haemophilia. If so, suspicion is aroused by the triviality or absence of causative trauma. Blood often fills the joint, in either sex, after direct contusion without fracture; or it may come on, apparently spontaneously, in the elderly, presumably as the result of rupture of an intra-articular vein.

The patient states that after a trivial injury, some overuse, or for no reason, the knee suddenly became very painful and swollen, filling up in a few minutes. The speed of appearance of the effusion and the severe pain by far exceed that caused by clear fluid; for blood fills the joint rapidly and is a strong irritant. About half of all haemophiliac articular effusions occur at the knee.

Signs

In severe cases the patient walks in on crutches, his knee bent up, unable to put foot to ground. The knee is hot and distended to its utmost with fluid. Examination reveals 45 degrees limitation of extension, 90 degrees limitation of flexion. This limitation of movement is unaltered after some weeks in bed. Aspiration reveals the cause of the trouble at once. If haemophilia is suspected, a vial of Russell viper venom for local application should be at hand in case oozing from the skin puncture proves troublesome.

In less marked haemarthrosis, the patient can hobble along, but palpation of the joint shows it to be warm and very tense with fluid, far more so than when the effusion is clear. Examination shows considerable limitation of movement of the capsular pattern and aspiration confirms the diagnosis.

Intra-articular Adhesion

History

This is a rare and remarkable condition. After what appears an unexceptional sprain or operation at the inner side of the knee (e.g. the removal of an osteoma at the medial femoral condyle), the knee progressively stiffens almost painlessly, in spite of vigorous physiotherapy. The patient complains of inability to flex the knee, e.g. in walking upstairs; this increases as the days go by, but there is hardly any discomfort. After, say, a fortnight, the knee retains 90 degrees of flexion range; after a month, only 45 degrees.

Signs

This uncommon disorder is brought to mind when, after an injury, the joint is cold, not swollen, devoid of intra-articular fluid, and yet on examination has a full range of extension and 90 degrees to 135 degrees limitation of flexion. The discrepancy between such gross limitation of movement and the absence of local articular signs is diagnostic. The radiograph does not reveal a Stieda-Pellegrini shadow. No amount of forcing while the patient lies supine is effective. However, if the patient is turned to lie prone and the knee forced towards flexion (see Vol. II) there is a loud sound as of tearing silk and full flexion is achieved at once.

Subsynovial Haematoma

History

This is merely the result of a severe blow on the front of the thigh, just above the knee, followed by pain, swelling and disablement.

Signs

The knee is swollen and warm; if aspirated the fluid is often blood-stained. Extension is of full range and only slightly painful; flexion on the other hand is at least 90 degrees limited. Resisted extension is painless. These findings indicate a localized articular lesion affecting the front only

z

of the joint; palpation reveals a haematoma lying between the femur and the suprapatellar pouch. During the first few days, aspiration, not of the fluid in the joint, but by passing the needle backwards till it reaches bone, confirms this diagnosis. Later, the blood coagulates and cannot be withdrawn.

Posterior Capsular Lesions

Capsular Strain

History

The patient describes a severe hyperextension sprain of the knee from which he has never fully recovered, the joint swelling and aching for several days after exercise. The pain is behind or all over the knee, not on one side only as in a ligamentous injury.

Signs

If there has been recent exertion, the knee is warm and contains fluid. Examination shows that only full passive extension hurts. Stretching the anterior cruciate ligament is painless. Occasionally, the radiograph shows one or two linear calcified streaks at the posterior aspect of the joint.

Capsular Rupture

Long-standing rheumatoid arthritis of the knee with chronic distension of the joint with fluid weakens the posterior ligaments, which may rupture during exertion. The fluid now extravasates into the upper calf, causing sudden pain at the back of the knee. The venous return is impeded and the foot becomes very oedematous in a manner suggesting venous thrombosis. The sudden onset and the swelling at the popliteal space and upper calf should lead to immediate aspiration of the swelling (if it is fluctuant) or *via* the knee joint itself (if fluctuation in the calf cannot be detected).

Osteoarthritis

Although minor degrees of osteophyte formation do not give rise to symptoms unless a loose body forms and moves, gross osteoarthritis causes pain as soon as articular cartilage wears through. This is apt to happen if the patient suffered repeatedly from attacks of internal derangement due to a torn meniscus that was never excised. Alternatively, a marked valgus deformity has been present since youth, the result of rickets or an old mal-united fracture, and the shearing strain on the joint has worn one cartilage through (on the outer side in genu valgum). The knee is often affected in osteitis deformans.

Osteoarthritis of the knee is considered very common. It is not; it is rare; and is frequently incorrectly diagnosed. What inaccurately receives this label is monarticular rheumatoid arthritis or an impacted loose body, each occurring in a middle-aged or elderly patient with osteophytes mis-leadingly visible radiologically: a normal phenomenon at that age.

In uncomplicated osteoarthritis, the characteristic features are a cold joint, devoid of synovial thickening, and a hard and painless end-feel. Osteophytes can often be seen and palpated. Extension is a few degrees limited, the movement ending abruptly by bone hitting bone. Flexion may be 60 or 90 degrees limited, the movement again coming to a sudden dead stop. An attempt to increase range is not so much painful as felt to be quite impossible owing to bony contact. In gross osteoarthritis, marked limitation of movement of the capsular pattern combines with the intermittent creaking of bone against bone. The same signs without any discomfort indicate a neurogenic arthropathy, nearly always tabetic.

Chondrocalcinosis

Pseudo-gout is brought to mind when recurrent attacks of pain and limited movement come on suddenly without apparent cause, lasting one to four weeks. This is too long for palindromic rheumatism and too short a duration for the other types of rheumatoid arthritis or gout itself (un-treated). Examination of aspirated fluid reveals crystals of pyrophosphate rather than urates. Faires and McCarty (1962) showed that both sodium-urate and calcium-pyrophosphate crystals caused acute arthritis when injected into the knee-joint. Attacks of pseudo-gout also occur in patients with chronic renal failure who are kept alive by intermittent dialysis (Caner and Decker, 1964), since uric acid dialyses less readily than urea. Their analysis showed that the knee contained calcium and phosphate with negligible amounts of urates. Sooner or later, linear calcification of articular or meniscus makes its appearance radiographically and settles the diagnosis.

UPPER TIBIO-FIBULAR JOINT

This joint is examined at the same time as the knee. It is seldom affected, but a blow may strain the ligaments holding the head of the fibula to the tibia. A spontaneously appearing lesion is rare.

The patient complains of localized pain at the outer side of the knee, just below the joint-line. On examination the knee-joint is normal, but when resisted flexion and lateral rotation are tested, contraction of the biceps elicits the pain by pulling the fibula backwards, especially if the movement is carried out with the knee at a right-angle. When the biceps tendon is examined for tenderness, none is found. This rare disorder is then brought to mind, and the tibio-fibular ligament—usually the anterior—is tender. One infiltration of hydrocortisone is usually curative.

DISORDERS OF QUADRICEPS MECHANISM

1. Recurrent Dislocation of the Patella

History

If an accurate history is not obtained, dislocation of the patella is easily mistaken for meniscal trouble at the knee; for both are a type of internal derangement. However, the condition begins in childhood, between the ages of eight and fifteen, i.e. before the age of rupture of a meniscus. The youngster complains that the knee suddenly and painfully gives way; he falls to the ground and feels that something is out of place at his knee; he straightens his leg, there is a loud click and his knee is serviceable once more. The knee swells and hurts afterwards for some days. Sooner or later, the incident recurs.

Signs

Examination may show a genu valgum deformity or poor development of the lateral condyle of the femur. With rare exceptions, the dislocation is outwards. The disorder is distinguished by the following tests: (a) the infrapatellar tendon is elongated and the patella correspondingly hypermobile; (b) for some weeks after an attack, tenderness is present at the medial aspect of the patella; (c) the patella is pushed laterally with the leg in full extension. As the patella approaches the position where it will slip over the lateral femoral condyle, the patient suddenly contracts his quadriceps muscle and brings the patella back. If the patella were not apt to dislocate, the patient would have no fear of such pressure and thus would not use the quadriceps muscle to avert displacement.

2. Patellar-femoral Arthritis

History

In young patients, the knee is merely stated to ache anteriorly walking upstairs, after a long walk or ski-ing. Elderly patients complain of the same anterior ache but also say that the knee grates loudly. Walking upstairs hurts more than on the flat.

Signs

Examination on the couch reveals nothing since this tests only the unaffected tibio-femoral joint; even moving the patella up and down against the femur does not cause more than a commonplace feeling of roughness. The patellar-femoral joint must be examined during weight-bearing, when the pull of the quadriceps applies the patella strongly to the femoral condyles. Hence, it is only when the patient is asked to stand and bend his knees that the familiar pain is brought on and the examiner's hand placed on the patella feels the marked crepitus.

If this sign is found in young patients without a history of trauma, the cause is chondromalacia patellae; if it follows an injury, flake fracture of the articular surface of the patella is probably responsible. In either case, loose bodies may form; then it is attacks of internal derangement that bring the disorder to light. If the loose body present in the joint has no osseous centre, X-rays reveal no abnormality.

If crepitus is found in middle-age, it may be caused by osteoarthritis affecting the patellar-condylar joint. An old stellate fracture leads to enlargement of the whole patella and incongruity of the opposed joint surfaces. Naturally, localized osteoarthritis supervenes.

3. Lesions of the Quadriceps Bellies

History

The patient makes a correct diagnosis himself, stating that while running or jumping he was brought up short by feeling something give way painfully at the front of his thigh. Afterwards he could walk only slowly and with a limp.

Signs in Minor Rupture

The hip-joint is normal. The knee-joint is normal too except that flexion is slightly or greatly restricted, depending on the size of the rupture. If the patient is asked to lie prone (thus keeping his hip extended) marked limitation of knee-flexion is found when the two sides are compared; for the upper end of the muscle remains taut in this position. Resisted extension of the knee hurts but is not weak. The tender area and the haematoma are palpable, usually at mid-thigh. This condition has been called 'cricket-leg' and mistakenly attributed to rupture of the sartorius muscle.

Signs in Major Rupture

This occurs just above the suprapatellar tendon and may amount to complete separation. The swelling just above the knee is obvious, and palpation reveals the gap in the muscle. Resisted extension is very weak as well as painful; sometimes the patient cannot voluntarily straighten the knee against the mere resistance of the weight of the leg.

Adherence

When the belly of the quadriceps muscle has become adherent to the mid-shaft of the femur at the site of a fracture, limitation of flexion at the knee to 90 degrees is a commonplace. The other knee movements are of full range—i.e. the extra-articular type of limitation of movement is present.

Weakness of the Quadriceps Muscles

If both muscles are weak and wasted, but there is no pain on resisted extension of the knee, the rest of the nervous system must be examined. If no other abnormality is found, the diagnoses to be considered are:

1. Spinal tumour or metastases at the third lumbar level.
2. Myopathy.
3. Myositis.

The electromyogram is helpful and if myositis is suspected biopsy should be undertaken. In myositis and sarcoidosis, granulomatous foci are seen, and in the former case treatment by cortisone arrests the disease.

4. Lesions about the Patella

Fracture

A patient with a fractured patella may walk in complaining merely of pain in the knee following either a fall on to the front of his knee (stellate fracture) or indirect violence (transverse fracture). If the capsule enclosing the patella is not ruptured, displacement is avoided and disability is often slight.

Signs

The knee is warm to the touch and is tense with blood. The passive movements hurt and are much limited by the haemarthrosis. Resisted extension is markedly weak as well as painful. This association of articular with quadriceps signs shows that the lesion partly involves the joint, and partly that section of the quadriceps mechanism overlying the knee, in other words, the patella. Local tenderness and radiography are confirmative.

Tendinitis

This occurs at three sites: at the suprapatellar tendon, at the quadriceps expansion to either side of the patella, and at the infrapatellar tendon. The history is merely of pain at the front of the knee on walking, especially upstairs. It is uncommon except in athletes, ballet dancers and the one-legged; the latter are very apt to strain the patellar mechanism as they step downstairs.

Signs
The knee-joint is normal; only resisted extension is uncomfortable. Palpation reveals the site of the lesion. The tendons are always affected at the teno-periosteal junction and the same applies to the quadriceps expansion which becomes strained only at its insertion at the edge of the patella.

Apophysitis

Boys aged 10 to 15 may develop osteochondritis of the tibial tuberosity (Schlatter's disease) or, rarely, of the lower epiphysis of the patella. In either case, local pain elicited by a resisted extension movement is the only positive finding; the site of tenderness is distinctive. The age of the patient should lead to radiography. Spontaneous recovery often takes two years.

5. Strained Ilio-tibial Band

This lesion appears confined to athletes. While running, he notices an increasing pain at the outer side of his knee, and usually has to drop out of the race. He rests a week, then runs again. This time the pain comes on sooner and is more severe; the next day, walking hurts. Thereafter, he cannot run fast or far.

Examination reveals no lesion of the knee-joint or its ligaments, but discomfort is felt when extension and lateral rotation are carried out against resistance. Resisted flexion is painless. The tender spot is found at and just below the joint-line, between the infrapatellar tendon and the fibular collateral ligament.

DISORDERS OF MUSCLE

Hamstrings

When the knee-joint is normal but resisted flexion of the knee hurts in the thigh, there is a lesion of the hamstrings. If it affects the muscle bellies and is of any severity, straight-leg raising is limited. Pain on resisted lateral rotation incriminates the biceps muscle. The area of induration of muscle suffused with blood is tender and swollen. If the pain is at the knee, the bicipital tendon close to the head of the fibula may be at fault. Should resisted medial rotation hurt at the knee, strain of the semi-membranosus tendon at the groove on the tibia is a possibility.

It must not be forgotten that there exist two disorders in which resisted flexion of the knee hurts without any disorder of the hamstring muscles. In each, the resisted movement hurts if the knee is (as is usual) bent to a right-angle for this test. If the resisted movement is carried out with the knee almost fully extended, no pain is evoked.

1. Strain of the Posterior Cruciate Ligament

Contraction of the hamstrings pulls the tibia backwards on the femur, painfully straining the affected cruciate ligament. The pain, however, is felt within the knee-joint, and articular signs are present.

2. Strain of the Upper Tibio-fibular Joint

If the biceps muscle contracts while the knee is bent, the head of the fibula is drawn backwards, straining the ligaments that attach it to the femur. Tenderness is absent at the biceps tendon but present at the upper tibio-fibular ligament.

Strained Popliteus Muscle

The patient sprains the back of his knee in an undistinctive way; the position of pain suggests a lesion of the posterior cruciate ligament.

Examination shows that the knee-joint itself is normal, but that resisted flexion and resisted medial rotation hurt posteriorly. The semimem-branosus and semitendinosus tendons are not tender; only the popliteus remains.

Tenderness is sought along the muscle from the emergence of the tendon under the lateral ligament of the knee, at and just above the joint-line, to the back of the upper tibia.

The tendon responds well to massage or hydrocortisone, the belly to deep massage only.

BURSITIS AT THE KNEE

Prepatellar bursitis causes pain felt at the front of the knee, chiefly on kneeling. The knee and its muscles are normal. Pinching up the tissues between patella and skin reveals a fluctuant swelling. Local heat without redness suggests haemorrhage into the bursa; aspiration is diagnostic. Local heat accompanied by reddening of the skin means a septic bursitis. Bilateral bursitis is said to be an occasional manifestation of tertiary syphilis.

The semimembranosus bursa seldom communicates with the joint. A bulging bursa does not give rise to symptoms, though a swelling at the back of the knee and pain felt there invite the patient to associate the two. In case of doubt, it should be aspirated and the patient thus shown that emptying the bursa does not alter the pain. The knee should be re-examined at once while the bursa, which soon fills up again, is empty.

THE RADIOGRAPH

Radiography is not often informative at the knee-joint; indeed, as elsewhere, its value is largely negative. Evidence of osteophyte formation, unless gross, affords no guarantee that the symptoms are due to osteo-arthritis. Bennett, Waine and Bauer's (1942) careful post-mortem and radiological research in normal subjects showed that superficial fraying of the articular cartilage begins at the knee-joint during a person's twenties. Roughening and splitting at the weight-bearing areas follow, but extensive erosion has to occur before the radiological appearances alter. Lipping, they found, appears during most people's forties. It is clear from these painstaking observations no less than from clinical experience that, except in gross disease, the clinical examination of the knee, not the inspection of the radiograph, alone decides the presence or absence of arthritis. If arthritis is present clinically, the radiograph may assist the attempt to determine the type of joint lesion present. Even here its value is limited, for in early rheumatoid and inflammatory arthritis the appearances are normal. Alternatively, such arthritis may come on at an age when osteophyte formation is already visible; the radiograph is then misleading. Later on, arthritis is shown as a general decalcification of the bone-ends; finally, secondary disorganization of the joint with osteophyte formation is seen, but the lesion remains clinically rheumatoid.

Erosion of cartilage is shown as a thinning of the joint line. Ossification and calcification in capsule or ligament may be relevant findings.

Meniscal deposits in pseudo-gout show well. Loose bodies within the joint are visible on the radiograph only if they contain bone or are foreign, e.g. glass. Fractures, osteochondritis dessicans, abscess in the bone, tuberculous disease, neoplasm and osteitis deformans are clearly shown.

In soft tissue lesions, or in rupture or cyst formation of a meniscus, the radiographic appearances are normal. Air-arthrography can disclose the split in a meniscus or an otherwise invisible loose body.

TREATMENT AT THE KNEE

Nearly all the lesions of the knee respond well to treatment. Accurate diagnosis with accurate physiotherapy gives the happiest results.

Treatment of Arthritis

Early osteoarthritis causes no symptoms to speak of unless a small fragment of cartilage becomes impacted between the articular surfaces. If osteoarthritis is gross enough itself to cause symptoms, no conservative treatment helps and hinge-arthroplasty may be required.

Monarticular rheumatoid arthritis often clears up after two to four intra-articular injections of 5 cc. hydrocortisone suspension, not only in the early case, but even after some years' increasing arthritis. If hydrocortisone is ineffective in what appears a monarticular rheumatoid case, Reiter's disease or chondrocalcinosis should be considered.

The arthritis that heralds or complicates spondylitis ankylopoetica responds well to hydrocortisone. Psuedo-gout is best treated by phenylbutazone (200 mg. four times a day during the acute phase).

In advanced villous arthritis, X-ray therapy or synovectomy should be considered if hydrocortisone fails.

Reiter's arthritis is intractable, although tetracycline is usually given for the urethritis.

Treatment of Ligamentous Sprain

The principle of treatment is the attainment of healing in the presence of adequate movement. This is achieved by methods differing according to the time that has elapsed since the accident.

Acute Stage

During the first few days after a sprain, hydrocortisone injection is the treatment of choice and shortens the acute phase by aborting excessive

local reaction to injury. The site of the tear should be infiltrated with
1 or 2 cc. of suspension of hydrocortisone as soon as the patient is seen.
A thin needle two cm. long suffices. The patient walks away. A few days
later he should attend for the treatment suited to subacute sprain.

Subacute Stage

If several days have elapsed since the accident, deep massage should be
given at once to the site of the minor tear in the ligament. This is essential
in the coronary ligaments, for they do not span the joint. Hence, adequate
movement cannot be imparted to the tibio-meniscal joint by merely
moving the knee—the wrong joint—and recovery takes months if this
method is adopted alone. But it is quite simple to move the ligament by
drawing the finger to and fro across it (see Vol. II); indeed, this way of
maintaining or restoring mobility is the essential measure in coronary
sprain. Similar considerations apply to the tibial collateral ligament when
traumatic arthritis prevents flexion at the knee-joint; the ligament cannot
therefore be put through its full range. Thus unwanted scars soon bind
the ligament down. Friction imitates the normal behaviour of the ligament, moving it to and fro over the bone at a time when the bone cannot
be adequately moved to and fro under the ligament, thus hindering the
formation of adhesions. In either case the friction is followed by gentle
forcing of movement to the point of discomfort but not of pain. Deep
massage allows a large increase in movement to be obtained almost
painlessly each day. The patient repeats the movements actively and is
taught to walk slowly and carefully without a limp. Treatment should be
continued until the range of movement at the knee is full and without
discomfort.

Treatment which omits friction to the site of the tear may take months
instead of weeks.

Chronic Stage

This stage is never reached if the patient receives early adequate treatment early on.

The principle of treatment is to restore a full range of movement to the
ligament by rupturing scar tissue binding it abnormally to bone. Deep
friction to the affected part of the ligament moves it to and fro; forcing
movement by a sharp jerk completes the mobilization. General anaesthesia is scarcely ever necessary. The sequence of events is illustrated in
Fig. 117. Intra-articular adhesion is treated by a special manipulation (see
Vol. II).

When the posterior cruciate ligament is the site of chronic strain, in all
the cases encountered so far the lesion lay at the posterior attachment to
the tibia. Infiltration of 2 cc. hydrocortisone suspension must, therefore,
be aimed at this point. The patient lies prone and the level of the joint-line
identified. A needle 5 cm. long is inserted from one or other side, so as to
avoid the popliteal artery. The centre of the back of the tibia is palpated
with the tip of the needle, which is moved upwards until resistance is lost

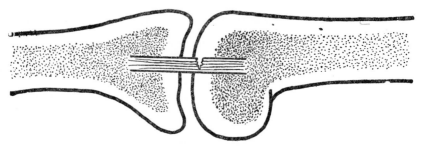

(*a*) The patient rests with the knee held in extension. An adherent scar forms at the site of the tear, binding the ligament to bone and restricting mobility.

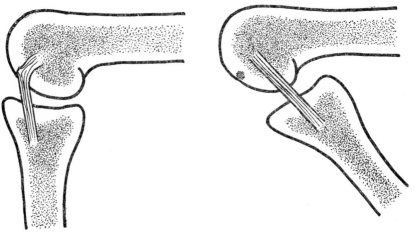

(*b*) Limitation of flexion results from scarring.   (*c*) Forcing full flexion at the knee frees the
As flexion proceeds the ligament becomes pro-   ligament from its abnormal attachment and a
gressively deformed and over-stretched.   full range of movement is restored to the joint.

Fig, 117. Chronic sprain of medial collateral ligament (diagrammatic)

as it penetrates the knee-joint. The needle is then moved back to the
previous point, just below the articular surface of the tibia, and the tissues
here infiltrated. One well-placed injection is curative.

Chronic strain of the anterior cruciate ligament is rarer and more
difficult to treat, since the lesion may lie at either end of this ligament. If

the patient feels the pain posteriorly, the medial aspect of the lateral condyle should be infiltrated by a posterior oblique approach. If he feels it right inside the knee, the anterior attachment just in front of the tibial spine should be injected. To this end, the knee is bent to a right-angle and the needle inserted just below the lower pole of the patella and aimed at the centre of the upper surface of the tibia. In a difficult case, both approaches may have to be made.

Lengthening of Ligaments

If this has occurred, permanent disability results. After sprain of the cruciate ligaments, the knee should be spared all strains until the traumatic arthritis subsides; this takes at least six months unless the ligaments can be correctly infiltrated with hydrocortisone. If permanent lengthening results in sufficient disability, an operation depressing the tibial spine and thus indirectly shortening the ligament is indicated. Alternatively, the middle third of the patellar tendon and patella itself can be used to replace the lengthened ligament (Jones, 1963). In minor cases, continued strengthening of the quadriceps muscle helps to stabilize the joint. Lengthening of the medial collateral ligament gives rise to an increased range of movement towards valgus at the knee, but remarkably little disability; treatment is thus seldom required. Surgery has nothing to offer in Stieda-Pellegrini's disease; the treatment is expectant.

Treatment of Effusion

Haemorrhage

Blood in the joint must be aspirated at once, and the remaining blood-tinged synovial effusion aspirated a few days later. Blood stays in the knee joint for months, causing severe arthritis owing to irritation of synovial membrane and its errosive action on articular cartilage. In haemophilia, the presence of blood tends to dilate the blood-vessels with which it lies in contact, thus leading to increased tendency to bleed; this enhances the liability to disintegration of cartilage. Hence aspiration should be carried out as soon as the patient is seen, in consultation with the haematologist. The cryo-precipitate method of preparing anti-haemophilic globulin by freezing and thawing results in a much greater concentration of the missing factor than was previously possible. Out-patient injection of 20 ml. of this precipitate replaces the large infusions that used to need in-patient treatment.

A subperiosteal haematoma lying under the suprapatellar pouch should also be aspirated, to obviate months of disablement otherwise. If, as is apt to happen in the late case, the blood is no longer fluid, deep effleurage should be given all over the suprapatellar pouch for an hour daily for as many weeks as proves necessary, otherwise limitation of flexion can continue for more than a year.

Clear Fluid

This designates the presence of an articular lesion at the knee and is a sign common to many disorders; it is a result, not a cause. 'Synovitis' at the knee is thus a symptom, not a diagnosis, and no reasonable treatment can be based on a diagnosis of 'synovitis of the knee'. Aspiration of a clear effusion is a waste of time; it is tapped only when a needle is inserted to discover whether an effusion is of blood or synovial fluid. The treatment of a clear effusion is to discover its cause (e.g. a sprained ligament, rheumatoid arthritis, internal derangement, gout) and to deal with that.

An effusion into the prepatellar bursa makes it impossible for the patient to kneel. It should therefore be aspirated at once. If due to haemorrhage it seldom returns. If a prepatellar bursa keeps filling up, and the provision of a soft rubber kneeling mat is ineffective, it should be excised.

Treatment of Intra-articular Displacement

The immediate measure is to reduce the displacement.

Ruptured Meniscus

In the usual bucket-handle tear, it is the more deeply placed fragment that becomes displaced towards the centre of the joint, the superficial piece remaining in place on account of its continued attachment to the coronary ligament. The manipulation is therefore designed to allow the luxated fragment to slip back, over the dome of the femoral condyle, towards its proper bed. General anaesthesia is usually necessary, but it is often worth trying first without, especially in recurrent cases (see Vol. II).

Splintage and conservative treatment after reduction are useless, since cartilage, having no blood-supply, cannot unite; the after-treatment is that of an acute coronary sprain.

Recurrent Displacement of Meniscus

Bonesetters, in particular the late Sir Herbert Barker, claim to cure this condition. Very occasionally they appear to succeed, but not by causing the fractured surfaces to join; this is impossible. Really forcible manipulation may complete the rupture in the meniscus and force the loosened half into the intercondylar notch. In this position, it no longer interferes with the articulating surfaces and if it stays there the patient has no more trouble, it is 'cured'. But this happy result is obtained only rarely and manipulation for recurrent dislocation is scarcely worth while. What bonesetters do in fact cure is chronic sprain, i.e. adherent scars, at the tibial collateral ligament, and for the chronic stage of these conditions forced movement is indubitably the correct treatment. The question is one of diagnosis. It is clearly undesirable and time-wasting, repeatedly to manipulate a joint when there is every chance that it will finally require operation. Recurrent dislocation of either meniscus must be treated by excision. This is the only certain means of preventing the osteoarthritis which supervenes early, as the result of the repeated severe sprains to which this accident subjects the joint.

Cyst formation at the meniscus can be treated by acupuncture; if the cyst contains fluid, cure may follow, since any puncture hole in cartilage remains patent indefinitely. Should this simple treatment fail, the entire meniscus should be excised, since many cystic menisci are also torn.

Loose Bodies

The one or more loose bodies that are found in young persons' knees should be removed as soon as possible, since the more attacks of internal derangement the knee suffers, the sooner osteoarthritis is likely to set in.

Having an osseous centre, their position is revealed by the radiograph; since they may move, this should be taken immediately before the operation.

Impacted Loose Body complicating Osteoarthritis

Such loose bodies are not suited to excision for a variety of reasons. They are usually wholly cartilaginous, and are thus not revealed by radiography. Being so small, it is doubtful if air-arthrography would help either. The patient is old and the degenerate state of his joint precludes exploration. Manipulative disimpaction must, therefore, be carried out as often as the loose body moves and causes symptoms. Manipulation as for a dislocated semilunar cartilage is unsuccessful, because this type of loose body does not move unless the joint surfaces have been separated first. Thus the principle governing manipulation for this type of displacement is performance during: (a) ligamentous relaxation (i.e. in flexion); (b) strong traction (see Vol. II).

Recurrence is apt to follow kneeling or keeping the knee well bent for some time and the patient should be warned against this.

Treatment of Patellar Lesions

Recurrent dislocation is treated by operation in which the infrapatellar tendon is shortened and the tuberosity re-sited medially. Intra-articular silicone oil provides the only conservative treatment for patellar-femoral arthritis. In severe cases, the patella can be excised.

The tendons above and below the patella and the ilio-tibial band at the tibia recover both with hydrocortisone and deep massage. The quadriceps expansion responds only to deep massage, given by a special technique (see Vol. II).

Fractured patella without separation requires aspiration of the haemarthrosis; with separation, the tear in the quadriceps expansion on either side should be sutured, and/or the patella wired. It is safe to wait until the haemarthrosis has been dealt with and the traumatic arthritis has subsided.

Treatment of Tendons

A localized lesion is best infiltrated with hydrocortisone. When the lesion is extensive, deep massage is preferred. If this cures, well and good; if a small point remains, this can be infiltrated. Tendons are nearly always strained at their teno-periosteal junction; hence, the treatment—whether massage or injection—should be directed to this point (see Vol. II).

Treatment of Muscles

Major rupture requires operative suture. In minor rupture, as soon as the patient is seen, the lesion is infiltrated with 50 cc. 0·5 per cent procaine. The next day, deep massage and faradism are given to the muscle while it is held fully shortened so that the belly moves but no strain falls on the healing breach. This involves considerable flexion at the knee and full extension of the hip when the hamstrings are partly torn.

The tendency to recurrence is considerable if the patient goes back to athletics too soon. Especially after a lesion of the hamstrings, the patient should continue treatment for a week after he is clinically well, and should not run hard for a month after the accident. Zinc sulphate may well prove to hasten union in these cases.

Treatment of Genu Valgum

If this persists beyond the age of ten, and the medial malleoli lie 5 cm. apart or more, stapling the medial femoral epiphysis should be undertaken without delay. Correction takes about a year, whereupon the staple is removed.

After growth of bone has ceased, prophylactic supracondylar osteotomy is indicated. Even if no symptoms have yet arisen, by middle-age, years of weight-bearing concentrated on the outer condyle of femur and tibia will lead to complete erosion of the meniscus and of articular cartilage there. Loss of tissue leads to gross arthritis with increase in the deformity and to pain from elongation of the medial ligament at the inner side and to bone impinging against bone at the outer side of the knee. If this has already occurred, some relief can be gained by throwing as much of the patient's body weight as possible on to the inner side of the knee. To this end he wears heels with a $\frac{1}{4}$-inch inner wedge.

25

The Leg and the Ankle

The conditions that affect the leg are very simple. Diagnosis is seldom difficult. The only disorder which commonly gives rise to pain in the calf only without local cause is primary postero-lateral protrusion of nuclear substance at the fifth lumbar level. The root-pain is constant and remains unaltered by, e.g., standing on tip-toe. This finding naturally suggests that the pain is referred to the calf from a lesion at the proximal end of the first and second sacral segments.

Two conditions at the calf give rise to a characteristic history. Intermittent claudication presents as pain in the calf coming on after the individual has walked a certain distance, disappearing as soon as he rests and recurring as soon as he has again walked for the critical distance. In 'tennis-leg' the pain in the calf comes on abruptly as the patient rises vigorously on tip-toe. Usually during a game of tennis, he feels a sudden pain resembling the lash of a whip at mid-calf and at once finds that pain prevents his putting one heel to the ground and that he has to hobble on tip-toe.

It must be remembered that the 'growing pains' felt in the legs both by normal and by rheumatic children give rise to no local signs. Constitutional signs and a raised erythrocyte sedimentation rate should be sought. Neither do the severe pains in arms and legs starting in childhood that characterize diffuse angiokeratoma corporis.

Gait

This should be observed as the patient walks in.

In children who fall easily, a minor degree of spastic diplegia may be present. Various minor deviations of the lower limbs from the normal are often invoked to explain the child's instability—an idea that only inspection of gait corrects.

THE BONES

Inspection reveals the shape of the bones; palpation discloses the nature of their surface, sometimes warmth.

Both tibiae are curved inward at birth: the result of the ordinary intra-uterine position. This bowing becomes gradually obliterated and by the age of two the tibia has straightened. Now knock-knees replaces the previous bow-legs. This developmental genu valgum reaches its maxi-mum at about four years of age and it is not until the age of six that the legs are once more as aligned as at the age of two.

In almost every child, a slight *outward rotation* in the course of the tibia comes on during growth. This makes the mid-line of the foot point slightly laterally to the sagittal axis of the knee. In consequence, adults 'turn their feet out'. However, this twist may become exaggerated. If it is towards lateral rotation, the youngster is bad at games; for, when the foot is not kept in line with the direction in which the individual moves, he loses an inch or two at every stride he takes. Short calf muscles, especially when associated with a plantaris deformity of the forefoot, prevent use of the foot in the sagittal plane, and the child tends to turn his foot more and more outwards; lateral rotation is forced on the growing tibia which, in due course, becomes shaped that way.

Occasionally the twist is reversed, and during growth, for no clear reason the tibia grows towards *inward rotation*. This is called 'pigeon-toes', but it is a misnomer, since the deformity arises not in the foot but in the course of the tibia.

Genu valgum in children persisting after the age of six is often the result of congenital inversion of the forefoot. Nowadays, genu valgum due to Vitamin-D deficiency is almost as rare as renal rickets.

A varus deformity of the tibia with rounding of its anterior edge occurs in osteitis deformans. The front of the leg is often warm. The patient is elderly and the bowing is of recent onset. Radiography confirms the diagnosis.

Traumatic periostitis of the subcutaneous surface of the tibia may prove rather obstinate, the patient presenting himself after he has forgotten the blow. He will, however, indicate the right place, where tenderness of the periosteum together with irregularity of its surface will be found. Some-times fluctuation from effused blood can be elicited. Post-traumatic osteoporosis occurs, the foot becoming a deep purple when dependent. Syphilitic periostitis of the tibia is very rare nowadays. In dermatomyositis atrophic glossy skin becomes attached to hard and immobile muscles, contracture of which prevents movement at the ankle joint.

Treatment

If the child is suffering from rickets, this must, of course, be treated. Apart from that, the tibia vara of babies and genu valgum of young children should be left to correct itself. If the genu valgum is secondary to inversion of the forefoot, this must be energetically treated at once. If genu valgum persists after the age of ten, it should not be allowed to continue; for arthritis of the knee with gross erosion of the lateral tibial and femoral condyles ensues in middle-age. The medial femoral epiphysis should be stapled at about the age of ten. If the patient is seen later, after bone growth has ceased, femoral osteotomy is required. Rotation in the course of the tibia can be corrected only by osteoclasis, which is best postponed until the child is at least eight years old. The subsidence of traumatic periostitis is hastened by deep effleurage. Blood is absorbed very slowly from under the periosteum and is apt to leave thickening that remains tender for months. Aspiration is therefore indicated if fluctuation can be elicited. In osteitis deformans, Rich (1960) found that sodium fluoride (20 mg. thrice daily) relieved pain and reversed the negative calcium balance, but he reported that it had to be continued for two or three months before the improvement was noted. However, in 1964, toxic optic neuritis was reported in one case so treated.

THE MUSCLES AND TENDONS

Painful Plantiflexor Muscles

The muscles are examined next. First the patient stands and is asked to rise on tip-toe. Then he lies supine and dorsiflexion, eversion and inversion are tested against resistance. Note is made whether the movement is painful or painless, strong or weak.

If rising on tip-toe hurts, the calf muscles are at fault. In such cases, the following test distinguishes between the soleus and gastrocnemius muscles. The patient lies prone and plantiflexion of the foot is resisted, first with his knee fully extended, then while flexed to a right-angle. Bending the knee relaxes the femoral extremity of the gastrocnemius muscle but does not alter the strain on the soleus muscle; hence, abolition of pain when the movement is tested during knee-flexion incriminates the gastrocnemius muscle. This is the likelihood, nearly all minor ruptures occurring in the belly of this muscle.

If the upper calf is swollen after a severe strain during athletics or a direct blow, a haematoma should be sought and, if fluctuant, aspirated.

When, however, the upper calf is swollen, in the absence of any injury, in a patient with long-standing rheumatoid arthritis at the knee, posterior capsular rupture with extravasation of synovial fluid into the upper calf has taken place (described by Morant Baker in 1877 as a chronic synovial cyst). Tait, Bach and Dixon (1965) have shown by arthrography that the fluid escapes between the semimembranosus and semitendinosus tendons on one side and the quadriceps muscle laterally. If so, the venous return from the foot is much embarrassed and the foot becomes oedematous in a manner suggesting venous thrombosis. The diagnosis can be confirmed by contrast arthrography and aspiration is required at once.

Tennis-leg

This disorder has for years been regarded as a ruptured plantaris tendon, but the physicial signs present at once show this ascription to be false. The patient describes sudden pain in the calf and hobbles in, tip-toeing on the affected side. Examination reveals pain on plantiflexion against resistance but no weakness. Dorsiflexion at the ankle is markedly restricted, owing to localized spasm of the muscle about the ruptured fibres. Bending the knee increases the range of dorsiflexion obtainable at the ankle; an instance of the constant length phenomenon. Were the plantaris tendon ruptured, the foot would not be fixed in plantiflexion nor would resisted plantiflexion be painful. Palpation of the calf reveals either (a) a tender area in the gastrocnemius muscle, usually some two inches above the musculo-tendinous junction and rather to the inner side of the belly, or (b) in more severe cases, a palpable gap in much the same situation about half an inch wide.

Treatment

As soon as the patient is seen, whether it is the same day or some weeks later, local anaesthesia should be induced at the site of the partial rupture. The exact spot is difficult to find; for gentle pressure over the site of a lesion in the deeper part of the muscle naturally does not disclose tenderness, whereas strong pressure is apt to hurt throughout the belly. It is thus best to locate the spot approximately and then use 50 ml. of 0·5 per cent procaine solution for the infiltration. The pain ceases and a much greater range of dorsiflexion of the foot becomes possible within a few minutes of a successful injection. This must *not* be tested with the patient standing, since this may lead to further tearing. The patient is taught to move his foot up and down as he lies on the couch, restoring the range actively without the strain of weight-bearing falling on the muscle. While he lies there practising this movement, a cork platform should be made and fitted into the shoe. The extent of muscle above and below the breach can contract and relax normally, but the mid-part is in spasm about the tear; hence, the muscle is shortened for the time being. A raised heel enables him to use the unaffected parts of the muscle without straining the healing breach. The first day he may need a raise of 3 to 4 cm. and at each attendance the thickness of the platform is revised; its height is reduced until after, say, a week it becomes unnecessary.

The next and following days, the patient attends for deep massage to the area of the lesion, and, if he is an athlete, faradism to the muscle while the knee is held fully flexed and the foot plantiflexed. The muscle then moves fully without any strain falling on it at the extreme of contraction. When this treatment is instituted during the first few days after the accident, patients can expect to be playing tennis again at the end of ten days; without immediate active treatment, the disability lasts for six weeks to six months or more. Rest and over-exertion, as in all muscular injuries, are both equally harmful. In chronic cases, scarring should be broken up by deep massage and mobility increased by the same faradism with the muscle held in the shortened position. When a palpable gap exists in the muscle-belly, tip-toe exercises during weight-bearing should be avoided for three weeks.

Teno-synovitis of the Tendo Achillis

The patient complains of pain at the heel, felt only during movement, and present ever since some unaccustomed exertion, perhaps in heel-less shoes. He states that rising on tip-toe hurts at the back of the heel.

If, as is common, the lesion is a teno-synovitis, no movement hurts except resisted plantiflexion of the foot. The site of the lesion is usually at mid-tendon. Occasionally, the strain occurs level with the upper border of the calcaneus; if so, full plantiflexion of the foot squeezes the affected part of the tendon against the posterior aspect of the tibia; hence this movement hurts slightly too.

The tendon is carefully palpated and it will be found that the lesion lies always at the inner or outer or both aspects of the tendon, sometimes on the anterior surface and scarcely ever on the posterior surface. Since the effective treatment for this disorder is deep transverse massage (and massage acts where it is applied and not elsewhere), if the anterior tenderness is not sought and treated, the case will be unjustly regarded as refractory to friction. This is a rarity; the commonplace is massage inadequately given. My experience with hydrocortisone is disappointing; the lesion may be too extensive for thorough infiltration, and even a successful injection is often followed by relapse a few weeks or months later. By contrast, recovery after friction is nearly always permanent: an important matter to athletes.

Teno-vaginitis of the Tendo Achillis

This takes three forms, rheumatoid, gouty and xanthomatous.

Rheumatoid or Gouty Teno-vaginitis

The contrast between the slight symptoms and the marked signs is striking. The patient complains mainly of pain when his heel catches against an object. Examination shows that rising on tip-toe is scarcely uncomfortable. Yet the tendon is warm to the touch, swollen, and very tender. There is no crepitus. Erosion of bone visible radiographically at the calcanean insertion of the tendo Achillis has been described in rheumatoid disease. Infiltration with hydrocortisone is very successful in rheumatoid cases, and butazolidine or indomethacin is indicated in gout.

Xanthomatous Teno-vaginitis

The tendo Achillis is a fairly common site for xanthomatosis. Both heels hurt during walking. Both tendons can be seen to be thickened and palpation reveals enlargement and a diffuse nodularity. The diagnosis becomes clear when similar nodules are seen and felt at the extensor tendons on the dorsum of both hands. Occasionally, similar swellings form on the tendons crossing the dorsum of the foot, and quite large deposits may form on the bone at the upper part of the ulna and tibia.

Clofibrate 0·5 g. thrice daily should be given for some years and regression has been reported (Roper, 1964); doubtless Bengal Gram will now be tried too.

Intermittent Claudication

Claudication is, of course, merely a local manifestation of a general condition and the cerebral and coronary arteries are naturally apt to be affected too, particularly if the patient is diabetic. Women are seldom affected by claudication in the calf. The name was first used in 1831 by a veterinary surgeon called Bouley to designate a form of limping in horses, and Charcot described a case in 1858.

The phenomenon is dependent on the anatomical fact that two long arteries supply the gastrocnemius muscle. They follow its whole length, without forming anastomoses. This is a different pattern of blood-supply from: (a) the soleus muscle, which receives a number of branches entering at intervals all the way down; (b) the tibialis anterior and extensor hallucis bellies which are supplied by a series of anastomotic loops derived from a succession of vessels (Blomfield). Owing to this exceptional arrangement of its nutrient arteries, the gastrocnemius muscle is more susceptible than others to ischaemia as the result of arteriosclerosis. Claudication in early middle-age suggests endarteritis obliterans; in youth, coarctation of the aorta or an aberrant slip of muscle compressing the artery.

History

The history is characteristic. An elderly patient reports that pain in one calf is brought on by exertion and relieved by rest. A similar history may be given by a patient with the mushroom phenomenon, but standing still does not then relieve his pain, he must sit down. In very early claudication, the patient finds that walking some hundred yards brings the pain on, but that walking on farther, no less than resting, abolishes the pain. In the former event, continuation of the stimulus to vasodilatation has clearly enhanced the flow sufficiently to prevent the products of muscular metabolism from remaining at a painful level. Later, the symptoms can no longer be abolished by walking on; the patient is forced to rest each hundred yards or so to let the metabolites reach a concentration below the threshold of pain. He can then walk on another similar distance. Sooner or later, pain at night is apt to appear, relieved by allowing the limb to cool outside the bed-clothes. When the muscles become warm, their metabolic requirement rises, just as it does during walking, to the point at which the possible arterial flow becomes inadequate. Pain at rest suggests that gangrene will come on within three to six months (Martin, 1960).

Claudication is usually felt unilaterally. If the state of his arteries enables a man to walk, say, a hundred yards with his left leg and a hundred and ten yards with his right, he never gets to the point of experiencing right-sided claudication.

If the anterior tibial artery is narrowed—a rarity— the intermittent claudication is felt at the front instead of the back of the leg. Ischaemia of the muscles of the sole is a not uncommon cause of elderly patients' 'foot-strain'.

Signs

If plantiflexion is tested against resistance as the patient lies on the couch, neither weakness nor pain is elicited. If he is asked to plantiflex and dorsiflex his foot quickly and repeatedly, the familiar pain is brought on. Dependent, the foot is a dusky red. If it blanches on elevating the limb, the distal extent of the arteries of the leg and foot is shown to be patent. If not, the whole arterial tree is affected and gangrene must be anticipated. Pulsation in the dorsalis pedis, posterior tibial and popliteal arteries is usually absent on both sides. If the femoral arteries do not pulsate either, aortic occlusion or coarctation should be considered and aortography performed.

Treatment

Vasodilator and anticoagulant drugs, Buerger's exercises and physio-therapy are all valueless. Indeed, vaso-dilator drugs are harmful, since they dilate arteries that are not diseased elsewhere in the body, thus diminishing blood-pressure generally and reducing the flow through the sclerotic arteries. Smoking should be forbidden and great care taken of the skin of the feet. A raised heel gives the muscles rather less to do and the adoption of a steady slow pace brings requirement and supply closer to equilibrium. If the symptoms warrant, the gastrocnemius may be divided at its insertion into the tendo Achillis. This leaves the soleus muscle, with its satisfactory arrangement of arteries, intact and is to be preferred to mere tenotomy of the tendo Achillis. Crushing the motor nerve to the gastrocnemius is an alternative (Reid, Watt & Grey, 1963) via incision in the popliteal fossa.

Sympathectomy warms the foot but seldom increases the walking distance materially, but varicose or ischaemic ulcers often heal quickly after the operation.

In recent years, the treatment of choice has become the restoration of a patent artery by surgery. Cockett began in 1952 with grafting but now (Cockett & Maurice, 1963) performs a rebore. If the femoral pulse is absent, the operation has an excellent result; if the femoral pulse is present and the popliteal absent, and the arteriogram shows the sural arteries to be patent, operation is again indicated. If the occlusion lies at or distal to the popliteal bifurcation, the condition is clearly insusceptible to arterial surgery.

Venous Claudication

Those who suffer from permanent obstruction to the venous return from a lower limb develop what Cockett et al. (1967) termed venous claudication. Exertion increases the venous pressure in the affected leg, thus exerting backpressure against the arterial flow. Discomfort in the calf after walking some way results.

Nocturnal Cramp

This wakens elderly patients and can be most troublesome. It has some connection with disc lesions for it often follows sciatica and is felt on the affected side only. In other cases, no cause is discernible. It may be a most troublesome sequel to section of the posterior root at the fifth lumbar or first sacral level (Sicard & Leca, 1954). The patient can sometimes precipitate an attack of cramp in the calf by stretching his leg out fully. Patients describe a ball of contracted muscle that travels along the belly, and mention various positions in which the limb is fixed during the attack; a common one is extension at the knee, plantiflexion at the ankle and extension at the toes. Such a position involves coordination between several groups of muscles and must therefore be initiated centrally. I regard cramp, therefore, as caused by an epilepsy of the anterior horn cells of the spinal cord.

Quinine diminishes the excitability of skeletal muscle by increasing its refractory period (Harvey, 1939). Five grains taken at bed-time should be continued for some months, after which it may be found that the tendency has passed and there is no relapse. If it does, the patient should try out for himself the minimum dose that prevents the cramp. Should quinine fail, carisoprodol 0·5 gm. taken last thing at night should be tried; it can be continued indefinitely. It relaxes skeletal muscle and has a central analgesic effect as well. If the attacks of cramp follow sciatica, residual bruising of the nerve-root may be the focus whence the attack originates. Epidural local anaesthesia is then often successful in mitigating or abolishing the attacks.

Weak Plantiflexor Muscles

Painless weakness is best detected by asking the patient to stand on each leg in turn and rise on tip-toe. Apart from upper motor neurone lesions, peroneal atrophy and direct injury to the sciatic nerve, the common cause of weakness unaccompanied by increase in pain when the calf-muscles contract is a fifth lumbar disc lesion causing a first and second sacral root-palsy.

Rupture of the Tendo Achillis

This simple condition usually remains undiagnosed until too late, cursory examination resulting in its being dismissed as some sort of sprained ankle. The patient states that while playing, say, squash, his foot suddenly hurt and gave way. The pain was momentary, but he found at once that he could only hobble on a flat foot. He limped home and, when examined as he lay on a couch, active plantiflexion was found not to be lost. Since the plantaris, flexor longus hallucis and digitorum muscles all remain intact, the supine patient can just voluntarily plantiflex his foot. Had the movement been tested against the slightest resistance, gross weakness would have been revealed. The pain in the calf and fixed equinus of a patient with a minor tear in his gastrocnemius muscle contrast with the absence of pain, inability to plantiflex strongly and excessive dorsiflexion range at the ankle characterizing rupture of the tendo Achillis. When the patient lies prone, the defect in the tendon is easy to feel; a half to three-quarter-inch gap is palpable at, or slightly above the middle of the tendon.

Treatment

If the rupture is discovered within ten days of the accident, contracture of the calf-muscles is not yet too great to prevent operative suture.

After this period has elapsed, spontaneous organization of the haematoma with eventual fibrous repair should be awaited. This takes several months during which the patient should make no effort to rise on tip-toe. The thickened tissues at each side of the enlarged tendon should be massaged twice a week, for two or three months even in long-standing cases. Alleviation, not cure, may be expected. For the rest of his life, the tendon remains twice its original width; the fibrous swelling at the point of rupture never disappears and some residual disability is permanent. This may amount merely to some aching towards the end of a round of golf, but other patients are permanently unable to run, or to walk any distance without pain.

Short Plantiflexor Muscles

Shortening forms parts of a talipes equino-varus deformity in babies. If the equinus position of a baby's feet can be overcome by strong resistance, diplegia is present. In some children the calf-muscles are short as an isolated phenomenon; if so, it usually escapes detection. In due course the mother complains of the child's gait, mentioning his feet, not his calves. She notices that the youngster turns his feet out too much, stands tilted backwards and runs conspicuously slower than his schoolfellows. She is right. Inability to bear weight properly on the heel because of equinus, forces the lad to twist his foot into lateral rotation; hence, when he runs, instead of landing on his heel and taking off from the forefoot held in line with the movement of the body, he takes off from a foot oblique to this line. Hence he may lose several cm. of forward movement at each step. Moveover, standing on his heels involves his remaining tilted slightly backwards; he is not properly poised above his centre of gravity. In consequence, muscular force in excess of the minimum has to be expended during standing; the child therefore complains that prolonged standing is tiring. If, as is common, a plantaris deformity of the forefoot complicates the short muscles, he cannot bear adequate weight on his heels and mid-tarsal hypermobility and, later, painful strain results.

On examination dorsiflexion at the ankle joint is painlessly limited to the horizontal line—what is often well described as equinus to 90 degrees —since the calf muscles will not stretch farther.

Treatment of Equinus Deformity

In children, the treatment is temporarily to provide the shoe with a raised heel to protect the mid-tarsal joint, and to teach the following exercises. For stretching the soleus muscles: the child should perform a knee-flexion exercise barefoot, keeping the heel on the ground. For stretching the gastrocnemius muscle: the patient stands with the foot fully dorsiflexed at the ankle by pressure against a wall, the heel remaining on the ground; he should then lean forward vigorously keeping the knee in full extension. When the calf muscles have lengthened, which takes some months of hard work, the raised heel on the shoe can be discarded.

In adults, the process of stretching out the calf muscles is too tedious, and shortening can be adequately compensated by raising the heel of the shoe and increasing the obliquity of its upper surface. Elongation of the tendo Achillis by subcutaneous tenotomy followed by six weeks' immobilzation in a plaster case is the alternative.

THE DORSIFLEXOR MUSCLES

The strength of dorsiflexion on the two sides is compared; pain on this movement is noted. Normal dorsiflexor muscles easily overcome the examiner's resistance. This movement elicits pain in lesions affecting the anterior tibial and extensor longus hallucis and digitorum muscles. A resisted extension movement of the hallux and then of the toes picks out the offending muscle.

Myosynovitis of the tibialis anterior muscle is an interesting condition, with only one other parallel in the body—myosynovitis with crepitus of the bellies of the abductor longus and the extensores pollicis muscles in the forearm. It is an uncommon disorder except in army service, when recruits march unaccustomed distances in boots. The resisted dorsiflexion movement hurts above the front of the ankle; further testing shows the long extensor muscles of the digits to be unaffected, and palpation fails to reveal any tenderness of the anterior tibial tendon itself. If the examiner now puts his finger on the outer aspect of the junction of the middle with the lower third of the tibia, crepitus on movement is felt at the musculo-tendinous junction of the anterior tibial muscle close to the bone.

At the ankle, teno-synovitis (sometimes with crepitus) of the extensor longus hallucis or digitorum is a rarity and is an uncommon sequel to a sprained ankle. Shortening of these muscles complicates a pes cavus deformity, eventually fixing the toes in the clawed position.

Weakness of the muscles dorsiflexing the foot is a common finding in upper motor neurone lesions, anterior poliomyelitis and lumbar disc lesions at the fourth level.

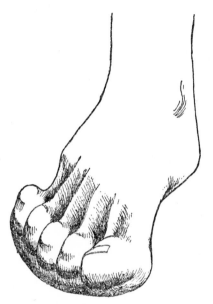

FIG. 118. Pes cavus. The foot is short and broad. The extensor tendons of the toes stand out holding the toes clawed. The toes have corns and a large callosity has formed under the metatarsal heads.

The extensor hallucis muscle may develop ischaemic contracture or become adherent after a fracture in mid-tibia; the constant-length phenomenon results. In these cases, each time the foot is plantiflexed, the big toe has to extend; it is forced against the upper of the shoe and becomes extremely sore. Tenotomy under local anaesthesia level with the first metatarso-phalangeal joint gives permanent relief.

Treatment

Lesions of the bellies of these muscles respond well to both local anaesthesia and deep massage. Their tendons respond to deep massage and to hydrocortisone.

TIGHT FASCIAL COMPARTMENT

Symptoms superficially resembling intermittent claudication result from a tight fascial compartment for the dorsiflexor muscles in the leg. In minor cases, the patient states that, after walking say half a mile, he becomes unable to dorsiflex his foot voluntarily, and has to stump along flexing his knee to get his foot off the ground. Alternatively, he may develop a drop-foot after kicking a football about for ten minutes. The weakness is devoid of discomfort. After a short rest, the muscle recovers. In these cases examination in the resting state reveals nothing, and the arteries at the ankle pulsate normally. After the causative exertion, the tibialis anterior muscles are found temporarily paralysed, the pulses still remaining palpable.

The cause is a tight fascial compartment. The contents of the anterior tibial compartment lie in an inelastic space. The bellies of the anterior tibial, extensor hallucis and digitorum muscles are confined by the tibia, fibula, interosseous membrane and superficial fascia. The normal increase in bulk due to increased blood flow during exertion may cause such swelling that the lumen of the anterior tibial artery is temporarily occluded. The muscle is paralysed, but regains its strength in a few minutes. If, however, the minute vessels in the belly itself become silted up with cells (Harman, 1948), the disorder may become irreversible. The swelling may also trap the superficial peroneal nerve at its exit through the fascial foramen at mid-leg and cause pins and needles at the inner four toes.

Severe cases are encountered. A healthy young man develops pain at the front of the mid-leg after some exertion; within a few hours it is intense. Redness and oedema of the skin now appear over the belly of the tibialis anterior muscle. If the fascia is not divided at once, ischaemic necrosis may ensue, contracture or even complete paralysis resulting. If so, the power to dorsiflex foot and toes is permanently lost.

The anterior tibial syndrome may also result from thrombosis or embolism of the anterior tibial artery in older patients. This is quite a different condition, caused by primary arterial occlusion, not a tight fascia. D. C. Watson (1955) gives a good review of the literature and describes two cases caused by arterial disease; Freedman and Knowles (1959) describe five more such cases.

Treatment

This consists in removal of the fascia at the front of the tibial belly; if necrosis is impending, the operation is urgent.

THE EVERTOR MUSCLES

If resisted eversion of the foot hurts, the peroneal muscles are affected. Tendinitis here occurs anywhere from the lower fibula to the cuboid and fifth metatarsal base; the site of tenderness defines the position of the lesion. Peroneal tendinitis is one cause of continued disability after a sprained ankle. Since the pain is at the outer side of the ankle, it is naturally ascribed to post-traumatic adhesions and the foot is mobilized and exercised in a way that unintentionally makes the condition worse. Testing the resisted movements gives the clue at once.

The peroneal tendons may get loose in their groove on the posterior surface of the fibula and slip forwards over the malleolus, thus giving rise to a 'snapping ankle'. This is usually not painful or much of a disability; when the foot is plantiflexed the tendons jump back again. Mucocoele of the peroneal tendons results in swelling leading eventually to considerable aching. The glairy fluid can be made to fluctuate from above to below the malleolus. Ganglia occur in connection with these tendons, above as well as below the ankle.

Spasm of the peroneal muscles results, not from intrinsic defect, but from arthritis of the talo-calcanean and mid-tarsal joints, which are thereby fixed in valgus and abduction respectively. Hence the term 'spasmodic pes planus' is a misnomer.

Weakness of the peroneal muscles is caused mainly by upper motor neurone lesions, peroneal atrophy and disc protrusions at the fifth lumbar level. Unreadiness to bring them into play results in recurrent varus sprain at the ankle.

Treatment

Peroneal tendinitis responds well to massage; the lesion is seldom localized enough for an injection of hydrocortisone (see Vol. II). Mucocoele has been treated merely by puncture of the tendon-sheath with a tenotomy knife followed by digital expression of one or two ounces of mucus. This procedure has to be repeated about once a year.

THE INVERTOR MUSCLES

These are the anterior and posterior tibial muscles. If a resisted inversion movement hurts, and dorsiflexion does not, the posterior tibial muscle is at fault. The tendon is palpated throughout its extent until the site of the lesion is found.

'Shin-soreness'

Athletes use this word for pain in the leg caused by running. Examination shows that the usual cause is a lesion of the posterior tibial or peroneal muscles at the musculo-tendinous junction. It is an overuse phenomenon, responding well to deep massage. Rarely, the radiograph reveals a stress-fracture.

Treatment

A posterior tibial tendinitis caused by ordinary overuse recovers with a few sessions of massage. However, in older patients it may result from years of overuse, secondary to a valgus deformity at the heel, especially if the cause is fixed inversion of the forefoot. The pain goes on indefinitely. They are curable only by a combined approach: a support to correct the lack of parallel between hindfoot and forefoot (Fig. 133) combined with massage to the affected extent of tendon (see Vol. II). Neither measure alone suffices.

THE NERVES OF THE LEG

Saphenous and Deep Peroneal Nerves

The saphenous nerve may suffer compression at its exit from the deep fascia just below the inner condyle of the tibia. In addition to paraesthesia at the inner ankle and along the medial border of the foot, ill-defined aching is felt along the subcutaneous border of the tibia.

Either nerve may suffer direct contusion at the point where its terminal part crosses the front of the ankle joint. If so, after the blow, the patient complains of pins and needles at the dorsum of the distal part of the foot, especially at the adjacent borders of the big and second toe in the case of the superficial peroneal nerve. If the saphenous nerve has suffered contusion at the front of the ankle, the inner aspect of the dorsum of the foot as far as the supero-medial aspect of the hallux tingles; sharp neuralgic twinges may be felt when the nerve is stretched by flexion of the hallux. Hirschfield called this the 'tarsal tunnel syndrome' (1960, personal communication) and found procaine curative. Whichever nerve is affected, combined plantiflexion and inversion of the foot stretch the bruised nerve and bring on or accentuate the tingling. The tender extent of the nerve usually lies level with the ankle joint. Lam (1962) has described another lesion as the 'tarsal tunnel syndrome'. The patient complained of pins and needles along the medial border of the foot and two and a half inner toes. Operation showed the peroneal nerve to be caught up by a slip of the flexor retinaculum, division of which was curative. Contusion of the medial terminal branch of the deep peroneal nerve occurs at the ankle; the dorsum of the outer foot and three outer toes become paraesthetic. In such a case, inversion of the foot during plantiflexion causes a twinge of pins and needles.

The superficial peroneal nerve issues from the deep fascia at the junction of the middle and lower third of the leg; it is compressed there when the tibialis anterior swells inside a tight fascia, also idiopathically, in a manner similar to meralgia paraesthetica. It divides into two branches, one supplying the inner three toes, the other the outer three toes; hence, in this case the dorsum of the whole foot and all the toes tingle.

Treatment

This consists of the diagnostic injection of procaine, which is always required to make sure the correct area of nerve has been found. Should this fail therapeutically but show that the right spot has been chosen, hydrocortisone is substituted.

Common Peroneal Nerve

This nerve is exposed to a blow or to sustained pressure at the point where it winds round the lateral aspect of the neck of the fibula. It can be compressed by sitting with the legs crossed or by keeping the knee pressed against e.g. the side of a desk. Since the nerve supplies the tibialis anterior extensor haelucis and peroneal muscles, drop-foot results and the outer foot and calf go numb.

Spontaneous recovery may take a month or two and how to avoid the causative posture is explained to the patient.

Tibial Nerve

This is compressed by sitting with the knees half-crossed, the patella of the nether knee squeezing the tibial nerve against the posterior aspect of the tibia. There is seldom appreciable weakness but the heel and sole may remain numb for a couple of months.

The causative posture must be avoided.

THE ANKLE JOINT

This is a simple joint allowing two movements in only one plane: plantiflexion and dorsiflexion. The range of dorsiflexion is limited by the length of the calf-muscles. These are at their most extensible in babies in

AA

whom the dorsum of the foot can often be laid against the leg with ease. Plantiflexion is limited by the engagement of the heel, *via* the tendo Achillis, against the back of the tibia. The talus is held in place by the tibio-fibular mortice, which in turn depends on the inferior tibio-fibular ligament for its effectiveness.

Examination

Five movements are required: two primary for the joint and three accessory for ligaments. For the joint: the range of plantiflexion and dorsiflexion is ascertained, compared with the other side and the production or not of pain noted. The end-feel has particular diagnostic importance. Both extremes are soft at a normal joint, since compression of the insertion of the tendo Achillis against the back of the tibia, and full stretching of the calf muscles, can have nothing abrupt about them. In arthritis, the joint itself is felt to come to a dead stop with a hard end-feel.

The *capsular pattern* is rather more limitation of plantiflexion than of dorsiflexion. However, in patients with a short calf muscle, this may limit dorsiflexion before the extreme of the possible articular range is reached, thus disguising the hard restriction of dorsiflexion. In such a case, a clinical diagnosis of arthritis at the ankle joint rests on the discovery of limited plantiflexion with a hard end-feel.

For the ligaments: the deltoid ligament is stretched by a combined eversion and plantiflexion movement, and the anterior fasciculus of the lateral ligament by inversion during plantiflexion. The inferior tibio-fibular ligament is stretched by a strong varus movement applied to the talus *via* the calcaneus. Hence, varus at the heel is vigorously forced when a sprung mortice is suspected.

The following disorders occur:

Equinus

Limitation of dorsiflexion as an isolated finding designates short calf muscles and often complicates a pes cavus deformity, thus rendering the plantaris posture of the forefoot more unfortunate than ever. Equinus at the ankle joint may result in mid-tarsal strain in children and adults. Since they cannot dorsiflex at the ankle joint, they are forced to carry out this movement at the next available joint—the mid-tarsal. Since, too, the child with fixed equinus can best get his heel to the ground by rotating the limb laterally, he tends to turn his feet out more and more, thus gradually developing a considerable outward rotation deformity in the course of the tibial shaft.

In a child, an equinus deformity that disappears on strong pressure characterizes cerebral diplegia.

Treatment

In children this consists of stretching the soleus and gastrocnemius muscles out separately—the first by active knee flexion exercises with the heel flat on the ground; the second by placing the fully dorsiflexed foot against a wall and then leaning forwards with the knee fully extended. It may take months.

Adults should have the heel raised and the obliquity of its upper surface increased, or the tendo Achillis lengthened by operation.

Arthritis at the Ankle

This is present when both dorsiflexion and plantiflexion are limited. In early cases, plantiflexion may be found limited alone, if the calf muscles are too short to allow the foot to reach the extreme of range at the ankle joint.

The rheumatoid conditions, which so often affect the other tarsal joints, conspicuously avoid the ankle joint. I have seen psoriatic arthritis at this joint; it responds very well to intra-articular hydrocortisone. The only common condition is osteoarthritis, almost always the result of mal-union of a tibio-fibular fracture. If a shearing strain is put on the joint by mal-union with angulation at the fracture, osteoarthritis will certainly supervene.

Repeated severe sprains—e.g. in rugby footballers—may in the end set up osteoarthritis, sometimes with ligamentous ossification visible on the radiograph. Osteoarthritis shows up well on the radiograph.

In osteoarthritis, conservative treatment is seldom satisfactory. In early cases, intra-articular hydrocortisone may help; mobilization under anaesthesia may bring several months' relief. Fitting the patient's shoes with a higher heel may enable him to walk without fully dorsiflexing his foot, thus avoiding the painful extreme of movement. If the symptoms warrant, arthrodesis should be performed without delay, or the condition goes on getting worse indefinitely.

Limitation of movement without arthritis occurs after the ankle has been immobilized for months in the treatment of tibio-fibular fractures. In such cases, strong daily forcing, supplanted by the patient's active exertions, in due course restores an adequate range of movement.

Loose Body in Ankle Joint

The patient complains that, some time after a severe sprain of the ankle, he has suffered bouts of twinges at the ankle, usually on pointing the foot to go downstairs. Severe momentary pain prevents his stepping on to that foot; he gives it a shake and the disability ceases, only to be repeated some time later.

Examination and radiography reveal nothing, since the subluxation is momentary only and the fragment cartilaginous, merely showing that no other cause for the twinges is present. Differential diagnosis is difficult between a sprung mortice and a loose body in the talo-calcanean joint. Treatment is difficult too, for the attempt must be made to shift the loose fragment to a position within the joint whence it does not subluxate (see Vol. II). Since no displacement exists at the time of the manipulation, the usual clinical criteria that help guide the manipulator towards the correct way to deal with internal derangement are absent.

Unstable Mortice

The patient states that some years previously he sprained his ankle severely. He recovered in due course, but then found that he could no longer rely on his foot which has turned over easily ever since, with a sudden click and momentary severe pain at the ankle. After some moments, he walks on again; the ankle merely feels sore for a day or two afterwards. The cause is permanent lengthening of the inferior tibio-fibular ligament.

When the ankle joint is examined, nothing is detected at first, but when valgus and varus movements are tested at the talo-calcanean joint, the click is reproduced at the ankle when varus is forced hard. If this movement is repeated with the examiner's fingers palpating the two malleoli, they can be felt to move apart, and if a radiograph is taken while strong varus pressure is exerted at the heel, the increased distance apart of the lower ends of tibia and fibula can be seen.

Treatment
The bones must be wired together again.

Sprain of the Anterior Tibio-talar Ligament

This is an uncommon injury and is caused by a pure plantiflexion stress. Chronic aching often results, which may last many years, but is never severe and only prevents vigorous use. Examination shows that full passive plantiflexion hurts at the front of the ankle; all other movements are painless. Palpation involves pushing the tendons aside and searching for the tender spot at the talo-tibial ligament. Massage or hydrocortisone injection is permanently effective. Manipulation is useless.

Sprain of the Posterior Talo-fibular Ligament

Sprain of the posterior fasciculus of the fibular collateral ligament is rare. The diagnosis is made with some difficulty; for the only painful movement is apt to be passive eversion of the foot, which compresses the tender ligament between the tip of the fibula and the everted calcaneus. If then the movement intended to stretch the deltoid ligament hurts at the *outer* side of the heel, this lesion is recalled.

One injection of hydrocortisone into the tender ligament gives lasting relief.

Anterior Periostitis

This disorder, the reverse phenomenon of dancer's heel, is a rarity. It is caused by a dorsiflexion strain that forces the neck of the talus against the anterior margin of the tibia. The ballet-dancer lands flat on her foot, then bends her knee and feels an immediate pain at the front of the ankle. Examination shows full passive dorsiflexion to hurt at the front of the ankle, i.e. something is pinched. Passive plantiflexion does not hurt, thus exculpating the anterior ligament.

An injection of hydrocortisone is curative and the dancer is fit to perform two days later. Prophylaxis consists of slightly raising the heel of the ballet shoe.

Jumper's Sprain

An athlete, landing on his heel as he takes off to jump, may force his foot into dorsiflexion and eversion. As a result, the supero-lateral aspect of the anterior margin of the calcaneus hits against the edge of the fibula, producing a traumatic periostitis there. After that, every time he takes off the pain reappears, felt clearly at the outer side of the ankle.

Examination reveals nothing, since the ligaments and muscles are not affected. Forcing the everted foot into dorsiflexion is the only way to reproduce the pain. Palpation reveals localized tenderness at the anteroinferior surface of the fibula, but no corresponding tenderness on the calcaneus.

One or two injections of hydrocortisone bring relief, but the athlete must avoid repeating the same trauma, if necessary by wearing a 0·5 cm. inner wedge within his shoe.

SPRAINED ANKLE

'Sprained ankle' is the general name for a variety of traumatic lesions occurring at what the patient calls his ankle. Several conditions may legitimately be described under this heading; each may exist alone, but combined lesions predominate. Moreover, one structure may recover, leaving chronic disability due to another.

The talus is slightly wedge-shaped, larger anteriorly. Hence in dorsiflexion the bone is gripped in the tibio-fibular mortice; force applied to it is likely to cause a fracture or lengthening of the inferior tibio-fibular ligament. In plantiflexion, the bone does not fit closely in the mortice and force can produce enough movement to sprain ligaments. Strong inversion during forced plantiflexion is the way an ankle becomes sprained.

Sprained ankle may be classified according as the causative stress is towards varus or valgus, and according to the length of time that has elapsed since the accident.

Varus Sprain

This is as common as valgus sprain is uncommon. The stresses imposed on the tarsus by a varus sprain are: (1) plantiflexion at the ankle joint, stretching its outer side and the extensor longus digitorum muscle; (2) varus at the talo-calcanean joint, stretching the fibulo-calcanean ligament and the peroneal tendons; (3) medial rotation and adduction at the mid-tarsal joint, stretching the ligament at the outer aspect of the calcaneo-cuboid joint. Exceptionally the cubo-fifth-metatarsal or cubo-navicular joints suffer as well. Thus, injury to one or more of these structures may correctly be described by the patient as a sprained ankle.

Examination in Varus Sprain

This must include:
1. Five passive movements at the ankle joint.
2. Two passive movements at the talo-calcanean joint.
3. Six passive movements at the mid-tarsal joint.
4. The four resisted movements—dorsiflexion, plantiflexion, inversion, eversion.

The site of the lesion is deduced from the pattern that emerges when these passive and resisted movements are tested. Once the site of the sprain has been outlined by this examination, tenderness of the appropriate structure is sought. In recent severe cases, gross oedema often gives rise to such generalized tenderness that palpation yields no information; if so, the diagnosis is arrived at purely by inference from a study of the response to these movements. The affected sites, in order of descending frequency, are:

(a) The fibular origin of the fibular collateral ligament of the ankle; (b) the talar insertion of this ligament; (c) the outer fibres of the calcaneo-cuboid joint-capsule; (d) the upper extent of the fibulo-calcanean ligament; (e) the peroneal tendons; (f) the tendon of the extensor longus digitorum. The commonest lesion is a combined sprain of the fibular collateral ligament and the capsule of the calcaneo-cuboid joint.

If examination shows the tendons to be affected as much as, or more than, the ligaments, the customary treatment of a sprained ankle by early ambulation is inadvisable. The patient should rest as much as he can for a few days until massage has cleared up the tendinous strain.

Treatment of Varus Sprain

This depends on the time that has elapsed since the accident.

Acute Stage

During the first twenty-four hours after a ligamentous sprain, immediate injection of hydrocortisone is indicated. The necessity for

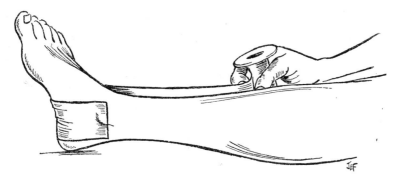

FIG. 119. Strapping for protection of fibulo-calcanean ligament. The strapping begins at the medial malleolus and holds the heel in full valgus by firm application at the outer side of the lower leg.

accurate diagnosis is now obvious, since infiltration has to be performed at some definite point. Deep effleurage is a great aid to precision; for, after the physiotherapist has removed most of the oedema, tenderness is elicited and bony points defined much more easily. If a haematoma of any size has formed, this is aspirated immediately before the injection. Two c.c. of hydrocortisone give little latitude in the choice of where to inject. Strapping may be applied to prevent recurrence of the swelling and for the moral support that it gives the patient. The patient walks out and attends the following day for the treatment described below as appropriate to the subacute stage. The sooner after the injury the infiltration is made, the more spectacular the results. In tendinitis, at this stage, the lesion is too diffuse for injection of hydrocortisone to be practicable. Massage is given daily to the tendon over the whole of its affected extent.

Subacute Stage

Massage is used to move the ligament in imitation of its normal behaviour, followed by gentle passive movements, which become stronger as recovery advances. Massage consists in the first place of effleurage to reduce oedema. There follows a very few minutes' deep friction to the actual site of the tear in each ligament. This eases the pain further, disperses local effusion and moves the affected structure to and fro over subajacent bone. Movement is then increased passively in each direction, the range of each affected joint being gently forced to the point of discomfort but not of pain. The movements at the ankle, talo-calcanean and mid-tarsal joints are each performed to the limit of the possible range. Unless the physiotherapist is unthinkably rough, no danger of overstretching the sprained ligaments results from these movements, since an excessive range is adequately prevented by observing the patient's reaction. The main difficulty is to get him to realize how much greater the painless range is than he believes. Active movements follow the passive movements at once; they further the effect of the friction in preventing scar tissue from forming abnormal adherence. Finally, the patient departs, walking slowly and carefully with proper heel-and-toe gait. Walking with the foot held stiffly has no therapeutic value.

If a tendon is affected alone, no treatment is required other than deep massage and the avoidance of such exertion as causes pain.

Chronic Stage

The foot is quite adequate for ordinary purposes but is apt to swell and ache after vigorous or prolonged use. This means that scars were allowed to form abnormal attachments as the result of healing in the absence of enough movement; alternatively, the ligamentous sprain has recovered leaving a chronic tendinitis.

The treatment of adhesions about a ligament is naturally their manipulative rupture. This is quite easy and very seldom requires anaesthesia. One sharp twist (see Vol. II) stretching out the talo-fibular and calcaneo-cuboid ligaments suffices. There is a tiny crack, and the patient is cured. No after-treatment is necessary.

Chronic tendinitis requires deep massage to the affected part of the tendon. Until well, the patient should avoid such exertion as causes pain. If a small stretch of tendon remains refractory to friction, an injection of hydrocortisone suspension is given there.

Recurrent Varus Sprain

The patient states that his ankle turns over easily; it lacks stability and is thus subjected to a succession of minor sprains. If the examiner can reproduce the sprain at will, with an audible click as varus is forced at the heel, lengthening of the inferior tibio-fibular ligament should be suspected. However, the mortice is found stable.

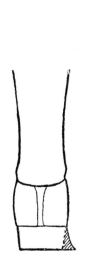 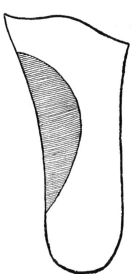

FIG. 120. Heel floated at outer side. For recurrent varus sprain of ankle.

FIG. 121. Valgus support. The thickness lies at the inner side of the mid-tarsal joint.

The recent case should be treated on the lines suggested above, but the sprain in recurrent trouble is seldom severe. The patient is usually a girl in her teens, and on examination the peroneal muscles are not weak; when the ankle starts turning over, they are merely brought into play too slowly to prevent the sprain. It would seem that, as time goes on, the reflex becomes more rapid. Meanwhile, repetition is best prevented by floating out the heel of the patient's shoes (Fig. 120).

If the peroneal muscles are weak, it must be remembered that at times the first complaint in an upper motor neurone lesion may be recurrent varus sprain at the ankle. Sciatica leading to a fifth lumbar root-palsy naturally leaves the patient liable to sprain his ankle for the duration of the peroneal weakness.

Valgus Sprain

When this rare condition is encountered, the foot should be examined in an endeavour to discover why the stress took the unusual direction. Usually the patient stands with a valgus deformity of his heel and abduction of the forefoot. Hence, every time he puts his foot to the ground, he overstretches the damaged tibio-navicular or tibio-calcanean ligaments. For this reason, sprains of the anterior and middle fasciculi of the deltoid ligament are apt to go on hurting for many months, even years, since the patient strains the ligament anew at every step.

Treatment

This is twofold. The heel and forefoot must be so supported that strain during weight-bearing is removed from the affected fasciculus. To this end a support is prescribed—thick at the inner aspect of its calcanean and mid-tarsal extent (Fig. 121). When this is fitted, the calcaneus assumes the neutral position during weight-bearing (thus relaxing the tibio-calcanean ligament) and the cessation of abduction of the forefoot spares the tibio-navicular ligament. Hydrocortisone suspension injected into the affected areas of ligament now hastens cure, but is ineffective unless the support is fitted first. Manipulation is contra-indicated.

The posterior tibial tendon is often also affected. If a resisted inversion movement hurts, the affected area of tendon must be given massage. If a localized extent of tendon remains troublesome, it is infiltrated with hydrocortisone suspension.

26

The Foot

The patient can usually point fairly accurately to the site of a lesion in the foot. Pain is hardly ever referred to the foot only; but pain in the foot unaltered by standing or walking does raise this possibility.

EXAMINATION

Examination of the joints and muscles of the foot comprises: (1) inspection; (2) testing the five passive movements at the ankle joint; (3) testing the two passive movements at the talo-calcanean joint; (4) testing the six passive movements at the mid-tarsal joint while the heel and ankle joints are held still; (5) testing the passive movements at the metatarso-phalangeal and interphalangeal joints; (6) testing the resisted movements.

After the foot has been examined with the patient lying, it should be inspected again while the patient stands. The general posture of the foot, and the changes in shape caused by weight-bearing, are noted. If the examination standing is conducted first, the physician does not yet know what is wrong with the foot and he cannot therefore yet assess the bearing of any alterations in shape and colour he may find.

It is quite possible for a foot to hurt and yet to appear normal on clinical examination. This implies that the momentary stress imposed by manual testing of various movements does not suffice to evoke pain. This is particularly apt to occur in athletes and ballet-dancers who get pain after, say, fifteen minutes exertion, i.e. after strain far greater and more prolonged than any examiner can impose on the foot by mere clinical testing. In such cases, inspection of the shape of the foot, and of the changes it undergoes when bearing weight, shows where this undue strain falls and by corollary where it must be diminished. Inspection of the patient's worn shoes is often a help in showing where he bears most weight. Moreover, it reveals whether they suit his foot or not.

THE HEEL

The conditions giving rise to pain at the heel can be grouped under nine headings.

Traumatic Periostitis and Fracture

Blows on either side of the calcaneus may set up a traumatic periostitis at its subcutaneous surfaces; subsidence of the swelling and pain is hastened by deep effleurage. Minor flaking or cracks are uncommon and require no treatment. More severe fractures give rise to local pain and tenderness associated with bruising at the anterior part of the sole and require up to two months' complete avoidance of weight-bearing. Fractures involving the surface of the calcaneus articulating with the talus set up a painful and intractable osteoarthritis. Arthrodesis is better performed early than late; for disabling symptoms continue indefinitely. Osteitis deformans may attack the calcaneus.

Subcutaneous Nodules

Posteriorly, nodules may form in the subcutaneous fascia. When these get pinched between the calcaneus and the back of the shoe, severe pain results. On examination, tender nodules the size of a small pea can be felt slipping to and fro under the finger. No conservative treatment avails except the provision of shoes with a gap posteriorly. Division of the nodules by subcutaneous tenotomy under local anaesthesia gives results as good as excision.

Plantar Fasciitis

Overstrain

The patient complains of pain at the inner aspect of the sole of one or both heels when walking and standing, quickly relieved by avoiding weight-bearing. The most characteristic symptom is severe pain at the heel on first getting up to walk after sitting. During standing, the normal shape of the foot is partly maintained by the muscles; prolonged weight-bearing tires the muscles which eventually prove unequal to the burden. Strain, soon becoming painful, then falls on the plantar fascia instead.

Patients with Dupuytren's contracture at the palm sometimes develop similar swellings, but without contracture in the plantar fascia. They cause no symptoms.

Examination of the joints and muscles of the foot is negative. Tenderness is sought and found at the inner part of the front of the calcaneus, at the origin of the plantar fascia. Various other spots are palpated first, to ensure that psychogenic symptoms are detected.

Calcanean Spur

Continued overstrain of the fascia may result in the periosteum being pulled away at its origin from the calcaneus.

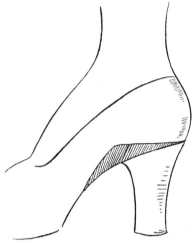

FIG. 122. Platform. The upper surface of the heel of the shoe is rendered horizontal by a wedge, thicker anteriorly. The plantar fascia is relaxed, because the forefoot drops into greater plantaris.

Since periosteum is the limiting membrane of bone, the gap becomes filled by new growth of bone as also occurs in osteophyte formation at the lumbar joints. The fact that the patient has, or did at one time have, strain on his plantar fascia now becomes visible on radiography. The presence of a calcanean spur on the X-ray photograph cannot determine whether the patient has symptoms or not. Spurs may develop painlessly; painful plantar fasciitis may not be associated with a visible spur. Once a spur has formed, it is permanent; hence radiography may disclose spurs, the pain from which ceased years previously. If history and clinical examination show painful strain to exist at the origin of the plantar fascia, radiography is of no particular assistance.

Treatment

This is very simple, spur or no spur; it consists in taking the strain off the plantar fascia. The less the angle between hindfoot and forefoot, the more the fascia is relaxed. Hence, all that need be done is to stand the patient on wooden platforms of different thickness, until the minimum height of heel that abolishes the symptoms is found. Provided the upper surface of the heel of the shoe remains horizontal, the higher the heel the more must the forefoot drop towards plantaris when he stands (Fig. 122). This shortens the distance from metatarsus to heel and relieves the fascia from strain. Thus, a height of heel can be found that affords immediate relief. The short flexor muscles in the sole are now energetically treated with faradism and exercises until their strength is once more adequate to protect the fascia from undue stress. The soreness leaves the fascia very slowly and it is often six months before a patient can return to his ordinary shoes without experiencing recurrence.

Occasionally, return to ordinary shoes provokes pain again each time it is attempted. In a woman, this is not of much account, but a man may not wish to wear a raised heel indefinitely. If so, hydrocortisone may be injected into the fascial origin and the patient warned of two days' considerable after-pain. The plantar skin is too thick to be capable of surface sterilization; hence the puncture must be made in the thin skin at the inner side of the heel. Alternatively, tenotomy of the fascial origin at the calcaneus under local anaesthesia is required, followed by a couple of days in bed. Exercises for the short flexor muscles are carried out from the outset. It is a very successful little operation.

Superficial Plantar Fasciitis

The pain is felt all over the posterior part of the sole, usually bilaterally. Curiously enough, the pain may be constant, felt even in bed, although worse during weight-bearing.

Examination shows the whole inferior surface of the heel to be uniformly tender, including the half-inch around the edge of the heel that does not touch the ground.

The only effective treatment is an injection of 10 c.c. 0·5 per cent procaine between the superficial plantar fascia and the surface of the calcaneum. The solution diffuses over the whole area forming a large tense swelling. The patient walks away and is usually pain-free by some days later, even after months or years of hitherto intractable symptoms.

Venereal Fasciitis

Gonorrhoea

The pain is in both heels and is constant, unrelieved when the patient rests. The patient, if he is honest, admits to a recent attack of gonorrhoea. A few days in bed should be advised to avoid strain on the fascia while the primary infection is being energetically treated.

Reiter's Disease

When plantar fasciitis is present with disease of joints as well, the association with non-gonococcal urethritis should be recalled. Mason (1964) states that plantar fasciitis occurs in 20 per cent of all such cases, and is characterized by a fluffy appearance of the spur, designating periostitis. Csonka (1958) also reported that 21·6 per cent of patients with non-gonococcal urethritis develop plantar fasciitis.

TENDINOUS LESIONS

These will merely be enumerated, having been considered in the previous chapter.

Teno-synovitis of the tendo Achillis from overuse.

Teno-vaginitis of the tendo Achillis due to rheumatoid disease, gout or xanthomatosis.

Rupture of the tendo Achillis.

Teno-synovitis of the peroneal and posterior tibial tendons. Mucocoele of these tendons.

BURSITIS

A bursa is normally present between the tendo Achillis and the tibia. If it becomes tender, pain is elicited when it is squeezed between the tendon and the tibia at the extreme of passive plantiflexion at the ankle. Bursitis is distinguished from lesions of the tendon itself by the fact that rising on tip-toe is painless. One or two injections of hydrocortisone are curative.

Another bursa may form at the centre of the inferior aspect of the calcaneus. It lies superficial to the mid-part of the origin of the plantar fascia. A heel support scooped out centrally is required, i.e. shaped like a horse-shoe.

An adventitious bursa may form between the skin and the posterior aspect of the calcaneus in women who wear shoes too incurved at their upper edge posteriorly. The back of the shoe must be altered and a rubber pad can be introduced at the lower half of the back of the calcaneus, keeping the upper half away from the shoe. Excision is seldom necessary.

LESIONS OF THE FIBULO-CALCANEAN LIGAMENT

Sprain

This is one of the possible lesions in a sprained ankle. The varus movement at the talo-calcanean joint is of full range and painful; the valgus movement full and painless. Tenderness is sought along the ligament, and hydrocortisone is injected, then friction given to this point in the standard way.

Rupture

This is signalled when an excessive range of varus movement is found on testing the talo-calcanean joint. Strapping (Fig. 119) is applied holding the joint in valgus and kept on for a month. By then, union will have occurred. Associated lesions are dealt with in the ordinary way, but varus movements must be avoided.

If a recent rupture passes unnoticed, permanent lengthening of the ligament results for which the patient must wear a floated heel (Fig. 120) indefinitely. Alternatively, a new ligament can be formed by fixing the tendon of the peroneus brevis through holes bored in the neck of the talus and the lower end of the fibula.

LESIONS OF THE TALO-CALCANEAN JOINT

The joint allows movement in only two directions—varus and valgus. The capsular pattern consists of increasing limitation of varus range and ultimate fixation in valgus.

Talipes Equino-varus

A varus position of the calcaneus on the talus forms part of the club-foot deformity. Correction and the maintenance of correction by Denis-Browne splintage should be instituted as soon after birth as possible.

Immobilizational Stiffness

Marked limitation of movement results from the immobilization imposed on the tarsal joints by the treatment in plaster of some tibio-fibular fractures. The joint is stiff, but there is no muscle spasm when the joint is forced.

Mobilization of the joint is technically difficult; for there is no lever. Whether performed manually or under anaesthesia by means of a Thomas's wrench, the small size of the calcaneus affords very little purchase. Many months' repeated forcing by the physiotherapist eventually brings its reward. Restoration of a full range is not essential; a slightly limited range is compatible with good function.

Osteoarthritis

This follows fractures of the calcaneus involving the surface articulating with the talus. Intractable pain results, curable only by arthrodesis.

Loose Body in the Joint

This is suggested by a history of twinges. The discomfort is produced by movement at the talo-calcanean joint, and not at the ankle joint. Alternatively, the patient may complain of bouts of painful fixation at his heel and, if he attends during an attack the heel will be found fixed in valgus by muscle spasm.

Manipulative reduction must be attempted, but seldom proves permanent.

Subacute Traumatic Arthritis

Recovery after a sprained ankle is unduly delayed by pain in the heel and mid-foot. Examination shows limitation of varus movement at the talo-calcanean joint maintained by muscle spasm. The mid-tarsal joint is also usually affected. Local warmth is often detectable if the patient has recently walked a distance.

This condition is often mistaken for post-traumatic adhesions; for there is chronic pain after an injury and the radiograph shows that the bones are not damaged. If the limitation of movement at the talo-calcanean joint is missed, such patients may well be treated by mobilization under anaesthesia for supposed adhesions, which leads to aggravation for 1–2 months. Patients in whom a subacute traumatic arthritis has been exacerbated by manipulation are often regarded as hysterics, but in psychological disorders the heel is fixed in varus, not valgus.

Treatment consists of one or two injections of hydrocortisone into the joint. Since the heel is held in valgus, the simpler approach is at the inner side. The lower edge of the medial malleolus is identified, and 2 cm. below lies the prominence of the sustentaculum tali. The needle is inserted at this level and passes to about 1 cm. before striking bone. The point of the needle is then manœuvred up and down slightly until the spot is found where resistance ceases and the needle passes another 1 cm. and lies intra-articularly. Two c.c. of the suspension are injected here. This treatment seldom fails, but if it does, several months immobilization in plaster is indicated.

Monarticular Rheumatoid Arthritis

There is no history of injury and the disorder is often bilateral. In addition to the limitation of movement towards varus by muscle spasm, local heat and synovial thickening are palpable. The mid-tarsal joint is usually also affected. It is a rheumatoid manifestation, often accompanied by the typical changes in other joints. In young men, Reiter's disease and ankylosing spondylitis are possible alternative causes; in elderly men, gout should not be forgotten. In rheumatoid arthritis, hydrocortisone injected into the joint destroys the pain within a day and, even if the range does not increase, the patient can by this means be kept comfortable for many months, even years.

Dancer's Heel

During their training, ballet dancers develop hypermobility towards plantiflexion at the ankle joint as the result of work *sur les pointes*. Consequently, bruising of the periosteum at the back of the lower tibia may be caused from repeated pressure by the upper edge of the posterior surface of the calcaneus. Athletes may bruise the periosteum in the same way; less often, one plantiflexion strain may have this result.

The pain is felt at the back of the heel and is reproduced by full passive plantiflexion at the ankle, which presses the calcaneus against the area of traumatic periostitis.

Two or three injections of hydrocortisone stop the tenderness, but the dancer must have the mechanism of the disorder explained, so that she takes care not to repeat the causative trauma by repeatedly over-pointing the foot again.

Calcanean Apophysitis (Osgood)

Between the ages of six and twelve years, apophysitis may occur, often bilaterally. The bone is slightly tender and the radiographic appearances characteristic. I have seen a child in whom a piece of radio-translucent glass lying against the periosteum gave rise to what at first appeared to be an apophysitis. Spontaneous recovery occurs in a year or two, often with the development of a slight permanent prominence at the posterior aspect of the calcaneus.

THE MID-TARSAL JOINT

The talo-navicular and calcaneo—cuboid joints comprise the mid-tarsal joint. Movement is possible in six directions: dorsiflexion and planti-flexion, adduction and abduction, lateral and medial rotation. On account of the obliquity of the joint-surfaces, dorsiflexion at the mid-tarsal joint is accompanied by abduction of the forefoot with consequent stretching—often painful—of the calcaneo-navicular ligament. Hence excessive dorsiflexion strains on the mid-tarsal joint should be avoided.

When movement at the mid-tarsal joint is tested, the heel must be pulled down and held still. This precaution prevents movement at the ankle and talo-calcanean joints from complicating the clinical picture.

Five different conditions affect the mid-tarsal joint.

Mid-tarsal Strain

If power in the musculature of the sole becomes insufficient to maintain a sufficient degree of plantaris of the forefoot during weight-bearing, the mid-tarsal ligaments become painfully strained. This is particularly likely to occur in patients who already have an over-arched foot or an equinus deformity at the ankle. In such cases, weight-bearing dorsiflexes, and therefore abducts, the forefoot at the mid-tarsal joint; this stretches the capsular ligaments, the calcaneo-navicular ligament and the plantar fascia. At first the plantiflexion-dorsiflexion range of movement increases and the foot becomes wobbly; later on discomfort (mid-tarsal strain) appears, pain occurring at the extreme of passive range, especially rotation.

Treatment

This consists of three measures: (1) raising the heel of the shoe, so as to allow the forefoot to adopt a more plantigrade position during weight-bearing; (2) exercises (faradic and resisted) to the short flexor muscles in the sole so that they become adequate to take the strain and thus relieve tension on the ligament; (3) mobilization of the mid-tarsal joint, to ensure that the full range of movement can be achieved painlessly. Although the range of movement at the joint is excessive, repeated strains, followed by healing of minor ligamentous ruptures, have led to the formation of adhesions and consequent discomfort at the extreme of range. This is the only example in the body of manipulation being required at a joint which already possesses an excessive range of movement. Faradism to the short flexor muscles and exercises follow.

Mid-tarsal Osteoarthritis

Unless gross and the result of fracture or of an old navicular apophysitis (Kohler), osteoarthritis causes no symptoms. It results in osteophytes

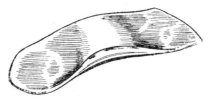

FIG. 123. Steel support. This is accurately moulded to the sole of the foot and prevents as far as possible all movement at the tarsal joints.

visible and palpable at the dorsum of the foot and equally visible on the radiograph. Osteoarthritis at the mid-tarsal joint is largely a misnomer, based on mistaken deduction from radiological appearances. If the ligaments are strained—whether osteoarthritis shows on the radiograph or not—the treatment for mid-tarsal strain applies. If gross disturbance of the anatomy of the foot has really led to marked osteoarthritis causing symptoms, a steel support moulded accurately to the sole of the foot (Fig.123) minimizes movement as far as possible at the disorganized joints. Arthrodesis is a last resort.

Mid-tarsal Ligamentous Contracture

After immobilization in plaster for fractures of the lower leg, middle-aged patients may complain months or some years later that, although they can walk short distances in comfort, they cannot run or ski without immediate pain. Limitation of movement at the mid-tarsal joint has become permanent owing to ligamentous contracture. This has proved resistant even to mobilization under anaesthesia, which has already been carried out, usually several times, without benefit.

Examination discloses considerable limitation of movement at the mid-tarsal joint, without muscle spasm. This indicates structural contracture. The shortened ligaments on the dorsum of the foot are tender.

Treatment

After all the tender ligaments have been adequately infiltrated with hydrocortisone suspension, pain ceases, usually permanently, although there is no increase in the range of movement. The foot does not become quite normal, but running and ski-ing once more become possible with, at most, slight discomfort.

Subacute Arthritis in Adolescence
(Spasmodic Pes Planus)

This disorder has for years been known as 'spasmodic pes planus' because the sign that first drew attention to the condition was spasm of the peroneal muscles. The name originated with a past generation of orthopaedic surgeons, but muscle spasm is never primary. In this instance, the spasm results from arthritis, and is not intermittent, but continuous. The name is misleading and should be abandoned.

This overuse arthritis occurs almost exclusively in boys between the ages of twelve and sixteen. The talo-calcanean and mid-tarsal joints of both feet are affected together. Little or no pain results; the patient's mother is the person who usually complains. The boy stumps in with a clumsy gait and is found either to have a long thin foot or to be overweight and have some degree of pes cavus—in other words, a foot so shaped as to be easily overstrained.

The condition is not common except in districts where a large number of factories exist and boys fresh from school are put to work (e.g. at a lathe) that entails standing all day. Such overuse is the aetiological factor. On examination, valgus deformity of the heel and abduction deformity of the forefoot are seen to be maintained by spasm of the peroneal and extensor longus digitorum muscles. When the patient stands, the tendons are seen as a prominent tight band behind and below the lateral malleolus. Passive inversion at the heel and tarsus is prevented by muscle spasm. A mere valgus position of the heel and abduction of the forefoot during weight-bearing do not suggest this uncommon condition; the diagnosis is justified only when muscle spasm restricts movement at, or long-standing spasm has led to contracture fixing, these two joints. The radiograph reveals no abnormality.

Untreated, the slight symptoms cease at the end of two years and the foot becomes permanently but painlessly fixed in the deformed position. An ungainly gait results; that is all. No troubles ensue in later life.

Conservative Treatment

Early Case

Movement at the joint has not been entirely lost and the patient experiences discomfort on standing for some time but walking is painless and in the absence of weight-bearing there is no aching. The essence of treatment is relief from weight-bearing and support for the joint.

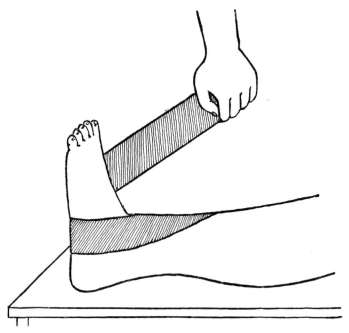

Fig. 124A. The foot is held at right-angles to the leg. The strapping is applied first to the inner side of the leg, and is brought round the outer side of the mid-tarsus.

The lad therefore requires (a) a sedentary job, (b) a bicycle, (c) a wedge on the heels of his shoes and (d) strapping of the joint. He is told never to stand for one instant if he can help it. If he sits at home, sits at work and travels everywhere on a bicycle, weight-bearing is practically completely avoided. Nevertheless he remains able to get about satisfactorily.

The heels of his shoes are fitted with inner wedges; these tend towards a varus position of the calcaneus. Non-elastic strapping is applied freshly each week to support the affected joint. The strapping should be put on while the foot is held at a right-angle and as far over towards varus as possible. First the strapping is fixed to the inner aspect of the lower leg, then carried round the mid-tarsus, then fixed to the outer aspect of the

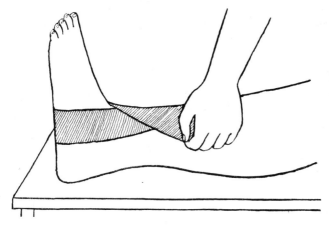

B. Strong tension is exerted as the strapping is applied to the inner side of the mid-tarsus and fixed to the outer side of the leg. This inverts the forefoot as much as possible.

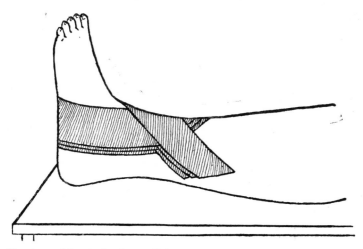

C. Three layers of strapping have been applied.

FIG. 124. Strapping for mid-tarsal joint.

lower leg during strong traction (Fig. 124). The patient is kept under observation and in the course of six to twelve months usually regains a full range of movement and loses his deformity. Recurrence is improbable.

Late Case

There is no movement at the talo-calcanean joint which is fixed by peroneal spasm in the position of valgus; little or no movement is possible at the mid-tarsal joint.

The leg and foot should be encased from below the knee to the toes in a plaster cast while the foot is held in the varus position. In most cases, this position can be attained by blocking the peroneal nerve at the point where it winds round the neck of the fibula. The nerve-trunk is identified by palpation and local anaesthesia induced. Paralysis of the peroneal and extensor longus digitorum muscles results and the bar to varus movement is thus abolished. The plaster cast is kept on for six weeks, when it is removed and the measures indicated for the early case instituted.

Fixation

If paralysis of the evertor muscles does not permit movement towards varus, structural contracture of the ligaments about the talo-calcanean and mid-tarsal joints has occurred. The decision must now be taken whether to allow the deformity to continue in the knowledge that it will remain as a fixed deformity, painless but unsightly, or to perform arthrodesis. This leads to fixation in a good position, but is scarcely worth while.

Subacute Arthritis in Middle-age

The patients are usually stout women. The muscular spasm and limitation of movement are less pronounced than in adolescence. Overuse is a much commoner cause than an isolated sprain. Examination reveals that muscular spasm partly restricts an inversion movement at the talo-calcanean and mid-tarsal joints, usually unilaterally. The radiological appearances are normal. If only one joint is affected, it can be successfully infiltrated with hydrocortisone. If the lesion is too diffuse, treatment by rest, tilting the heel and strapping in the varus position nearly always leads to eventual subsidence of the arthritis. Cases that have persisted for two or three years are not uncommon; without treatment the condition appears to continue indefinitely without much alteration. Six months of this modified rest are usually required; for some years afterwards the patient should guard against renewed overuse. Mobilization under anaesthesia is contra-indicated.

Monarticular Rheumatoid Arthritis

Arthritis, usually bilateral, sets in for no apparent reason at the talo-calcanean and mid-tarsal joints. If the arthritis is at all severe, the patient can scarcely hobble a few steps and attends in a wheel-chair. Sleep is disturbed.

In severe cases, the foot is markedly oedematous, warm to the touch and movement at these two joints is very much restricted. If the oedema allows, synovial swelling is palpable at the dorsum of the foot. The usual cause is a rheumatoid type of disorder, but in young men gonorrhoea, Reiter's disease and ankylosing spondylitis should be considered, and in elderly men, gout.

Immobilization in a plaster cast is required at once in rheumatoid arthritis. This is followed within a few days by complete relief from pain, the patient being able to walk short distances without discomfort. He can return to sedentary work. The plaster cast has to be kept on for at least a year. In practice the patient requests its removal or it becomes loose after some months; in either case the pain returns and another cast has to be applied. Recovery usually takes one or two years. If not, rather than allow the patient to continue indefinitely in pain, arthrodesis is recommended.

Hydrocortisone, so useful when a joint can be accurately infiltrated, is scarcely practicable over such a large extent, especially as the inferior ligaments are difficult to locate precisely.

THE CUNEO-FIRST-METATARSAL JOINT

Osteoarthritis

Goodfellow's (1965) research on hallux rigidus showed that this resultsd from a previous osteochondritis. It is thus highly probable that the cause of bilateral osteoarthritis at the cuneo-first-metatarsal joint also appearing in adolescence is also osteochondritis.

The onset is usually insidious. The patient, usually a girl, finds that if she wears shoes that lace tightly across the dorsum of her foot, localized pain arises at the site of a small bilateral projection. Palpation reveals this to be an osteophyte at the cuneo-first-metatarsal joint; radiography confirms this. By the age of sixteen, the osteophytes may have become quite large, and in a man wearing laced shoes is a sufficient embarrassment for removal to be requested.

Rarely, the onset is sudden, both joints becoming tender and swollen for about a week. After this severe phase has subsided, the girl finds she has a small prominence, previously absent, on each foot.

The condition is harmless. Recurrent pain is due to pressure of a lace-up shoe squeezing the skin against the osteophytes. In men, or for cosmetic reasons in girls, the bony prominences can be chiselled away.

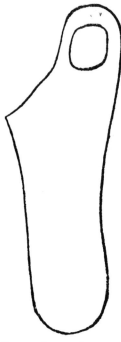

FIG. 125. Support for sesamoid-itis. The hole in the support corresponds to the first metatarso-phalangeal joint.

Treatment

If the arthritis is acute, a few days' rest is advised, with weight-bearing only in a high-heeled court shoe, no part of which touches the joint. Spontaneous recovery from the pain is a certainty. Avoiding pressure on the now prominent joint and wearing a heel high enough to make the plantiflexion deformity innocuous keep the patient's foot comfortable. A felt ring about the bony outcrop enables the girl to wear lace-up shoes.

It is important that the patient should not be told without adequate explanation that she has 'arthritis' in her feet. This is alarming to patient and parents, who, when the onset is so early in life, naturally envisage eventual crippledom.

Osteoarthritis of the cuneo-first-metatarsal joint may lead to fixation of the joint with considerable plantaris deformity. This may in turn result in metatarsalgia affecting the first metatarso-phalangeal or the sesamoid-metatarsal joint. If so, a support (Fig. 125) must be prescribed to take weight off the head of the bone.

Gout

This rarely attacks this joint before the big-toe. Warmth, reddening of the skin and pain at night suggest the diagnosis.

Loose Body

Athletes may complain of sudden twinges at this joint during a sprint. These are recurrent and disabling in race after race.

Examination shows that the twinges appear not to arise from the ankle or the talo-calcanean joint, and that no actual subluxation of the metatarsal bone itself on the cuneiform occurs when the patient rises on tip-toe.

Sustained traction on the joint of 9 kg. (20 lb.) for 30 minutes two or three times a week (see Vol. II) is curative; presumably internal derangement is the cause.

THE METATARSAL SHAFTS

Short First Metatarsal Bone

Much is made of atavistic shortening of the first metatarsal bone. Such shortening is compatible with full painless function of the foot, and the cause of pain should be sought elsewhere.

Marching Fracture

The feature that should bring this condition to mind at once is unilateral localized warmth and oedema lying in a circular patch over the metatarsus. The condition has been ascribed to 'fatigue' of the bone, and may occur rarely at other parts of the skeleton. As a rule, there is no history of injury or of an audible crack, not even always of excessive walking.

Children are almost as liable to marching fractures as adults; my youngest patient was aged six.

Examination during the first month after the pain began reveals: (a) local warmth; (b) oedema over the dorsum of the forefoot; (c) tenderness of the metatarsal shaft and of the interosseous muscles on each side of it. Clearly the two halves of the bone cannot move on each other without straining these muscles (cf. fractured rib). The tenderness is therefore more diffuse than is expected from the fracture as such, and it is not always easy to decide which of the metatarsal bones has broken. The fracture is most often at the neck of the second or fourth metatarsal bone but may lie anywhere. Stress fractures appear not to occur at the first and fifth metatarsal bones.

After two or three weeks, the tumour caused by callus becomes clearly palpable, especially when the distal part of the shaft has broken. Diagnosis is then easy, and may be confirmed by radiography. Since appreciable displacement does not occur, and no callus is visible during the first two or three weeks, and the tiny crack may not show on the radiograph of a recent case, it is well to wait until the third week before having X-rays taken.

Abortive cases occur, in which the periosteal reaction round the neck of the bone is indicated by a faint fusiform shadow, visible only on one side of the bone. Such an appearance suggests a partial crack not extending through the whole shaft, but the condition is nevertheless painful.

Differential Diagnosis

Circular elevation on the dorsum of the foot caused by a tendency to oedema and a shoe with a narrow strap across the dorsum may be seen, but this is bilateral, painless, not warm and absent on waking.

Localized warmth, swelling and tenderness at the dorsum of the distal part of the foot occur in: (a) Gout. The recurrent history in an elderly man is suggestive; the skin over the joint is at least slightly red. (b) Gonorrhoea, when the rheumatoid type of response has occurred. (c) Rheumatoid arthritis. This is usually multiple, and the disorder has persisted for too long. A marching fracture recovers spontaneously in six weeks. (d) Freiburg's arthritis of the second metatarso-phalangeal joint. (e) Reiter's disease usually affects several metatarso-phalangeal joints simultaneously, and also a large joint. (f) Ringworm. If a small crack exists between two toes owing to infection with the fungus, local cellulitis may occur with swelling, warmth and reddening at the dorsum of the foot. Inspection of the interdigital clefts makes the diagnosis clear. (g) Morton's metatarsalgia. If a patient with this disorder is seen within a few hours of an attack, the vascular reaction that follows gives rise to local warmth but no oedema. (h) Tuberculosis. This is a rarity at the cuneo-metatarsal joint. Swelling and warmth were present in the one case that I have encountered, but there was no oedema of the forefoot.

Treatment

The bone is firmly enough united to be painless in six weeks, whether the fracture was partial or complete. Mal-union need not be feared. There is no necessity for the patient to stop walking during the period of union; his forefoot should merely be firmly bound to diminish movement at the fracture and to enable the other metatarsal shafts to splint the broken bone. Even so, weight-bearing is bound to hurt a little; it is for the patient to do as much as he will in these circumstances.

Persistent pain after the six weeks have elapsed originates not at the fracture but at the interosseous muscles, strained by the abnormal stresses. They should be treated by deep massage (see Vol. II). Full recovery seldom takes longer than a fortnight.

SPLAY-FOOT

When this causes symptoms, these are due to painful over-stretching of the transverse interosseus ligaments, whereby the metatarsal bones are given excessive horizontal play. Other conditions, particularly weakness of the short flexor muscles of the toes, are also usually present. Such weakness should be treated energetically and the foot bound.

Localized splaying indicates a ganglion lying between two metatarsal heads. When the patient stands, an excessive interval is seen between two toes and palpation reveals that a semi-solid tumour keeps them apart. Since the tumour is thick and loculated, often composed partly of fibro-lipomatous material, attempted aspiration seldom diminishes its size or the patient's symptoms. Excision is indicated.

THE TOE JOINTS

The First Metatarso-phalangeal Joint

This joint is normally capable of 30 degrees of flexion and 90 degrees of extension; it is the latter movement which is important. As he walks, an individual has to extend the big toe of his hinder foot to at least 45 degrees when his other foot goes forwards, more if high heels are worn. Hence in men osteoarthritis remains painless until half the range of extension has been lost, whereas women suffer much earlier.

Arthritis in Adolescence

The cause of osteoarthritis at the first-metatarso-phalangeal joint long remained obscure. Since the disorder was unprovoked, bilateral and appeared in adolescence, this suggested a constitutional factor. However, in 1965 Goodfellow presented his research into the aetiology of hallux rigidus. He showed that the cause was the same osteochondritis dessicans as occurs at other joints during adolescence, and included in his paper radiographs and microscopical section of excised tissue.

In a youngster aged fifteen to twenty, large osteophytes gradually form at the dorsum of both first metatarso-phalangeal joints. Patients are nearly always male. The onset is slow and unprovoked by overuse or injury. At first, compensation is achieved in such young patients by the development of hyperextensibility at the interphalangeal joint. Within a few years the joint fixes in the neutral position and a hallux rigidus has developed; now pain at every step is inevitable due to bone being forced against bone at the dorsum of the joint. Examination shows a fixed big toe, little or no range of extension remaining, and gross dorsal osteophytes.

Conservative treatment consists in the prescription of a rocker (Fig. 126) whereby the patient can adopt a normal gait, pivoting over the rocker instead of forcing his osteoarthritic joint towards extension. If this does not suffice, operative removal of the base of the proximal phalanx is indicated. Alternatively, a steel sole prevents movement at the metatarso-phalangeal joint, but the gait is less natural.

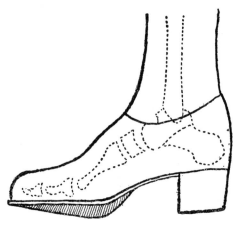

FIG. 126. Rocker. For the relief of hallux rigidus. Instead of extending at the first metatarso-phalangeal joint, the forefoot rocks over the thickened sole.

Arthritis in Middle Age

Osteoarthritis at the first metatarso-phalangeal joint also occurs between the ages of forty and sixty; this cannot be the result of osteochondritis. Sometimes a heavy weight falling on the joint stimulates the degeneration. In men, symptoms begin when only 45 degrees of extension range remain, but a woman, with her higher heels, gets pain when 30 degrees range has been lost. Since aggravation is slow, no symptoms may arise for years.

Treatment

The arthritis itself causes no symptoms unless the joint is overstrained by being forced into extension with each step the patient takes. In minor cases, or if the cause was one long walk, the disorder is really a traumatic arthritis. The result of such overuse can be abolished by intra-articular hydrocortisone. The pain caused by the injection is considerable for twelve hours; the patient is then comfortable, but must be careful in the future.

Good results can also be achieved by traction. The foot is fixed and a Japanese finger-stall applied to the hallux. Twenty pounds traction for twenty minutes on, say, 6 to 8 occasions, is an average. Afterwards, recurrence must be avoided by a rocker fitted to the sole of the shoe (Fig. 126). Alternatively, a strong spring can be incorporated in the sole of the shoe, lying at the medial side and extending from the waist to the anterior of the sole. This impedes extension at the affected joint.

Gout

This occurs typically at the big toe in elderly men. The attacks are unprovoked, recurrent, alternate from one foot to the other and for at least some years leave the joint normal between attacks. The joint swells and becomes warm to the touch. Soon the skin becomes red, owing to the accumulation of plasma kinins in sufficient concentration to cause vasodilatation. Eisen (1966) showed that phagocytosis of the micro-crystals of urates in the inflammatory effusion caused release of proteolytic enzymes activating kininogen. This change in colour should not be awaited because, sepsis apart, no other condition causes spontaneous swelling and warmth of the joint. The radiograph is no help in the early case, showing nothing or perhaps, on account of the patient's age, a little osteoarthritis—misleadingly. The punched-out areas appear only after some years.

The best drug is indomethacin (6 tablets of 25 mg. the first day, 3 the next) which aborts the attack in about 24 hours. Butazolidine comes a close second, 200 mg. four times the first day and then gradually diminishing also stops the pain in a day or two. Colchicum has been superseded. In the absence of drug treatment, an attack of gout in the big toe may well take a month or two to subside. Between attacks, the excretion of urates has to be enhanced by aspirin, probenecid (Benemid) tablets or sulphin-pyrazone (Anturan) tablets (100 mg.) 3 times a day.

Pseudo-gout also attacks the big toe. McCarty and Hollander (1961) examined the crystals in synovial fluid from gouty patients and found that, in a small proportion, the crystals were not urates but calcium pyro-phosphate. However, the response to butazolidine is satisfactory in these cases too. Curry and Swettenham (1965) report that more than one type of crystal can often be isolated from the aspirated joint fluid in cases of calcified joint cartilage, and the position is not yet clear.

Metatarsalgia at the First Joint

This is uncommon. The cause is an excessively small angle between forefoot and hindfoot, usually as the result of a pes cavus deformity or secondary to osteoarthritis at the cuneo-first-metatarsal joint. Intra-articular hydrocortisone quickly abates the traumatic arthritis.

Sesamo-metatarsal Arthritis

Bruising of the sesamoid bone of flexor longus hallucis tendon may also result; with pain elicited by resisted flexion of the big toe. The position of the tender spot alters with flexion and extension of the hallux. A patient with a cavus foot, particularly if the calf-muscles are also short, may come down too hard on his forefoot at each step, setting up a traumatic arthritis at the sesamo-first-metatarsal joint. An injection of hydrocortisone abolishes the reaction to overuse. Then, raising the heel of the patient's shoe while keeping its upper surface horizontal and fitting a support (Fig. 125) serve to relieve pressure.

The Outer Four Metatarso-phalangeal Joints

Pain at the plantar aspect of the forefoot is called metatarsalgia.

Chronic Metatarsalgia

This affects the middle three toes and arises in the following conditions, in which an excessive proportion of the body-weight falls on the forefoot. Normally the forefoot should bear only one-third of the total, and that third should be distributed between the pads of the toes and the metatarso-phalangeal joints. When the digital flexor muscles contract adequately, the metatarsal heads are relieved of much pressure, which falls on the flexed toes instead.

In the six conditions listed below there is pain felt at the plantar aspect of the forefoot on standing and walking, relieved by rest. Although the tenderness is always spoken of as 'of the metatarsal heads', it is not the articular cartilage which is tender, but the plantar aspect of the capsule of these metatarso-phalangeal joints. Since this capsulitis is essentially traumatic and due to excessive pressure, no irreversible changes have taken place and relief from bearing too much weight on the forefoot leads to full recovery.

1. *Pes Plantaris*

In patients with a pes plantaris deformity—especially if there is also a slight equinus—too much pressure is borne by the forefoot (Fig. 127), with the result that the plantar aspect of the capsules of the metatarso-phalangeal joints, especially the second, third and fourth, develops traumatic tenderness.

2. *Pes Cavus*

Hyperextension at the metatarso-phalangeal joints, which often accompanies a pes cavus deformity, is caused by shortening of the extensor longus hallucis and digitorum muscles. In such a case the toes bear none of the body-weight, and metatarsalgia with a large callosity under the heads of the middle three metatarsal heads is almost inevitable (Fig. 118).

3. *Weak Flexor Muscles*

This is the commonest single cause of pain in the foot. If the short muscles in the sole weaken as the result of rest in bed during an illness, or

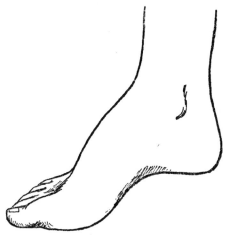

FIG. 127. Pes plantaris. Note the dropped forefoot without any other deformity.

are suddenly given too much exertion, they prove inadequate. Since they cease to flex the toes properly at each step, excessive weight is repeatedly thrown on to the metatarso-phalangeal joints instead; pain results.

4. *Results of Wearing High Heels*

In all ready-made shoes, high heels possess an oblique upper surface. The patient stands on an inclined plane, sliding down on to her forefoot all the time. High heels, the upper surface of which is horizontal, or nearly so, are free from this defect and should be worn with comfort by all women with a plantaris forefoot.

Treatment

This consists of the avoidance of excessive weight-bearing at the forefoot. Active and passive measures can be taken. The former consist of so strengthening the short flexor muscles of the sole by faradism and exercises that the toes flex properly at every step and do not tire after standing or walking. Prophylactic foot-exercises, after a long stay in bed or debilitating illness are an obvious precaution. A support (Fig. 128) is provided which stops short just behind the heads of the metatarsal bones and ensures that the shafts of these bones bear more weight than the joints themselves. A heel with a horizontal upper surface hinders the foot from sliding forwards and enables weight to be borne on the hindfoot as well as the forefoot (Fig. 130).

BB

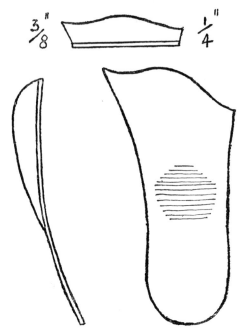

FIG. 128. Support for metatarsalgia. The thickness lies just behind the heads of the metatarsal bones, the shafts of which are thus made to bear the greater weight.

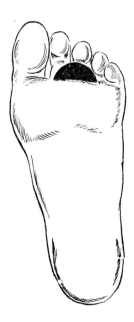

FIG. 129. Dancer's meta-tarsalgia. Semilunar anterior support making the proximal phalanges of the three middle toes bear more weight.

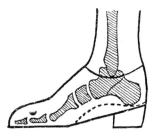 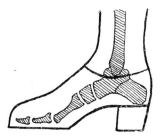

(a) Note how the central part of the sole of the foot is out of contact with the shoe, and how the pressure of the heel on an inclined plane pushes the body-weight on to the forefoot. (b) Note how the shoe fits the sole of the foot and how weight-bearing on the heel is devoid of forward stress.

FIG. 130. Shoes with (*a*) oblique heels and (*b*) horizontal heels

5. Local Injury

Traumatic arthritis at a metatarso-phalangeal joint is rare. It can result both from violence applied to the toe straining the joint indirectly and from a direct blow. Limited movement results which continues for many months but responds very well to one intra-articular injection of hydro-cortisone. The joint is very sore for twelve hours, then complete lasting relief is to be expected.

6. Dancer's Metatarsalgia

A dancer who does much tip-toe work (not *sur les pointes*) may bruise the pad of fibrous tissue in the sole lying anterior to the second, third and fourth metatarso-phalangeal joints. When this happens, he must be made to bear more weight at the plantar surface of the toes. To this end his ballet shoes are fitted with a small semilunar pad (Fig. 120) which ensures that the joints are spared as much weight as possible.

Chronic Metatarsalgia due to Structural Change

Freiburg's Osteochondritis

This disorder is confined to the head of the second metatarsal bone, and was first described by Freiburg in 1914. My youngest patient was fourteen years old and had had a fortnight's pain. Examination showed localized arthritis of the second metatarso-phalangeal joint. At first, local swelling and warmth are present, together with limitation of flexion and extension at this joint. At this stage, Freiburg's disease is difficult to distinguish from a marching fracture. Radiography gives no immediate help, since it takes a month from the onset of pain for the characteristic radiographic change to begin to show at the head of the bone, and it often takes three weeks for a marching fracture to become visible.

Spontaneous recovery from the subacute arthritis takes a year. By that time, the joint recovers an adequate, but not full, range of movement, and the head of the bone is permanently enlarged. Palpation reveals the increase in size and a prominent ridge on the bone at the dorsal aspect of its articular edge. Sooner or later, metatarsalgia due to the bony enlargement ensues. In due course, osteoarthritis supervenes and, by the time the patient is forty or fifty, the joint may become fixed in a manner analogous to hallux rigidus and excision of the metatarsal head become necessary. In the early case, Smillie's (1967) operation restores the blood supply and prevents subsequent deformity.

Rheumatoid Arthritis and Gout

In advanced cases, the toes become fixed in the clawed position. Metatarsalgia inevitably results, and is largely relieved by a support.

Pressure on Nerves at the Forefoot

Pressure on nerves here causes acute twinges of pain, but no loss of conduction is discernible. Hence the diagnosis is made largely on the history.

Bruising of the Second Digital Nerve

This nerve passes forwards at the lateral side of the plantar aspect of the first metatarso-phalangeal joint, and can easily be palpated there as a thick strand. It bifurcates just distal to the joint, supplying sensation to the adjacent borders of the first and second toes. In view of its exposed position, it is surprising that it is so seldom injured. Stepping on a sharp stone, or a puncture wound at the place where the nerve crosses the joint may be followed by persistent bruising of the nerve. Consequently, the patient gets sharp painful twinges on walking followed by a few seconds' pins and needles.

Treatment

The patient should wear a thick rubber pad under the forefoot for three to six months; this may prevent the twinges. Hydrocortisone suspension should be injected about the affected extent of nerve at once. A long thin needle is introduced between the dorsum of the foot, the metatarso-phalangeal joints and thrust in until it is felt to impinge against the plantar skin. Its point can be felt, and steered towards the tender extent of nerve.

A neuroma requiring excision seems not to occur at the first interspace.

Acute Metatarsalgia (Morton)

This condition was described by Morton in 1876 and before that by Durlacher in 1845 (Kemp, 1949). The history is characteristic.

The patient complains that, as he walks, he is suddenly seized with agonizing pain at the outer border of his forefoot. He has to stop still and stand on his good foot; he takes his shoe off and rubs the painful area. After some minutes the pain ceases but the foot becomes warm and stays so for several hours. When the pain has gone, he is able to walk on comfortably. He may experience two attacks in a week then none for a year; recurrences are very variable and tend to become more frequent. Between attacks, there are no symptoms or physical signs.

The disorder comes on between the ages of fifteen and fifty, and is much commoner in women. The aetiology was first put on a firm basis by Betts (1940), who ascribed it to nipping between the bones of a fibrous swelling of the fourth digital nerve proximal to its point of division. Resection of the nerve was curative. This view has been amply confirmed. Although the fourth and fifth toes are those usually affected, an occasional case between the third and fourth toes is encountered.

Examination is wholly negative. An attempt to reproduce the attack by moving the heads of the metatarsal bones against each other during compression fails. Cutaneous analgesia at the affected toes is absent. Palpation of the sole fails to reveal the tumour on the digital nerve. The diagnostic points are therefore: (a) the history of severe momentary bouts of pain at the outer forefoot followed by long periods of freedom, and (b) the absence of any discernible disorder at the foot.

Treatment

Conservative treatment consists merely of altering the alignment of the metatarsal heads. If the nerve is nipped in the fourth interspace, the patient

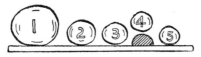

Fig. 131. Support for Morton's metatarsalgia. The small pad alters the alignment of the fourth metatarsal head on the fifth. Painful nipping of the digital nerve is then obviated.

is prescribed a support elevating the head of the fourth bone (Fig. 131). This keeps the bones slightly out of line and prevents pinching. Since it is arguable whether the swelling on the nerve is the cause or the result of a series of nippings, it may well be that such a support prevents the later formation of the enlargement that aggravates the condition. Occasionally, the patient finds this support uncomfortable and may prefer one supporting the third and fifth bones. The effect is the same in respect of the alteration in position of the fourth bone in relation to its neighbours—merely down instead of up.

Should conservative treatment fail, the sole of the foot should be explored and the nerve with its neuroma excised.

THE TENDONS OF THE FOOT

Disorders of the tendons are few and obvious.

A ganglion or a xanthoma may form at the dorsum of the foot in connection with a tendon.

The extensor hallucis and digitorum muscles become shortened in pes cavus, leading to clawing of the toes, i.e. fixation in extension at the meta-tarso-phalangeal joints and flexion at the interphalangeal joints. Tenotomy under local anaesthesia may be required. Teno-synovitis of the extensor hallucis or digitorum tendons at the front of the ankle is uncommon; it leads to pain elicited by resisted extension of the big or the four little toes. Massage cures in so few sessions that hydrocortisone is seldom required. In dancers, gross crepitus is often present at the flexor hallucis tendon at its course at the back of the ankle. It is due to overuse and, although the crepitus may even be audible, symptoms seldom ensue. If pain is provoked when the tendon moves, deep massage is rapidly curative. Rupture of the flexor longus hallucis at its insertion leads to a flail distal phalanx and is an appreciable disability; for the big toe keeps catching when the patient walks without shoes. Arthrodesis is indicated. Ischaemic contracture of the extensor hallucis longus after fracture is rare. In such a case, when the foot is plantiflexed, the big toe is forced into extension and is bruised against the upper of the shoe. Tenotomy under local anaesthesia is curative.

A plantaris deformity of the forefoot may induce excessive weight-bearing on the joint between the head of the first metatarsal bone and the sesamoid bone in the flexor hallucis longus tendon. Hydrocortisone and a support (Fig. 125) to relieve this joint of stress are required.

Weakness of the extensor hallucis muscle is a common result of fourth or fifth lumbar disc lesions.

THE HALLUX

Fractured Terminal Phalanx

Several days' severe pain results from the tense subungual haematoma that forms after fracture. Puncture of the nail with a red-hot needle allows the blood to exude and affords immediate relief; it also largely prevents subsequent sepsis.

A collodion splint should be applied and kept on for a month. In factories where workmen are apt to drop weights on their big toes, shoes with steel toe-caps should be worn to prevent this common industrial accident.

THE TOE-NAILS

Ingrowing Toe-nail

In this condition the two sides of the nail of the big toe press into the flesh and may cause severe pain. This can occur only if the nail is stiff and curved. When pain begins for this reason, the patient seeks relief by paring away the sides of the nail. This aggravates the condition, since the flesh is no longer held away from the sides of the nail by a full width distally.

In treatment, all that is required is to pare away the centre of the convex surface of the nail with a knife until it is quite thin and has lost its rigidity. The edges of the nail are then no longer held pressed against the sides of the bed. Thinning is maintained until a nail of full width has grown beyond the full extent of the bed. If now the patient cuts the nail straight across, he seldom has further trouble. If he does, he must keep the nail thinned and flexible indefinitely, or submit to operation. Amputation of the whole nail bed and the distal half of the terminal phalanx gives a very good result.

Dancer's Toe-nail

A similar condition causes dancers great trouble at the second and third toes. If a nail is stiff and curved, it forces itself into the flesh of the toe when she rises *sur les pointes*. Scraping the nail so as to keep it thin removes the disability at once.

Onychogryphosis

Brown discoloration and great thickening of the nail occurs in onychogryphosis. Removal only leads to the growth of another identical nail. The chiropodist, by using a burr, can keep the nail thin and the patient comfortable. The alternative is amputation of the distal half of the terminal phalanx.

Nipped Flesh

An uncommon cause of pain that may escape detection is such an excessive degree of flexion of the toes during weight-bearing that the pad of the toe at the free edge of the nail becomes nipped. A piece of felt placed under the bases of the toes prevents the toes from bending over too far.

ISCHAEMIA OF THE FOOT

In advanced ateriosclerosis, the circulatory defect may show itself at the sole rather than in the calf-muscles, particularly when the posterior tibial artery is affected. Alternatively, the nutrition of the toes may suffer. Claudication in the short flexor bellies is usually called cramp by the patient and comes on when the metabolic requirement is increased on walking or when the feet get warm in bed.

The foot, especially the toes, is a dusky red colour when the patient stands. The circulation returns slowly after an area of skin has been blanched by pressure. Elevation of the limb for a minute or less leads to rapid blanching of the foot; on dependency the redness returns equally soon. The foot feels cold both to the patient and the examiner. No pulsation is palpable at the posterior tibial or dorsalis pedis arteries, which the radiograph may show to be calcified. The patient, lying on the couch, is asked to flex his toes repeatedly as quickly as he can. This soon induces pain in intermittent claudication.

No treatment is of much avail. Sympathectomy warms the foot but seldom stops the muscles claudicating.

DEFORMITIES OF THE FOOT

Congenital Deformities

Equinus

The triple deformity of talipes equino-varus (equinus at the ankle, varus at the talo-calcanean, adduction at the mid-tarsal joint) is familiar. But when one of these deformities occurs alone it may initially be overlooked. A pure equinus deformity results from short calf-muscles. An equinus deformity that disappears on pressure, only to reappear when this is released, may be the first sign to be noted of a cerebral diplegia.

Metatarsus Varus

This is an uncomplicated adduction deformity of the forefoot, some-times accompanied by a hallux varus.

Metatarsus Inversus

This is an uncomplicated inversion deformity of the forefoot at the mid-tarsal joint, and in children is a common cause of valgus deformities at the knee and the heel (Plate 61). In this condition, on walking, the outer side of the forefoot reaches the ground first. Then, as the patient's weight

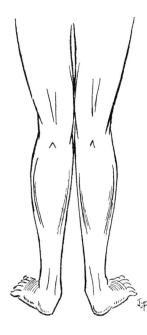

FIG. 132. Genu valgum deformity secondary to congenital in-version of the forefeet.

comes on to it, it rotates towards eversion until flat on the ground, thereby bringing the hindfoot with it and inducing a valgus deformity at the talo-calcanean joint—its worst posture. The hindfoot may also carry the leg with it and throw it slightly out of the vertical. Thus a genu valgum deformity develops in due course (Fig. 132).

Talipes Calcaneus

There is often a valgus deformity of the heel as well as limitation of plantiflexion range at the ankle. It has usually recovered spontaneously by the time the child has begun to stand; if not, manipulation and strapping holding the heel in varus, are indicated.

Pes Planus

The congenital variety is rare. There may be calcaneo-navicular fusion. A steel support (Fig. 123, p. 726) may help.

Hammer Toe

There is a fixed flexion deformity at the proximal interphalangeal joint with hyperextension at the distal joint. This would be symptomless but for the wearing of shoes, pressure against which causes a painful corn on the prominent joint.

Aquired Deformities

Pes Cavus

This deformity begins to be noticeable at the age of eight and progresses steadily until growth ceases at about the age of twenty; it then remains stationary. The foot is short, broad and thick (Fig. 118, p. 704), and the angle between the forefoot and hindfoot is abnormally small, sometimes even approaching a right-angle. The toes are clawed (i.e. held in full extension at the metatarso-phalangeal joints and in flexion at the inter-phalangeal joints) because of the increased tone, leading to structural shortening, that develops in the extensor longus hallucis and digitorum muscles as a result of an attempt to compensate for the weakness of the interosseus and lumbrical muscles. A large callosity nearly always forms under the heads of the middle three metatarsal bones because—the toes not being used in walking—they transmit excessive pressure to the under-lying skin.

Pes Plantaris

By this is meant an over-arched foot, i.e. one in which the angle between the hindfoot and the forefoot is diminished (as in cavus deformity) but the foot and toes are otherwise normal (Fig. 127, p. 739). In women, a minor degree of this condition is very common and not necessarily the result of wearing high-heeled shoes. Adolescent girls, who have worn low heels all their lives, may nevertheless develop a plantaris deformity which results in painful strain until compensated by raising the heel of the shoe.

In pes plantaris, the stress of weight-bearing first induces a greatly increased range at the mid-tarsal joint, particularly dorsiflexion-planti-flexion. Initially, there are no symptoms. Sooner or later the muscles of the sole of the foot prove unequal to the task of maintaining the plantaris position of the forefoot during weight-bearing. Excessive stress then falls upon (a) the ligaments at the mid-tarsal joint (mid-tarsal strain); (b) the plantar fascia; (c) the metatarsal heads (metatarsalgia). Thus, three separate lesions may develop according to where in the foot the major stress falls.

This is the type of foot that is often called 'flat'. It is not; it is over-arched, and flattens towards the normal shape only with pain.

Pes Planus

When excessive dorisflexion takes place at the mid-tarsal joint, two further deformities arise: valgus at the heel and abduction at the forefoot. The calcaneo-navicular ligament, the mid-tarsal ligaments, and the plantar fascia are all over-stretched; the first becomes painful, tender and prominent. Finally, shortening of the various joint-capsules may occur, thus fixing the foot in the deformed position. The deformity is now no longer reducible and cannot profitably be treated by conservative measures. Not all flat feet hurt; those that do not should be left alone.

Hallux Rigidus

This is the late result of an adolescent osteochondritis at the first metatarso-phalangeal joint.

Hallux Valgus

If the weight-bearing surface of the heel of a shoe is oblique, the foot tends to slide forwards during weight-bearing. Since most shoes taper at the toes, the first and fifth toes are squeezed towards the midline of the foot at each step. The big toe is forced farther and farther towards the valgus, and once this has begun, the pull of the flexor and extensor tendons increases the deformity. Shine (1965) found in St. Helena that hallux valgus was present in only 2 per cent of unshod islanders, but in 16 per cent of men and 48 per cent of women who had always worn shoes. The deformity is symptomless unless complicated by arthritis, bursitis or pressure of the skin over the prominent bone against the upper of the shoe.

Treatment of Deformities of the Foot

In the treatment of any deformity here, two alternatives exist: either to force the movement that cannot be performed until good passive and active over-correction is obtained, or to compensate for the deformity by alterations to the shoe. Exercises, supports and strapping are used to prevent relapse. Both methods may be employed together.

Plantaris Deformity

Compensation is secured by raising the heel of the patient's shoe, while keeping its upper surface horizontal (Fig. 130). The short muscles in the sole must be strengthened so that their tone may keep the forefoot in the plantaris position during weight-bearing and diminish movement at the mid-tarsal joint. Furthermore, their increased power takes pressure off the metatarso-phalangeal joint and tension off the plantar fascia.

Planus Deformity

The valgus element that occurs in this condition can be corrected by giving the heel of the patient's shoe a $\frac{3}{16}$ inch inner wedge, to push his heel over into a varus position as he takes weight. Since the abduction deformity is secondary to excessive dorsiflexion at the mid-tarsal joint, plantiflexion should be encouraged here by providing the patient's shoe with an anterior wedge (Fig. 130, p. 741) to the heel (as long as he has no equinus deformity) and by strengthening the short flexor muscles of the sole of the foot and the tibialis anterior and posterior muscles. If these measures do not suffice, a support, thick at the inner aspect of the mid-tarsus, becomes necessary (Fig. 121, p. 715).

Cavus Deformity

A *child* may be seen whose foot has the typical shape but no symptoms have yet arisen. The progressive nature of the deformity should be explained and the importance of maintaining full length of the extensor longus hallucis and digitorum muscles, and full strength in the small muscles of the sole, must be emphasized. To this end, the child himself, or an adult, should stretch the toes out daily, until full flexion is reached and maintained. Resisted exercises towards toe-flexion follow. The heel should be kept at a height adequate to compensate for the plantaris element in the deformity. If this is done, and the child kept under observation, say, yearly until the age of twenty, no symptoms need ever arise.

In adults with fixed deformity of the toes, division of the extensor longus tendons is an essential preliminary to reduction of the clawing. This is very simply done under local anaesthesia. There is practically no after-pain and the patient walks home immediately after the tenotomy. He must keep stretching his toes out towards flexion for the next few days to prevent the tendons uniting without lengthening. If only two tendons are cut at a time, a cradle (Fig. 134) is applied. Measures to strengthen the short flexor muscles of the sole by faradism and exercises are vigorously pursued daily, during which the flexion range at the metatarso-phalangeal joints is maintained. A support (as for metatarsalgia) is often also required.

In advanced cases, the fitting of a thick support to raise the heel and take weight off the metatarsal heads may prove the only practicable measure. Open operation is sometimes necessary.

Deformities of the Forefoot

Forcing the mid-tarsal joint towards eversion or abduction (for meta-tarsus inversus and varus deformities respectively) calls for great strength,

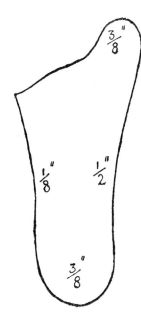

FIG. 133. Support for metatarsus inversus. The support is thick all along its inner side and is prolonged under the first metatarso-phalangeal joint, so as to enable weight-bearing to take place while the forefoot remains inverted.

even in the treatment of children. For the forcing of an eversion move-ment, the hands should be clasped about the patient's forefoot (see Vol. II) and a series of twists given of gradually increasing range. The ligamentous fibres limiting movement must be stretched out and broken; hence the mobilization should be continued at each session until at least one strand is heard to part. Treatment must continue for a year or two.

In adults, a suitable support (Fig. 133) is required.

Hammer Toe

Hammer toe can be straightened by merely breaking the plantar aspect of the capsular fibres by force; local anaesthesia suffices. The toe must be kept straight in a cradle for a week or two afterwards. A cradle consists of strapping passed under the toes on either side and over the one affected, so placed as to hold the proximal interphalangeal joint in extension (Fig. 134). If this procedure fails, arthrodesis is indicated.

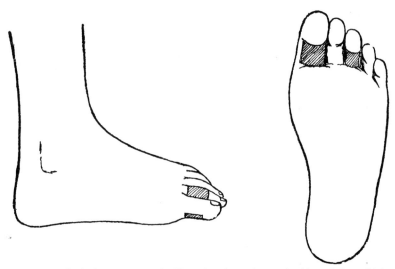

FIG. 134. Cradle for hammer toe. The illustration shows the proximal interphalangeal joint of the second toe held in extension by the strapping.

Hallux Valgus

Children should wear shoes with a straight inner border for prophylaxis. If alteration of the shoe to relieve pressure on the bunion does not suffice, the base of the proximal phalanx may be excised.

Hallux Rigidus

A rocker or a built-in steel in the sole relieves symptoms if some extension range remains. If not, the base of the first phalanx is excised.

SUPPORTS

The main purposes for which supports are prescribed are as follows:

1. *To Ensure Plantiflexion at the Mid-tarsal Joint*

If the height of a heel is raised without a change in the angle of its upper surface, plantiflexion occurs at the mid-tarsal joint. The same object is achieved when the heel is kept the same height but the angle of its upper surface altered to approach more nearly the horizontal. Good plantiflexion must be ensured here in order to maintain the reduction of a pes planus deformity. Again, the essence in the treatment of pes plantaris deformity and of plantar fasciitis is to allow increased plantiflexion during weight-bearing (Fig. 129).

2. To Diminish Pressure on the Metatarsal Heads

A thick platform stopping short of the metatarsal heads encourages weight-bearing by the whole extent of the metatarsal shafts and takes much of the weight off the metatarso-phalangeal joints (Fig. 128, p. 740). A metatarsal bar, which crosses the shoe just behind the heads, makes the necks of the metatarsal bones bear the great weight; it is much less satisfactory.

3. To Diminish a Pes Planus Deformity

The inner aspect of the mid-tarsus is kept raised by a support, thick under this area (Fig. 121, p. 715).

4. To Prevent Movement at the Mid-tarsal joint

When there is a mid-tarsal arthritis, pain is elicited towards the extreme of every movement. The application of a well-fitting steel to the sole of the foot prevents movement as far as is possible.

5. To Compensate for Metatarsus Inversus

This deformity may be discovered for the first time in middle age, perhaps because of a secondary posterior tibial teno-synovitis. The support must enable the heel to maintain the mid-position during weight-bearing; that is, it must allow the forefoot to remain inverted and yet in contact with the ground. It is therefore made like a wedge, thick at the inner and tapering to nothing at the outer border of that forefoot. It must project under the first metatarso-phalangeal joint almost as far forward as the interphalangeal joint. At the heel the support is level (Fig. 133).

6. For Sesamoiditis at the First Metatarso-phalangeal Joint

A support taking the weight off the joint by providing thickness at the metatarsal neck often suffices. It should take the form of a ring, thick in front of, as well as behind, the sesamoid bone (Fig. 125). The heel of the shoe should be raised, to encourage weight-bearing posteriorly.

7. For Calcanean Bursitis

The support is $\frac{3}{8}$ inch thick and made of non-porous rubber in the shape of a horseshoe.

8. *For Strain of the Plantar Fascia*

As an alternative to raising the heel of the shoe, a heel-pad may be fitted within the shoe. It should be of hard rubber and 1 cm. thick anteriorly, tapering to nothing at the back of the shoe, so that the upper surface of the heel now lies horizontal.

9. *For Morton's Metatarsalgia*

The alignment of the metatarsal heads is altered by raising the fourth on a small dome (Fig. 131). Occasionally, the patient prefers the third and fifth bones raised, leaving the fourth relatively depressed (Fig. 135).

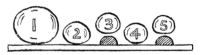

FIG. 135. Alternative support for Morton's metatarsalgia. Instead of raising the fourth metatarsal head (see Fig. 131) the third and fifth are supported and the fourth allowed to sink down.

ALTERATIONS AND ADDITIONS TO THE SHOE

The following are commonly required:

An Inner Wedge

When a reducible valgus deformity at the talo-calcanean joint is present, a varus position of the calcaneus during weight-bearing can be secured by an inner wedge to the heel of the shoe: $\frac{3}{16}$ inch thick for adults, $\frac{1}{8}$ inch for children (Fig. 136). An inner and an anterior wedge can often be advantageously combined.

An Anterior Wedge

This renders horizontal the oblique upper surface of a heel and the shoe thus properly adapted to a foot with a plantaris deformity (Fig. 122, p. 719) Shoes with a horizontal heel are the most comfortable for nearly all women; it is therefore the more surprising that women's shoes always have an oblique heel—which looks no more elegant, increases the apparent length and diameter of the foot, and hence are so shaped that the waist of the shoe is not in contact with the sole of the foot. All women with a tendency to plantaris shaping of the forefoot ought to wear horizontal heels; these have several important advantages: (a) the patient can take weight directly on the heel; (b) the waist of the shoe lies against the tarsus and some weight can be borne there; (c) plantiflexion at the mid-tarsal joint is assured; and (d) as there is no tendency for the foot to slide forward, metatarsalgia is prevented.

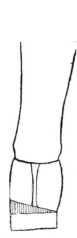

FIG. 136. Inner wedge to heel of shoe

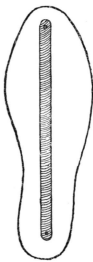

FIG. 137. Steel sole. For preventing all movement at the tarsal joints. Useful in congenital pes planus

Raising the Heel

When a horizontal heel is to be supplied, it must be the right height. For this purpose, blocks of wood of various thicknesses are placed under the patient's heel while standing with forefoot on the ground. The most comfortable height is measured and the thickness of the sole of the shoe added to this figure. Hence the same height will not apply for thin and walking shoes.

When compensation for an equinus deformity is required, the heel is raised and the obliquity of its upper surface increased.

A Floated Heel

If recurrent varus sprain of the ankle is to be prevented, broadening the base of the shoe on its outer side is effective (Fig. 120, p. 715).

A Rocker

A hallux rigidus deformity can be rendered symptomless and natural gait restored by a device that avoids extension of the hallux, i.e. a rocker. In theory, a ridge built into the sole of the shoe at the metatarso-phalangeal joint-line would best ensure this, but, as the joint itself is tender, the maximum thickness is better placed a short distance behind this point. Surgical shoe-makers usually put the projection too far back. This, or the fact that the rocker is too low, is the fault when full relief is not obtained. The patient must wear shoes with a rocker constantly and permanently (Fig. 126, p. 736). A metatarsal bar can be used as a rocker if it is put straight across the sole instead of obliquely, and *at*, rather than behind the metatarsal heads.

A Steel

In a congenital pes planus deformity nothing can be done, particularly if there is calcaneo-navicular fusion, except to make an entire steel sole so that as little movement as possible occurs at all the joints of the foot (Fig. 137). The same measure can be used for hallux rigidus, but a rocker or a spring in the sole of the shoe is much better.

27

Psychogenic Pain

Patients with pain devoid of organic basis naturally gravitate to the orthopaedic physician, since it is he who normally deals with patients whose symptoms give rise to few or no physical signs. If the patient is examined by the methods here described, it is difficult for imagined disorders to escape detection at the first attendance. Broadly, patients with genuine pain which is doubted are fewer than those who have partly or wholly carried off the deception.

The fact that patients with every type of obscure pain reach an orthopaedic physician for diagnosis and treatment provides him with many interesting problems. While it is no substitute for a diagnosis to regard every patient with a symptom the source of which is not immediately apparent as suffering from an imaginary disorder, much confusion results from believing too much. An open mind accepts and registers as they appear disorders not previously familiar. The difficult balance between excessive scepticism and credulity must be maintained.

Nothing is more disheartening to a physiotherapist than to treat, apparently endlessly, a patient whose malady has not been clearly defined, who never improves and never stops coming. By contrast, the short course of stimulating measures applicable to patients with psychogenic pain can be confidently—and therefore effectively—instituted when the patient's symptoms are known not to have an organic basis.

'Psychological Basis of Rheumatism'

Much has been written about a psychological basis for what has been misnamed 'rheumatic' pain. This is an inverted attitude towards the disorder present; for a pain devoid of physical cause should not be called rheumatic. There is another attitude in such cases—namely, to discard such labels as 'fibrositis' or 'rheumatism' for patients whose complaint has no organic foundation and to substitute a diagnosis of psychogenic pain.

Criterion of Cure

In many of the lesions discussed in this book, the patient's uncorroborated statement may provide the chief, at times the only, criterion of the results of treatment.

If a patient states that manipulation of his back has made him better or worse, it is almost useless for the doctor to offer a contrary opinion. Hence, it is important to avoid active methods of treatment unless patient and doctor are, so to speak, on the same side. If, no matter what is done, the patient (on account of his attitude of mind) will probably allege aggravation, it is essential to avoid any measure that he could credibly suggest made him worse. It may, therefore, be unwise to treat a patient who is psychoneurotic with a grievance or is enmeshed in a compensation claim, even when he clearly has a minor lesion which can be remedied easily.

When the patient's attitude appears to be more important than the minor organic lesion, the almoner's view on how the patient is likely to react to treatment, even if effective, is valuable. Sometimes it is best to warn a patient, his doctor and his solicitor, before any treatment begins, that measures to achieve relief may on the one hand upset the patient's psyche or, if they prove successful, may on the other hand damage his position in law.

EXAMINATION IN CASES OF SUSPECTED PSYCHOGENIC PAIN

A necessary preliminary to this examination is to bear in mind and face the implications of four not uncommon prejudices.

1. *Confusion between the Unknown and the Inconsistent*

The practitioner should not assume that a condition which he has not encountered before, does not exist. Indeed, his opinion is likely to be sought in just those cases of unwavering complaint which have defied elucidation. Sooner or later, one meets one of the rarer causes of pain in a patient referred for an opinion. If the patient's symptoms do not transgress the segmental boundaries, and if his responses to diagnostic movements are consistent, an organic lesion must be present. It should be remembered that, particularly in affections of a nerve-root, pain may be present in the virtual absence of physical signs. If the patient's history, symptoms, progress and responses conform closely to the known patterns and to the segmentation of the limb, his story is credible. As a rule, it is only when a condition is seen for the second or third time and the similarity between patients' stories and signs—or lack of signs—becomes apparent, that the examiner is confident that he is dealing with a real entity.

2. Suspicions engendered by the Patient's Manner or by the Diffuseness of his Pain.

A patient who has seen several practitioners without avail naturally feels under suspicion, perhaps begins to suspect himself, and so may develop the demeanour of a suspect. According to his temperament, he may become prolix and emphatic, or sullen, or apologetic. It is not so much the way he says it, as the remarkable sequence of events and sensations that he describes which should raise the question of psychogenic pain. Even so, the extrasegmental way in which pain radiates from the dura mater must be taken into account. The presence of pain in an apparently normal limb is not a reason for suspecting the patient's veracity, but rather for considering whether and whence the pain may be referred.

3. Suspicions based on the Results of Treatment

The fact that expert and apparently adequate treatment has not been followed by cure, is not evidence that the patient's ills are imaginary. Many common painful disorders are entirely unrelievable in the absence of an exact diagnosis implemented by equally exact treatment. For example, unless the doctor can inject hydrocortisone, or the physiotherapist give massage, accurately, a diagnosis of supraspinatus tendinitis remains purely academic.

4. Bias towards the Employer

A doctor, like any other individual, tends towards sympathy for those who come to him for help. Hence, when he sees a patient—particularly a private patient—his natural reaction is to side with him. Equally, when a doctor is retained by an insurance company, his instinct is to protect their interests. It takes a conscious effort to be perfectly impartial in these cases. Nevertheless, a dispassionate view is the essence of an examination to decide whether or not the patient's symptoms are psychogenic; and, when an organic lesion has led to excessive disablement, to assess the proportions of each factor. No medical man should feel that he is acting *for* or *against* the patient; he is there to establish certain facts, to report on his findings and to draw reasoned conclusions.

The History

The examiner should listen to the history with care, from the time when the symptoms began. Attention should be directed to the circumstances leading up to its first appearance, and the patient should be asked to point to its exact site then, and to indicate the area to which it has since spread.

Such diligence may elicit a coherent account from a patient apt to ramble or unable to explain himself well. By contrast, patients with psychogenic pain are apt to embroider, and their symptoms may be heard to come and go in the most improbable ways or to diffuse farther and farther as the tale continues. Radiation may be alleged which grossly transgresses the rules that referred pain keeps within one dermatome and does not cross the midline. Thus, unilateral pain may spread to both limbs, or a pectoral pain travel down to the lower abdomen.

Patients with psychogenic symptoms are disinclined to describe them; for, without necessarily being fully conscious of the fact, they are dimly aware that they do not quite know what they should say. Instead, they enlarge on the degree of suffering and disablement and embark on a long list of doctors consulted, diagnoses made, and ineffective treatments received. When repeatedly brought back to the point, i.e. what the symptoms were that made them seek medical advice, they become increasingly restive. They are irritated, implying that the listener must be a very inadequate physician not to realize that such intense suffering drove the patient to seek help. When pressed to describe the exact position of the pain, its variation and spread, what makes it better or worse and so on, these questions are resented. This attitude provides a strong contrast to the patient with organic disease who is only too glad to find a doctor who listens attentively and inquisitively.

Then there are a number of sequences that the experienced physician recognizes: for example, pain in the back radiating to the lower limb, the backache easing when the root pain becomes severe; the painful shoulder preventing the patient from lying on that side at night because of pain in the upper limb. Certain accounts characterize certain disorders, but in neurosis none of the recognizable patterns emerge.

It is always more difficult to be sure that there is no organic cause for a pain than that there is; hence, the ability to listen without losing patience and to adopt a sympathetic manner often repays the examiner well. Moreover, the patient who is allowed to go on talking, as well as contradicting his own earlier statements, may advance irrelevances that afford a clue to the true origin of his symptoms.

Inspection

Little is to be expected from inspection; for should this reveal obvious abnormality, the question of purely psychogenic symptoms hardly arises. Difficulties are encountered when a patient knows that he has a deformity, perhaps postural since adolescence or the result of past disease or fracture, and makes use of it to give colour to his story.

The mere fact that the patient can walk in and sit down shows certain muscles not to be paralysed and indicates that movement exists at the joints of the lower limbs. The patient may be well-nourished and show none of the facial expression that designates sleepless nights and severe pain.

The gait may reveal a limp or small shuffling steps or a joint held stiffly for which no limitation of joint movement, loss of muscle power or impairment of nervous control can later be found. Joints assume a characteristic posture when diseased, whereas psychogenic stiffness characteristically results in fixation in quite different positions, e.g. medial rotation at the hip, full extension at the knee, varus at the heel. Sometimes the wrong joint is held fixed; for example, a patient with lumbar pain may hold the neck and thoracic spine to one side, while the lumbar spine remains vertical. In true lumbar deviation, the list is seen there, with a compensating curve in the other direction above. Again, disorders of the cervical spine do not cause the scapula to be held elevated by contraction of the trapezius muscle.

Examination of Movements

The responses on examination of patients with organic lesions form a pattern. If a new pattern results, one must consider whether it is impossible or conceivable. During a resisted movement, pain may be felt at a site other than the muscle being tested. A complaint of pain on all the resisted movements at the scapula, shoulder, elbow and wrist joints is self-contradictory, since it would identify the lesion as situated in a dozen different places. However, the fact that every resisted shoulder or hip movement hurts is consistent with acute internal derangement of a cervical or lumbar intervertebral joint, and, in such a case, direct examination of the neck or lumbar movements must reveal a severe disorder. If, therefore, little abnormality is detected here, the reality of the symptoms is in great doubt. Except at a few sites, and then in a known manner, limitation of movement at a joint is also accompanied by proportionate limitation in the other directions. Pain on a resisted movement is accompanied, except in rare instances, by a full range of movement at the joint, and the extremes of such movements as neither stretch nor squeeze the affected tissue are always of full range and painless. Weakness of some resisted movement may be alleged, whereas the visible bulk of the relevant muscle shows that it is strong; or a muscle may have full power when tested in one way, but appear paralysed when tested by a different method. Alternatively, the mere fact that the patient walked in and sat down may show that the weakness is not organic. The muscles that are alleged to be weak may transgress the known patterns and, if pins and needles or numbness are present, they may occupy an inconsistent area of skin.

Patients assume that the first act of the examiner after listening to the history is to request them to make a movement which causes pain. A part of the body, as far distant as is reasonably possible from the allegedly affected area, should be chosen; if the knee or shoulder is said to hurt, for example, trunk movements may be tried first. It is remarkable how few psychoneurotic patients possess the strength of mind to resist this invitation.

The Essence of Examination is to Give the Patient Plenty of Scope

If inconsistencies are to be revealed, a large number of movements must be tested so that a congruous or an incongruous pattern can emerge. Trial of a series of active, passive and resisted movements at a number of joints, accompanied by a request to be told whether each hurts or not, is very confusing to a patient without organic disease. He cannot know, nor work out quickly in his mind, which movement he should say is painful and which not, which limited and which not. He is, therefore, apt to guess wildly, his random answers forming a pattern inconsistent with any one lesion. Or he may say that every movement at several joints sets up pain; this is too much. Suspicion is aroused if the patient allows the examiner's tone of voice to influence his response to movements, or by a pause followed by a glance at his face that appears designed to read the answer in his countenance. More difficulty is presented when every movement is said to leave the pain unaltered, for this is a perfectly possible finding in visceral pain (since the wrong parts are being examined) or in some cases of pressure on a nerve.

There is one remark which crops up again and again. When the series of movements is tested, ordinary patients say that such-and-such a movement hurts whereas another does not. The idea that any movement should be quite painless is repugnant to many neurotic patients and, instead of declaring some of the movements to be painless, they say 'not too bad'. If this phrase keeps recurring, the physician should be on his guard.

Positive Inconsistencies

The doctor who deals with the moving parts is in a happy position when the question of psychogenic pain arises. The physician who deals with dyspepsia or debility or headache cannot go further than to sum up the patient's character and, when every test proves negative, supposes that the trouble is caused by neurosis. The orthopaedic physician bases his diagnosis on the discovery of positive inconsistencies, and thus treads on much firmer ground. It is not the fact that nothing can be found to account for a pain that enables him to decide that the symptoms possess an emotional origin; it is the contradictions that pile up as the examination proceeds. Indeed, I have found (rather to my annoyance, for everyone likes to think himself a good judge of his fellow men) that when a patient appears quite sincere while he recounts the history but examination suggests psychogenesis, the examination is the better criterion. The opposite also holds; a nervous patient may by his manner suggest neurotic symptoms and yet examination may show a neat pattern that is clearly organic.

To uncover inconsistencies, the patient must be given plenty of opportunity. A large number of movements must be tested, some relevant to a pain at the site described, many not. If lumbar pain is alleged, the resisted movements of the neck make a good starting point.

Inconsistencies are:

Between the patient's appearance and his degree of suffering.

Between his description of his symptoms, even taken at their face value, and his disablement. He can sit at home and walk out shopping but cannot travel to work.

Between the site of pain and the way it has spread.

Between the site of the pain and the movements he cannot perform. In extreme cases, pain in the back may prevent raising the arms above the horizontal.

Between the site of pain and the movements reported to hurt.

Between his symptoms and his posture and gait.

Between what he can do and the physical signs. For example, the patient who cannot abduct the arm at all, but possesses a full range of movement at the shoulder joint when it is examined passively, together with full strength in the abductor muscles tested with the arm by the patient's side, has shown that he refuses to carry out a movement that he can in fact perform.

Between one set of physical signs and another set. If pain in the arm is brought on by neck movements, the lesion must be cervical. Hence the shoulder, elbow and wrist movements will not exacerbate the pain (although they may demonstrate a root-palsy), and vice versa.

Between the results of the same movement carried out in different ways or a second time. A patient who sits normally must possess 90 degrees range of flexion at the hip and knee.

N.B. It is important to realize that the range of straight-leg raising is not necessarily the same as the range of trunk-flexion, for, in the former case, the body-weight is not borne by the joint, whereas in the latter the joint is compressed. In consequence, it is a common finding in lumbago that the patient cannot bend forwards and yet has a full range of straight-leg raising.

The valid comparison in this connection is between trunk-flexion and sitting up with the legs out straight; for in both cases the joint is identically squeezed. This finding is medico-legally important; hence, it must be demonstrated in the way that is fair to the patient.

Between a finding of limitation in one direction and the range in other directions. There are many known patterns, but this may not fit with any.

Between the signs put forward and the site of alleged tenderness.

Between the site of tenderness at one moment and another.

Between the lesion possibly present and the fact that there is any tender point at all. If arthritis at the hip or shoulder is suspected, there is no relevant tenderness.

Doubtful Cases

Naturally, difficult cases abound especially when a minor ache is elevated into a disabling disease by neurosis. If the almoner's interview also proves uninformative, the next step is to record all the patient's responses. He should then be ordered a fortnight's indifferent treatment chosen for its known lack of effect on whatever the possible lesions are: e.g. heat or faradism. At the end of this period he may state himself to be cured; this is strong evidence of absent organic lesion. If not, he should be examined again, the same movements being tried, this time in a different order. When a series of movements is tried in rapid succession at several joints, patients seldom remember at this interval of time which were and which were not originally said to hurt. Should the responses tally closely on the two occasions, his complaint should be taken seriously and detailed examination repeated in an attempt to establish the source of his pain.

It is never the mere absence of physical signs that provides a confident diagnosis of psychogenic pain. On the other hand, the patient who alleges the presence of signs that contradict each other himself supplies the evidence of his own mental state.

Local Anaesthesia

In local anaesthesia, the examiner has another means of detecting unreal pains. The nature of the solution should not be explained; it suffices to say that the examiner wishes to give an injection. Patients anxious to make the worst of their case are often tempted into saying that the infiltration has made the pain worse. This is impossible. Again, the induction of local anaesthesia cannot fail to abolish local tenderness. It must be remembered, however, that if local anaesthesia does not remove a pain felt at the infiltrated area, this is perfectly consistent with an organic lesion situated elsewhere and referring pain to this spot.

Radiography

Although it is a sad waste of material, this examination should not be omitted. An unexpected positive finding is a great rarity, for soft-tissue lesions which alter the radiological appearances are usually advanced enough to make the clinical diagnosis easy. The presence of some trivial abnormality, e.g. an osteophyte or a diminished intervertebral joint space, must not be regarded as proving a patient's symptoms to have an organic cause.

FINDINGS IN SUSPECTED PSYCHOGENIC PAIN

The possible findings on examination conducted on these lines fall into four main groups.

1. Absence of Organic Lesion

In obvious cases the history is remarkable; the disability is out of proportion even to the alleged symptoms; the responses to diagnostic movements conflict; clear inconsistencies are detected; acute tenderness is diffuse. If the patient appears to have a conscious belief in the reality of his symptoms, he is regarded as suffering from a psychogenic disorder. If he does not even believe in them himself, he is termed a malingerer. The examination reveals only the absence of organic basis for the patient's pain; the study of his state of mind during this time may or may not allow an opinion on how far he believes in his own symptoms. No hard and fast line can in any case be drawn; cases at each extreme are clearly enough defined but they merge at a centre about which self-deception changes to conscious assumption. No objective test can distinguish psychoneurosis from malingering. An emphatic but cheerful description of non-organic symptoms characterizes assumed pain; bland indifference to a serious disability denotes hysteria; normal examination-findings in an apathetic patient who clearly maintains a hopeless view that he will never get better, signify endogenous depression.

2. Organic Lesion with Psychogenic Overlay

These are difficult cases requiring much patience and clinical experience to disentangle. The symptoms and physical signs, though largely correct in quality, are grossly excessive in quantity. Moreover, mixed in with and obscuring the genuine factors are unbelievable complaints and alleged signs. Much time and considerable repetition of the examination may be required to enable the real lesion to emerge after it has been distinguished from the welter of unfounded symptoms. In such cases, it is often wise to convert the patient to a more reasonable frame of mind by a fortnight's indifferent treatment from a physiotherapist. She, by imparting her unemotional and commonsense attitude, can nearly always get a patient so to collect himself that, at the next examination, it is hard to believe that there could have been any difficulty in arriving at a diagnosis.

It is well to remember that psychogenic signs may over-shadow organic signs. For example, a patient with 10 degrees limitation of abduction at the shoulder, who refuses to move his arm from his side at all, conceals a genuine sign, which only assiduity and repetition will reveal. Although the patient has brought the misdiagnosis of himself, unfairness results if such a patient is regarded as suffering from a purely psychogenic disability. Treatment by suggestion is apt to be powerless in the presence of real—however minor—pain; in contrast, relief of the genuine lesion, by depriving the patient of the basis for his malady, is sometimes curative alone. Even if it is not, he is now responsive to psychotherapy.

3. Pain in Neurotic Patients

Another difficulty appears with the psychoneurotic patient who happens to develop a painful condition. His excessive distress and nervous behaviour on giving his history conflict with the simple and consistent pattern that, to his own and the examiner's surprise, is discovered on examination. The hypersensitive state present must be allowed for when treatment is ordered, but there is seldom any need for treatment of his mental state with which, as long as no painful disorder has upset its balance, he has coped quite well for years.

4. No Physical Signs Detected

There always remains a very small group of patients in whom no decision is possible. The history is credible and the response to movements unhelpful but constant on repetition and devoid of inconsistency. Tenderness may be absent and local anaesthesia unavailing. Sometimes, repeated examinations may enable a decision to be reached in the end; in a very few cases the decision is never really reached.

Elderly patients with, for example, a minor disc lesion at an osteophytic spinal joint, may have no clear signs to explain their brachial, thoracic or sciatic pain. In due course, such signs do sometimes develop; only analogy with these cases enables an early diagnosis to be made. In other cases also of irritation of the sheath of a sciatic nerve root, the pain may be felt at, say, the calf only and, even if this possibility is kept in mind, investigation may at first reveal nothing. Paraesthesiae in one hand may be the first symptoms of protrusion of a cervical intervertebral disc, or of the thoracic outlet syndrome, or of compression in the carpal tunnel; at first, all signs may be absent. Pain in the groin or iliac fossa may be caused by dural compression at a low lumbar level, without necessarily physical signs. When perineal pain arises from pressure on the fourth sacral root, it is exceptional for any physical signs to exist at all.

In such cases, the fault clearly lies with the examiner rather than the patient; an examination delicate enough to detect his organic disorder does not exist. It is wise, after repeated endeavour has failed to detect the lesion, local anaesthesia has proved negative, and a short course of such treatment as suggested itself has failed, to confess to the patient that one has been unable to arrive at a diagnosis. In fairness, one should add that one has no doubt that the symptoms are genuine, that since clinical examinations and radiography have all failed to disclose a source, it is most unlikely to be anything serious; that he is welcome to come and be seen again at any time; that further treatment is clearly a waste of time equally for the patient and doctor; that, should a diagnosis ever be made, or any method of treatment prove effective, he should certainly report it.

TREATMENT OF PSYCHOGENIC DISABILITY

Hospital Practice

It is unreasonable and impractical to refer all patients with minor psychogenic trouble to the psychologist. Moreover, simple suggestion of the type that physiotherapy supplies often succeeds in dispelling symptoms, at any rate for the time being. My endeavour in these cases is to get the patient back to work with the least possible delay. The first essential is to bring the patient over to co-operate with the doctor and so enable the former to declare that he is cured without loss of the very self-esteem that the symptoms are unconsciously designed to protect. Nothing, therefore, can be more unfortunate in its results than a cursory examination followed by a brusque statement that there is nothing the matter with the patient and that he is fit to return to work at once. This engenders immediate dislike of the doctor, who is at once regarded as unsympathetic and incompetent (and rightly so; for there *is* something the matter, although not what the patient believes); indeed, this attitude is tantamount to asking the patient to admit to others and—far worse—to himself, that he is shamming: a situation that he naturally resents. Such a statement, then, only induces in the patient an added determination to prove by unwavering complaint that his disablement is genuine.

After a sympathetic hearing and a thorough examination, the patient's confidence will have been won and a pleasant relationship established. Finally the examiner confidently announces that the patient will receive a fortnight's treatment which it is hoped will put him on the road to recovery. To say that cure is certain is too strong and annoys the patient by its disparaging suggestion of a minor malady.

Full physical examination, especially the diagnostic movements, has another advantage. If detailed notes are kept, and they are lying on the table before the doctor, it dawns on the patient when he comes up for examination at the end of a fortnight that, if he states he is no better, he will be put through all these movements again. A large factor in obtaining 'cure' may be provided by the patient's unwillingness to be asked questions to which he suddenly realizes he has now forgotten the answers. This explains those cases in which the physiotherapist has, so she reports, not affected the allegations of pain; yet the patient walks in next day beaming, declaring he is well.

This friendly atmosphere abolishes the patient's stubbornness and readiness to take offence. The physiotherapist with her faradic battery continues in the same strain. On the one hand, she applies faradic stimulation of increasing strength to whatever area the patient alleges is painful or weak, after which the patient practises the hitherto impossible or painful movement. On the other, she too maintains a persistent pleasant and encouraging manner. Her conversation should turn on the patient's life and circumstances, and emphasize the advantages to him of getting well. The patient, swayed in the same direction by such pleasant people and such disagreeable measures, more often than not declares himself well after a week or two of such treatment. In a series, seventy-six of one hundred and seven patients seen in my department in 1943 and regarded as suffering from purely psychogenic symptoms declared themselves well and returned to work at the end of two or three weeks. Compensation cases are not included in this series.

Treatment should not be continued for longer than two weeks. A fortnight's stimulating physiotherapy may induce a patient to state that he is cured; if not, prolongation of treatment is merely added evidence to all of the presence of organic disease. Hence, the remaining patients must be taken off physiotherapy and the decision reached whether they should be discharged or referred for psychological investigation, or sent to an institutional rehabilitation centre. Consideration of the patient's age, work-record in the past; responsibilities, apparent character and social value determine the result; obviously the almoner's investigations bear strongly on these points. This residue of patients, otherwise reasonably sound human beings, for whose relief these superficial measures have not sufficed, are troubled by deep unconscious motives that require a psychiatrist.

It may well be argued that this is a most superficial approach to a deep-seated psychological frailty and that nothing has been done to prevent recurrence of symptoms later or to build up the patient's strength of will. This is true; but even the best psychologist cannot evoke character of which the patient is constitutionally devoid. Moreover, that a psychologist should spend many hours in the attempt to build with such inferior material is a great deal to ask. Hence, the rough and ready method outlined here, since it so often results in the patient's speedy resumption of his proper activities, may be regarded as a reasonable pragmatic approach, however unsound theoretically. Of patients relieved of psychogenic symptoms, less than 10 per cent return with further allegations during the next two years—at any rate to the same hospital.

Private Practice

In private practice, the situation is rather different; for the patients are less suggestible; there is no almoner; the physician has more time. The diagnosis, and the reasons for arriving at this conclusion, should be stated at once, and the patient asked without further ado if, in view of this finding, he would like psychiatric advice. It is explained that both pent-up tension and depression can give rise to sensations that are interpreted as painful in such states of emotional tone. It is remarkable how many patients immediately agree that this ascription is correct, even though they may have insisted on physiotherapy and osteopathy for years. With this agreement, a talk on how to avoid the now-overt emotional strain follows; often simple constructive proposals can be made for patient, spouse and doctor. Some patients find the diagnosis hard to accept. If so, I ask them to see a psychiatrist and, if he considers this mistaken, offer then to examine them again. Some patients reject the diagnosis and merely leave the consulting room unconvinced. For this reason, it is always best to set out the basis for the opinion by talking to the patient in the presence of the nearest relative. The diagnosis is then communicated to the patient's family, who have usually suspected that neurosis was present, but in the absence of support have been unable to take suitable steps. Once the relations know the situation, they can direct their sympathy into more useful channels.

In children, it is best to talk to the parents alone. Psychological symptoms of the sort seen by the orthopaedic physician commonly arise in two sets of circumstances: (i) when the child wants to direct his parents' attention to himself, since he has concluded that they like or value a younger brother or sister more; (ii) when a child resents his parents' decision being forced on him, particularly in the choice of a career. The situation is usually fairly simple; to discover why the child thinks his parents prefer his sibling or where the parents are being inflexible and disregarding the child's wishes about his own future. If they (a) alter their attitude or (b) ignore the child's complaints, symptoms gradually cease. If the parents wish to make a face-saving provision for the child, a week or two's stimulating physiotherapy may be justified.

There is one subtle device that can be used by patients with psychogenic troubles to discredit the physician who makes the diagnosis. Only by proving him incompetent can the patient hope to regain relatives' sympathy. A few days after the consultation, the patient becomes 'much worse', and may be brought for a second consultation, which serves only to confirm the original opinion. The patient goes at once to a healer, masseur or lay-manipulator who naturally says that all sorts of lesions are present. He now gives 'treatment' which the patient allows to be effective. The patient remains well, unwilling to risk illness again, and sings the other man's praises, while writing aggrieved letters to the physician.

THE ALMONER'S PART

It would be absurd to send all patients with psychogenic symptoms straight to the psychologist. He would find his department overwhelmed by trivial cases. Moreover, many such patients are so weak charactered that his skill and time are inadequately rewarded, even when alleviation, often ephemeral, results. It is amply justifiable in the first place to turn such patients over to the combined efforts of the almoner and the physiotherapist.

The work of a conscientious and understanding almoner supplies a vital part in the treatment of psychogenic pain; for she represents the patient's link with the outside world. She must possess aptitude and human understanding, and be the sort of person whose evident sympathy encourages confidences. She must have enough time to give special attention to those cases in which a doubtful diagnosis has been reached of pain devoid of organic basis or complicated by a neurotic overlay. Almoners find some of the most interesting problems in their work with this type of case. During inquiries into domestic, workaday and financial circumstances, factors may come to light that serve to explain the alleged disability. In doubtful cases, the discovery by the almoner of the presence or absence of conscious or unconscious motives lends weight to, or detracts from, the tentative diagnosis. Her conversation also enables her to help in dividing patients into the relatively deserving and undeserving. Some patients seek relief from unpleasant situations only on severe provocation; in such cases, the almoner can get in touch with employer or Labour Exchange, visit the home or arrange for various forms of assistance or convalescence. Others allege symptoms for the most unworthy reasons; in these cases, it would be an abuse to bring such facilities to the patient's aid. The almoner can also help in cases where the nature of the domestic background indicates that a short talk by the doctor with a member of the patient's family is desirable.

TRAUMATIC NEURASTHENIA

This is neurosis after an accident leading to the idea of disordered function. Such cases are often sent for a medico-legal opinion. Neurosis is noticeably uncommon after severe fractures or injuries sustained at home or during games and sport, whereas after car smashes or accidents at work emotional reactions often follow, since claims for compensation then arise. It is interesting to note that in France and in the Iron Curtain countries, where compensation is payable for bodily injury but no account is taken of emotional shock, traumatic neurasthenia is almost unknown. For that reason, some authorities prefer the term 'compensation neurasthenia'.

Traumatic neurasthenia is a self-engendered disorder, at least at first: the voluntary perpetuation of the shakiness that almost everyone feels immediately after escaping from what he realizes might have been a serious accident. It is kept in being by a wish to make the most of the incident, and is further maintained by the anxieties and delays of litigation.

Cases that come to the Courts are seldom settled until several years after the accident and, during the whole of this time, the patient has to lend colour to his claim by keeping off work, including such work as he could easily carry out, even if all his allegations were well-founded. This financial loss leads to real worry over his chances of eventual reimbursement, which now sets up well-grounded anxiety, augmented by the strains of protracted negotiation. These negotiations, unhappily, are not concerned with how best to speed the patient's recovery, but with reconciling different opinions on what is the matter with the patient, how long it may be before he recovers, and how much compensation he deserves. By now, his preoccupation may well have become very real, though it is centred on the possible result of litigation, not on the original injury; hence, a time comes when traumatic neurasthenia begins to possess a factual basis.

The insurance companies benefit from delay, and the law moves slowly. The prospect of another medical examination in six months' time, and very likely another, equally inconclusive, six months after that, and so on, engenders an exasperation that leads patients to wish for an early settlement on almost any terms. When, however, this manœuvre fails, the doctor's efforts to prevent the case dragging on from year to year usually prove futile.

Depression

Depression precipitated by injury is not traumatic neurasthenia. In patients liable to periods of depression, an accident may bring on such a state. Alternatively, the depressed patient who sustains, say, a fracture may, in that state of mind, decide that he will never recover, or his unavoidable absence from his business may give rise to ideas of impending financial ruin.

Such patients, when examined, do not allege a series of inconsistent signs of the neurasthenic type. Their signs are just what they ought to be, but it is clear that the construction that they put on their disorder is deeply coloured by their mood.

Such patients benefit from monoamine oxidase inhibitor drugs.

Treatment

The treatment of traumatic neurasthenia is obvious but not simple; to bring to an end the litigation that maintains it. As soon as the suit is settled, the neurasthenia ceases to serve any purpose and it abates quickly in nearly every instance. Even if the case goes against the plaintiff, however disgruntled he may feel he nearly always sets about earning his living again, though not necessarily at his original work. A few weeks' stimulating physiotherapy may save his face and speed 'recovery'; alternatively, training for a different job may prove acceptable.

It is wise, therefore, not to treat such patients until the suit is settled. Most of them have had endless physiotherapy and often osteopathy, and it is a waste of time and money, and would be a source of justified exasperation for trained staff, to give individual treatment. Reference to she occupational therapy department is rational but of little avail.

Reference to a group, e.g. a back-class, may be justified if the question of a minor organic lesion arises and the physician wishes to examine again soon. At least, it wastes no-one's time, not even the patient's; for he is not working. Even so, treatment in an exercise class is 'treatment', and lends colour to the patient's allegations. Moreover, the doctor who has ordered this measure finds himself embarrassed if he later has to appear in Court and state that, in his view, no organic lesion is present.

It is best, therefore, to write to the family doctor setting out the findings, and ask him to press for early settlement. If patients insist, I see them again and examine them again at intervals for as long as they care to keep coming, but I do not order any treatment.

Miller's (1961) classic paper on 'Accident Neurosis' must be read by all interested in the subject; it is entertainingly written as well as most informative. Of fifty patients with this disorder, he found only two who had not returned to work by two years after the legal suit was concluded, whether favourably or unfavourably. He found that workmen were much more prone to neurosis than employers, and that the likelihood of neurasthenic symptoms bore an inverse proportion to the severity of the injury.

THE RADIOGRAPH IN MEDICO-LEGAL CASES

In patients complaining of persistent pain as a consequence of some accident, a decision on the relevance of radiographic abnormalities is beset by many pitfalls. In my view, in nearly every case the clinical findings take precedence over X-ray changes. Rarely, the photograph may show an overriding lesion that clinical examination did not detect; then only is it diagnostic taken alone.

Much unfairness results from excessive reliance on radiography. For example, slight symptomless wedging following injury to a vertebral body may be regarded as clear proof of allegedly severe pain, and some patients, after being made aware of the radiographic abnormality, trade on this knowledge. By contrast, patients in real pain, but with a normal X-ray picture, may receive scant consideration.

Comparison of the clinical and radiological evidence leads to four main types of conclusion.

1. *The Radiograph Confirms the Clinical Findings or is itself Diagnostic*

In such cases, there is happily no conflict of evidence and the X-ray photograph lends precision to the clinical diagnosis. Alternatively, it may reveal a lesion almost impossible to detect clinically, e.g. early tuberculous caries, a vertebral fracture without a kyphos.

To assess the degree of disability set up by the lesion is a purely clinical task, as is the prognosis.

2. *The Radiograph Confirms the Past Occurrence of an Injury but is not clearly Relevant to the Patient's Symptoms*

Difficulty may arise in determining whether the injury in question or some previous accident caused the abnormality detected on the radiograph. Pictures taken soon after an accident reveal the difference between recent and long-standing bony changes, but after a time no limiting date can be given. It must not be forgotten that bony abnormalities, both congenital and acquired, may be revealed by chance on a radiograph taken for some other reason. The history may disclose that a vertebral fracture occurred several decades ago; produced only transient stiffness then and no symptoms since. Hence, the presence of such an abnormality does not afford unequivocal evidence of the presence of pain. Once bony union is complete, wedging of a vertebral body cannot itself cause pain, let alone unilateral pain. Equally, fracture of a vertebral transverse process does not give rise to bilateral pain or pain lasting longer than a month. The most that can be said of such evidence of damage to bone is that the accident was evidently severe. In such cases, if a soft tissue lesion explains the symptoms, the radiographic appearances largely corroborate the patient's contention that it is the result of injury.

The radiograph may show some condition like osteoarthritis at an age when this is a common finding. The presence of osteophytosis at, for example, the shoulder does not protect against tendinitis or bursitis.

Judges have been led to believe that osteophyte formation at the vertebral joints is a painful disorder, as it is, say, at the hip. This enables counsel to aver that the patient's backache is the result of exacerbation of a naturally occurring disease, or that the osteoarthritis visible radiographically shows that he would have developed backache, with or without injury, in due course. These preconceptions suit defendants very well and are thus perpetuated. In consequence, the expert witness may have to clear the air somewhat in order to make his evidence comprehensible.

3. *The Radiograph is Uninformative*

Normal radiographic appearances cannot be held to preclude the existence of organic disorder any more than every visible abnormality indicates the presence of pain. Few painful soft tissue lesions give rise to radiographic signs. Only clinical examination can reveal lesions such as tennis-elbow, supraspinatus tendinitis, monarticular rheumatoid arthritis, displacement of a fragment of intervertebral disc, early gout, ligamentous sprains, or rupture of the meniscus at the knee-joint, to mention only a few common conditions.

4. *The Radiograph is Misleading*

Shadows may be seen on the radiograph that suggest a diagnosis which clinical examination shows to be false. Small opacities in a ligament, tendon or bursa are not evidence that any pain in that region arises from the structure to which attention has been drawn. Small areas of calcification in, for example, the supraspinatus tendon or the tibial collateral ligament of the knee are often accompanied by perfect function. Quite large areas of calcification of the subdeltoid bursa may be wholly symptomless. Again, an appreciable degree of osteophyte formation at joints such as the intervertebral, knee or tarsal is consistent with normal function. Osteophyte formation at the sacro-iliac joint shows commencing ossification of the ligaments and proves the joint to be stable and painless. X-ray evidence suggesting osteo-arthritis in the joint of a sacralized fifth lumbar transverse process has never in my experience given rise to symptoms. Such instances could be multiplied and emphasize the paramount importance of clinical examination.

28

Manipulation: Medical and Lay

Manipulation has a bad name. This is to a large extent deserved, since manipulation is apt to be carried out as a tentative measure adopted as a last resort for lack of an alternative rather than because a positive indication, based on a clear pathological concept, has emerged. Its advocates claim too much for manipulation, thus affording its opponents a good reason for pouring scorn on a useful treatment. It is ridiculous that medical men should be swayed by laymen's absurd hypotheses into holding strong opinions for or against manipulation, advocating it warmly for a displaced cartilage in the knee and not for a fragment of cartilage displaced within a lumbar joint. Like all other treatment, manipulation should be prescribed or withheld on a basis of the lesion present, not of emotional bias.

Lay manipulators' untenable claims for the virtues of manipulation do not worry the public. For example, an elderly man's headache is wrongly attributed to hyperpiesis, when it is in fact due merely to ligamentous contracture at the upper two cervical joints with normal reference of pain within the first and second cervical dermatomes. Treatment for the hyperpiesis has no effect, but a layman cures the headache by manipulating the cervical joints. Patient, and probably the manipulator too, are ignorant enough to suppose that hyperpiesis has been relieved by manipulating the neck. The same applies to patients with root-pain felt at the front of the trunk as a result of a thoracic disc lesion, in whom a mistaken diagnosis of angina, renal disease, chronic appendicitis, etc., has been arrived at, and manipulation has proved curative after other methods (including laparotomy) have failed. These diagnostic errors naturally lead the public and these laymen themselves to suppose that spinal manipulation can cure visceral disorders. It is events like these that give rise to the strong divergence of opinion between doctors and the public on the subject, for the doctor asks for scientific evidence, whereas the public wants a cure, and will naturally believe any hypothesis, however ill-founded, if treatment apparently based on it brings relief. It is such claims that have delayed the acceptance of manipulation by the medical profession and have given doctors such a bad impression of lay manipulators. It is not their work that is bad, for some of it is good, but it is their idea of what to treat, what can be expected of manipulation, and how it achieves its effect, that outrages a doctor's scientific attitude.

Most of the spinal manipulation carried out in this country today is performed by laymen. There are believed to be some three thousand such persons, of whom two hundred are on the osteopathic register, and there are also forty medical men practising osteopathy and two chiropraxy. The patient with a lesion requiring manipulation seldom gets it from his own doctor or from an orthopaedic surgeon unless the displacement is visible radiologically, as in fracture or dislocation. On his friends' insistence, he visits a layman who may well make a mistaken diagnosis (e.g. primary muscle spasm or perhaps a bone out of place) but then proceeds to give the correct treatment with dramatic relief. No wonder our newspapers carry reports on the miracles of lay-manipulation, and will go on doing so as long as the medical profession in general maintains a negative attitude towards a treatment that is so easily learnt that even the largely untutored make a success of it.

In the past, doctors have correctly pointed out that lay manipulators' dogma is demonstrably false, and have regarded that as good enough. Alas, it is not. The remedy is for doctors to show that they are conversant as much with the indications for, as with the abuses of, manipulation, and are as ready to have it carried out within the medical sphere in suitable cases as they are bound to discountenance its use in the unsuitable case. One important error in logic must be avoided—to abhor manipulation because of a dislike of lay manipulators. Obviously, no doctor can approve of a person who, wishing to treat patients, neither follows the medical curriculum first and secures a medical qualification, nor takes the normal course of a medical auxiliary. But there are many of these, and they have only stepped into a therapeutic hiatus that has been left wide open by medical men. The way to prevent lay manipulation from flourishing is the acceptance by the medical profession of this method as a normal medical treatment. Indeed, the more a doctor dislikes such treatment by laymen, the more he should see to it that suitable patients are manipulated within the medical sphere. Nevertheless there are still some doctors who carry prejudice against lay manipulators so far (though their numbers are diminishing) that they extend their dislike of everything to do with manipulation to those medical men who are trying to bring a useful medical treatment back within the medical ambit.

Every doctor knows of successful manipulation by laymen in sincere patients previously treated—mostly alas by physiotherapy—without avail under the highest medical auspices. These patients cannot be written off as a group of mere hysterics; indeed, they include doctors themselves. Some are hysterics, of course; but many more are people anxious to get well and return to work quickly who have followed their friends' advice when it became plain to them that the medical profession had nothing to offer. This group, however small a proportion of laymen's clients that it comprises, bears witness to medical neglect of a simple therapy. As a result doctors now find to their discomfort that they have been virtually ousted from a field they once scorned to occupy.

Manipulation is a respectable and logical method of treatment, effective in a restricted series of disorders, important because these disorders are so common and form so high a proportion of cases of industrial absence from work.

MANIPULATION

This is a method of treatment. It consists of different kinds of passive movement performed by the hands in a definite manner for a prescribed purpose. Its use does not involve the operator in any particular belief in the causes and treatment of all disease; he is merely treating the patient with one particular disorder in what he believes is the best way. Fractures and dislocations often require manipulation for the reduction of the displacement, and the same applies when a loose fragment of cartilage has become displaced within a joint, blocking movement.

Definition

In the past, definitions of manipulation have been framed too much with osteopathy in view. Definitions suited to a healing system confining itself to the spine and based on the idea of replacing a subluxated vertebra are too narrow. The osteopath points out quite correctly that the spinal joints possess an active range of movement of so much, a passive range of slightly more, and are capable of being forced a little farther still by manipulative overpressure. Hence, so far as osteopathy goes, manipulation consists in applying such overpressure to a spinal joint.

Unfortunately, a definition based on this excludes a great many orthopaedic medical manœuvres. When, for example, manipulative reduction is carried out at the neck or knee, the loose fragment often shifts long before the extreme of even the active range is reached. Nor, in either of these instances, is it a case of forcing the movement found to be painful; many manœuvres, especially when carried out during traction, are effective when a movement already known to be painless is performed. Neither is it necessarily a question of restoring full range to a joint at which limitation exists; it is often directed merely to making the extreme of such movement as is present, painless instead of painful. No power on earth will restore a full range of movement to an osteoarthritic neck; when the osteophytes engage, the bony block is felt and further forcing is useless. The aim of treatment in such cases is to secure pain-free stiffness.

Over-pessure can be carried out at a spinal joint, but not necessarily at a peripheral joint. For example, there is no difference in the active, passive and overpressure range in extension at the elbow joint, where these three ranges are the same, since in each case movement ceases when the olecranon engages against the back of the humerus. When reduction is attempted at the wrist by gliding the proximal on the distal row of carpal bones, a movement incapable of active performance is carried out. Rocking the tibia and rotating two adjacent thoracic vertebrae simultaneously in opposite directions are other examples of manœuvres that do not apply overpressure at the extreme of range.

Manipulation is simply defined as: *passive movement with a therapeutic purpose, using the hands.* The fact that it has a definite aim transforms a passive movement into manipulation. It is not the mere moving of a joint passively this way and that; it is a series of macœuvres with a defined purpose carried out with variations in technique dependent on the lesion present, the joint affected and the result to be achieved.

Types of Passive Movement

Confusion exists on the different purposes of passive movement; in particular, what part of it is covered by the term 'manipulation'.

Manipulation for reduction in such conditions as fracture, dislocation, displaced meniscus at knee or jaw, strangulated hernia, breech presentation, or retroverted uterus is not considered here. No controversy exists about terminology, and the manœuvres required, together with their indications, are set out in standard textbooks. In fact, the word 'manipulation' is often omitted in these connections. A fracture or dislocation is 'reduced'; hernia is treated by 'taxis' and the position of the uterus or foetal malpresentation is 'corrected'.

The different types are set out below:

1. *Passive Movement in Examination*

This is required when the range of movement at a joint, or how far a ligament or a muscle or a nerve-root will stretch has to be ascertained; in either case, it is important to note if pain is provoked at the extreme of the possible range—limited, normal or excessive. During the movement, abnormal sensations of diagnostic importance may be imparted to the examiner's hand, e.g. crepitus. How the extreme of range makes itself apparent in degrees of softness or hardness—the 'end-feel'—whether pain and limitation of movement come on together or separately, is often most informative. The examining hand is constantly alert to receive information from the tissues it is handling and, during manipulation, as the extreme of range is approached.

2. *Passive Movement without Forcing the Joint*

The purpose is the maintenance of mobility. It is often required in recent sprain. A strained ligament at the ankle, for example, may set up enough pain to make the patient hold his talo-calcanean and mid-tarsal joints immobile, although they are not themselves affected. Passive maintenance of range is the best treatment for the first few days. Again, a recent hemiplegic's shoulder will become stiff and painful unless passive movement is instituted immediately. The joint is normal; the purpose of any forcing required is to overcome muscle hypertonus; range has to be maintained until the patient can move the joint for himself. This type of movement can also be used to show an uncertain patient how far his joint will actually move, or to teach him the postural sense of what the movement feels like.

3. *Passive Movement with Sudden Forcing*

Adhesions can be ruptured by a sharp jerk carried out at the extreme of range. The position that best stretches the adhesion is ascertained and sudden overpressure is exerted farther in the same direction. This type of forced movement is often called 'mobilization' (which is a description of the result), but it is also common to talk of the manipulative rupture of an adhesion. Anaesthesia is often desirable.

4. *Passive Movement with Slow Forcing*

A contracture, congenital or acquired, can often be overcome by maintaining a series of strong stretches. The joint is moved as far as possible in the direction of limitation, then pressed on farther and held there as long as is reasonable. Release is equally gradual. This is the type of forcing required in torticollis, talipes equinovarus or osteoarthritis at hip or shoulder.

This sort of stretching is not, in daily medical usage, called mobilization or manipulation.

5. *Passive Movement for Reducing a Displacement*

The essential difference between manipulation for internal derangement and the other sorts of passive movement is the indirect manner of attaining a stated intention. In this sort of manipulation, an increased range of movement and diminution in pain are achieved, not by forcing movement in the direction in which it is restricted, but by a series of far more subtle manœuvres which experience has taught afford benefit in this type of disorder. The reduction of an intra-articular displacement is attempted purely on a basis of what has been found effective in similar cases. The likelihood of such reduction is, of course, enhanced if the loose fragment is given room to move; hence, manipulation with this intention is often best performed during distraction of the joint surfaces. One passive movement—traction—is then the adjuvant to another type of passive movement.

The manœuvre that is carried out is seldom the one towards the direction of limitation, certainly not in early stages of attempted reduction. For example, if a patient cannot bend forwards because of lumbar pain, no effort is ever made to force flexion at the lumbar joints; for there is nothing to stretch out; the joint is blocked. The pattern of which movements are painful and which not, which are limited and which not, often helps to indicate which manœuvre is most likely to succeed and thus determines technique. The first manœuvre to be attempted is chosen on a basis of three, sometimes conflicting, criteria: (1) The likeliest to succeed. (2) The least painful. (3) The most informative. The experienced manipulator distinguishes different types of end-feel as the joint he is treating approaches the extreme of range and his hand is ready instantly to increase or relax the power of his movement, depending on the sensations imparted to his hand. Working on a basis of trial, end-feel and effect, the manipulator continues his series of manœuvres, repeating or abandoning a particular technique on a basis of result and of end-feel. If difficulty arises, strong forcing during maximal traction may be required, or if no progress is made the whole attempt may be abandoned early. Anaesthesia is contra-indicated because the patient must be examined afresh after each manœuvre; he reports any change in symptoms; the manipulator notes any change in signs. In this way the loose fragment can be watched changing (or not) its position as the manipulator proceeds and pointers appear towards what to do next and whether to go on or stop. Moreover, as the extreme of manipulative range is reached, different feelings are imparted to the manipulator's hand that also guide him in judging his next step. For example, a stone-hard stop tells him that further force in that direction is useless; a soft stop encourages him to repeat the same movement more firmly. Manipulative reduction succeeds in a very few sessions, or not at all; no one should receive weekly manipulation for many months on end.

The reduction of internal derangement may take place without full range in any direction being reached. For example, at the neck or knee, when a rotary manipulation during strong traction is begun, a click may be felt long before the extreme of range is reached. If this click is shown by examination to have effected reduction, no more need be done. Again, in central posterior cervical protrusion, reduction is often secured by strong traction with only a few degrees of rotation added.

Passive movement for the reduction of internal derangement consists of a sequence of calculated manœuvres. It is the type of passive movement that is most often required and calls for much more skill and judgement than the other types. The strength of the manœuvre varies from scarcely any to the use of considerable, albeit controlled, force. It is carried out so as to influence the joint whence the symptoms originate, and consists of a series performed without anaesthesia, usually during traction, chosen in a sequence that depends on repeated examination of the patient and on what the manipulator feels at the end of his stroke, continued—not necessarily at one session only—until all movements at the affected joint become (if possible) painless. Technique also varies with the size and position of the loose fragment, with due regard for the age, size, tolerance and per-sonality of the patient. Thought, care, knowledge, clinical sense and manual skill—all are essential for this type of manipulation, which is not primarily a question of muscular power, and even less of merely forcing the joint the way it will not go.

The term 'manipulation' is best reserved for that branch of therapeutic passive movement which is concerned with a series of manœuvres carried out for reduction in internal derangement, and in which primary forcing of a joint towards the restricted range plays no part.

6. Traction

Distraction of the bone ends serves two purposes.

(1) Traction is a most effective adjuvant to manipulation for internal derangement. When the articular surfaces separate, a loose body pre-viously impacted becomes free to move, and the discomfort of the mani-pulation is greatly reduced. Moreover, a centripetal stress is now acting on the contents of the joint: a particularly desirable factor when dis-placement beyond the articular edge is present at an intervertebral joint, and a great safeguard against the increased protrusion that manipulation without traction can produce.

(2) Traction can also be used alone, in order to create a negative pressure within a joint. For example, in nuclear protrusion at an intervertebral joint, especially in the lumbar region, the protrusion consists of soft material which cannot be shifted by manipulation. Sustained traction results in suction, which, aided by distraction of the bone ends and tauten-ing of the posterior longitudinal ligament, slowly returns the protrusion to its proper place. The traction lasts half-an-hour and is given daily for about two weeks, strong force being required (40 to 80 kg.). Occasionally

lesser force is required continuously for some days during recumbency. Lesser force then suffices (5 kg. for the neck and 20 kg. for the lumbar joints).

Pure traction, even when applied manually, is seldom called 'manipulation'.

SPINAL MANIPULATIVE TECHNIQUE

The intention throughout is to do something to the affected tissue that the patient cannot do for himself. The patient can, let us say, turn his neck by using his own muscles; weight-bearing and muscle pull then combine to exert a *centrifugal* stress on the articular contents during the movement. When the same rotation movement is carried out passively during strong traction, a *centripetal* force acts on the joint and the contrary effect is exerted on the tissues within the joint. It is for this reason that exercises, or orthopaedic surgical manipulation under anaesthesia may have an effect opposite to that of orthopaedic medical manipulation, although to all appearances the same movement is carried out; the difference lies in whether the movement is carried out while centrifugal or centripetal force is acting on the intra-articular contents. In such cases, the orthopaedic medical manœuvre may be as strongly indicated as the surgical type of manipulation is contra-indicated. This is understandable; for the surgeon wishes merely to restore the range of movement by mobilization under anaesthesia and the osteopathic and chiropractic techniques were originally devised to shift one vertebra on another. Had it turned out that it really was the bone that was displaced (and not a fragment of disc), osteopathic and chiropractic methods might have proved the best.

Many of the adverse opinions on the effects of manipulation, especially of the cervical joints, are correctly founded on the results of manœuvres carried out when the joint is subjected to centrifugal instead of centripetal force. The opinions are justified, so far as they go, but should not be extended to include a type of manipulation that has the opposite effect to that correctly held to be dangerous.

1. The Patient's Posture

For a number of manipulations, the joint is placed in a special position. This involves the patient, the affected part, the manipulator and his assistants adopting postures that facilitate the movement required and enable the patient to relax. When manipulation during traction is required, as occurs so often in orthopaedic medical manipulation, the physiotherapist must synchronize with the manipulator. Since no two people manipulate exactly alike, this involves individuals practising as a team.

2. Positioning the Joint

Since manipulation is a movement of small amplitude often performed at the extreme of range, the patient's joint is usually taken passively into this position until the resistance of the tissues to further movement can be felt by the manipulator. He is then able to make the minor jerk that constitutes the manipulation proper. Hence, in manipulating a neck at which 90 degrees of active rotation range is present, the positioning will involve 90 degrees of movement and the manipulation perhaps 5 degrees more. Manipulation must not, therefore, be thought of as a huge movement involving 95 degrees of movement, even though, in some cases, the pause between positioning and applying the extra force is barely perceptible to the onlooker. During manipulation of a lumbar joint, however, the distinction is more obvious; for the trunk may well be rotated to full range and held there for a second or two before the extra force is applied.

A movement may be employed that can also be carried out voluntarily by the patient's own muscles, or a movement outside the patient's active range may be required. For example, full flexion at the knee cannot be performed actively, but may well have to be forced therapeutically.

3. The Direction of the Movement

Since the vertebrae move at three joints simultaneously, the intervertebral and the two facet joints, it is best to force movement at the joint between the vertebral bodies in a manner suited to the inclination of the articular surfaces of the facet joints. This is a point well insisted upon by osteopaths. Side-flexion of the neck involves rotation towards the same side on account of the inclination of the facet joint surfaces. Hence a larger range is secured, for example, when cervical side-flexion to the left is forced during traction if some rotation to the left is also allowed. Again, when cervical rotation is forced during traction, the manipulator may lower his body as the extreme of range is approached so as also to obtain some side-flexion towards the same side .

4. Direction Indolore

Should the forcing be towards the deviation or towards correction?

Maigne, probably the best-known manipulator in France and the author of the best known French book on osteopathic technique, has laid down the rule that all spinal manipulation must be carried out in the direction of the deformity and in the direction that has been found painless. Adherence to this rule, he states, makes it almost impossible to do harm by manipulation. Doubtless, this is an excellent precaution if manipulation is to be performed in the osteopathic manner on patients regarded on ostoepathic grounds as needing manipulation, but is far from valid when orthopaedic medical methods of diagnosis and manipulation are employed. Moreover, it seems probable that manipulation even with his proviso could well do harm if a really unsuitable case were chosen for manipulation. In fact, when the lumbar spine deviates towards the painful side, reduction is clearly encouraged by a manipulation that includes side-flexion away from that side, giving the loose fragment room to move.

5. The Type of Pressure

A sharp jerk is suited to breaking adhesions or to shifting a small fragment of cartilage, whereas maintenance of substantial pressure is suited to slowly squeezing a nuclear bulge.

6. Single or Repetitive Movement

During an attempt at manipulative reduction, moving the joint quickly to and fro several times may be the best method for inducing a small fragment loose within a joint to shift its position. Moreover, rhythmical movements of increasing amplitude may, after a while, relax the patient enough to enable a sudden thrust to be used at the exact moment when the manipulator feels the proper degree of tissue resistance.

7. Multiple Forces

Some manipulations are carried out while several forces act on the joint at once. For example, when manipulative reduction is attempted for a loose body in the knee, the knee is bent to a right-angle and strong traction is applied. Then alternate rotations are forced during increasing movement towards extension of the joint—four separate forces in all.

8. The Effective Movement

This may be at mid-range, towards the extreme of range or only when strong overpressure is applied. Naturally, the technique varies with the diagnosis, the intention, the manipulator's expectations, and what he can perceive happening within the joint as he moves it. In a difficult case, several different techniques are employed and the result of each is assessed by immediate re-examination after each manœuvre. In this way, the manipulator is guided towards the measure most beneficial in that particular lesion. The change in the physical signs indicates best what to do next, and perhaps what to avoid.

9. The Force Employed

This varies with the lesion and the patient's sensitivity to pain. The first time a manœuvre is attempted, it is done fairly gently, to get the feel of the joint and to judge the patient's reaction. Subsequent manipulations are carried out more strongly on a basis of: (1) What, on re-examination, the result is seen to have been; (2) what the joint felt like at the range to which it was taken last time; (3) what the manipulator feels as the joint approaches full range. At that instant, the different types of end-feel tell him what to do within the next split second. The operative hand receives sensations which determine how much farther he takes the joint.

REDUCTION

Successful manipulation has two different results; objective and sub-jective reduction.

Objective Reduction

In fractures and dislocations, reduction is an objective phenomenon. No one asks the patient anything; he can contribute nothing to the manœuvre; indeed, he is often anaesthetized. The same applies to the reduction of a torn cartilage at the knee; the manipulator feels the loose part click into place, and the block to extension is suddenly abolished. The torn piece of meniscus can be only 'in' or 'out'; it cannot perch half-way on the apex of the curve of the femoral condyle. This is a *set* manipulation: the manipulator is master of the situation and anaesthesia may be essential; it is always an advantage, never a disservice.

Subjective Reduction

This is performed principally at the spinal joints and the situation is entirely different, for reduction is a subjective phenomenon. Even if the manipulator feels a click, he has no means of knowing whether this is relevant or not, beneficial or harmful, except by cooperation with the patient. The loose fragment can occupy a number of different positions and seldom shifts back into place with only one noticeable click. It often has to be edged back little by little as judged by the alteration in symptoms and physical signs with each adjustment.

The manipulation has to be carried out without anaesthesia, the conscious patient helping throughout. The physical signs are ascertained, a manœuvre is performed and the result is assessed there and then, any change (a) in the degree or location of pain being reported by the patient, and (b) in physical signs being noted by the examiner. For example, if a cough hurts, or straight-leg raising is limited, or a lumbar movement is painful, this is tested afresh after each manipulative attempt. In this way, the manipulator is guided towards the correct technique, and at the same time warned if any manœuvre has had an adverse effect. The manipulator decides to go on or stop, which measures help and which do not, what to repeat and what to avoid, entirely on a basis of what he and the patient *mutually* discover. However skilled, no one can decide in advance the exact way in which he should manipulate a displaced fragment of disc, although experience enables him to make a shrewd guess. He merely knows how to set about his task, performs the manœuvre most likely to afford benefit, assesses the result, and carries on from there according to results. He cannot tell, unless the patient is conscious, when a painless range of movement has been restored to the affected joint; for this may not be full anatomical range, but as far as that particular patient's joint will ever move now. Many patients with a past disc lesion causing no symptoms and requiring no treatment possess a lumbar joint fixed with some permanent deformity which it would be futile, indeed dangerous, to try to alter. Under anaesthesia, the manipulator has no means of being warned that the manœuvre is causing aggravation. Hence, he would find himself in a difficult position medico-legally if the patient alleged that harm had been done and it transpired that anaesthesia had been employed for an attempt at spinal reduction. The essence of this type of manipulation is that it is *not set*, and is effective and safe only when the patient's conscious cooperation is secured throughout.

OSTEOPATHY AND CHIROPRACTICE

Osteopathy was, and to a large extent still is, a system of healing based on the notion that nearly all diseases arise in the first place from spinal derangements, whose correction, by corollary, constitutes both the prevention and the cure. Hence, the difference between medical manipulation (merely a method of treatment) and osteopathy is that osteopathy is an alternative system of medicine, in opposition to the one that doctors everywhere adopt. Medical manipulation affords merely one way of dealing with suitable lesions of the joints; osteopathy is regarded as suited to visceral disorders too. It is this tenet of osteopathic dogma that enables its adherents to manipulate the vertebral column for a variety of non-spinal diseases. This brings them into conflict with a mass of medically-established facts; it leads to fruitless manipulation for a large number of unsuitable conditions, and gives doctors good reason to deride osteopathy.

Whereas osteopaths palpate for lack of spinal mobility, chiropractors palpate for spinal displacement, but they too claim to be able to influence visceral disease by altering autonomic tone and indeed to cure many medical conditions.

There is no doubt that, without realizing it, osteopaths and chiropractors too, have been reducing spinal disc displacements for a great many years. Indeed, there must be few doctors who do not, at regular intervals, meet patients with disc lesions which have been relieved by an osteopath or a chiropractor (often after rest, physiotherapy and corsetry had failed). Doctors no longer dispute this fact, and it is high time that in general they accepted—and preferably also practised—spinal manipulation in suitable cases, however much they deplore osteopathic and chiropractic theory.

MAITLAND'S MOBILIZATIONS

This method of manipulating the spinal joints is set out in Maitland's book (1964). In part, the technique resembles the rhythmic movements that osteopaths perform under the name 'articulation'. However, they comprise gentle manual oscillations induced by the operator's hand held at each spinal level in turn, more in the chiropractic manner. He may well have taken a good leaf out of each book.

These mobilizations have a number of advantages, especially for physiotherapists.

1. First and foremost, the use of this technique involves no belief in the theories of any sect, and even allows for differences in opinion among medical men. Maitland creditably goes out of his way not to get involved in the essentially medical question of diagnosis. He ascertains the presence of certain clinical signs and his mobilizations serve to abolish these signs. This is a laudable policy, for it keeps physiotherapists out of academic arguments between medical men on the exact nature of the pathological

entity present. They are thus able to get on with their work of getting the patient well without appearing to take sides in a medical controversy, thereby antagonizing at least one medical faction to the point where patients needing manipulation are denied it. The physiotherapist does not hold herself out as able to reduce a disc lesion, but, if a patient with lumbago cannot bend forwards, she is prepared to manipulate his back until he can do so fully without pain. In this way he hopes that doctors will allow patients to be put right within the medical sphere although their arguments on the theorectical aspect of such cases are not yet concluded.

2. These mobilizations are graded into five degrees of diminishing gentleness; the first so mild as scarcely to have any effect, the fifth quite strong. Here is thus a progression that allays a young student's anxiety on first treating patients and engenders patients' confidence, especially if they feared some strong and painful manœuvre. Relaxation is secured and results can be gradually achieved.

3. They involve gradually getting the feel of the articular movements during a time when no attempt to reach full range at the joint is being made. The patient can thus state if unreasonable discomfort is being provoked before much has yet been done. This is very different from the attitude of orthopaedic medicine, viz., examination has shown that the lesion is suited to spinal manipulation, let it be carried out then without further ado. Clearly, the St. Thomas's techniques are more direct, but they involve the employment of clear diagnostic criteria.

4. They can lead to more direct techniques. If gentle manipulation has helped somewhat, the physiotherapist becomes sure that manipulation is the correct treatment. She can then increase her strength, passing on confidently to orthopaedic medical manœuvres.

5. They require no assistant, whereas the St. Thomas's manipulations for the neck and thorax involve two assistants.

6. They return to within the physiotherapist's competence acute lesions in which the symptoms are so severe that our type of manipulation cannot be borne. This applies in particular to acute lumbago (which the orthopaedic physician relieves at once by inducing epidural local anaesthesia), when any attempt at the ordinary manipulation provokes such pain that neither osteopath nor orthopaedic physician would dream of attempting manipulation. If the injection is unobtainable, these gentle techniques persevered with for a long time provide the only helpful measure that a physiotherapist can adopt.

7. They are strongly indicated in cases of aching in the neck or trunk in which the spinal movements provoke scarcely any symptoms. For example, central spinal discomfort may continue after a fractured vertebra

has united, and the active movements of the joint may not aggravate it, whereas the passive movements are a little uncomfortable. Ordinary manipulation is apt to aggravate such lesions, though they often respond well to traction. Oscillation is a good alternative.

Maitland's Mobilizing Techniques

The method consists of antero-posterior pressures and releases given to the affected joint as the patient lies prone. In the neck and lumbar spine, lateral oscillations can also be employed. First, each spinal joint is tested in turn in order to ascertain where pain is provoked or resistance encountered; treatment is correctly concentrated at this level. The manipulator places both thumbs on the tip of the appropriate spinous process and applies his oscillations at the rate of about two a second. Movement is generated by alternately flexing and extending both elbows synchronously, so that a series of little thrusts is delivered to the bone. As a result, the joint is extended slightly at the same time as the bone is pressed anteriorly. An antero-posterior glide is imparted during slight extension. The elasticity of the tissues brings the joints back to the neutral position again, ready for the next little thrust.

A number of variations exist. The thrusts can be applied with different degrees of amplitude and force, and the pressure extending the joint can be fully or only partly relieved between thrusts. They can be applied centrally, on both sides, on one side, and from the lateral or postero-lateral aspect as well as, in the case of neck and lumbar region, to the transverse process. The joint may be supported in side-flexion or rotation (or both) before the mobilizations are begun. These oscillations are used without traction and many hundreds are given at one session. The patient is examined at short intervals during the session, to enable the manipulator to assess the result of his treatment so far. He continues or alters his technique in accordance with the change, or absence of change, detected.

These mobilizations clearly provide the physiotherapist with a useful addition to the St. Thomas's methods and, better still, with an introduction to them. She gains confidence from using gentle manœuvres and, if the case responds well—albeit in longer time—need seek no further. They cannot be expected to be as quickly effective in considerable displacement; but having gained confidence in carrying out the oscillatory techniques, she does not hesitate to pass on to stronger measures if they are seen to be required. Ending with more forcible manœuvres is very different from having to plunge straight into effective manipulation in a case where the physiotherapist is uncertain of her skill or of the exact lesion present.

BONESETTING

This craft started centuries ago and continues now. The manipulators who call themselves bonesetters are largely uneducated countrymen who have an inborn flair for manipulation, or come from a family that has practised manipulation for generations. The bonesetter does not set bones in the meaning of today, i.e. reduce dislocations or fractures, but manipulates, alleging that he adjusts minor bony subluxations only.

Bone setters regard the click as the fragment shifts, or the snap as the adhesion ruptures, as evidence that 'the bone has been put back'. But they have the advantage of not professing any cult; they have no theories on disease; they merely manipulate to the best of their ability those who come to visit them. There is a certain rough honesty here, even if their idea of what occurs is mistaken, and their infectious belief in their own powers appears quite sincere.

WHO SHOULD MANIPULATE?

Spinal manipulation means different things to different people. To most lay manipulators it implies the restoration, without anaesthesia, of mobility to all the joints of the spine, whether or not the lesion present is connected with the spine and whether or not the patient's symptoms could conceivably arise from a spinal lesion at the manipulated levels. The osteopath and the chiropractor seek evidence of disorder, or even of predisposition to a disorder, in palpating the spinal joints for minor degrees of restricted movement or of displacement and for areas of muscle tension.

In general, to the orthopaedic surgeon, manipulation implies mobilization under anaesthesia with discovery of the result when the patient is questioned and examined next day.

To the orthopaedic physician, it implies a series of passive movements performed at a spinal joint, without anaesthesia, in the treatment of a lesion that previous examination has shown to be spinal, each manœuvre being followed by re-examination of the patient. Ideally, the session of manipulation continues until pain on all movements has ceased. Whether or not a full range of movement has been restored to the affected spinal joint is immaterial. The physician stops also if he judges that he has done enough for one day. Clearly, therefore, an opinion on the advisability and likely effect of manipulation must differ not only from lesion to lesion, but also from one sort of manipulator to another when confronted with an identical lesion.

Orthopaedic Surgeons

All orthopaedic surgeons manipulate for fractures and dislocations. They also manipulate, necessarily under anaesthesia, joints rendered stiff by immobilization or trauma. A few have made a special study of spinal manipulation, but most carry it out as a side-line to their more important work. As so much of their manipulation of joints is to bring about the rupture of adhesions, they are apt to carry forward this idea of capsulo-ligamentous stiffness to their spinal work, manipulating in a way better adapted to breaking adhesions than to reducing internal derangement. Many are disappointed with the results and with the occasional case of aggravation; the tendency is thus towards a gradual abandonment of spinal manipulation.

Laymen

Most of the manipulation done in this country today is carried out by laymen; when it comes to spinal manipulation, nearly all of it is so performed. The number of lay manipulators 30 years ago was estimated at three thousand and it has certainly increased since. There is probably one such layman to each 8 to 10 family doctors. Of these, a high proportion are entirely self-styled. This would not be considered a suitable situation in any other profession, and it is deplorable that any patient anxious to get well and return to work should today be forced, at his own expense, to go to someone who claims that he is a manipulator whatever his education or competence, at a time when the State sets out to provide all medical care free of charge. Had he needed any treatment other than manipulation, he would have experienced no difficulty in obtaining it from an expert within the Health Service. This situation is well known to all doctors, and costs the Health Service millions of pounds in unnecessary days off work, compensation cases and neuroses.

Physiotherapists

The physiotherapy profession provides ethical personnel accustomed to working with doctors. They know how to use their hands and have special knowledge of the way joints move and muscles work. In 1965 their curriculum was expanded to bring in manipulation, including that of the spinal joints. Doctors should, therefore, insist on manipulation by physiotherapists within the Health Service rather than let their patients drift off to laymen outside the Service. This has been the policy at St. Thomas's since 1939, and the Chartered Society should foster the growing tendency for doctors to look to physiotherapists for informed manipulation, ethically conducted.

The Family Doctor

In general, when a doctor is faced with a displacement, his first thought is whether or not an attempt at reduction should be made. In dislocations, many fractures, early strangulated hernia, breech presentation, retroverted uterus, or meniscal displacement at the knee or temporo-mandibular joint, the question comes up at once. Indeed, any medical man who, dealing, say, with a Colles's fracture, made no effort at reduction would soon find himself in medico-legal trouble. Yet reduction by active methods appears scarcely to figure in medical thought when a diagnosis of a displaced fragment of cartilage in an intervertebral joint has been reached. In the olden days, before Mixter and Barr (1934) and Cyriax (1945) had ascribed sciatica and lumbago respectively to such displacements, the conditions were thought to be caused by neuritis and muscular inflammation ('fibrositis'); in consequence, manipulation appeared illogical. Now, however, that the discal pathology of these symptoms has become so widely accepted, reason demands the abandonment of traditional treatment directed to the muscles and the institution of measures that directly affect the joint. But it is commonplace for the patient, when told he has a disc displacement and in answer to the question of the possibility of replacement, to be told that nothing active can be done. The likelihood is that the patient is advised rest, heat, massage or exercises. Alternatively, he may get his neck put in a collar or his trunk encased in plaster or a corset without previous reduction.

No wonder the family doctor is nonplussed about disc lesions and dismayed equally when, in some cases, laymen manipulate with dramatic success and in others with aggravation. Should he play safe and advise inaction, thus perhaps wasting weeks or months of an impatient sufferer's time, with consequent avoidable pain and financial loss, or should he turn a blind eye to lay manipulation, let him risk it and hope for the best? Neither the medical consultant nor, if he talks to him, the lay manipulator can help in his dilemma; for the one tends to be as sceptical as the other is oversanguine. Moreover, neither is likely to have much awareness of the points in the history and physical signs that determine whether manipulation is indicated or contra-indicated. The decisive factors are the duration, size, consistency and position of the displacement, the age and nature of the patient himself, coupled with the type of manipulation that is contemplated, i.e. surgical, under anaesthesia; osteopathic or chiropractic; medical orthopaedic.

'EMPTY AT THE TOP'

A curious situation exists putting manipulation in an anomalous position. Since the teaching schools other than St. Thomas's do not offer medical students a grounding in these methods, such doctors as do decide to practise it have to learn it as best they can after qualification. They are forced to come to St. Thomas's Hospital as unpaid clinical assistants or to go to the London College of Osteopathy, which has now forty medically qualified graduates, or to learn it out of Stoddart's, Maigne's or my own illustrated book.

The doctor who takes up manipulation is usually a good general practitioner. He has found that a group of his patients, in despair after ordinary medical measures have failed and after the consultants at one or more hospitals have not been able to help either, have wandered off to lay manipulators who cured a proportion of them. A minority of doctors, finding that their patients need a certain type of treatment and that it is unobtainable *via* the Health Service, meet the challenge and decide to carry it out themselves. They do not know how to set about this worthy endeavour and must try and hope. A certain number have a natural aptitude, find the work interesting and rewarding and so persevere until they become competent, with little or no guidance, while carrying on as family doctors. After a time, they become known for this work, and more and more patients come to them from far and wide. In due course, they develop a part-time practice in manipulation, soon acquiring rooms in the Harley Street area. Some continue in this way; others finally shift to full-time manipulative practice. These doctors are now 'specialists' in the eyes of the public, with rooms in the accepted area, plenty of patients who praise their skill, and so on. They are not so in the eyes of the medical profession; for they do not have the academic qualifications nor the hospital appointments which normal consultants all possess, and they have no opportunity to teach medical students. Naturally, if a method of treatment is seen to be practised as a speciality almost entirely by doctors who do not conform to their colleagues' ideas of professional respectability, a slur falls on the method. But it is not these doctors' fault that the manipulative branch of medicine is empty at the top; it is so understaffed, and the disorders responding are so common, that today it cannot be entered modestly in the accepted way. The doctor cannot serve an apprenticeship (where would he find a post and a teacher?); he can only be a specialist from the start, since *any* knowledge of this branch of medicine is so far in advance of no knowledge whatever that pressure of patients forces him to start at the top.

TEACHING MANIPULATION

It is a sad fact that a physiotherapist or a doctor who wants to learn manipulation in England today has really nowhere to go. The osteopaths offer a two-year course to physiotherapists and a nine-months' course to doctors, but on both courses they get embroiled in theories about osteopathic lesions, autonomic effects, etc.

Manipulation is not difficult to learn; the difficulty is to determine what cases do and do not respond to manipulation. Doctors do not learn this at osteopathic colleges, since there the net is spread too wide, and they cannot come in droves to St. Thomas's Hospital. Since the finances of the Health Service are so much the poorer for the lack of orthopaedic physicians at the hospitals of Britain, it is remarkable that the Ministry of Health has not by now pressed for the creation of an Institute of Orthopaedic Medicine.

All medical students are grounded as a matter of course in the simpler techniques that are appropriate to everyday medical practice. There is only one exception: manipulation. Since hardly a day passes without the family doctor seeing at least one patient who needs a simple manipulation, most often for an early disc displacement, it is obvious that this is one of the methods which every doctor needs to know. Yet, today, students are taught nothing of these methods. Though they are so often required, they are very seldom applicable to the cases that require admission to the wards, where the bulk of the tuition is carried out, and out-patient manipulation is seldom available at a teaching hospital.

Who Should be Taught Manipulation?

Doctors and Medical Students

Obviously, not all doctors wish to manipulate, any more than all of them want to aspirate a pleural effusion or remove the appendix. But they have all, while undergraduates, seen aspiration and abdominal surgery carried out and thus possess no prejudices based on ignorance of this sort of work. Medical students, in short, should also have been shown manipulation in action (as they are at St. Thomas's), and have it explained to them when and when not it is called for, and how it can be obtained. Some will want to do it themselves and there should then be house-physician posts and registrarships and an institute for postgraduate courses to teach the subject in detail to those who want to become proficient. In other words, all doctors should know a little about manipulation, and some (certainly one on the staff of every teaching hospital) should know a great deal.

Doctors' present uncertainty about the indications for and against manipulation, not to mention their natural prejudice against an unknown method, is easily avoidable by undergraduate tuition, supplemented by demonstrations. A patient with lumbago should be shown to the students, the physical signs pointed out and a session of manipulation given there and then, so that they can see how the signs regress during reduction. They can then be in no doubt about the effect of manipulation and will have no prejudice against it in their graduate years. Until this policy is followed at our teaching hospitals, doctors' and physiotherapists' uncertainty will continue to provide large numbers of cases for lay manipulators. It is clearly undesirable that patients should be driven to find some layman as best they can, at their own expense, at a time when the State has taken over the provision of all necessary medical care. Moreover, less than no guarantee exists that the manipulator, once unearthed, has any competence whatever. There are less than three hundred names on the osteopathic register, so the seeker's chances of running into a manipulator with any sort of training must be scarcely one in ten. This unhappy situation is well known to all family doctors, and there is undoubtedly a need for a much larger number of skilled manipulators than exist in this country at present.

If some grounding, however sketchy, were given to medical students in the indications for, contra-indications of, and manner of, manipulation, there would soon be enough adequate manipulators to go round.

Letting doctors know about manipulation would help to bring about the proper use of such trained manipulators as do exist. Once doctors realize that it is a rational treatment, they will countenance, even encourage, its performance.

Physiotherapists

It is ridiculous that there should exist four varieties of spinal manipulation—osteopathy, chiropraxy, Maitland's mobilizations and the methods taught at St. Thomas's. There is a good deal of overlap, and all four have their successes. The only set of medical auxiliaries undoctrinaire enough to allow themselves to be grounded in the best parts of all these four methods are the physiotherapists, and the only physiotherapist who maintains this attitude in his teaching is Kaltenborn in Norway. His approach is truly eclectic and offers an example that our schools in Britain might well copy. Physiotherapists are the very people to carry out manipulation, for the patients needing this treatment have been sent to them for years, though hitherto for traditional measures.

The advantages of manipulation by physiotherapists are manifold. Firstly, manipulation would be restricted to patients who had been selected by medical men as suffering from lesions likely to benefit. Secondly, manipulation would be carried out by educated and ethical persons, who had been taught the work and examined in it properly. Thirdly, manipulation would be obtainable within the Health Service. Fourthly, the number of visits per patient required by a doctor in some disorders would be greatly lessened. Instead, let us say, of visiting a patient with lumbago treated by bed-rest six times in a month, by asking a physiotherapist to go round to manipulate, he might well need to go to his home only once. Fifthly, if the patient were off work for only a few days instead of for several weeks it would save him and the sickness funds a great deal of money. Sixthly, the tendency to regard disc lesions as a good opportunity for prolonged invalidism, compensation for injury and lawsuits would not arise. These attitudes start after some weeks' recumbency, when the patient has had time to ponder his position. The doctor's matter-of-fact attitude and the prompt response to adequate treatment would afford no encouragement to traumatic neurosis.

It can be argued that an occasional difficult case in a large strong man may be beyond a girl's capabilities; this is true, but it would also be beyond the powers of a small, old or frail doctor or osteopath. Moreover, there are male physiotherapists, to whom the profession would become much more attractive if they were all trained as skilled manipulators. There is every advantage in physiotherapists dealing with all except the most resistant cases (and most are very easy) and leaving that small remainder to be dealt with by the medically-qualified expert.

Who Should Teach Manipulation?

Only those who practise manipulation should teach it. Clearly, medical men who employ this measure with discrimination and skill are the best placed to give useful tuition. There should be one such at every hospital in the country and all our teaching hospitals should give a course of not less than six set lectures a year to medical students followed by a demonstration at each of, say, manipulative reduction of a cervical and a lumbar displacement; of the induction of epidural local anaesthesia; of injection of hydrocortisone into joints and tendons.

This is what is done at St. Thomas's. Six voluntary formal lecture-demonstrations are given each year and are well attended; there is daily teaching at out-patient clinics, and a weekly teaching-clinic for medical students to which they are allocated as duty in one of the special departments. Here too, they see immediate manipulative reduction, hydrocortisone and epidural injections, and, more important, the clinical examination leading to these measures. The fact that most medical students become friendly with physiotherapy students plays quite a big part in the education of the former in clinical examination of the moving parts and the virtues of manipulation! The result is that these young doctors go out into the world, not knowing how to manipulate, it is true, but without prejudice against it. They know it can be done; they have seen it done; they have in their notes a series of indications and contra-indications to which they can refer. Asking a physiotherapist to carry out manipulative reduction at a spinal joint appears to them perfectly reasonable. To them its employment has become a decision like any other in medicine, and emotion no longer plays a part.

An important point in teaching medical manipulation is that it cannot usefully be taught as just a series of manœuvres. This is the main fault of the books on osteopathy which have appeared recently. They merely set out techniques. Far more important is a description of the clinical examination that makes for a clear diagnosis and indicates whether manipulation is required or not and, if not, what alternative measure should be employed. Moreover, any book on manipulation should give equal emphasis to contra-indications as to indications. No such osteopathic book exists. The osteopath, concerned as he is with dealing with those spinal joints at which he perceives movement to be limited, continuing until he is satisfied that a proper range has been restored, has little need to consider other clinical signs or even the effect of his manipulations on the patient's symptoms. Orthopaedic medicine, on the other hand, demands a clear view of the whole clinical picture; then one manœuvre is performed, followed by a further examination to establish the result; then another manœuvre, and so on. The manipulator is thus guided towards an effective technique. It is to be regretted that even recent books on manipulation do not deal with the subject in this way. They teach technique, but give no real guidance on how the clinical examination of the moving parts is best carried out, still less when and when not to manipulate on the basis of what such examination reveals.

Osteopaths should certainly not be allowed to teach their theories to medical students, since their ideas on pathology and on the effects of manipulation and its indications are not suited to those who (a) have medical examinations to pass; (b) have not yet acquired enough basic knowledge to enable them to evaluate dogmatic statements of dubious accuracy. In particular, the layman's habits of manipulating spinal joints at a level whence the symptoms present could not originate, and for supposed autonomic effects, would hopelessly confuse any medical or physiotherapy students. However, it is desirable that medical and physiotherapy students or graduates should learn osteopathic or chiropractic techniques, provided the theory was omitted, and this is what is done in Scandinavia.

THE SCANDINAVIAN ACHIEVEMENT

The first country outside England to foster manipulation by physiotherapists was Norway. After a visit to St. Thomas's in 1952, the physiotherapist Kaltenborn devoted his considerable energies to getting the physiotherapists' charter enlarged to include manipulation. His application was backed by doctors and secured approval from the Norweigan Health Authorities in 1957. The same year, a physiotherapeutic association of manipulation was founded, and in 1962 a similar association of medical men. Under the wise medical leadership first of Schiotz and now of Koefoed, the advantages of manipulation were put before their Scandinavian colleagues again and again. In due course, prejudice was abated and the medical men of Norway, Denmark, Sweden and Finland looked at the matter scientifically and in large measure approved. In 1962, Hult gave a lecture in Stockholm on the results of employing a St. Thomas's graduate at his hospital.

With doctors' participation, Kaltenborn began courses on the localization of lesions and on manual treatment for doctors and physiotherapists alike in 1962. As from 1964, all physiotherapy students were examined in these techniques at their qualifying examinations. In 1966 the book by, and for, doctors and physiotherapists was published, entitled *Manipulation av Ryggraden* by Brodin, Bang, Bechgaard, Kaltenborn and Schiotz, and in 1967 Kaltenborn's next illustrated book for physiotherapists appeared (*Fgigjoring a Ryggraden*, i.e. 'Freeing of the Spine').

To give some idea of Kaltenborn's indefatigable determination to get manipulation accepted on a sound basis, it suffices to say that, in the twelve months ending May 1967, he gave 11 courses in Norway, 12 in Sweden, 3 in Denmark and 1 in Iceland. They were attended by 180 doctors from all over Europe (of whom I was one) and 809 physiotherapists (counting a participant at more than one course as a fresh individual). It is evident that one dedicated physiotherapist with enlightened medical support has, in the course of only fifteen years, reversed the entire medical climate in Scandinavia in respect of manipulation and has secured widespread medical approval for his work for physiotherapists. (In consequence, there is only one lay osteopath practising in the whole of Norway.) At his courses, he teaches what he has found best in osteopathy, chiropraxy and orthopaedic medicine without a trace of fringe indoctrination. He tells me that he uses the orthopaedic medical approach to clinical examination and prefers osteopathic manœuvres. This is very satisfactory; for the clinical examination is what matters; manipulation done one way or the other is less important than how to identify the patient requring manipulation. The physiotherapists who have learnt from him are now teaching in most of the schools in Scandinavia. He has four grades of instruction, some for doctors only, some for physiotherapists, some for both. There is no doubt in my mind that the high standard of tuition that is today obtainable in Norway far surpasses that offered to physiotherapists in any other country in Europe.

References

ANDERSON, H. G. & DUKES, C. (1925). Treatment of haemorrhoids by submucous injections of chemicals; with a description of the pathological change produced. *Brit. med. J., 2;* 100.

ARMSTRONG, J. R. (1965). *Lumbar Disc Lesions.* 3rd Ed. Edinburgh: Livingstone.

ARONSON, H. A. & DUNSMORE, R. H. (1963). Herniated upper lumbar discs; *J. Bone Jt Surg., 45A,* 311.

BAKER, H., GOLDING, D. N. & THOMPSON, M. (1963). Psoriasis and arthritis. *Ann. intern. Med., 58,* 909.

BARBOR, R. (1964). Treatment for chronic low back pain. *Proc. IVth int. Congr. Phys. Med. (Paris).*

BARLOW, T. G. (1962). Early diagnosis and treatment of congenital dislocation of the hip. *J. Bone Jt Surg., 44B,* 292.

BARNETT, C. H. (1963). Effects of age on articular cartilage. *Research Reviews, 1963/4,* 183.

BARR, J. S. & CRAIG, W. M. (1946). Ruptured intervertebral disk. *J. nerv. ment. Dis., 103,* 688.

BARRY, P. J. & KENDALL, P. H. (1962). Corticosteroid infiltration of the extradural space. *Ann. phys. Med., 6,* 267.

BECHGAARD, P. (1966). Late post-traumatic headache and manipulation. *Brit. med. J., 1,* 1419.

BENEKE, R. (1897). *Zur Lehre von der Spondylitis deformans.* (Beitr. z. wissensch.) Med. Festschrift an der 59 Versammlung deutscher Naturforscher und Ärzte. Braunschveig.

BENNETT, G. A., WAINE, H. & BAUER, W. (1942). *Changes in the Knee joint at Various Ages.* New York: Commonwealth Fund.

BENSON, R. & FOWLER, P. D. (1964). Treatment of Weber-Christian disease. *Brit. med. J., 2,* 615.

BERNHARDT, M. (1896). Ueber eine wenig bekannte Form des Beschäftigungsneuralgie. *Neurol. Centralbl., xv,* 13.

BOHM, E., FRANKSSON, C. & PETERSEN, I. (1956). Sacral rhizopathies and sacral syndromes. *Acta chir. scand.,* 216.

BOLDREY, E., MAASS, A. & MILLER, E. R. (1956). Role of atlantoid compression in etiology of internal carotid thrombosis. *J. Neurosurg., 13,* 127.

BONNEY, G. (1956). Arterial disease as a cause of pain in the buttock and thigh. *J. Bone Jt. Surg., 38B,* 686.

BOWRIE, E. A. & GLASGOW, G. L. (1961). Cauda equina lesions associated with ankylosing spondylitis. Report of three cases. *Brit. med. J., 1,* 24.

BRAIN, W. R. (1963). Some unsolved problems of cervical spondylosis. *Brit. med. J., 1,* 771.

—— & WILKINSON, M. (1967). Cervical Spondylosis. London: Heinemann.

——, WRIGHT, A. D. & WILKINSON, M. (1947). Spontaneous compression of both median nerves in carpal tunnel: 6 cases treated surgically. *Lancet, 1,* 277.

BREWERTON, D. A., NICHOLS, P. J. R., LOGUE, V., MANNING, C. W. F., MARTIN-JONES, M., MASON, R. M., NEWELL, D. J. & SANDIFER, P. H. (1966). Pain in the neck and arm; a multicentre trial of the effects of physiotherapy. Arranged by the British Association of Physical Medicine. *Brit. med. J., 1,* 253.

BRODIN, H., BANG, J., BECHGAARD, P., KALTENBORN, F. & SCHOITZ, E. (1966). Manipulation av Ryggraden. Scandinavicen University Books.

BROWN, W. M. C. & DOLL, R. (1965). Mortality from cancer and other causes after radio-therapy for ankylosing spondylitis. *Brit. med. J. 2,* 1327.

BROWSE, N. L. (1965). *Physiology and Pathology of Bed-rest*. Thomas: Springfield, Ill.

BULL, J. W. D. & ZILKHA, K. J. (1968). Rationalising Requests for X-ray films in neurology. *Brit. med. J., 2,* 569.

BURKE, G. L. (1964). *Backache from Occiput to Coccyx*. MacDonald: Vancouver.

BYWATERS, E. G. L. (1968). Case of ankylosing spondylitis. *Brit. med. J., 1,* 412.

—— & ANSELL, B. M. (1958). Arthritis associated with ulcerative colitis; a clinical and pathological study. *Ann. rheum. Dis., 17,* 169.

CAMPBELL, A. M. G. & PHILLIPS, D. G. (1960). Cervical disc lesions with neurological disorder. *Brit. med. J., 2,* 481.

CAMPBELL, D. G. & PARSONS, C. M. (1944). Referred head pain and its concomitants; report of preliminary experimental investigation with implications for post-traumatic 'head' syndrome. *J. nerv. ment. Dis., 99,* 544.

CARP, L. (1932). Tennis elbow (epicondylitis) caused by radio-humeral bursitis; anatomic, clinical, roentgenologic and pathological aspects with suggestions as to treatment. *Act. Surg., 24,* 905.

CAUSSADE, G. & QUESTE, P. (1909). Traitement de la sciatique par injection epidurale de cocaine. *Soc. med. Hôpit.*

CHANDLER, G. N. & WRIGHT, V. (1958). Deleterious effect of intra-articular hydrocortisone. *Lancet, 2:* 661.

CHARCOT, J. M. (1858; quoted by Miller, H. 1967). Three great neurologists. *Proc. roy. Soc. Med., 60,* 399.

CHARNLEY, J. (1960). Surgery of the hip joint: present and future developments. *Brit. med. J., 1,* 1, 821.

CLARK, C. J. & WHITWELL, J. (1961). Intraocular haemorrhage after epidural injection. *Brit. med. J. 2,* 1612.

CLEVELAND, D. A. (1955). Use of methyl-acrylic for spinal stabilisation after disc operation *Marquette med. Rev., 20,* 62.

COCKETT F. B. & MAURICE, B. A. (1963). Evolution of direct arterial surgery for claudication and ischaemia of legs. A nine-year survey. *Brit. med. J., 1,* 353.

——, THOMAS, M. L. & NEGUS, D. (1967). Iliac vein compression; its relation to ilio-femoral thrombosis and the post-thrombotic syndrome. *Brit. med. J., 1,* 214.

COHEN, P. (1966). Myelomatosis treated with sodium fluoride. *J. Amer. med. Ass., 198,* 583

COLLIS, J. S. (1963). *Lumbar Discography*. Thomas: Springfield, Ill.

COOMES, E. N. (1959) in *The Innervation of Muscle*, COËRS, C. & WOOLF, A. L. p. 74–79. Blackwell Scientific Publications: Oxford.

—— & SHARP, J. (1961). Polymyalgia rheumatica. *Lancet, 2,* 1328.

COPE, S. & RYAN, G. M. S. (1959). Cervical and otolith vertigo. *J. Laryngol. Otol., 73,* 113.

COTUGNO, (1764). *De Ischide Nervosa Commentarius.*

COUDERE, A. (1896). Etude sur un nouvel accident professionel des maîtres-d'armes dû à la rupture probable et partialle du tendon epicondylien. Thèse de Bordeaux.

CROW, N. E. & BROGDEN, B. G. (1959). The 'normal' lumbo-sacral spine. *Radiology, 71(6),* 72, 97.

CSONKA, G. W., (1958). The course of Reiter's syndrome. *Brit. med. J., 1,* 1088.

CURREY, H. L. F. & SWETTENHAM, K. V. (1965). Synovial fluid in gout. *Brit. med. J., 2,* 481.

CURTIS, A. C. & POLLARD, H. M. (1940). Felty's syndrome; its several features, including tissue changes, compared with other forms of rheumatoid arthritis. *Ann. intern. Med., 13,* 2265.

CYRIAX, J. (1936). Pathology and treatment of tennis elbow. *J. Bone Jt Surg., 18,* 921.

—— (1938). Rheumatic headache. *Brit. med. J., 2,* 1367.

—— (1941a). Sacro-iliac strain. *Brit. med. J., 2,* 847.

—— (1941b). *Massage, Manipulation and Local Anaesthesia*. London: Hamilton.

—— (1942). Perineuritis. *Brit. med. J., 1,* 578.

—— (1945), Lumbago: the mechanism of dural pain. *Lancet, 2,* 427.

—— (1947). *Rheumatism and Soft-tissue Injuries*. London: Hamilton.

—— (1948). Fibrositis. *Brit. med. J., 2,* 251.

—— (1949a). *Osteopathy and Manipulation*. London: Crosby Lockwood.

—— (1949b). Pressure on the nerves of the neck and upper limb. *St Thom. Hosp. Rep., v,* 67.

CYRIAX J. (1950a). Thoracic disc lesions. *St Thom. Hosp. Rep., vi*, 171.

—— (1950b). Treatment of lumbar disc lesions. *Brit. med. J., 2*, 1434.

—— (1952). Zervicale bandscheibenschäden. *Medizinische*, 485, 489.

—— (1953). *Disc Lesions.* London: Cassell.

—— (1955a). Les Manipulations Vertébrales. Premières journées internationales de kinésithérapie. Bruxelles.

—— (1955b). Spinal disc lesions: assessment after 21 years. *Brit. med. J., 1*, 140.

—— (1956). *Hydrocortisone in Orthopaedic Medicine.* London: Cassell.

—— (1957a). Statistics on conservative treatment of lumbar disc lesions. *Rpt. Internat. Congr. Occup. Hlth, Helsinki, i*, 124.

—— (1957b). *The Shoulder.* London: Cassell.

—— (1958a). Lumbar disc lesions; conservative treatment. *S. Afr. med. J., 32, 1*, 1.

—— (1958b). Diagnosis at the shoulder. *S. Afr. med. J., 32, 1*, 62.

—— (1958c). Soft-tissue injuries in athletes. *Med. sportiva, xii*, 249.

—— (1959a). Esame funzionalenelle lesioni delle parti non scheletriche dell'apparato locomotore. *Atti. Soc. lombarda Sci. med.-biol., xiv*, 829.

—— (1959b). Indications for and against manipulation. In *Die Wirbelsäule in Forschung und Praxis,* Vol. 13. Junghanns: Oldenburg.

—— (1959e). Use and misuse of physiotherapy. *Med. Press*, 505.

—— (1960). Clinical applications of massage. In *Massage, Manipulation and Traction,* by Licht. New Haven, Conn: Licht.

—— (1965–69). *Textbook of Orthopaedic Medicine. I.* Diagnosis of Soft Tissue Lesions, 5th ed. II. Treatment by Manipulation and Massage, 7th ed. London: Ballière, Tindall & Cassell.

—— (1966a). Manipulation. *Clin. med. Chicago, 73*, 37.

—— (1966b). Manipulative Surgery. In *Clinical Surgery,* Rob. C. & Smith, R. London: Butterworth.

—— & GOULD, J. (1953). Pain in the trunk. *Brit. med. J., 1*, 1077.

—— & TROISIER, O. (1953). Hydrocortisone and soft-tissue lesions. *Brit. med. J., 2*, 966.

DANDY, W. E. (1929). Loose cartilage from intervertebral disc simulating tumour of spinal cord. *Arch, Surg., 19*, 660.

DAVIDSON, J. A. (1962). Assessment of hypnosis in pregnancy and labour. *Brit. med. J., 2*, 951.

DAVIES, D. V., BARNETT, C. H., COCHRANE, W. & PALFREY, A. J. (1962), Electron microscopy of articular cartilage in the young rabbit. *Ann. rheum. Dis., 21*, 11.

DE BEURMANN (1884). Note sur un signe peu connu de la sciatique. *Arch. physiol. Norm. Path., 3*, 375.

DEJERINE, J. (1906), Sur la claudication intermittente de la moelle épinière. *Rev, neurol., 14*, 341.

DE QUERVAIN, F. (1895). Uber eine Form von chronischer Tendovaginitis. *Korresp.-Bl. schweiz, Artz., 25*, 389.

DE SÈZE, S. (1955). Les attitudes antalgiques dans la sciatique disco-radiculaire commune. Etude clinique et radiologique; interprétation pathogénique. *Sem. Hôp. Paris, 31*, 2291.

DILLANE, J. B., FRY, J. & KALTON, G. (1966). Acute back syndrome; a study from general practice. *Brit. med. J., 2*, 82.

DUCKWORTH, J. (1966). Personal communication.

EDGAR, M. A. & NUNDY, S. (1966). Innervation of the spinal dura mater. *Neurol. Neurosurg. Psychiat., 29*, 530.

EDSTRÖM, G. (1944). Rheumatism as public health problem in Sweden; field studies of population in certain districts during summer of 1943. *Upsala Läk.-Fören. Fösh., 49*, 303.

EISEN, V. (1966). Urates and kinin formation in synovial fluid. *Proc. roy. Soc. Med., 59*, 302.

ELSBERG, C. A. (1916). Diagnosis and treatment of surgical diseases of the spinal cord and its membranes. Philadelphia & London: W. B. Saunders.

EVANS, J. G. (1964). Neurogenic intermittent claudication. *Brit. med. J., 2*, 985.

FAJERSZTAJN, J. (1901). Uber das gekreuzte Ischiasphänomen; ein Beitrag zur Symptomatologie der Ischias. *Wien. klin. Wschr., 14*, 41.

FALCONER, M. A. (1953). Surgical treatment of intractable phantom-limb pain. *Brit. med. J., i*, 299.

DD

FELDBERG, W. (1951). Physiology of neuromuscular transmission and neuromuscular block. *Brit. med. J., i,* 967.

FÉRÉ, G. (1897). Note sur l'epicondylalgie. *Rev. Méd. Paris, xvii,* 144.

FERNSTRÖM, U. (1957). Lumbar intervertebral disc degeneration with abdominal pain. *Acta chir. scand., 113,* 436.

—— (1960). Discographic study of ruptured lumbar intervertebral discs. *Acta. chir. Scand., 258,* 1.

—— (1964). Diskprotes av metall vid lumbal diskruptur. *Nord. Med., 71,* 160.

FILTZER, D. L. & BAHNSON, H. T. (1959). Low back pain due to arterial obstruction. *J. Bone Jt Surg., 41B,* 244.

FLAVELL, G. (1956). Reversal of pulmonary hypertrophic osteoarthropathy by vagotomy. *Lancet, 1,* 260.

FOERSTER, O. (1933). Dermatomes in man. *Brain, 56,* 1.

FORD, F. R. (Baltimore) & CLARK, D. (1956). Thrombosis of basilar artery with softenings in cerebellum and brain stem due to manipulation of neck; report of 2 cases with one post-mortem examination. Reasons are given to prove that damage to vertebral arteries is responsible. *Bull. Johns Hopk. Hosp., 98,* 37.

FORESTIER, J. & ROTES-QUEROL, J. (1950). Senile ankylosing hyperostosis of spine. *Ann. rheumat. Dis., 9,* 321.

FORST, J. J. (1881). *Contribution à l'Etude Clinique de la Sciatique.* Thése de Paris. 49p. 40. No. 33.

FREIBURG, A. H. (1914). Infraction of the second metatarsal bone, a typical injury. *Surg. Gynec. Obstet, xix,* 191.

FREUND, H. A., STEINER, G., LEICHTENTRITT, B. & PRICE, A. E. (1942). Peripheral nerves in chronic atrophic arthritis. *Amer. J. Path., 18,* 865.

FRYKHOLM, R. (1951a). Lower cervical nerve-roots and their investments. *Acta chir. Scand., 101,* 457.

—— (1951b). Lower cervical vertebrae and intervertebral discs. Surgical anatomy and pathology. *Acta chir. Scand., 101,* 345.

GARDEN, R. S. (1961). Tennis elbow. *J. Bone Jt Surg., 43B,* 100.

GIBSON, H. J., KERSLEY, G. D. & DESMARAIS, M. H. L. (1946). Lesions in muscle in arthritis. *Ann. rheum. Dis., 5,* 131.

GILL, G. G., MANNING, J. G. & WHITE, H. L. (1955). Surgical treatment of spondylolisthesis without spine fusion; excision of loose lamina with decompression of nerve roots. *J. Bone Jt Surg., 37A,* 493.

GILLESPIE, H. W. & LLOYD-ROBERTS, G. (1953). Osteitis condensans. *Brit. J. Radiol., 26,* 16.

GLORIEUX, P. (1937). *La Hernie Posterieure du Ménisque Intervertébral.* Paris: Masson.

GOODFELLOW, J. (1966). Aetiology of hallux rigidus. *Proc. roy. Soc. Med., 59,* 821.

GRANIT, R., LEKSELL, L. & SKOGLUND, C. R. (1944). Fibre interaction in injured or compressed region of nerve. *Brain, 67,* 125.

HACKETT, G. S. (1958). *Ligament and Tendon Relaxation.* Springfield, Ill.: Thomas.

HAMBY, W. B. & GLASER, H. T. (1959). Replacement of spinal intervertebral discs with locally polymerizing methyl methacrylate; experimental study of effects upon tissues and report of a small clinical series. *Neurosurg., 16,* 311.

HARLEY, C. (1966). Extradural corticosteroid infiltration; a follow-up study of 50 cases. *Proc. Brit. Assoc. phys. Med., London, 9,* 22.

HARMAN, J. B. (1951). Angina in analgesic limb. *Brit. med. J., 2,* 521.

HARRISON, M. H. M., SCHAJOWICZ, F. & TRUETA, J. (1953). Osteoarthritis of hip: study of nature and evolution of disease. *J. Bone Jt Surg., 35B,* 598.

HART, F. D. & GOLDING, J. R. (1960). Rheumatoid neuropathy. *Brit. med. J., 1,* 1594.

HELFET, A. J. (1963). *Management of Internal Derangements of the Knee.* Philadelphia: Lipincott.

HENDERSON, W. R. (1967). Trigeminal neuralgia; the pain and its treatment. *Brit. med. J., 1,* 7.

HENDRY, N. G. C. (1958). The hydration of the nucleus pulposus and its relation to intervertebral disc derangement. *J. Bone Jt Surg., 40B,* 132.

HENSON, R. A. & PARSONS, M. (1967). Ischaemic lesions of the spinal cord: an illustrated review. *Quart. J. Med., 142,* 205.

HERFORT, R. & NICKERSON, S. H. (1959). Relief of arthritic pain and rehabilitation of chronic arthritic patient by extended sympathetic denervation. *Arch. phys. Med., 40*, 133.

HIRSCHFELD, P. F. (1962). Die Konservative Behandlung des lumbalen Bandscheibenvorfalls nach der Methode Cyriax. *Deut. med. Wschr., ix*, 299.

HOCKADAY, J. M. & WHITTY, C. W. M. (1967). Patterns of referred pain in the normal subject. *Brain, 90*, 481.

HOHMANN, (1933). Das Wesen und die Behandlung des sogenannten Tennis-ellenbogens. *Munch. med. Wschr., 80*, 250.

HOLLING, H. E., BRODEY, R. S. & BOLAND, H. C. (1960). Pulmonary osteoarthropathy. *Trans. Ass. Amer. Phycns., 73*, 305.

HULT, L. (1954a). *The Munkfors Investigation.* Copenhagen: Munksgaard.

—— (1954b). *Cervical, Dorsal and Lumbar Spinal Syndromes.* Copenhagen: Munksgaard.

ILLOUZ, G. & COSTE, F. (1964). Le signe du trepied dans l'exploration clinique des sacro-iliaques. *Presse méd., 72*, 1979.

ISDALE, I. C. (1962). Femoral head destruction in rheumatoid arthritis and osteoarthritis. A clinical review of 27 cases. *Ann. rheum. Dis., 21*, 23.

JEPSON, E. M. (1961). Hypercholesterolaemic Xanthomatosis. Treatment with a corn-oil diet. *Brit. med. J., 1*, 847.

JOHNSTON, A.W. (1960). Acroparaesthecia and acromegaly. *Brit. med. J., 1*, 1616.

JOSEPH, J. (1964). Electromyographic studies on muscle tone and the erect posture in man. *Brit. J. Surg., 51*, 616.

KELLGREN, J. H. (1938). Observations on referred pain arising from muscle. *Clin. Sci., 3*, 175.

—— (1939). On distribution of pain arising from deep somatic structures with charts of segmental pain areas. *Clin. Sci. 4*, 35.

KINMONTH, J. B. (1952). Physiology and relief of traumaticarterial spasm. *Brit. med. J., 1*, 59.

KLEINBURG, S. (1951). *Scoliosis: Pathology, Etiology and Treatment.* London: Baillière.

DE KLEYN, A. (1939). Some remarks on vestibular nystagmus. *Confin. neurol. Basal, 2*, 257.

KONSTAM, P. G. & BLESOVSKY, A. (1962). Ambulant treatment of spinal tuberculosis. *Brit. J. Surg., 50*, 26.

KOPELL, H. P. & THOMPSON, W. A. L. (1963). Peripheral entrapment neuropathy. Baltimore: Williams & Wilkins.

KOVACS, A. (1955). Subluxation and deformation of cervical apophyseal joints; contribution to aetiology of headache. *Acta radiol. Stockh., 43*, 1.

LASSÈGUE, (1864). Consideration sur la sciatique. *Arch. gen. Med., 2*, 558.

LEWIS, T. (1942). *Pain.* New York: Macmillan.

LINDAHL, O. (1966). Hyperalgesia of the lumbar nerve roots in sciatica. *Act. orthop. scand., 37*, 367.

LIPSON, R. L. & SLOCUMB, C. H. (1965). The progressive nature of gout with inadequate therapy. *Arth. & Rheum., 8*, 80.

LORIMER (1884). Discussion: The nosological relations of chronic rheumatic (rheumatoid) arthritis. *Brit. med. J., 2*, 269.

LUSCHKA, H. (1850). *Die Nerven des Menslischen Wirbelkanales.* Tübingen.

McCARTY, D. J. & HOLLANDER, J. L. (1961). Identification of urate crystals in gouty synovial fluid. *Ann. intern. Med., 54*, 452.

McCUTCHEN, C. W. (1964). Lubrication of joints. *Brit. med. J., 1*, 1044.

McGILL, D. M. (1964). Tarsal tunnel syndrome. *Proc. roy. Soc. Med., 57*, 1125.

MAGILL, H. K. & AITKEN, A. P. (1954). Pulled elbow, *Surg. Gynec. Obstet., 98*, 753.

MAGNUSON, P. B. (1944), *Ann Surg., 119*, 878.

McGUIRE, R. J. & VALLANCE, M. (1964). Aversion therapy by electric shock: a simple technique. *Brit. med. J., 1*, 151.

MAIGNE, R. (1960). *Les Manipulations Vertébrales.* Paris: Expansion Scientifique Française.

MAITLAND, G. D. (1964). *Vertebral Manipulation.* London: Butterworth.

MAKIN, M. (1960) Relationship between vesical mucosa and bone induction. *Brit. med. J., 2*, 1518.

MALAWISTA, S. E., SEEGMILLER, J. E., HATHAWAY, B. E. & SOKOLOFF, L. (1965). Sacro-iliac gout. *J. Amer. med. Ass., 194*, 954.

MARTIN, J. P. (1965). Curvature of the spine in post-encephalitis parkinsonism. *J. Neurol. Neurosurg. Psychiat., 28*, 395.

MARTIN, P. (1960). Atherosclerosis of the arteries of the limbs. *Proc. roy. Soc. Med.*, *53*, 31.

MASON, R. M. (1964). Spondylitis. *Proc. roy. Soc. Med.*, *57*, 533. June.

——, MURRAY, R. S., OATES, J. K. & YOUNG, A. C. (1958). Prostatitis and ankylosing spondylitis. *Brit. med. J.*, *i*, 748.

——, ——, & —— (1959). A comparative radiological study of Reiter's disease, rheumatoid arthritis and ankylosing spondylitis. *J. Bone Jt Surg.*, *41B*, 137.

——, OATES, J. K. & YOUNG, A. C. Sacro-iliitis in Reiter's disease. *Brit. med. J.*, *2*, 1013.

MATHESON, A. T. (1960). Cauda equina syndrome. *Brit. med. J.*, *1*, 570.

MATHEWS, J. A. (1968). Dynamic discography: a study of lumbar traction. *Ann. phys. Med.*, *7*, 275.

MATTHEWS, B. F. (1952). Collagen/chondroitin sulphate ratio of human articular cartilage related to function. *Brit. med J.*, *2*, 1295.

MATHUR, K. S., KAHN, M. A. & SHARMA, R. D. (1968). Hypocholesterolaemic effect of Bengal gram; a long-term study in man. *Brit. med. J.*, *1*, 30.

MENGERT, W. F. (1943). *Southern Med. J.*, *36*, 256.

MENKIN, V. (1943). Chemical basis of injury in inflammation. *Arch. Path.*, *36*, 269. September.

—— (1956). *Biochemical Mechanisms in Inflammation.* Thomas: Springfield, Ill.

MIDDLETON, G. S. & TEACHER, J. H. (1911). Injury of the spinal cord due to rupture of an intervertebral disc during muscular effort. *Glasg. J.*, *76*, 1.

MILLER, H. (1961). Accident neurosis. *Brit. med. J.* *1*, 919.

—— (1966). Polyneuritis. *Brit. med. J.*, *2*, 1219.

MILLS, G. P. (1928). Treatment of tennis elbow. *Brit. med. J.*, *1*, 12.

MINEIRO, J. D. (1965). *Coluna Vertebral Humana.* Lisboa: Soc. Indust. Grafica.

MIXTER, W. J. & BARR, J. S. (1934). Rupture of intervertebral disc with involvement of spinal canal. *New Engl. J. Med.*, *211*, 210.

MOBERG, E. (1967). Surgery of the rheumatoid hand. *Brit. med. J.*, *1*, 696.

MONDOR, H. (1939). Tronculite sous-cutanèe subaiguë de la paroi thoracique antèro-latèral. *Mem. Acad. Chir.*, *65*, 1271.

MONRO, A. (1788). *Description of All Bursal Hucosae of Human Body.* Edinburgh: Elliott.

MORRIS, H. (1882). Rider's Sprain. *Lancet*, *2*, 557.

MORRISON, L. R., SHORT, C. L., LUDWIG, A. O. & SCHWAB, R. S. (1947). Neuromuscular system in rheumatoid arthritis; electromyographic and historical observations. *Amer. J. Sic.*, *214*, 33.

MURRAY, I. P. & SIMPSON, J. A. (1958). Acroparaesthesia in myxoedema; a clinical and electromyographic study. *Lancet*, *1*, 1360.

NACHEMSON, A. (1959). Measurement of intradiscal pressure. *Acta orthop. scand.*, *28*, 269.

—— (1960). Lumbar intradiscal pressure; experimental studies on post-mortem material. *Acta orthop. scandinav. Suppl.*, *43*, 1.

—— (1962). Some mechanical properties of the lumbar intervertebral discs. *Bull. Hosp. Jt Dis. N.Y.*, *xxiii*, 2.

—— & MORRIS, J. M. (1963). *In-vivo* measurements of intradiscal pressure. *J. Bone Jt Surg.*, *46A*, 1077.

NEVIASER, J. S. (1945). Adhesive capsulitis of shoulder; study of pathological findings in periarthritis of shoulder. *J. Bone Jt Surg.* *27*, 211.

NEWMAN, P. H. (1968). The spine, the wood and the trees. *Proc. roy. Soc. Med.*, *61*, 35.

NICHOLS, P. J. R. (1960). Short-leg syndrome. *Brit. med. J.*, *1*, 1863.

NORTHFIELD, D.W. (1963). The cerebro-spinal fluid. *N.Z. med. J.*, *62*, 167.

OATES, G. D. (1960). Median-nerve palsy as complication of acute pyogenic infections of hand. *Brit. med. J.*, *1*, 1618.

ORTOLANI, M. (1937). Un segno poco noto e sua importanza per la diagnosi precoce di prelussazione congenita dell'anca. *Pediatria*, *45*, 129.

OSGOOD, R. B. (1922). Radiohumeral bursitis, epicondylitis, epicondylalgia (tennis elbow). *Arch. surg. Chicago*, *iv*, 420.

PALLIS, C. A. & SCOTT, J. T. (1965). Peripheral neuropathy in rheumatoid arthritis. *Brit. med. J.*, *1*, 1141.

PAGET, J. (1867). Cases that bonesetters cure. *Brit. med. J., 1, 1.*

PARVES, L. R. & GRAHAM J. R. (1965). Headache Rounds. 36.

PAUWELS, F. (1959). New guides for the surgical treatment of osteoarthritis of the hip. *Rev. chir. Orthop., 45, 681.*

PEARCE, J. & MOLL, J. H. (1967). Conservative treatment of natural history of acute lumbar disc lesions. *J. Neurol. Neurosurg. Psychiat., 30, 13.*

PRATT-THOMAS, H. R. & BERGER, K. E. (1947). Cerebellar and spinal injuries after chiropractic manipulation. *J. Amer. med. Ass., 133, 600.*

PRINGLE, B. (1956). Approach to intervertebral disc lesions. *Trans. Ass. industr. med. Offrs, 5,* 127.

RAAF, J. & BERGLUND, G. (1949). Results of operations for lumbar protruded intervertebral disc. *J. Neurol. Neurosurg., 6, 160.*

REEVES, B. (1966). Arthographic changes in frozen and post-traumatic stiff shoulder. *Proc. roy. Soc. Med., 59, 827.*

REID, J. D. (1958). Ascending nerve roots and tightness of dura mater. *N.Z. Med. J., 57, 16.*

REID, W., WATT, J. K. & GRAY, T. G. (1963). Selective nerve crush in intermittent claudication. *Brit. med. J., 1, 1576.*

REMAK, E. (1894). *Beschaftigungsneurosen.* Wien: Urban & Schwarzenberg.

RIBBERT, H. (1895). Ueber die experimentelle Erzengung einer Ecchondrosis Physalifora. *Verh. Kongr. inn. Med., xiii, 455.*

ROB, C. G. & STANDEVEN, A. (1958). Arterial occlusion complicating thoracic outlet compression syndrome. *Brit. med. J., 2, 709.*

RODWAY, H. E. (1957). Education for childbirth and its results. *J. Obstet. Gynaec. Brit. Emp., 64, 545.*

ROMAGNOLI, C. & DALMONTE, A. (1965). Semeiological contribution to sciatic pain in hernia of disc. *Gazzetta Sanitaria Bologna, 24.*

ROPER, B.W. (1964). Essential hypercholesterolaemic xanthomatosis. *Brit. med. J., 2, 990.*

ROSTON, J. B. & HAINES, R.W. (1947). Cracking in metacarpo-phalangeal joint. *J. Anat., 81,* 165.

RUNGE, F. (1873). Zur Gevese und Behandlung des Schreibekrampfes. *Berl. klin. Wschr., x, 245.*

RUSSELL, W. R. (1959). Treatment of intractable pain. *Proc. roy. Soc. Med., 52, 983.*

———, MILLER, H. & O'CONNELL, J. E. A. (1956). Discussion on cervical spondylosis. *Proc. roy. Soc. Med., 49, 197.*

RYDER, H. W. & OTHERS. (1953). Mechanism of change in cerebrospinal fluid pressure following induced change in volume of fluid space. *J. Lab. clin. Med., 41, 428.*

SCHIOTZ, E. H. (1958). Manipulasjonsbehandling av columna under medisinskhistorisk synsvinkel. *T. norske Laegeforen., 359, 429, 946, 1003.*

SCHMITT, J. (1921). Bursitis calcarea am Epicondylus externus humeri. *Arch. orthop. Unfall-Chir., xix, 215.*

SCHREGER, G. B. (1825). *Debursis Mucosis Subcutaneis.* Erlangen: Palmand Enke.

SCHWARZ, G. A., GEIGER, J. K. & SPANO, A. V. (1956). Posterior inferior cerebellar artery syndrome of Wallenberg after chiropractic manipulation. *Arch. intern. Med. Chicago, 3, 352.*

SCHWARTZ, H. G. (1956). Anastomoses between cervical nerve roots. *J. Neurosurg., 13, 190.*

SCOTT, P. D. & MALLINSON, P. (1944). Hysterical Sequelae of injuries. *Brit. med. J. 1, 450.*

SEMMES, R. E. (1964). *Rupture of the Lumbar Intervertebral Disc.* Thomas: Springfield, U.S.A.

SEWARD, G. R. (1966). Pain from dental disease. *Brit. med. J., 2, 509.*

SHARP, J. & PURSER, D. W. (1961). Spontaneous atlanto-axial dislocation in ankylosing spondylitis and rheumatoid arthritis. *Ann. rheum. Dis., 20, 47.*

SHINE, I. B. (1965). Hallux valgus. *Brit. med. J., 1, 1648.*

SICARD, A. (1901). Les injections medicamenteuses extra-durales par voie sacro-coccygienne. *C. R. Soc. Biol., Paris, 53, 396.*

——— (1954). Le chirurgien devant des douleurs du bas du dos. *Sem. Hôp. Paris, 30, 2793.*

———, BOUREAU, M. & LECA, A. (1958). Hernies du troisième disque lombaire. *Presse méd., 66, 1809.*

SMITH, L. & BROWN, J. E. (1967). Treatment of lumbar intervertebral disc lesions by direct injection of chymopapain. *J. Bone Jt Surg. 49B, 502.*

SMITH, M. J. & WRIGHT, V. (1958). Sciatica and the intervertebral disc. *J. Bone Jt Surg., 40A*, 1401.

SMITH, R. A. & ESTRIDGE, M. N. (1962). Neurological complications of head and neck manipulations. *J. Amer. med. Ass., 182*, 528.

SOUTHWORTH, J. D. & BERSACK, S. R. (1950). Anomalies of lumbo-sacral vertebrae in 550 individuals without symptoms referable to low back. *Amer. J. Roentgenol., 64*, 624.

STARY, O. (1956). Pathogenesis of discogenic disease. *Review of Czechoslovak Medicine, ii*, 1.

—— (1959). *Nektere Otazky Patogenesy Diskogenni Nemoci.* Praha.

STEARNS, M. L. (1940). Studies on development of connective tissue in transparent chambers in rabbit's ear. *Amer. J. Anat., 67*, 55.

STEINBERG, V. L. & PARRY, C. B. (1961). Electromyographic changes in rheumatoid arthritis. *Brit. med. J., 1*, 630.

STILWELL, D. L. (1956). Nerve supply of vertebral column and its associated structures in monkey. *Anat. Rec., 125*, 139.

STODDARD, A. (1959). *Manual of Osteopathic Technique.* London: Hutchinson.

STRANGE, F. G. ST. C. (1966). President's address: Debunking the disc. *Proc. roy. Soc. Med., 59*, 952.

SUDECK, P. (1900). Uber die acute Entzündliche Knockenatzophie. *Arch. klin. Chir. Berlin, 62*, 147.

SUTOW, W. W. & PRYDE, A. W. (1956). Incidence of spina bifida occulta in relation to age. *J. Dis. Child., 91*, 211.

SUTTON, R. D., BENEDEK, T. G. & EDWARDS, G. A. (1963). Aseptic bone necrosis and corticosteroid therapy. *Arch. intern. Med., 112*, 594.

SWEETNAM, D. R., MASON, R. M. & MURRAY, R. O. (1960). Steroid arthropathy of the hip. *Brit. med. J., 1*, 1392.

SYMPOSIUM ON CLINICAL PROBLEMS OF PRACTICE. (1967). The Sair Back. *J. Coll. gen. Practit., xiii*, 60.

THEOBALD, G. W., MENZIES, D. N. & BRYANT, G. H. (1966). Critical electrical stimulus which causes uterine pain. *Brit. med. J. 1*, 716.

TODD, T. W. & PYLE, S. I. (1928). Quantitative study of vertebral column by direct and roentgenoscopic methods. *Amer. J. phys. Anthropol., 12*, 321.

TROISIER, O. (1962). *Lèsions des Disques Intervertébraux.* Paris: Masson.

VAINIO, K. (1967). Surgery of the rheumatoid hand. *Brit. med. J., 1*, 696.

VAISHNAVA, H. P. & RIZVI, S. N. A. (1967). Osteomalacia in Northern India. *Brit. med. J., 1*, 112.

WASSMANN, K. (1951), Kyphosis juvenilis Schuermann—occupational disorder. *Acta orthop. scand., 21*, 65.

WHITTY, C. W. M. & WILLISON, R. G. (1958). Some aspects of referred pain. *Lancet, 2*, 226.

WILKINSON, M. (1964). Anatomy and Pathology of cervical spondylosis. *Proc. roy. Soc. Med., 57*, 159.

WILSON, D. G., (1962). Manipulative treatment in general practice. *Lancet, 1*, 1013.

WOLF, B. S., KHILNANI, M. & MALIS, L. I. (1956). Sagittal diameter of bony cervical spinal canal and its significance in cervical spondylosis. *J. Mt Sinai Hosp., 23*, 283.

WOOLF, A. L. & TILL, K. (1955). Pathology of the lower motor neurone in the light of new muscle biopsy techniques. *Proc. roy. Soc. Med., 48*, 189.

WOOLSEY, C. N., MARSHALL, W. H. & BARD, P. (1941). Observations on cortical somatic sensory mechanisms of cat and monkey. *J. Neurophysiol., 4*, 1.

WRIGHT, V. & WATKINSON, G. (1965). Sacro-iliitis and ulcerative colitis. *Brit. med. J., 2*, 675.

YOUNG, A. C. (1967). Radiology in cervical spondylosis. In *Cervical Spondylosis.* London: Heinemann.

YOUNG, R. H. (1951). Results of surgery in sciatica and low back pain. *Lancet, 1*, 245.

ZITNAN, D., SITAJ, S., HUTTL, S., SKROVINA, B., HANIC, F., MARKOVIC, O. & TRNAVSKA, Z. (1963). Chondrocalcinosis articularis, section I. Clinical and radiological study. *Ann. rheum. Dis., 22*, 158.

ZIZINA, M. (1910). *La Douleur Controlateral dans la Sciatique.* Thèse de Montpellier, 2.

ZORAB, P. A. (1966). Chest deformities. *Brit. med. J., 1*, 1155.

Index

Index

Backache—*cont.*
  epidural injection and, 535
  intractable, 577–80
  posture and, 394–5
  sclerosing injections for, 578–81
  time factor in, 553
  undiagnosed, 498–9
Basilar syndrome, 140
Bed, traction in, 193–4, 529–30
Bed-rest, 524, 550–3
  epidural injection v., 536
  posture in, 388, 508
Biceps, of arm, 172, 223, 255, 258, 265, 269, 290, 300–3, 303
  of thigh, 649, 659, 682
Biconvex disc, 472
Bladder weakness, 413, 425, 477–9, 518, 559
  laminectomy and, 559
  manipulation and, 518
Bonesetters, 295, 513–14, 688–9, 791
Bony block, 239
Bornholm disease, 6
Brachial artery, 318
  plexus, 172, 173, 205–12
  traction palsy, 174
Brachialis muscle, myositis in, 293–5, 302
Breast, female, 386–7
Bronchus, neoplasm, 173, 327
Buckled end-plate, 560
Bunion, 752
Bursitis, acute, 242–3, 260, 285
  adhesive, 262
  adventitious, 721
  aspiration of, 286, 305
  calcanean, 721, 753
  calcified deposit in, 261, 285–6
  chronic, 253, 260–1
  crepitating, 262
  at elbow, 304–5
  gluteal, 497, 625–6, 627–30
  at hallux, 749
  haemorrhagic, 262, 286, 304, 630
  incomprehensible, 262–3
  ischial, 629
  at knee, 683
  psoas, 627–8, 630
  rheumatoid, 286
  septic, 305, 629–30
  subcoracoid, 223, 242, 245, 286–7

  subdeltoid, 223, 240, 242–3, 253, 257, 259–63, 284–6
Buttock, 623–32
  bursitis, 627–30
  claudication, 630–1
  psychogenic disorder, 631
  segmentation of, 51, 623–4
  sign of the, 456, 624–6
  tuberculous abscess, 631
  wasting of, 461

Calcanean apophysitis, 724–5
  bursitis, 721, 753
  fracture, 718
  spur, 719–20
  tendinitis, 696–7, 700–1
Calcification, at shoulder, 261, 285–6
Calf muscles, 694–7, 700–2
  claudication in, 692, 697–700
  short, 701
  weakness, 700–2
Calvé's osteochondritis, 372, 484
Capitate, subluxation of, 323, 325
Capsular lesions, clinical findings in, 102–9
Capsular pattern, 17, 105–9
  patterns listed, 107–9
  (*see also* under individual joints)
Capsulitis, adhesive, 222
  cervical spine, 198–9
  clinical findings, 102–9
  end-feel in, 102–4
  at shoulder, 222
Car seats, 567–9
Carotid artery, 190
Carpal bone, fracture of, 322, 324
  subluxation of, 323, 325, 336, 338
  ligamentous sprain, 324–5
  tunnel, 71, 172, 328, 333–8
  injection, technique for, 335
Carpus: *see* Wrist
Cartilage, costal, 377
  intervetebral: *see* Disc, intervertebral
  non-union of, 398 429, 550
Cauda equina, 413, 477–9
Causalgia, 67
Cervical disc lesions, 153–4, 164–200, 213
  anatomy, 164–6
  articular signs, 166–7
  arthrodesis, 189